Nutrition
During Infancy
Principles and Practice

second edition

EDITORS

Reginald C. Tsang M.B.B.S.
Department of Pediatrics,
Pediatric Bone Research Center,
University of Cincinnati Medical Center,
Cincinnati, Ohio

Stanley H. Zlotkin M.D., Ph.D.
Department of Pediatrics,
Division of Gastroenterology/Nutrition,
Research Institute,
The Hospital for Sick Children,
Toronto, Ontario

Buford L. Nichols M.D.
Children's Nutrition Research Center,
Department of Pediatrics,
Baylor College of Medicine,
Houston, Texas

James W. Hansen M.D., Ph.D.
Director, Nutrition and Metabolism,
Mead Johnson Nutritionals,
Evansville, Indiana

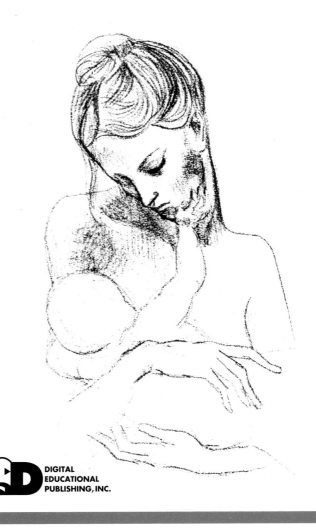

DIGITAL
EDUCATIONAL
PUBLISHING, INC.

Publisher
Digital Educational Publishing, Inc.
700 Walnut Street
Suite 450
Cincinnati, Ohio 45202

Toll Free 1.888.679.2300
Phone   513.345.6716
E-mail   info@DEPinc.com

Executive Producer
Timothy J. Mullican

Copy Editors
Emilie Copeland D'Agostino
Scott Schneider
Mary Silva

Graphic Design/Layout

Troy Hitch	Jenny Robinson
Scott Hosso	Scott Schneider
Lisa Klancher	Patrick Schreiber
Emiko Koike	Susan Young

Digital Image Processing/Photo Restoration
Richard Allendorf

Front Cover
The front cover illustration is a drawing by Pablo Picasso, 1904, Mother and Child and Four Studies of Her Right Hand (detail), black crayon on tan woven paper, 338 x 267 mm (1965.318 recto). Courtesy of The Harvard University of Museums (Fogg Art Museum). Bequest of Meta and Paul J. Sachs.

NUTRITION DURING INFANCY

ISBN 0-932883-09-5

Contents

Introduction

Nutrition During Infancy: Principles and Practice

In writing this book, the authors have taken a very special tack. The editors convened a group of world renowned experts to write a second edition of the well received book *Nutrition During Infancy: Principles and Practice*. The authors were "locked in a room" for two days to present their proposals for their respective chapters. Prior to arriving at the meeting, drafts of their manuscripts had been disseminated to all attendees and to external reviewers. In addition, two participating authors were chosen to be primary and secondary reviewers for on site review of each chapter.

Thus, as can be imagined, the authors' meeting was a very lively one that focused not only on the science of the book but also on textual presentation style. The authors were given explicit instructions to focus on "why a resident would want to read this book at 10:00 p.m.?"--admittedly, a challenging task. In fact, Dr. Louis Barness, guest reviewer invited to play the role of "official cynic", declared that it was a "nutty" proposal--what resident at 10:00 p.m. would read any book? However, it did appear that, as the process unfolded, even Dr. Barness, and Dr. Jack Filer, who was also invited to play the role of senior advisor, had to concede that a book written this way might just entice a resident at 10:00 p.m. to read it!

In order to attract the attention of this infamous resident, we decided after many brainstorming sessions of the editors, and in cooperation with the authors, to have many different ways of stimulating interest in the book. We created some lively, but practical titles that remind the reader that this is meant to be a practical book, and not just a collection of "facts, numbers, and tables" (which sadly is what most nutrition texts are perceived to be all about). With a practical clinical angle, we hope to attract the resident to consider nutrition in the clinical setting of the management of his/her patient on the wards, rather than as an isolated esoteric topic to be discussed at a seminar. "Bullets" or highlights of the chapter are placed in the beginning of most chapters, to remind the resident of the important issues in nutrition that pertain to direct clinical care, and in relation to a patient's general health.

We include a major theme diagram for most chapters that illustrates the flow of thought in the chapter and the key issues involved for that particular nutrient or subject. Throughout the text, interesting points will either be "boxed" or highlighted to draw attention, so that the enterprising, speed-reading resident could skim over and be reminded of important key points.

A very popular feature of the previous edition was the clinical case question and answer section of the chapters which allows readers to zoom in on practical lessons by the bedside. Often in nutrition texts there is an extensive discussion of pathophysiology and biochemistry, but the patient is often lost in the equation. The case history permits us to refocus to the individual patient, and clinicians can enjoy "sleuthing" through a series of facts and evidence to arrive at a logical conclusion and decision.

Throughout the chapters we have attempted to keep the presentations crisp and clear. In this, we are ably assisted by a team of artists lead by Timothy Mullican, DVM from the Observatory Group, Inc. in Cincinnati. The text is laced with a large number of graphs and figures in order to enhance the value and appeal of the text and make the text much more readable. Important points have been highlighted using modern artistic presentation styles, diagrams have been expertly illustrated and presented in attractive format, and eye-catching two-tone colors are used to enhance the impact of the book.

Throughout the text, we have included aphorisms and pithy quips from leading nutrition experts. These pearls of wisdom have been sprinkled through the text in order to capture the flavor of clinical medicine. The collected wisdom of decades of work in nutrition in infancy are often captured in these succinct remarks, by clinicians and nutritionists who are experienced in taking care of infants by the bedside. In clinical practice these principles are often learned at the feet of distinguished professors, but not all of us have the opportunity to work with this variety of distinguished professors; hence these quips were solicited widely and meant to be savored by a wide readership.

Nutrition history capsules have been retained in the book to remind ourselves of a history that is replete with interesting anecdotes and reminders of clinical acumen and scientific curiosity, which have been translated into clinical practice and care of infants.

We have also added sections which include global perspectives to reflect worldwide applications. In this, we were ably assisted by the international community of authors and reviewers to provide a wider perspective and information. During the authors' meeting, in particular, the international slant was emphasized to remind ourselves of different ways of examining nutrition problems. This is important especially as nutrition and its' approaches are widely divergent in different geographic areas, although the principles should transcend national boundaries.

Color plates have been included for illustrations of clinical problems that the authors felt might be diffi-cult to find in standard texts. In times past this approach was common; recently however, this custom seems to have been phased out, and the authors felt we should restore this fine tradition.

Because of the extensive nature of the reviews, we have chosen to include the names of the reviewers on the title page of each chapter, highlighting the important contributions that all reviewers had toward the excellence of the chapters. Reviewers were also given an opportunity of rebuttal or stating an alternative viewpoint within the text. This book is truly a collaborative effort of all concerned and participants threw themselves into the task with enthusiasm, generating a comprehensive yet readable text.

Finally, through the generous support from a Mead-Johnson education grant, we have been able to support several editors' planning meetings, the authors meeting, and some of the art work, so that we could keep the price of this book low in spite of the many special features of the book. We wish you happy reading, even at 10:00 p.m. If you have indeed been inspired by the book, we hope that you would write and inform us. If you dislike the book after reading it, we would like to hear from you on suggestions of improvement to make it more interesting, say at midnight (a future project?).

Reginald C. Tsang M.B.B.S.
Stanley Zlotkin M.D., Ph.D.
Buford Nichols M.D.
James Hansen M.D., Ph.D.

Preface

The art of nutrition dates back to antiquity; the science of nutrition has existed only for a few centuries. This book is an attempt to combine both the art and science of nutrition. The authors have taken on the challenge of communicating with nutritionists, nurses, pediatricians, and residents by producing a nutrition book that is informative, readable, entertaining, and, at times, provocative.

The book is a truly cooperative venture; authors were given opportunities to critique all manuscripts at a two-day intense session of "brainstorming."

Rather than traditional introductory remarks (which few persons read), we have chosen to introduce the book with a series of drawings by Dr. Wilhelm Camerer. Dr. Camerer's drawings illustrate the beginning of pediatric nutrition as a scientific discipline one hundred years ago. Born in 1842, Camerer unquestionably was one of the pioneers in scientific pediatric nutrition. He studied as a pupil of C. Vierordt who was the first physician to count red cells or measure hemoglobin. A practicing pediatrician, Camerer is credited with the discovery of anemia and pioneered the study of nitrogen balance and body composition in children. Based on the data he gathered while conducting metabolic balance studies on his own five children, he published, in 1896, an important treatise on "Metabolism and Energy Requirements of Childhood From Birth To Maturation." It is reported that he carried out the chemical analysis in the kitchen of his home. Camerer constructed the first tables for assessing growth and was the first to calculate the nutrient needs for growth. He spent many years studying the composition of human milk and charting the growth of 283 infants during their first year of life.

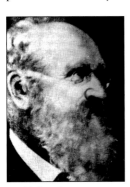

Wilhelm Camerer

This collection of drawings was first presented at a meeting of the German Academy of Pediatrics in Stuttgart, in September 1906.

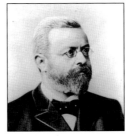

Otto Heubner

Otto Heubner M.D. (1843-1926) was trained in Internal Medicine in Leipzig. He was appointed the first full-time Chairman of Pediatrics at Berlin University and Director of the Children's Clinic at the Charite' Hospital. Heubner collaborated with Rubner in 1898-99 on studies of energy intake and expenditure by infants. The dietary ratio of kCal/kg body weight is still called the Heubner index in Europe. The Otto Heubner Prize is the highest award of the German Pediatric Society. Pioniere der Kinderheilkunde by J. Oehme, Hansisches, Lubeck 1993, 44 (Photo courtesy of NLM)

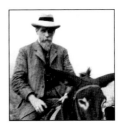

Max Rubner Ph.D.

Max Rubner Ph.D. (1854-1932) began his scientific career under a student of Liebig. His degree was from Voit's Munich laboratory where calorimetry was first applied in human investigations. Rubner's subsequent studies derived the standard values of 4.1, 9.3 and 4.1 kCal/g of protein, fat and carbohydrates. Rubner worked with the pediatricians Heubner and Langstein to carry out the first calorimetric studies of term and preterm infants. His *in vivo* work laid the foundation for subsequent in vitro studies of cell respiration which opened the pathway to modern enzyme biochemistry. J. Nutr. 48,1-12,1952 (Photo courtesy of CNRC)

Reginald C. Tsang M.B.B.S.
Cincinnati, Ohio

Buford L. Nichols M.D.
Houston, Texas

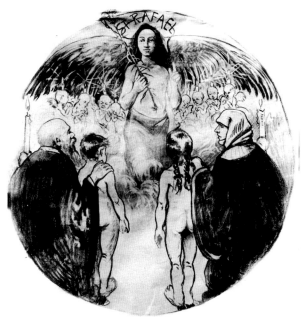

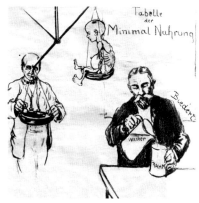

In this picture, Camerer, a Swabian knight, points out the high infant mortality that existed at the time of the birth of pediatric nutrition.

Weighing a malnourished infant. Note the infant's distended abdomen. Biedert, an early pediatrician, is mixing a formula composed of water and cream.

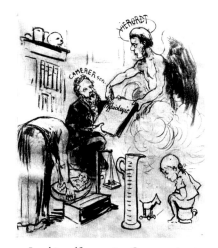

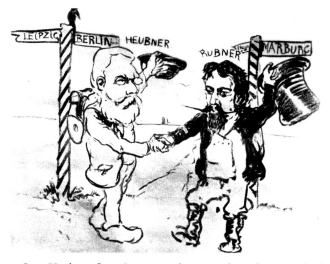

In this self-portrait, Camerer is pictured learning human physiology from Professor C. Vierdort at the Physiological Institute of the University of Tübingen in 1866. Camerer's wife is also depicted here, weighing one of their five children, while one of the other children collects samples for balance studies.

Otto Heubner from Leipzig and Max Rubner from Marburb meet in Berlin. As new faculty members associated with the Charity Hospital in Berlin, they collaborated on a report that contained information on the first quantitative investigations of infant energy metabolism, in 1898 and 1899.

In the next three sketches, Camerer introduces the three schools of German pediatrics: first, the school founded in Leipzig by Wünderlich, represented by Heubner; second, the school that was founded in Prague by Ritter von Rittershain, as personified by Keller; and third, the Munich school founded by Hauner and identified by Moro and Hamburger.

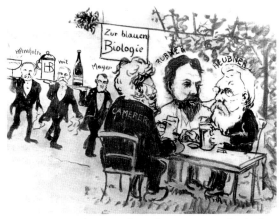

Camerer, Rubner, and Heubner meet at the biology tavern where they are waited on by the great geniuses of physiology, nutrition, and biochemistry: Helmholtz, Voit, and Mayer. This sketch represents the intellectual birth of scientific pediatric nutrition. Many early United States scientists trained under these scientific leaders.

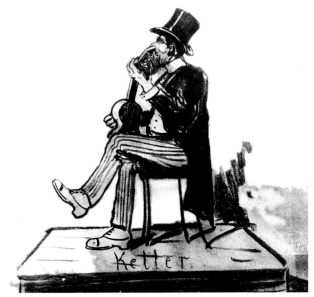

Keller trained at Breslau under Czerny, and also moved to Berlin. The picture implies that he lacks an adequate understanding of and interest in nutritional metabolism.

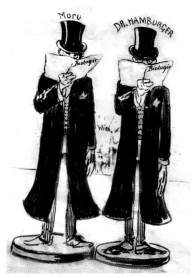

Camerer introduces two additional pediatricians, both from Munich: Moro and Hamburger. In this sketch, both are studying biology.

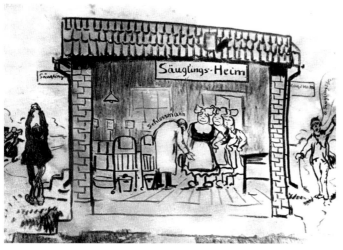

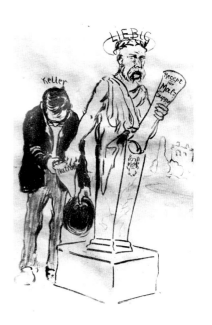

The Infants' Home. The doctor on the right is singing about the joys of working in the infants' ward, while Dr. Arthur Schlossman of Düsseldorf (center) is shown welcoming three wet nurses. He anticipates a liter of milk from each. To the left, Dr. Schlossman is greatly dismayed when one of the wet nurses leaves with her sweetheart. This scenario depicts the uncertainty over the supply of donated human milk, which leads to the next phase of pediatric nutrition.

Justus von Liebig, the venerated founder of the science of nutrition, is immortalized here in a statue complete with a halo about his head. In his left hand is the recipe for maltsoup, a partially hydrolyzed starch used in the first stage of beer-making and recommended as a food for infants in 1866. Many heralded this publication as the founding of scientific artificial infant-feeding. Liebig was a scientific grandchild of Lavoisier, and the first to study the composition of human milk. In this picture, Keller contributes a pinch of sodium bicarbonate to the maltsoup, which improved its acceptability to infants.

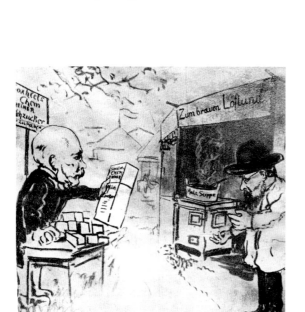

Two pediatricians promote their infant-feeding concepts. Soxhlet, the inventor of the method for terminal sterilization of infant formulas, promotes lactose and sucrose. Loflund is promoting various maltsoup preparations.

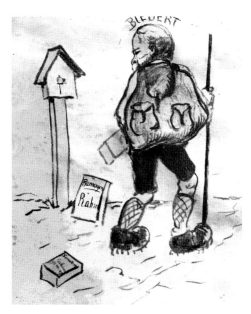

Biedert, who had studied with Liebig, is reintroduced. He was the first pediatrician to promote the theory that cow's milk casein was less digestible than human milk protein. In this picture, he derides the emphasis on carbohydrate and promotes an infant formula made with cream.

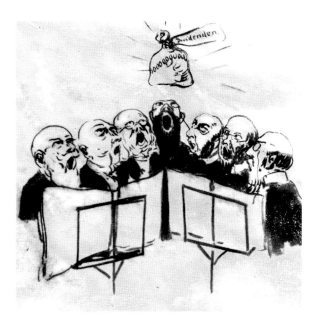

The industrialists are introduced. They discuss the uncertain qualities of mother's milk, and they rely on the unknown professor "Willig" to provide a testimonial that their formulas have miraculous powers. The Board of Directors sings the praise of formulas for their economic value, gazing at the purse of money that dangles over their heads.

Infant Feeding
By Dr. John Ruhräh
Lines Suggested by the Papers on Infant Feeding

Soranus, he of ancient Rome,
He had a simple trick
To see if milk was fit for sale,
He merely dropped it on his nail
To see if it would stick;
Yet spite of this the babies grew
As any school boy'll tell to you.

Good Metlinger in ages dark
Just called milk good or bad
No acid milk could vex his soul
He gave it good, he gave it whole
A method very sad;
Yet babies grew to man's estate
A fact quite curious to relate.

Time sped and science came along
To help the human race,
Percentages were brought to fame
By dear old Rotch, of honored name,
We miss his kindly face;
Percentages were fed to all
Yet babies grew both broad and tall.

The calorie now helped us know
The food that is required
Before the baby now could feed
We figured out his daily need
A factor much desired;
Again we see with great surprise
The babies grow in weight and size.

The vitamin helps clarify
Why infants fail to gain,
We feed the baby leafy food
Which for the guinea pig is good
A reason very plain;
And still we watch the human race
Go madly at its usual pace.

We have the baby weighed today
The nursing time is set,
At last we find we are so wise
We can begin to standardize
No baby now need fret;
In spite of this the baby grows
But why it does God only knows.

Away with all such childish stuff
Bring chemists to the fore,
The ion now is all the rage
We listen to the modern sage
With all his latest lore;
And if the baby fret or cry
We'll see just how the ions lie.

A hundred years will soon go by
Our places will be filled
By others who will theorize
And talk as long and look as wise
Until they too are stilled;
And I predict no one will know
What makes the baby gain and grow.

Contributors

Stephanie A. Atkinson Ph.D.
Department of Paediatrics,
McMaster University,
Hamilton, Ontario

Sandra J. Bartholmey Ph.D.
Nutrition Science,
Research and Development,
Gerber Products Company,
Fremont, Michigan

Helen K. Berry
Children's Hospital Medical Center,
Cincinnati, Ohio

Julia A. Boettcher M.Ed., R.D.
Mead Johnson Nutritionals,
Evansville, Indiana

A. Wesley Burks M.D.
Department of Pediatrics,
University of Arkansas for Medical Sciences,
Little Rock, Arkansas

Nancy F. Butte Ph.D.
USDA/ARS Children's Nutrition Research Center,
Department of Pediatrics,
Baylor College of Medicine,
Houston, Texas

Frank R. Greer M.D.
University of Wisconsin,
Madison, Wisconsin

James W. Hansen M.D., Ph.D.
Nutrition & Metabolism and
Mead Johnson Nutritionals,
Evansville, Indiana

Ferdinand Haschke M.D.
Department of Pediatrics,
University of Vienna,
Vienna, Austria

Judy Hopkinson Ph.D.
Children's Nutrition Research Center
at Baylor College of Medicine;
Houston, Texas

Kay James M.S., C.C.C.
Pediatric Therapy Center,
Houston, Texas

Stacie M. Jones M.D.
Department of Pediatrics,
University of Arkansas for Medical Sciences,
Little Rock, Arkansas

Berthold Koletzko, M.D.
Pediatrics Department
Kinderpoliklinik,
Ludwig-Maximilians-University of Munich,
Pettenkoferstr. 8a, D-80336 München, Germany

Winston W. K. Koo M.B.B.S.
Department of Pediatrics and Obstetrics/Gynecology,
Wayne State University School of Medicine,
Detroit, Michigan

Nancy D. Leslie, M.D.
Division of Human Genetics,
Children's Hospital Medical Center,
Cincinnati, Ohio

Kathleen J. Motil M.D., Ph.D.
USDA/ARS Children's Nutrition Research Center,
Department of Pediatrics,
Baylor College of Medicine,
Houston, Texas

Buford L. Nichols M.D.
Children's Nutrition Research Center,
Baylor College of Medicine,
Department of Pediatrics,
Houston, Texas

P.B. Pencharz M.B., Ch.B., Ph.D.
Departments of Pediatrics and Nutritional Sciences,
University of Toronto,
Toronto, Canada

Richard J. Schanler M.D.
Section of Neonatology and
USDA/ARS Children's Nutrition Research Center,
Department of Pediatrics,
Baylor College of Medicine,
Houston, TX

Reginald C. Tsang M.B.B.S.
Department of Pediatrics,
Pediatric Bone Research Center,
University of Cincinnati Medical Center,
Cincinnati, Ohio

D.C. Wilson M.D.
Departments of Pediatrics and Nutritional Sciences,
University of Toronto,
Toronto, Canada

J. Paul Zimmer Ph.D.
University of Alabama at Birmingham,
Birmingham, Alabama

Stanley H. Zlotkin M.D., Ph.D.
University of Toronto,
Department of Paediatrics,
Division of Gastroenterology/Nutrition,
Research Institute,
Hospital for Sick Children
Toronto, Canada

Forward

Infant nutrition must satisfy needs not only for life and growth but also for optimal mental and physical development. Nutrition of infants requires avoidance of deficiencies and toxins and hopefully helps prevent diseases later in life. For the first few months of life, milk from the infant's mother meets all of these criteria. Subsequently, requirements for optimal nutrition become more complex as the end results - what are we measuring and what should be measured - become more complex. Likewise, prenatally and perinatally goals now recognized to be influenced by nutrition include desirable growth and development of the fetus and obviating certain developmental anomalies and malformations.

Reading a list of nutrient requirements is boring and calculating nutrient consumption is best done with computers. But nutrition is an interesting subject. The editors of the present volume set for themselves the task of creating a volume which even the exhausted resident will find challenging and helpful even at 10 P.M. To accomplish this they have created a book with very readable text with fewer details than some texts and they have included some vignettes of historical interest. Information of practical application is made readily available by considerate and effective highlighting. The use of delightful visuals and occasional humor adds to the enjoyment of reading about nutrition of infants.

The establishment of good nutritional practices early in life may help avoid some of the problems related to nutrition which develop later. For example obesity, and delayed development may be traced to early approaches to diet and feeding practices. Nutrient deficiencies and imbalance can be eradicated. Hunger, which should have been totally eliminated, can at least be lessened with better utilization of nutritional knowledge.

Because of the recent enthusiasm and pronouncements of individuals with varied prejudices, agendas and beliefs the editors make one very important additional contribution. They clearly indicate what can and what cannot be expected from nutrition alone.

Lewis A. Barness M.D.
Professor of Pediatrics,
Department of Pediatrics,
College of Medicine,
University of South Florida,
Tampa, Florida

"Many books have been written on Pediatric Nutrition. The uniqueness of this volume is not only the science but also the clinical applications and the clinical experience that these top rate authors represent. I would not hesitate to strongly recommend this book for both clinicians and scientists with interest in pediatric nutrition."

Professor Chap-Yung Yeung, FRCP Lond, FRCP (C),
FRCP Ed, FRCP (Glasg), FRACP, FRCP I
The Unviersity of Hong Kong,
Department of Peadiatrics,
Queen Mary Hospital, Hong Kong

Nutritional disorders constitute the core health problem among infants and young children throughout the world. Unlike other mammals, the human infant is dependent and at the mercy of care takers for several years for meeting his essential health needs including nutritional requirements. Apart from adversely affecting the growth and development during early crucial years, undernutrition and deficiency of micronutrients is associated with increased vulnerability to a variety of disorders especially infectious diseases thus initiating a vicious self perpetuating cycle of malnutrition, infections and ill health.

Nutrition During Infancy: Principles and Practice is a comprehensive multi-author venture to provide current state-of-the-art information on a wide range of nutritional issues by an eminent team of international experts known for their outstanding contributions in the field of perinatal nutrition. Apart from conventional nutritional topics, the book covers a wide range of contemporary global concerns like role of microminerals in health and disease, food allergy, dietary management of systemic disorders and inborn errors of metabolism, enigma of weaning and challenge of commercially producing "human milk".

Apart from academic excellence and thoroughness of contents, the book is eminently readable and is replete with innovative ideas like catchy aphorisms, historical caricatures and humorous anecdotes. The clinical "pearls" and "bullets" of basic facts in bold print are easy on the cerebral cortex and are likely to leave lasting images on the memory lane. The excellent layout, clarity of print and artistic reproduction of diagrams, figures and line drawings are added merits. The documentation of representative clinical cases pertaining to various nutritional disorders in most chapters is the unique feature of the book for highlighting important messages of day-to-day practical relevance for the benefit of residents. Though the book is compiled by a galaxy of experts located in the developed world, its comprehensive contents encompass global concerns and perspectives with important messages of universal application. I have no doubt that *Nutrition During Infancy: Principles and Practice* will admirably serve the needs of pediatricians, nutritionists and public health doctors and nurses working both in the developed and developing world.

Dr. Meharban Singh M.D., F.A.M.S., F.I.A.P., F.A.A.P.
Former President,
National Neonatology Forum of India and
Neonatal Division,
All India Institute of Medical Sciences,
Ansari Nagar, New Delhi

Clinical Skills for Nutrition Evaluation

Stanley H. Zlotkin M.D., Ph.D.

University of Toronto, Department of Paediatrics,
Division of Gastroenterology/Nutrition, Research Institute,
Hospital for Sick Children

Reviewed by Buford L. Nichols M.D.

"What gets measured gets done."

Anonymous

Practical Points

- *Nutritional evaluation will help the clinician determine whether an infant's nutritional needs are being met by their 'normal' diet.*
- *The purpose of the baseline or screening nutritional assessment is to determine whether the infant is growing normally and whether normal eating habits are developing.*
- *If the infant has a normal growth rate, as indicated by sequential points along a growth channel, eats foods from each of the food groups, has no evidence of excess nutrient losses and follows a normal developmental pattern for eating, it is generally presumed that nutritional status is normal, that their nutritional needs are being met by their current diet. Further assessment of nutritional state would be unrevealing and therefore unnecessary.*
- *Infants whose nutritional needs are not being met by their diet would be assessed as 'not well nourished' by the baseline nutritional assessment. These infants need a detailed nutritional evaluation.*
- *The purpose of the detailed nutritional evaluation is to determine if nutrient deficiencies are present, to determine the possible causes of the abnormal nutritional status and to help direct nutritional therapy.*
- *The detailed evaluation should include a detailed history, assessment of food intake and eating behaviour, a physical exam looking for*

signs of nutrient deficiencies and appropriate anthropometry, and some specific diagnostic investigations.

Introduction

This chapter will describe the clinical skills and tools that are necessary to evaluate the nutritional state of the patient. Nutritional evaluation will help the clinician determine whether an infant's nutritional needs are being met by their "normal" diet. When used appropriately, it will also aid in the diagnosis of nutrition-related diseases and in determining individual nutritional needs.

The teaching of nutrition is new to most medical curricula and is not universally taught across North America. As such, many physicians do not have the experience nor confidence to incorporate nutritional evaluation into their assessment of the sick child. Nevertheless the principles which underlie the nutritional assessment as well as the assessment itself are quite straightforward. In this chapter, a clinical approach to nutritional evaluation will be described. The approach which can be simply and effectively used is generic in nature and can therefore be used to describe the nutritional status of infants with AIDS, cystic fibrosis, congenital heart disease or any acute or chronic disease.

Screening Nutritional Assessment

The process of screening an infant for nutritional status is similar to that used in the initial assessment of an infant's general medical state. The initial step in the medical evaluation involves obtaining baseline information through questions and physical examination and then comparing the answers (and findings) to nor-

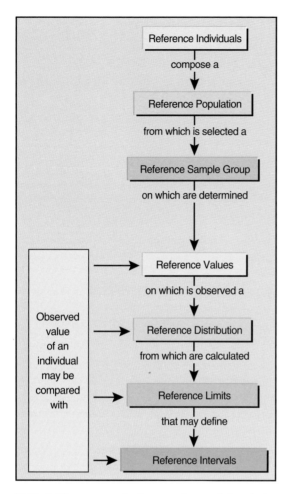

Table 1: The concept of reference values and the relationship of recommended terms.[1]

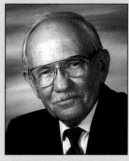

Arnold E. Schaefer Ph.D.
(1917-1992) a student of Conrad Elvehjem, the discoverer of nicotinic acid at the University of Wisconsin, directed the ICNND, the Interdepartmental Committee on Nutrition for National Defense, which was an outgrowth of U.S. military nutritional programs in and following World War II. His committee work began in 1955 with international nutritional surveys in 22 countries and was extended in 1967-68 to ten U.S. States . The surveys included examinations for clinical nutritional deficiency findings and some of the illustrations in our color atlas are photographs published in the survey manual. The results of the US surveys lead to laws establishing the Food Stamp Program, the Women's, Infant's and Children's (WIC) Program, and to enhancements of the School Lunch Program. These Federal programs, administered by the US Department of Agriculture, have had a significant benefit on contemporary infant mortality and child health. Kern, RA. Nutrition surveys co-sponsored by our government in foreign lands. Trans. Coll. Phys. Phila. 31: 98-119, 1963. Interdepartmental Committee on Nutrition for National Defense: Manual for Nutrition Surveys. 2nd ed. National Institutes of Health Bethesda, MD 1963

mative values. This comparison is most often a subconscious process by the time medical training is completed. Normative values for the clinical examination are primarily based on the practitioner's experience in examining "normal" children, while the symptoms are compared to normative data described in medical text books and literature. The physician usually continues to collect information about the infant until enough common features have been identified for classification into one of many categories ranging initially from "healthy with no obvious pathology" to "very sick with multiple pathologies." If a healthy infant is identified by this evaluative process, further evaluation is usually withheld. If a 'sick' infant is identified, then further evaluation is carried out.

Similar to the process used to assess baseline medical status, the baseline nutritional evaluation involves obtaining information by questioning about current and past health, usual food intake, anthropometric measurements and physical examination.

Baseline or Screening Nutritional Assessment

1. Direct questions about current and past health.
2. Determine typical dietary intake.
3. Take height, weight and head circumference measurements.
4. Have a good look at the patient.

The answers, findings and results are then compared to normative values. *For example, when taking the history, the most important questions are about past health, previous hospitalizations or operations since a child with previous hospitalizations or operations is more likely to have eaten poorly; an inquiry about emesis*

For each food item, indicate with a check mark the category that best describes the frequency with which you usually eat that particular food item.

Food item	More than once per day	Once per day	3-6 times per week	Once or twice per week	Once per month or less	Never
Milk	☐	☐	☐	☐	☐	☐
Formula	☐	☐	☐	☐	☐	☐
Nursing	☐	☐	☐	☐	☐	☐
Vegetable	☐	☐	☐	☐	☐	☐
Meat	☐	☐	☐	☐	☐	☐
Cereals	☐	☐	☐	☐	☐	☐
Cheese	☐	☐	☐	☐	☐	☐
Yogurt	☐	☐	☐	☐	☐	☐
Enter other foods not listed that are eaten regularly:						
1.........	☐	☐	☐			
2.........	☐	☐	☐			
3.........	☐	☐	☐			
4.........	☐	☐	☐			

Table 2: Abbreviated food frequency questionnaire. A few foods and food categories are shown as examples. A complete questionnaire might contain more than 100 items.

and stool pattern will assess the likelihood that excess nutrient losses are present. By measuring and plotting height and weight for age, and simply looking at the child, an initial classification of "normal" or "abnormal" nutritional status can be made. The process of comparing an individual child to population norms for growth, appearance and food intake is a baseline or screening nutritional assessment.

The purpose of the baseline or screening nutritional assessment is to determine whether the infant is growing normally and whether normal eating habits are developing. The baseline assessment is applicable to all patients in the pediatric age range. Assessment results must always be compared to some accepted "normal" standard. To conclude that a patient's nutritional status is "normal", one assumes that the patient's growth and eating habits fall within an acceptable normal range. Standards for normality by

definition must reflect the population as a whole, rather than individual values (Table 1).[1] Thus, standards for growth are established from populations of healthy growing children. "Normal" growth is described, for example, in standard growth charts derived from National Centre for Health Statistics (NCHS) cross-sectional data of American children.[2] The growth of an individual child, therefore, is compared to "normal" growth by sequential measurements and plots of height and weight at regular intervals. The NCHS charts are shown in the appendix.

Standards for nutrient intake for various ages, the RNI's (recommended nutrient intakes) are published by the Department of Health in Canada.[3] In the United States, equivalent standards are the RDAs (recommended dietary allowances) prepared by the Food and Nutrition Board of the National Research Council.[4] It is, however, not necessary to use the RDAs as

Name: Street Address: Town/City:				Date: Day of the week:		
					LAB USE ONLY	
Place eaten	Time	Description of food or drink. Give brand name if applicable	Amount	Day/meal Amount code	Food code	Code
Additional questions: Was intake unusual in any way? Yes (...) No (...) If yes, in what way? Do you take vitamin or mineral supplements? Yes (...) No(...) If yes, how many per day? (...) per week? (...) If yes, what kind? (give brand name if possible) Multivitamin Iron Ascorbic acid Other (list)						

Table 3: Sample data sheet for a twenty-four-hour record. From Gibson (6).

part of the baseline nutritional assessment. Nutrient intake in the baseline assessment is adequately assessed by using American Academy of Pediatrics or Canadian Paediatric Society guidelines which describe a nutritionally complete diet in general terms for infants.[5]

National food guides list foods according to food groups and recommend servings from each of the groups according to age. General food intake can be assessed using either a food frequency list or a 24-hour recall diet. The food frequency list is simply a record of the number of servings from each food group consumed by the child on a typical day (Table 2).[6] Such a list, for example, might show three portions of cereal/bread, three portions of dairy products, one fruit, one meat, and no vegetables. The 24-hour recall is a listing of the actual foods and portion sizes eaten the previous day (Table 3).[6] By comparing the data from one of these lists to the information from the food guides, one can estimate the normality of the child's food intake.

By four to six months, most infants are physiologically ready to handle solids (tables 4-7). Standards for the physiological progression of oral motor skills and the development of "normal" eating habits have been described by Illingworth[7] and codified by the American Academy of Pediatrics and the Canadian Pediatric Society in their published statements. These may be used to assess the normality of the child's eating behaviour. For example, an eighteen-month-old infant who is not yet eating any pureed foods would be defined as having abnormal eating habits.

In summary, therefore, if the infant has a normal growth rate, as indicated by sequential points along a growth channel, eats foods from each of the food groups, has no evidence of excess nutrient losses and

> *Never underestimate the wisdom of nutritional practices in traditional cultures.*
> Susan Henning Ph.D.
> Department of Pediatrics
> Baylor College of Medicine
> Houston, Texas

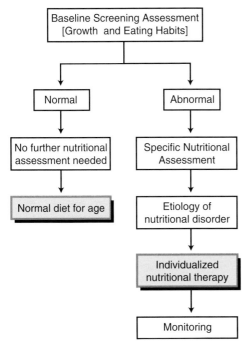

Figure 1: Assessment of nutritional status.

Age	Average Quantity Taken in Individual Feedings
1st and 2nd wk	2-3 oz (60-90 mL)
3 wk-2 mo	4-5 oz (120-150 mL)
2-3 mo	5-6 oz (150-180 mL)
3-4 mo	6-7 oz (180-210 mL)
5-12	7-8 oz (210-240 mL)

Table 5: Average quantity of feedings.

Age	Average No. of Feedings in 24 hr
Birth-1 wk	6-10
1 wk-1 mo	6-8
1-3 mo	5-6
3-7 mo	4-5
4-9 mo	3-4
8-12 mo	3

Table 4: Average daily number of feedings.

Physiologic Rationale for the Introduction of Solid Foods at 4-6 months

- The digestive system has developed sufficiently to permit good absorption of a variety of foods.

- The "extrusion reflex" useful for sucking and fixing the nipple in the mouth has gradually disappeared.

- The secretion of saliva has increased and facilitates the swallowing of solid foods.

- The neuromuscular coordination has improved; the tongue is now able to pass solids from the front to the back of the mouth.

- The mucosal barrier has matured and the risks of food allergies have diminished.

- The head control has improved; the baby can sit up; lean forward, turn away and send cues of satiety to the caregiver.

Table 6: Physiologic rationale for the introduction of solid foods at four to six months.

follows a normal developmental pattern for eating, it is generally presumed that nutritional status is normal, that their nutritional needs are being met by their current diet. Further assessment of nutritional state would be unrevealing and therefore unnecessary.

Detailed Nutritional Assessment

Infants whose nutritional needs are not being met by their diet would be assessed as 'not well nourished' by the baseline nutritional assessment. They would be characterized by one or more of the following features:

1) not following normal growth channels; 2) inadequate food intake or inappropriate food choice; 3) excess nutrient losses, or 4) retarded oral development. A more detailed nutritional assessment is warranted for this group of infants (Figure 1).

The purpose of the detailed nutritional evaluation is to determine if nutrient deficiencies are present, to determine the possible causes of the abnormal nutritional status and to help direct nutritional therapy. The most common causes of malnutrition are listed in Table 8. The assessment should include a detailed his-

Age (years)	Physical	Social/Personal
1–1-1/2	• grasps and releases foods with fingers • holds spoon but use poor • turns spoon in mouth • uses cup but release poor	• wants food other eating • loves performing
1-1/2–2	• appetite decreases • likes eating with hands • likes experimenting with textures	• ritual becomes important • displays food preferences • distracts easily

* Modified from A Joint Project of the Network of the Federal/Provincial/Territorial Group on Nutrition and National Institute of Nutrition. Promoting nutritional Health during the preschool years. Canadian Guidelines, 1989.

Table 7: Typical physical and social/personal characteristics related to eating during the second year of life.

1. Decrease in ingestion of food
-from, swallowing dysfunction or dysco-ordination -from, pain leading to anorexia -from, vomiting secondary to obstruction -from, nausea secondary to drug therapy -from, learned food aversion -from, purposeful or inadvertent withholding of food
2. Nutrient malabsorption and losses
-from, pancreatic insufficiency -from, hepatic dysfunction -from, rapid transit secondary to 'short bowel' -from, bacterial overgrowth -from, excess stool output -from, enteropathy (eg protein losing) -from, chronic parasitic infections
3. Increased nutrient needs (energy)
-from, chronic infection (increased energy expenditure and energy imbalance)

Table 8: Most common causes of malnutrition.

Specific Nutritional Assessment

1. **History -**
   - Medical
   - Surgical
   - Developmental
   - Drugs
2. **Diet -**
   - Food records
3. **P/E -**
   - Including Anthropometry
4. **Diagnostic Investigations**

Table 9: Specific nutritional assessment.

tory, assessment of food intake and eating behaviour, a physical exam looking for signs of nutrient deficiencies and appropriate anthropometry, and some specific diagnostic investigations (Table 9).

Detailed Nutrient Assessment - History

The nutrition history should include details regarding current and past medical or surgical conditions which may affect the patient's nutritional status. It should include a detailed functional inquiry and an assessment of possible nutrient losses through emesis and stool. A description of allergies which may limit the variety of foods eaten should be included. A list of medications should be compiled since complications of medications may affect hunger or nutrient absorption and excretion. A psycho-social inquiry including relevant environmental, social and family factors may suggest that behavioural issues are affecting nutrient intake.

Nutrient Intake

Malnutrition is most often the result of inadequate food intake. Food intake, however, should be verified before proceeding with further diagnostic evaluation or specific therapeutic intervention. Because neither the food frequency list nor the 24-hour recall are reliable for accurately assessing the nutrient intake of an individ-

Measurements + Common Error	Proposed Solution
All measurements	
Inadequate instrument	Select method appropriate to resources
Restless child	Postpone measurement Involve parent in procedures Use culturally appropriate procedures
Reading	Training and refresher exercises stressing accuracy Intermittent revision by supervisor
Recording	Record results immediately after measurement is taken Have results checked by second person
Length	
Incorrect method for age	Use only when subject is < 2 years old
Footwear and headwear not removed	Remove as local culture permits (or make allowances)
Head not in correct plane	Correct position of child before measuring

Child not straight along board and/or
    feet not parallel with movable board
	Have assistant and child's parent present:
	    don't take the measurement while the child is
	    struggling; settle child

Board not firmly against heels	Correct pressure should be practiced
Weight	
Room cold, no privacy	Use appropriate clinic facilities
Scale not calibrated to zero	Re-calibrate after every subject
Subject wearing heavy clothing	Remove or make allowances for clothing

Subject moving or anxious as a result
    of prior incident
	Wait until subject is calm or remove cause of anxiety
	    (e.g. scale too high)

Table 10: Common errors and possible solutions when measuring length, height, and weight. Modified from Zerfas AJ. (1979). In: Jelliffe DB, Jelliffe EFP (eds). Human Nutrition. A comprehensive Treatise, Volume 2. Nutrition and Growth, Plenum Press.

ual patient (these are designed to assess the mean intake of a group),[8] parents (or nursing staff on the ward) should be asked to keep a record of all food intake, portion size and manner of food preparation for three or seven days including at least one weekend day. This record would be analyzed by a dietitian for daily energy intake and the adequacy of the diet for meeting protein, vitamin and mineral needs according to the published standards (RNI, RDA).

Diets that are quantitatively normal are seldom limited in quality unless the variety of foods eaten is markedly restricted. An obvious example is iron deficiency anemia in infants who ingest large amounts of cow milk to the exclusion of other foods.[9] Diets that fail to meet energy needs may also be deficient in vitamins and minerals; however, deficient protein intake is not common in developed countries, but may be seen in developing countries or in refugee from these countries. Further history and physical examination will often clarify the reasons for inadequate energy intake.

Inadequate food intake may be due to anorexia associated with chronic disease, an underlying medical or surgical condition which interferes with chewing, swallowing, digestion, etc., or very rarely, failure of a parent to provide food to their child. Anorexia associated with chronic disease may be passive in origin (i.e. due to the disease or the treatment) or active if food refusal is a component of the anorexia. In children with chronic

Measurements + Common Error	Proposed Solution
Arm circumference Subject not standing in correct position Tape too thick, stretched, or creased Wrong arm Mid-arm point incorrectly marked Arm not hanging loosely by side during measurement, examiner not comfortable or level with subject, tape around arm not at midpoint: too tight (causing skin contour identation), too loose	Position subject correctly Use correct measurement Use left arm Measure midpoint carefully Correct techniques with training, supervision, and regular refresher courses. Take into account any cultural problems, such as wearing of arm band
Head circumference Occipital protuberance/supraorbital landmarks poorly defined Hair crushed inadequately, ears under tape or tension, and position poorly maintained at time of reading Headwear not removed	Position tape correctly Correct technique with training, supervision, and regular refresher courses Remove local culture permits
Triceps fatfold Wrong arm Mid-arm point or posterior plane incorrectly measured or marked Arm not loose by side during measurement Finger-thumb pinch or caliper placement too deep (muscle) or too superficial (skin) Caliper jaws not at marked site Reading done too early, pinch not maintained, caliper handle not fully released Examiner not comfortable or level with subject	Use left arm Measure midpoint carefully Correct technique with training, supervision, and regular refresher courses Ensure examiner is level with subject for measurement

Table 11: Common errors and possible solutions when measuring mid-upper-arm circumference, head circumference, and triceps skinfold. Modified from Zerfas AJ. (1979). In: Jelliffe DB, Jelliffe EFP (eds). Human Nutrition. A comprehensive Treatise, Volume 2. Nutrition and Growth. Plenum Press.

illnesses, there may be a significant psycho-social or "non-organic" component to the patient's refusal to ingest an adequate quantity of food.

Inadequate food intake because of faulty coordination of chewing, swallowing and breathing is particularly common in infants with various types of cerebral palsy.[10] Co-ordinated oromotor function is critical for establishing and maintaining adequate nutrient intake. Abnormalities in oromotor function can be initially detected through the history and verified by observing the child during feeding. Key points in the history include frequency of chest infections which may be secondary to tracheal aspiration of food; the time taken for each feeding period, since prolonged feeding periods are indicative of dysfunction; vomiting or nasal regurgitation; choking during feeding; the consistency of the food ingested since liquids are usually more difficult to swallow in the presence of oromotor dysfunction; and, general willingness to ingest food, since an aversion to eating is also likely to be associated with swallowing dyscoordination and chronic aspiration.

During a feeding session, the presence or extent of oromotor dysfunction can be determined by observing various characteristics of the infant's chewing, swallowing and breathing.[11] Gagging is associated with improper bolus formation such that some of the food or liquid in the mouth enters the pharynx prematurely. Nasal reflux indicates poor closure of the tongue against the soft palate and should not be present at any age. Tongue thrusting inhibits oral feeding and is abnormal beyond three months of age.[12] Drooling indicates poor lip and tongue control. Infants who cough and choke with feedings are likely aspirating food into the larynx. Poor oromotor function of any kind can limit the quantity or variety of food a child is able to tolerate and may lead to chronic malnutrition.

Although psycho-social anorexia and swallowing dysfunction are the two most common causes of malnutrition in infants, anorexia is a prominent characteristic of many chronic diseases, including chronic renal disease, chronic inflammatory diseases and many cancers. Examples from these categories are numerous. The tachypnea of bronchopulmonary dysplasia and congestive heart failure leave little time for the interruption of breathing necessary for swallowing. Infants who are fluid restricted invariably have limited intake (e.g. chronic renal failure, congestive heart disease, bronchopulmonary dysplasia). Medications, especially those associated with treatment of cancer can cause nausea and contribute to limited intake. In addition, digoxin may cause anorexia while some antibiotics are associated with abdominal pain, nausea and anorexia. Anticonvulsants may decrease level of consciousness thus interfering with food intake. In addition to the nausea, vomiting and general anorexia associated with many diseases or their treatment, prolonged periods of limited food oral intake during treatment may promote a behavioral indifference to eating or result in specific learned food aversions.

Although less common, inappropriate food choices by a parent on behalf of a infant may be a function of various socio-economic factors including education,

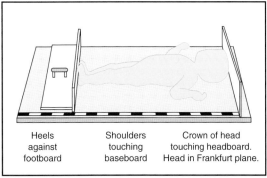

| Heels against footboard | Shoulders touching baseboard | Crown of head touching headboard. Head in Frankfurt plane. |

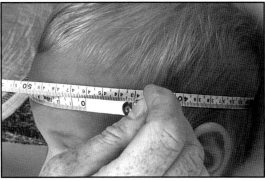

Figure 2: Correct methods for measuring the length of an infant and head circumference.

religion/culture and financial resources. These faulty food choices may result in specific nutrient deficiencies.[13, 14]

Whenever poor intake adequately explains growth failure, there is no need to pursue metabolic causes or to look for nutrient losses until the problems with intake have been addressed.

Anthropometry

Routine anthropometry in all patients undergoing a detailed nutritional assessment should include weight, height, head circumference (under age two years), fat folds and mid-arm circumference. These physical measurements, individually and in combination provide an indirect assessment of body composition. *By comparing the measurements taken on an individual patient to standards specific for age and sex, one can obtain an objective assessment of normality.*

The proper techniques for measuring length, head circumference and skin folds are shown in the follow-

Step 1. Plot the infant's length on a gender appropriate growth chart (see appendix).

Step 2. Determine length percentile.

Step 3. Determine the ideal weight-for-height (IBW). Determine the weight that corresponds to the same centile as that for actual height-for-age.

Step 4. Express actual weight as a percent of ideal weight-for-height (%IBW = actual weight/ideal weight-for-height x 100).

Table 12: Calculation of weight as a percentage of ideal weight-for-height.

% Expected Weight for Age	Classification	Category of Nutritional Status
>90%	Normal	Normal
76-90%	Mild malnutrition	1st degree malnutrition
61-75%	Moderate malnutrition	2nd degree malnutrition
≤60%	Severe malnutrition	3rd degree malnutrition

Table 13: The Gomez classification. Adapted from (16).

% Expected weight for age	Edema	
	Present	Absent
80-60%	Kwashiorkor	Underweight
<60%	Marasmic-kwashiorkor	Marasmus

Table 14: The Wellcome classification. Adapted from the Wellcome Trust Working Party (17).

Height for Age Degree of Stunting	Weight for Height Degree of Wasting			
Percent (Grade)	>90% (0)	80-90% (1)	70-80% (2)	<70% (3)
>90% (Grade = 0) 95-90% (Grade = 1)	Normal		Wasting	
85-90% (Grade = 2) <85% (Grade = 3)	Stunting		Stunting and Wasting	

Table 15: The Waterlow classification. Adapted from Waterlow (18).

Combination of Indices	Nutritional Status

Low wt/ht
   + low wt/age + normal ht/age
   + low wt/age + high ht/age
   + normal wt/age + high ht/age
	
	Currently underfed
	Currently underfed
	Currently underfed

Normal wt/ht
   + low wt/age + low ht/age
   + normal wt/age + normal ht/age
   + high wt/age + high ht/age
	
	Short, normally nourished
	Normal
	Tall, normally nourished

High wt/ht
   + normal wt/age + low ht/age
   + high wt/age + low ht/age
   + high wt/age + normal ht/age
	
	Currently overfed, short
	Obese
	Overfed, not necessarily obese

Table 16: The results of using various combinations of anthropometric indices and possible interpretations of the results.

ing pictures (Figure 2). The common measurement errors and possible solutions are listed in the following tables (Tables 10 and 11).

In adults, from the weight and height measurements, one can calculate the body mass index (BMI) (or Quatelet index). This index, expressed as weight/height^2 (kg/m^2) is a good indicator of relative fatness. It can be used to determine 'healthy' weights as well as to identify individuals at risk for complications associated with being overweight or underweight. Standardized percentile curves of body-mass index for children and adolescents have recently been published.[15] However none are available for infants. Determination of weight as a percentage of "ideal body weight for height" in infants is important because various indices are available which relate weight as a percentage of ideal weight-for-height to risk of malnutrition. Calculation of weight as a percentage of ideal weight for height is shown in Table 12.

To identify and classify malnourished individuals, the anthropometric indices can be compared with either predetermined reference limits or cutoff points

> *There is nothing that civilization has to offer which is better than the welfare of children.*
> *Above all I should recognize and try to get the world to recognize that the health and welfare of children depends on the education and affection of their parents rather than on material assets.*
>
> Primary Health Care Pioneer
> The Selected Works of
> Dr. Cicely D. Williams
> Naomi Baumslag, Editor
> World Federation of Public
> Health Associations
> and UNICEF

which can classify an individual into one or more 'risk' categories indicative of the severity of malnutrition and/or mortality risk. Unfortunately, there is no universally accepted classification system for describing risk of under- or over-nutrition in terms of type, severity or approximate duration. The most common classifications, for example, the Gomez, and the Wellcome classification do not take height into account and therefore cannot distinguish between wasting and stunting (Table 13 and 14).[16, 17] The Waterlow classification (Table 15) is an improvement over the previously mentioned classifications because it uses both height for age and weight for age as indices and the 50th percentile of the Harvard reference data as the reference point, but it too has its faults.[18] Its major drawback is its use of the 50th percentile height for age as the reference standard. An individual whose weight as a percentage of ideal weight-for-height is 100% may be classified as stunted, if their height is <90% of the 50th percentile of the Harvard reference data for height. In most situations (in North America) height measurements which are

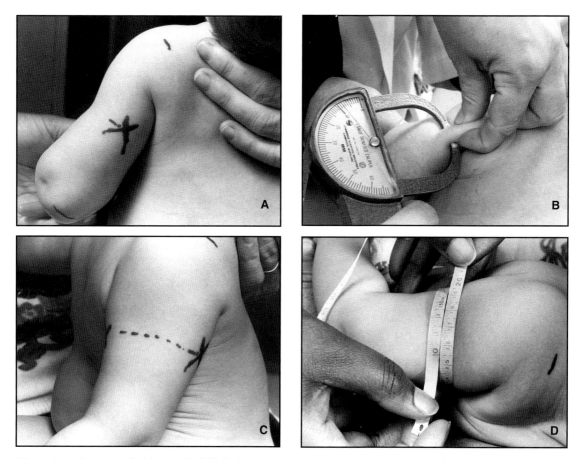

Figure 3: A. Location of mid-arm skinfold thickness measurement. B. Measurement of mid-arm skinfold thickness.
C. Location of upper mid-arm circumference. D. Measurement of upper mid-arm circumference.

<90% of the 50th percentile of the Harvard reference data for height are based on genetic predisposition, rather than chronic malnutrition. If one were to include values for parental height, the classification system would be improved.

Using the Waterlow classification, four broad categories of nutritional assessment are defined: normal; wasted; stunted and wasted; and stunted only. The reference limits selected for grades 1, 2 and 3 correspond approximately to 1, 2 and 3 standard deviations of height for age and weight for age of the Harvard reference data. By using this classification, one can distinguish between infants who are normal, wasted, stunted and wasted and stunted. These distinctions are potentially important since Waterlow and Rutishauser have suggested different degrees of intervention and response depending on the classification. For example, they suggested that infants who are wasted, or stunted and wasted, should receive the highest priority for nutrition intervention.

The World Health Organization has attempted to combine various combinations of anthropometric indices and possible interpretations of the results (Table 16). This table accurately describes the nutritional status of individuals based on weight and height, but does not distinguish the nutritionally stunted individual.

Standard deviation scores (SD score) also can be calculated for individual infants from reference data. For example, an infant with a length one standard deviation above the reference median for her age would have an SD score of +1, whereas an infant with a length two

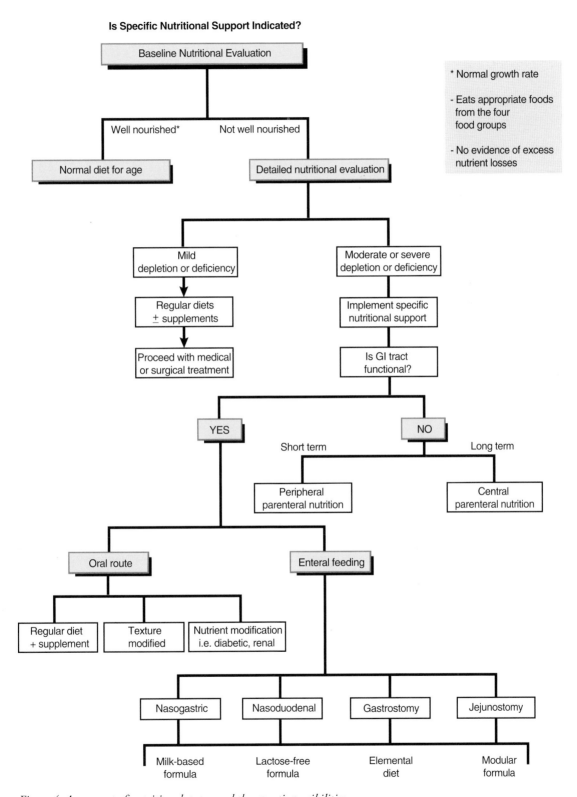

Figure 4: Assessment of nutritional status and therapeutic possibilities.

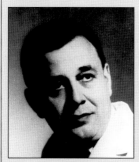

Tom D. Spies M.D.

(1902-1960) "was the epitome of the true physician who saw nutrition as the biochemical bridge between food and life." He directed the Nutrition clinic at Hillman Hospital, Birmingham, Alabama, where he used nicotinic acid to heal the scabrous incustations of pellagra. He pioneered in the use of folic acid for tropical sprue. He lead the fight to make multivitamin supplements available over the counter. A selection of his teaching slides are included in the color atlas of clinical nutritional deficiencies. J Nutr. 102, 1395-1399, 1972 (Photo courtesy of NLM)

standard deviations below the reference median for age would have a SD score of -2. Exact values for the standard deviation score of an individual can be calculated using the reference data provided in the appendix and the equation shown below.

$$\text{SD Score} = \frac{\text{Weight for subject} - \text{Median reference value of weight for height}}{\text{Median reference value} - \text{1 S.D. below median reference value}}$$

Although the reference data used to calculate standard deviation scores may vary, there is general agreement that scores of below -2 or above +2 reflect similar degrees of malnutrition or obesity irrespective of the anthropometric index used.

Changes in body composition in infants can be determined from measurement of subcutaneous fat (by triceps skinfold thickness) and muscle (mid-upper-arm circumference). They are useful in the initial evaluation of nutritional status and as a longitudinal reflection of change in body composition. These are particularly relevant when accurate length measurements are difficult to obtain or when changes in weight are difficult to interpret because of edema or ascites. Reference values (NCHS cross-sectional data) for infants are shown in the appendix. Proper technique for measuring these parameters are shown in Figure 3.

Physician Examination

Perhaps the most important component of the physical examination is the examiners subjective evaluation of "how the patient looks". We all have a sense of what an infant who is "too thin" looks like. Similarly, we all have a sense of what an overweight infant look like. From the history, the examiner should be in a good position to determine whether the infant is likely to be suffering from nutrient deficiencies, or not. In order to complete the physical examination, the infant must be examined totally unclothed. If severe malnutrition is suspected, the examination should be comprehensive, involving all components of the physical exam, including the neurological examination. If severe malnutrition is not suspected the examination need not be comprehensive, but should focus on specific parts of the body as indicated from the history.

For example, I recently saw a patient (five month old male infant) whose presented with weight loss, diarrhea, recent disinterest in feeding and a severe, unrelenting diaper rash. The history revealed that the infant had been born prematurely at 33 weeks gestation, had received expressed breast milk in the nursery and had been exclusively breast-fed since discharge. He was receiving an infant multivitamin preparation. My tentative diagnosis was zinc deficiency since human milk may not be an adequate source of zinc for the preterm infant born with limited zinc stores. For this physical examination, I concentrated on the examination of the skin, and observed, what I presumed to be the acrodermatitis diaper rash of zinc deficiency. I did not expect vitamin A deficiency, since the infant was receiving multivitamin drops which contained vitamin A. In situations where vitamin A deficiency are not suspected, a detailed examination of the eye for Bitot's spots or follicular hyperkeratosis would be of limited value. The physical examination should parallel the finding of the initial nutritional assessment.

Vitamin deficiencies are rare; however, in the appendix, we have compiled a colour pictorial index of signs of vitamin deficiencies which should be used as a reference should a vitamin deficiency be expected.

Index	Minimum Frequency	Indication
Anthropometry		
Weight	Every 3 months	Every 3 months
Height	Every 3 months	Every 3 months
Head Circumference	Every 3 months until 2 year	Every 3 months until 2 year
Midarm Circumference	Every 3 months	Every 3 months
Triceps Skinfolds	Every 3 months	Every 3 months
Nutritional Assessment		
Dietary Intake*	Yearly	Yearly
3-d Fat Balance†	As indicated	As indicated
Anticipatory dietary guidance	Yearly	Yearly
Laboratory Studies		
Complete blood count	Yearly	Yearly
Serum retinol	Yearly	Yearly
Serum α–tocopherol	Yearly	Yearly

Table 17: Nutritional status assessment. Adapted from (19).

Diagnostic Investigations

The final component of the specific nutritional assessment are the diagnostic tests. Two categories of tests may be used in the assessment. The first group are those tests which can be used to confirm a diagnosis or suspected diagnosis based on the initial nutritional assessment. For example, if based on the history, dietary assessment and physical examination the examiner suspects a protein losing enteropathy, then a serum total protein and albumin and 3 day stool collection for fat, protein and total energy would be useful to confirm the diagnosis. If iron deficiency is suspected from the initial nutritional assessment, then a blood hemoglobin, haematocrit, serum ferritin and free erythrocyte protoporphorin determination would help confirm the diagnosis.

The second category of tests are those which are most useful in determining the appropriate therapeutic intervention. Some of the tests that would be included in this category include a radiologic feeding study to determine the ability of the patient to swallow foods and liquids of varying consistency, esophageal pH probe to assess gastro-esophageal reflux, venogram to assess the patency of central veins, indirect calorimetry to determine resting energy needs, etc.

Tests which aim to assess body composition are particularly useful for monitoring the long- and short-term responses to nutritional therapy. Unfortunately, many of these tests remain in the domain of research, including for example bioelectric impedance, total nitrogen and total body potassium measurements, and double-labeled water studies of total energy expenditure.[19]

Once the initial nutritional assessment has been completed and the therapeutic intervention has been instituted, the final component of the nutritional therapy is monitoring the response to the intervention and the changing nutritional status of the patient. This may be accomplished using a similar set of procedures as outlined earlier in the section on the detailed nutritional assessment, but tailored to the specific condition of the patient in question. A recent consensus report on the use of the nutritional assessment in the management of cystic fibrosis exemplifies an appropriate use of the nutritional assessment in monitoring changes in nutritional status due to the chronic disease.[19] The assessment was used to monitor the effect of the ongoing disease process on nutritional status, as well as the response to appropriate nutritional intervention. As shown in Table 17, each of the tests and measurements is repeated at appropriate intervals to detect changes in the various parameters included in the assessment.

In summary, the extent and urgency of nutritional intervention for prophylaxis or nutritional rehabilita-

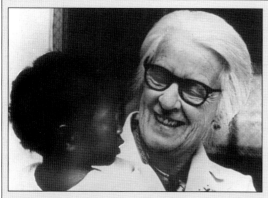

Cicely Williams M.D.

(1893-1994) studied under Osler at Oxford but parted company to lead the modern resurgence of primary care. While working on the Gold Coast of Africa she recognized a pediatric disorder kwashiorkor (local dialect for the sickness of the baby displaced from the breast). She recognized that this syndrome was due to protein deficiency. "Child heath must include the child, the whole child, and everything to do with the child, including the family and especially the mother....If you learn your 'nutrition' from a biochemist, you are not likely to learn how essential it is to blow a baby's nose before expecting him to suck." *Retired Except on Demand: The Life of Dr. Cicely Williams* by S. Craddock, Green College, Oxford, 1983 (Photo courtesy of Vanderbilt U.)

tion will depend on the nutritional status of the patient at the time of the initial assessment (Figure 4). The method of intervention which includes the route of nutrient delivery and the type of nutrients delivered will depend on the pathological findings identified during the nutritional assessment. Quite clearly, the nutritional evaluation is the key to determining nutritional therapy for the sick child.

Case History #1

Assume that you have been asked to see this patient to evaluate nutritional status and plan a nutritional strategy.

Patient JH was see in consultation at age 14 months (corrected). He was born at 32 weeks gestation with major perinatal complications. Briefly, he had RDS (respiratory distress syndrome), bilateral pneumothoracies, patent ductus arteriosis (PDA), hypospadius and a significant intraventricular hemorrhage. He was left with a difficult

to control seizure disorder, spastic diplegia, developmental delay, a VP shunt for mild hydrocephalus, and visual problems including far sightedness and astigmatism.

Since the newborn period he has had a very stormy course. At three months of age, due to recurrent seizures he had a feeding gastrostomy tube inserted. He had recurrent pneumonia secondary to aspiration that was associated with gastro-oesophageal reflux, for which he had received a Nissen fundoplication.

During this entire period of time he had seizures of varying types. At times they were generalized tonic - clonic and at other times focal seizures. He was treated with Phenobarbitol and Tegretol.

He was brought by his mother to clinic because she wanted permission to remove his gastrostomy feeding tube.

What are the important components about the history so far?

Teaching Point

The medical/surgical/social history is an important component of the nutritional assessment

What further information would you like to obtain?

To make a decision about the removal of the G-tube, further history was necessary. Information about his growth was obtained.

On the day that he was seen in consultation, he weighed 8.3 kg and his height was 73.5 cm.

What do you think about his growth? Use the growth charts in the appendix. What important information is still missing from your assessment?

Teaching Points:

Anthropometrics are an important component of the nutritional assessment. All data must be plotted before it can be interpreted.

You still need more information on feeding skills; feeding history; food intake history and more.

He receives a daily total of 760 ml of a nutritionally complete formula (1 kcal/ml) through his G-tube. JH's mother feels that her son feeds (orally) well enough to remove the G-tube, however, a report (which mom brought to clinic) of a recent barium swallow x-ray done at another hospital indicated aspiration of liquid barium after swallowing.

A detailed feeding history was obtained from JH's mother. There are days during which JH is capable of taking almost anything by mouth, including solids and liquids, without choking, coughing or any difficulty. There are also days when he is tired, has more seizure activity and is generally less able to respond to his environment. In the past, episodes of aspiration were invariably associated with these "bad" days.

What is your impression to this point? What would you like to do now?

Teaching Points:

The history is crutial for making a diagnosis

Current nutrient intakes (from G-tube) must be calculated.

The x-ray is often a very useful tool for nutritional evaluation.

On physical examination, he was noted to be very bright and alert (on this occasion). He was easily able to sit up straight and hold his head up on command although he would normally assume a slumped position supported by the table. We noted that JH was able to cough up secretions. We also noted that at the end of an absence seizure activity, he would cough.

He was fed. He was able to take solid foods and liquids without difficulty. He was able to close his lips on the spoon and transfer the food from the front to the back of his mouth without any difficulty and without any obvious aspiration. He had no difficulty initiating a swallow and no coughing, choking or sputtering. He had no increase in respiratory effort while being fed nor were there changes in auscultation of the chest following feeding.

JH's mother described the current feeding session as being "typical of a good day." She reiterated that it is only on "bad days" that he has trouble with his feeds (i.e. coughing, sputtering, etc. with feeds).

What is your interpretation of the information pro-

> Improved nutrition will do more to raise the standard of health and of living than any amount of medication, isolation mania, sanitary plumbing, prenatal mensuration and operating theatrical measures.
>
> Primary Health Care Pioneer
> The Selected Works of
> Dr. Cicely D. Williams
> Naomi Baumslag, Editor
> World Federation of Public
> Health Associations
> and UNICEF

vided above? Can you make a recommendation regarding JH's feeding or would you like further information or to perform further investigations?

Teaching Points:

Physical examination is an important component of the nutritional assessment.

Actually watching a child feed is often the most important part of the nutritional assessment.

JH was brought back to the Radiology Department on an "average day" for a radiologic feeding assessment. He was not having excess seizure activity, but was described by mother as being tired from going to bed too late the night before. The following was observed:

1. Barium coated solid foods were transferred from the front to the back of his mouth without difficulty. He was able to initiate a good swallow and there was no evidence of aspiration of barium into the trachea. The swallowing functions were well co-ordinated.

2. A very small amount of thin liquid barium was aspirated into the upper trachea with swallowing. This was expelled without coughing and did not continue into the lower airway.

Having gathered all this information about JH, what is your plan? Be specific!

Teaching Point:

A radiologic feeding study is often an important component of the nutritonal assessment. It will help to determine the most appropriate way of delivering nutrients to the patient.

These were the recommendations that were actually made for JH after the assessment was completed.

1. It is safe to feed JH semi-solids and items of thicker consistency. The consistency should be like pudding or even thicker. These foods should only be given to JH on 'good days'. These foods should be presented to JH in small amounts initially (two to three spoonfulls at a time) moving up in "two teaspoon increments" per week assuming that the foods are tolerated.

2. We recommended that liquids not be given by mouth (even on "average" days). The g-tube should be used to provide his fluid needs.

3. We encouraged dry swallows between mouthfulls of solid foods.

4. We encouraged thorough chewing of his foods and swallowing throughout the meal.

5. Since mid-day seems to be JH's best time of the day,

we recommended that the solid foods be fed at lunchtime and that the G-tube feeds be given after the meal only.

6. It was noted (from the feeding study and clinical observation) that JH did not always cough when there was liquid in his upper airway, although he would often cough without liquid in his airway. Thus a cough is not a good indicator of respiratory distress. Other signs of impending aspiration must be looked for, including increased respiratory effort, gagging, etc.

Historical Perspective...

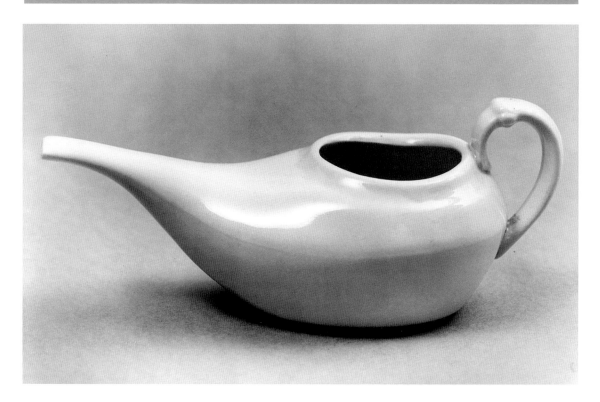

German pap boat, circa 1895 is made of Dresden China.

References

1. Grasbeck R, Siest G, Wilding P, et al. Provisional recommendations on the theory of reference values (1978). Part 1. The concept of reference values. *Clin Chem.* 1979;25:1506-1508.

2. Hamill PVV, Li TA, Johnson CL, Reed RB, Roche AF, Moore WM. Physical growth: National Centre for Health Statistics Percentile. *Am J Clin Nutr.* 1979;32: 607-629.

3. *Nutrition Recommendations.* Ottawa, Canada. Health and Welfare Canada. 1990: Canadian Government Publishing Centre.

4. *Recommended Dietary Allowances.* 10 ed. Washington, DC. Subcommittee on the 10th edition of the RDA's Food and Nutrition Board Commission on Life Sciences, National Research Council. 1989: National Academy Press.

5. *Canada's Food Guide Handbook.* Ottawa, Canada. Health and Welfare Canada: 1994. Ministry of Supply and Services.

6. Gibson R. Laboratory assessment of body composition. In: *Principles of Nutritional Assessment.* New York: Oxford University Press; 1990.

7. Illingworth RS, Lister J. The critical or sensitive period, with special reference to certain feeding problems in infants and children. *J Pediatr.* 1964;65:839-848.

8. Madden JP, Goodman SJ, Guthrie HA. Validity of the 24-hr recall: analysis of data obtained from elderly subjects. *J Am Diet Assoc.* 1976;68:143-147.

9. Wharton B. Which milk for normal infants? *Eur J Clin Nutr.* 1992;46 (Suppl 1):S27-S32.

10. Gisel EG, Patrick J. Identification of children with cerebral palsy unable to maintain a normal nutritional state. *Lancet.* 1988;1:283-285.

11. Sochaniwskyji AE, Koheil RM, Bablich K, Milner M, Kenny DJ. Oral motor functioning, frequency of swallowing and drooling in normal children and in children with cerebral palsy. *Arch Phys Med Rehab.* 1986; 67:866-874.

12. Stevenson RD, Allaire JH. The development of normal feeding and swallowing. In: *Development and Behavior: The very young child. Pediatric Clinic of North America,* Vol 6. Toronto: Saunders; 1991:1439-1453.

13. Sinatra FR, Merritt RJ. Iatrogenic kwashiorkor in infants. *Am J Dis Child.* 1981;135:21-23.

14. Pugliese MT, Weyman-Daum M, Moses N, Lifshitz F. Parental health beliefs as a cause of nonorganic failure to thrive. *Pediatr.* 1987;80:175-182.

15. Hammer LD, Kraemer HC, Wilson DM, Ritter PL, Dornbusch SM. Standardized percentile curves of body-mass index for children and adolescents. *Am J Dis Child.* 1991;145:259-263.

16. Gomez F, Galvan RR, Frenk S, Cravioto MJ, Chavezz R, Vazquez L. Mortality in second and third degree malnutrition. *J Trop Pediatr.* 1956;2:77-83.

17. Party WTW. Classification of infantile malnutrition. *Lancet.* 1970;2:302-303.

18. Waterlow JC. Classification and definition of protein calorie malnutrition. *Brit Med J.* 1972;3:566-569.

19. Ramsey BW, Farrell PM, Pencharz P, The Concensus Committee. Nutritional assessment and management in cystic fibrosis: a concensus report. *Am J Clin Nutr.* 1992; 55:108-116.

Managing Growth Faltering

Buford L. Nichols M.D.

Children's Nutrition Research Center,
Baylor College of Medicine, Department of Pediatrics,
Houston, Texas

Reviewed by Stanley H. Zlotkin M.D., Ph.D. and Steven Zeisel M.D., Ph.D.

Historical

The failure to thrive symptom complex was first described by Parrot, a founder of French Pediatrics in 1877. In his book entitled Athrepsia, *(Greek; neg. + nutrition) he described a syndrome which occurred in children less than three months of age which frequently was associated with "organic" (Greek; pertaining to an instrument or machine) autopsy findings. He also described a "primitive" form without demonstrable organic disease, now known as nonorganic failure to thrive. The physical findings in this syndrome included failure to gain weight, loss of weight, failure to gain length, loss of subcutaneous tissue and muscle mass, and a loss of host resistance leading to multiple acute infectious diseases. Parrot first described oral thrush as a complication of malnutrition in this book.[1]*

Failure to grow was distressingly common among hospitalized infants in the early days of pediatrics. In 1896, fewer than 20% of hospitalized young infants fed artificial formula would gain weight. Major improvements occurred when Huebner introduced Soxlet's method of sterilizing artificial formulas and Grancher's method of isolating individual young patients in glass cubicles at the new pediatric ward of the Charite Hospital in Berlin. With these reforms, in 1899, the number of infants who gained weight increased to 80% and the mortality in the ward fell from 75 to 17% of hospitalized admissions. This iatrogenic growth failure syndrome was called "Hospitalismus" by Huebner's disciple, Finkelstein.[2] These early European investigators were influential on American pediatrics. Since the first edition of Holt's American Textbook of Pediatrics in 1897, the syndromes of "failure to thrive" and "hospitalismus" have been presented in most American pediatric text books. These have been refined

over time as specific infectious, immunological, congenital, and genetic metabolic diseases have been recognized as organic contributors to this syndrome.[3]

During the last 50 years, the clinical definition of malnutrition in third world infants has led to a parallel international literature[4]. The organic forms of third world malnutrition have the same causes as the organic forms of failure to thrive and hospitalismus; and the sociological and psychological factors frequently associated with third world malnutrition are also found in the nonorganic failure-to-thrive syndromes.[4,5] For this reason, the present chapter includes all of the symptom complexes in a single heading: growth faltering. The clinical signs of growth faltering will be described. The criteria for early detection of growth faltering will be given. The role of anticipatory child health care in preventing growth faltering will be defined and the role of child nutrition programs in the process highlighted. Several specific subgroups of growth faltering will be described to help focus clinical attention on this symptom complex. Treatment and the criteria for response to management will be outlined. A summary of the clinical evaluation and the management will be provided.

Diagnosis

> Failure to thrive should be recognized on the basis of anthropometric criteria alone.[6]

Normal growth is an integrated functional outcome of a healthy child and family. Growth faltering should always be taken seriously and when detected, requires medical and/or behavioral intervention. The growth fail-

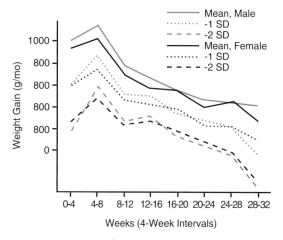

Figure 1: Incremental weight gains in males and females.

Diagnosis by Anthropometric Standards

The diagnosis of growth faltering is based on inadequate attained growth or on reduced growth velocity.[7]

> **Attained Weight Criteria**
> 1. Weight less than 80 to 85% of the 50th percentile of the NCHS growth standard; or
> 2. Weight for age less than the 5th percentile on the NCHS growth charts; or
> 3. Drop in weight of two or more percentile categories from a previously established growth channel; or
> 4. Z score of -2 below the normal 50th percentile.
>
> **Growth Velocity Criteria**
> 15-60 days: < 18 gm/d; and
> 61-270 days: < 12 gm/d; and
> 271-360 days: < 8 gm/d; and
> 361-540 days: < 5 gm/d; and
> Decrement   > 2 SD/90 d on velocity growth chart; and
> Loss of   > 1 SD Z score/90 d

ure is only visually apparent in extreme cases. The symptom complex is unchanged since Parrot's time. The responsible health care worker should recognize earlier stages of growth faltering and prevent the full expression of the classical syndromes of malnutrition, whether they are subsequently classified as athrepsia, infantile atrophy, pediatrophy, failure-to-thrive, hospitalismus, institutional growth retardation, decomposition, marasmus, marasmus infantilis, marasmus lactantium, kwashiorkor or protein calorie (energy) malnutrition. In this chapter, we focus on the milder disorders more prevalent than the full-fledged malnutrition syndromes described by these terms. This is with the intentional emphasis on preventing malnutrition and detecting early the acute and chronic disorders leading to malnutrition. We also emphasize that malnutrition is a physiological status of impaired metabolic functions, regardless of whether it is secondary to a physical illness or due to a dietary deficiency resulting from social or psychological disruptions of the home. Morbidity and mortality do not discriminate between these causal factors.

Growth evaluation focuses on objective anthropometry (the measurement of man) and clinical assessment. Growth measurement (see chapter on nutritional assessment) has become part of the anticipatory guidance offered in well child care and immunization clinics. The data available are most intensively clustered in the first six months of age and become infrequent after three years of age. This chapter focuses on the first two years of life, the period when early growth faltering is most commonly detected.

Because decline in rate of weight gain (velocity) is more sensitive than decline in linear or head circumference growth, and the presence of combined weight and length growth faltering is evidence of two or three month's chronicity, serial measurements of weight are essential for anticipatory guidance and provide the earliest warning of growth faltering at the breast. A drop in weight growth velocity is the earliest detectable sign of growth faltering.[8-10] Standards are given for breastfed infants in Figure 1.

> **Standards for Breast Feeders**
> 1. A fall below one standard deviation of normal growth velocity is indication for intense surveillance; or
> 2. A fall in growth velocity below two standard deviations from the normal mean is an indication for full investigation.

Clinical Assessment of Reduced Growth Achievement

In practice, the population most frequently demonstrating growth faltering is least likely to participate fully in health guidance. This frequently denies the use of velocity assessment to detect early growth faltering. In the child with achieved weight or height below the third percentile (approximately two standard deviations below normal), an investigation is indicated (Figure 2, a and b). It is necessary to know the birthweight to achieve full evaluation of small-for-gestational-age infants (Figure 2c) with growth faltering; for the same reason, allowance for premature delivery and perinatal complications is important.[11]

Confirmatory Catch-up Growth

The proof of non-organic growth failure is the response to dietary management. The nutritional and psychological aspects of this rehabilitation will be described subsequently. The diagnostic response to management is a systematic gain in weight followed by linear growth. In many infants with malnutrition, recovering weight gain is prompt and progressive; however, in others, especially when complicated by low serum albumin concentration and edema, a week or so of erratic daily weights precedes systematic weight gain. Finkelstein[12] called this the period of "hydrolability", when weight changes represent fluctuations in water balance. This period is extremely vexing in infants who have suspected formula intolerance. Personal experience and the recorded experience of other clinicians reveal that the equalization period requires close observation and step-wise regrading of the diet so that the objectives of energy requirement for growth are met as soon as possible.

> Catch-up weight gains on a caloric intake adequate for age should exceed 1.5 times the normal growth velocity for age (Figure 1).

Differential Diagnosis
Evaluation

While all infants with growth failure require a clinical evaluation, the extent need not always be exhaustive.

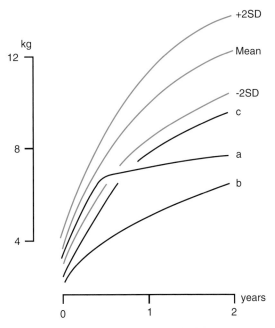

Figure 2: Common patterns of growth faltering.

Laboratory investigations are indicated, but only 0.8 to 1.4% of the investigations are positive.[17, 18] I find it useful to have a dietitian perform an analysis of dietary nutrient intake, to differentiate the hypermetabolic from hypometabolic cases. The presence of poor gain on a calorically adequate diet (hypermetabolic state) leads to a search for chronic infections, immunodeficiency (especially HIV), anemia, neoplastic or metabolic disorders and specific organ system failures. The general findings include a hyperdynamic heart, increased sleeping or resting pulse and postprandial sweating. The presence of specific symptoms and physical points to investigating specific organ systems.

In the hypometabolic patient, observing the infant's feedings is often diagnostic. Evaluating maternal-child interaction the infant's capacity to feed and the mother's response to the infant's communicative signals is valuable. The patience and skill of the mother and the interest of the infant are measures of the quality of the relationship. In the older infant, an inquiry into the environment and equipment for feeding can reveal an disorganized mealtime. In the case of the distracted or adversarial infant, a typical feeding should be observed in the clinic or the home. A search for "soft" neurological findings that impair feeding includes observing suckling mechanisms, and in older infants, observing spoon feeding to determine if lack of mouth-motor coordination is contributing to poor dietary intake. The duration of the feeding should be determined by history and direct observation. An abbreviated feeding period is often found in the presence of family disorganization and may correlate with poor coping within a family beset by crises. In this demanding environment, if a child has a difficult temperament, mouth-incoordination, or a chronic disease, growth faltering is common. Under these circumstances, the family's ability to cope with adversity determines the quality of the infant's growth. For formula-fed infants, it is necessary to evaluate the details of preparation of the formula and the method of feeding. In partially or fully weaned infants it is necessary to know what foods are prepared at home, and the quality of preparation, as well as the variety and amount of commercial baby foods fed.

Descriptive Classification (modified from Woolston,[13])

1. Organic
    a. Illnesses that cause malnutrition (example: malabsorption)
    b. Illnesses that contribute to malnutrition (example: mild heart disease)
    c. Illnesses that are concurrent with malnutrition (example: cleft lip)
    d. Illnesses caused by malnutrition (example: diarrhea due to carbohydrate intolerance)
    e. No illness
2. Developmental
    a. Delay of motor development
    b. Delay of cognitive development
3. Caretaker-Infant Interaction
    a. Homeostatic: (zero to two months) failure of adaptation to extra-uterine feeding cues
    b. Attachment: (two to six months) failure of psychological bonding
    c. Somato-psychological differentiation: (six to 36 months) failure to develop autonomy
4. Ineffective Feeding
    a. Maternal:
        1. Affective interaction with infant

2. Physical interaction with infant
3. Verbal interaction with infant
4. Specific feeding behaviors
5. Response to infant's cues (signals from infant to mother related to feeding)
6. Inadequate family and/or societal support systems
    b. Infant:
        1. Infant's general affect
        2. Interactive behavior with mother
        3. Eating behaviors
        4. Adverse family and/societal environment

Differential Diagnosis (modified from Kien,[14])

1. Failure to gain on adequate food intakes
    a. Maldigestion or malabsorption (examples: cystic fibrosis, Swachman-Diamond syndrome, celiac disease, liver disease, acute or chronic diarrhea, congenital heart disease,)
    b. Vomiting (examples: central nervous systems infections, tumors or other causes of increased intracranial pressure; metabolic disorders of amino acid, keto acid or organic acids; pyloric stenosis or other intestinal obstructions)
    c. Gastroesophageal reflux (examples: hiatal hernia, lower esophageal sphincter atony, bulimia, rumination)
    d. Elevated metabolic rate (examples: infection; major trauma; neoplastic diseases; hyperthyroidism; valvular insufficiencies and left-to-right shunts in congenital heart diseases; Myocardial myopathies, broncho-pulmonary dysplasia)
    e. Abnormal utilization of amino acids for protein synthesis (examples: metabolic disorders of amino acid, keto acid or organic acids)
2. Failure to gain due to inadequate food intakes (note overlap with 1.)
    a. Malabsorption (examples: cystic fibrosis; Swachman-Diamond syndrome; celiac disease; liver disease; acute or chronic diarrhea; congenital heart disease,
    b. Malignancies (example: cachexia of neoplastic diseases)
    c. Inadequate intakes (examples: marasmus, marasmic-kwashiorkor)
    d. Infection and inflammation (examples: congenital

rubella, toxoplasmosis, cytomegalovirus or human immunodeficiency virus infections, Crohn's disease, ulcerative colitis, juvenile rheumatoid arthritis, miliary tuberculosis, osteomyelitis, abdominal abscess)

e. Metabolic disorders (examples: metabolic disorders of amino acid, keto acid or organic acids)

f. Chronic and acute respiratory and/or cardiac insufficiency (valvular insufficiencies and left-to-right shunts in congenital heart diseases; myocardial myopathies; broncho-pulmonary dysplasia)

g. Sucking, swallowing and chewing disorders (examples: cerebral palsy; subdural hematoma; perinatal ventricular hemorrhage)

h. Neuro-psychiatric disorders (example: anorexia nervosa)

i. Chronic diseases of systemic nature (example: severe combined immunodeficiency)

3. Falure to gain due to non-nutritional disorders

a. Endocrine (example: craniopharyngioma)

b. Metabolic (example: azotemia)

c. Constitutional (example: intrauterine growth retardation)

Diagnostic Investigations

The nutritional evaluation and examination of the malnourished child are described in the chapter on Diagnosing Nutrition Disorders. Behavioral assessment of the child with growth faltering includes searching for characteristic findings such as a watchful, wary wide-eyed stare with overt gaze avoidance and poor eye contact. Some infants who are hypertonic arch backwards when held and demonstrate scissoring of the legs. Other infants are sad, listless and apathetic, and become irritable when held. These withdrawn infants spend much of the day sleeping or in self-play, and prefer objects to people. They are not responsive to physical affection. Older infants, often referred to as psychosocial dwarfs, manifest characteristics such as bizarre and voracious appetites, marked hyperactivity and severe speech delay.

1. Search for Organic Etiologies (modified from Kien,[14] and Wilson[15])

a. Malabsorption: sweat chloride; fecal fat; blood neutrophil count; intestinal biopsy; liver function

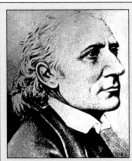

Marie-Jules Parrot M.D. (1839-1883) was the first Director of L'hospice des Enfants Assistes in Paris. He described "athrepsia" or marasmic malnutrition in 1875 and proposed that this nutritional state contributed to many infant diseases. He introduced direct sucking from the udders of donkeys as an alternative to maternal nursing. History of Pediatrics by F. H. Garrison and edited by I. A. Abt, Saunders, Philadelphia, 1965. (Drawing courtesy of R. LaPlane)

tests; stool for ova and parasites.

b. Vomiting: Investigation for central nervous system infections; CT scan; Upper GI series; esophagoscopy, gastroscopy and duodenoscopy; serum electrolytes, urea and albumin or retinol binding protein; blood glucose; plasma amino acids; lead screen; urine organic acids; urine toxicology screen.

c. Gastroesophageal reflux: esophagoscopy; intraesophageal pH monitoring; motility studies of suck and swallow.

d. Elevated metabolic expenditure: sedimentation rate; blood hemoglobin; white blood cell count and differential; total or basal energy expenditure; cardiac and pulmonary evaluation; search for arteris venous shunts.

e. Chronic infection: tuberculin test; congenital cytomegalovirus; congenital toxoplasmosis and human immunodeficiency virus titers;, cultures of blood, urine and stool; technetium scan of bone and abdomen.

f. Malignancy: organ scans, bone marrow examination.

g. Endocrine: bone age; thyroid function; somatomedin C levels; serum Zn levels.

2. Evaluation of Non-organic Etiologies (modified from Bithoney and Rathbun)16

a. Maternal-infant feeding interaction: richness of interaction, amount of eye and physical contact, sense of mutual pleasure, warmth and affection, consistency of response.

- Is the infant satisfied after a 15-minute intake at each breast?

- Are there eight or more wet diapers per day?

- Are the bowel movements characteristic of the normal breast-fed infant? Golden, salvelike, glistening, and of moderate volume?

- In the uncertain case, one should ask the mother to demonstrate her feeding technique.

NOTE: The infant should be weighed before and after feeding. The duration of feeding should be timed.

Table 1: Detecting early faltering at the breast.

b. Evaluation of mother and of infant relationship: responsiveness, self-regulatory capacity, frustration threshold and tolerance.

c. Maternal resources: expectations by mother, burden of infant's demands.

d. Family resources: marital stress; financial stress; disorganized life styles; highly dependent relationships; chronic physical and mental illnesses.

e. Maternal social isolation: family and neighborhood support; father's support; ineffective coping/compliance with medical and community support.

f. Pregnancy: adolescence, lack of birth control, perinatal complications, difficult pregnancy.

g. History of loss: death or abandonment in family; loss of self esteem; loss of the "expected child."

Special Syndromes
Growth Faltering at the Breast

Most mothers who discontinue breast-feeding or begin supplementing breast milk at an early age feel that their milk supply is inadequate for the infant's needs. In many cases the health provider can, by evaluating growth velocity, reassure the nursing mother that all is well and supplementation or weaning can be deferred. To provide this assurance, the health provider needs to understand growth processes of the normal suckling infant. Referring to the NCHS charts for growth are standard in this period, but not technically satisfactory because of the cross-sectional nature of the age group making up the NCHS standards, and the fact that those infants included in the database were fed primar-

ily evaporated milk formulas, a practice no longer prevalent in the developed countries (See Chapter 16, *Rationale for Breast-feeding*, Schanler, Butte).

Prospective studies of dietary intake and growth of infants fully fed at the breast are now available in the UK and the US.[17] A representative study is shown in Figure 1. Here the average one-month growth velocities are plotted, and two standard deviations calculated from a normal, advantaged "benchmark" population. These infants took in about 20 kcal/kg/day, fewer calories than the formula-fed "benchmark" population; yet the breast-fed and formula-fed infants gained weight at a similar rate for the first six months of life. Parallel studies reveal only a modest increase in body fat in breast-fed and greater lean tissue mass in the formula-fed infants.[18]

Many authorities on infant nutrition teach that breast-feeding may become inadequate after four months of age, and that supplementary food and gradual weaning is indicated between four and six months. This belief is based upon the assumption that supplementary foods will increase energy intake of the breast-fed infant. Studies indicate that in normal breast-feeders, supplementary foods replace energy from breast milk and do not increase the energy intake beyond that obtained from mother's milk alone.[19] The normally nourished formula-fed infant continues to consume a higher energy intake than the breast-fed when given supplementary foods.

The criteria for detecting growth faltering at the breast are given in Table 1. Recognition of this syndrome requires intervention (see chapter on Breast-feeding: How to make it work). Efforts can be made to increase milk output; however, interim feeding with banked human milk or formula is mandatory. Increased milk production is usually possible by counseling from an experienced breast-feeding consultant and use of a breast milk pump.

Many mothers are able to provide adequate nutrient intake for the nursing infant until after 12 months of age; others, because of a variety of problems such as return to work or social stress are not able to provide sufficient intake for normal growth. After four months of age, growth faltering should be managed by supplementation of maternal milk intake by infant formulas or baby foods.

Prevention of Faltering

Since Parrot, most authorities agree that growth faltering is more prevalent in less advantaged populations. These observations led to organized efforts to prevent growth faltering a century ago by the French Pediatrician Budin, and the creation of "Well Child Conferences" in 1892.

> Budin has said, "The consultation in the well-child clinic is worth just as much as the physician who conducts it, but no more."

Can growth faltering be prevented? Rathbun points out the discrepant high incidence of non-organic failure to thrive in the U.S. in comparison to its rare occurrence in the U.K. She attributes this anomalous difference to the systematic and centralized care under the National Health Care Scheme in the U.K. Prenatal care is provided to all and is widely used due to a careful tracking and outreach to all pregnant women. Routine postnatal care includes home visits, starting just after discharge from the maternity unit, by a mothercraft nurse. Careful attention is paid to establishing of successful and satisfying skills in breast-feeding, developmental and behavioral management, and nurturing the infant. The Well Child Clinics are a frequent locale for these services.[20]

Presently, more than 20% of all infants in the U.S. are cared for in public well-baby clinics where growth, maternal and infant nutritional status are evaluated and supplementary foods provided by the Womens, Infants, and Children (WIC) federal feeding program.[21] This and other government child health care programs are especially important in the public health care sector (Figure 3). In minority communities, half of all infants receive anticipatory guidance from public health care workers. Education concerning mothercraft and child feeding, including breast-feeding, continue to be a priority for improving child health in the U.S.

While the reasons are not understood, attendance in well baby clinics and participation in the WIC Program are rarely associated with successful maternal lactation (approximately 5%) when compared with that found in private practice (approximately 60% successful breast-feeding until four months of age). Nevertheless, the provision of supplementary foods through the WIC

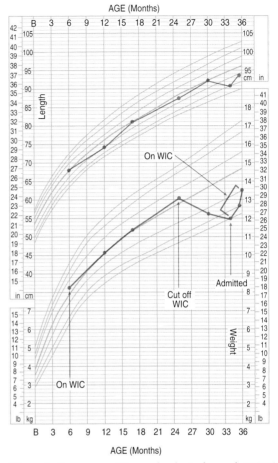

Figure 3: Boys zero to 36 months physical growth NCHS percentiles.

Program has improved birthweight and postnatal weight gain (Figure 3). The availability of prenatal iron supplements and iron-fortified formulas have resulted in reduced rates of anemia in WIC Program recipients during the second semester of life.[21] Providing of ready-to-feed formulas has reduced the incidence of acute diarrhea. In my experience, there has been a marked reduction in growth faltering and associated nutritional deficiencies, including feeding problems and chronic diarrhea, among participating WIC Program infants.

Family Disruption

Regardless of social status, growth faltering can occur if familial or societal disturbances and/or affective disorders are present. Unfortunately, social disturbances such as addiction to drugs or alcohol and unemployment or dislocation are associated with a high prevalence of family disorganization.[22-24] There is a recurrent complex of social crises associated with more prevalent growth failure in the infant. Family characteristics include low levels of maternal education, isolation from relatives, crowded housing, low income, and poor participation in government or agency programs. It is important to note that these same family characteristics are also associated with increased prevalence of child abuse. However, there are no predictive relationships between this cluster of family symptoms and the individual outcomes of growth faltering or child abuse. The cluster of crises associated with family disorganization demonstrates the need to address family structure as part of effective therapeutic intervention. Referral to social agencies and child welfare programs is mandatory for success of the health care team working with growth faltering.

Poor Feeders

Although major research attention has been given to family problems, problems of infant behavior are often present which contribute to non-organic growth faltering.[25,27] Investigators have discovered a high frequency of "soft" neurological signs in infants with this syndrome. These include hypotonia, inattention, disinterest, oral dysfunction, tongue incoordination, excessive salivation, excessive spitting-up, vomiting and rumination. In the face of family disorganization, these symptoms contribute to inadequate care-taking, to aversive interactions such as resistance or defiance by the infant, and inability of the family to cope with the increased demands for time and attention by a "difficult" infant. In many cases these interactions are intensified by congenital and acquired health problems. The management of poor feeding in the patient with organic failure to thrive is outlined in the chapter on Nutritional care of the Chronically Ill.

Milk Intolerance

The refeeding of malnourished infants is occasionally associated with occurrence of vomiting and diarrhea. Rosen von Rosenstein recognized this association in

> *On breast versus bottle feeding of infants, the pediatrician must ask how the parents have come to the conclusion of what to feed, and if breastfeeding is rejected, why. This is an opportunity for understanding the parents, and for education in the importance of breastfeeding.*
>
> Richard Grand M.D.
> New England Medical Center
> Boston, Massachusetts

the first textbook of pediatrics published in Sweden in 1772. At the turn of the century, German pediatricians recognized the specific dietary constituents contributing to this intolerance. In 1903, Moro reported the occurrence of cow milk protein hypersensitivity in a malnourished infant with recurrent diarrhea. Finkelstein, in 1905, demonstrated selective intolerance to milk sugar (lactose) in an infant with a similar clinical findings. Both reported that formula intolerance was overcome by changing the diet to eliminate either cow milk protein or lactose. An evolutionary refinement of the bacteriological and nutritional quality of formulas has led to less recurrence of diarrhea while refeeding malnourished infants since that time.

Cow milk protein hypersensitivity is frequently diagnosed in clinical practice. The diagnosis (see chapter on Recognizing and Managing Food Allergy) is based upon clinical judgement and usually is confirmed by improved formula tolerance following switching to a soy- or extensively hydrolyzed protein based preparation. Gastrointestinal symptoms are prominent in some infants with malnutrition. Contemporary investigators recognize an enterocolitis form of intolerance associated with explosive watery diarrhea, which probably represents acute type I hypersensitivity. There is also a more indolent, small intestinal form associated with altered jejunal morphology, which is probably a type III form of hypersensitivity.

This syndrome was called "intestinal decomposition" by Finkelstein;[28] this literally translates as "gut rot." Finkelstein found that there are symptoms of cow milk intolerance that can be ameliorated by reducing dietary milk sugar, and he demonstrated that nutritional rehabilitation is possible with a lactose-free cow milk diet when fed to most malnourished infants with chronic diarrhea (see chapter on Managing Dietary Carbohydrate Intolerance). Today, this disorder is suspected by a recurrence of diarrhea after feeding a calorically adequate feeding; it is confirmed by the presence of glucose and a pH less than 5.5 in a voluminous, mucus-laden, watery, green diarrheal stool.[28,29] These children invariably improve while fasting, which further exacerbates their malnutrition. In nine of 10 such infants, both the diarrhea and acidosis improve when alternate carbohydrates such as sucrose or small molecular weight starches are fed as a substitute for lactose in cow milk feedings.

The two concepts dominate our thinking concerning the pathogenesis of intestinal decomposition, now called intractable diarrhea, acquired carbohydrate intolerance, cow milk intolerance, and cow milk allergy. One concept is that allergy leads to a acquired carbohydrate intolerance; the other is that malnourished infants have a relative disability in their immune response to acute gastroenteritis. They develop a sub-acute or chronic course associated with small intestinal and colonic failure to digest and transport carbohydrates and their fermented products.[30,31] Is this distinction clinically relevant? Based upon the allergy concept, soy protein formulas and hydrolyzed protein formulas have been developed and are widely available in America. Based upon the concept of carbohydrate intolerance, a series of reduced or carbohydrate-free formulas are available allowing substitution of the various classes of dietary carbohydrates. Is there a unifying concept? Contemporary pediatric gastroenterologists are not of a single mind on this subject, but many believe that protein hypersensitivity is the etiologic factor leading to the small intestinal and colonic carbohydrate malabsorption of relapsing diarrhea. The mechanisms linking these two views are completely unknown.

Management of chronic dietary associated diarrhea follows Finkelstein's treatment algorithm, which substitutes one dietary component at a time. In contemporary practice, however, this first stage is less exact: soy formulas simultaneously substitute soy protein for cow milk proteins and replace lactose with a mixture of sucrose and glucose oligosaccharides. Persistent intolerance to soy formulas is not unusual. This leads to the suspicion of more complex intolerance. My clinical practice (see chapter on Managing Dietary Carbohydrate Intolerance) is to offer intravenous nutritional support if the carbohydrate intolerance is so severe that a 2.5% glucose solution added to a carbohydrate-free formula is not tolerated by nasogastric infusion. With exception of the intravenous nutritional support, management is essen-

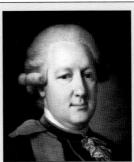

Nils Rosen von Rosenstein M.D. (1706-1773) published the first text of Pediatrics, in Swedish, in 1764. He describes artificial infant feeding by means of a "biberon" with a leather nipple. His classification of diarrhea lists 14 varieties; five were associated with malnutrition or feeding disorders. He is recognized by most historians as the founder of Pediatrics. The History of Pediatrics by G. F. Still, Dawsons, London, 1965 (Photo courtesy of CNRC)

tially identical to that outlined by Finkelstein in the early years of this century.

Can breast-feeding prevent food intolerance? Finkelstein taught that breast-feeding prevents intestinal decomposition and consequent failure to thrive. We have found that this is not always the case. The enterocolonic form of Type I hypersensitivity has been observed in rare instances when traces of whole allergens were transferred in mother's milk. In the specific case mentioned, the child improved when cow milk was removed from the mother's diet.[32] No cases of the form of growth failure associated with carbohydrate intolerance have been reported in breast-fed infants. Several investigators have reported that therapeutic benefit was observed when breast-feeding was reinstituted in these infants. We have found no specific benefits from giving 10% of required amounts of human milk to these infants.[33] In countries where infant formulas are not available, this syndrome is associated with weaning from the breast and feeding of supplementary foods at a later age. This suggests that human milk, fed in quantities sufficient to allow growth, postpones the age at which milk intolerance occurs to approximately one year, and demonstrates a protective effect.

Prevention of Growth Faltering Through Breast-feeding and Other Mothercraft Skills

Adequate family support systems, good mothercraft skills, and appropriate anticipatory guidance through well-child care are major factors contributing to adequate growth in healthy breast-fed and formula-fed infants. Nonetheless, growth faltering can occur in infants living under optimal circumstances, and normal growth occurs even in the most disadvantaged environment. The conclusion is that appropriate growth monitoring is an essential component of child health care and that systematic anthropometry is essential to early detection and to the monitoring of therapy of growth faltering.

Since the work of Rosenstein, breast-feeding has been recognized as an important factor in preventing growth failure. Unfortunately, it is not a universal antidote. Early detection of reduced growth velocity allows appropriate consultation with breast-feeding consultants and often results in full recovery. The management alternates of dietary supplementation or full weaning to an appropriate formula will usually provide equal correction of growth faltering.

Management

Growth faltering at the breast is managed by increasing maternal milk supply while at the same time supplementing the nutritional needs of the infant by cow milk formula. It is critically important to assure adequate hydration, as evidenced by frequent wet diapers, during the regrading of maternal milk intake. The combined use of services from an experienced breast-feeding consultant and an electric breast pump is usually effective in increasing maternal milk supply. The mother should continue to suckle the child during this period of three to five days, but management is dependent upon formula supplements until maternal milk supply is adequately increased. A prompt and gratifying improvement in the infant's interaction with the mother and catch-up growth constitute evidence that maternal milk supply has become inadequate.

In formula-fed and mixed-fed infants, the use of a surrogate mother is important in managing disturbed maternal-child interactions. A skilled relative or nurse can provide diagnostic as well as management assistance to the physician. A clear understanding of the

> *I hear a lot of parents talking about not allowing their babies to have cookies or other so called "junk food." If you give your child a chocolate cookie that is okay, it's not junk food. If you give him nothing but chocolate cookies all day, that's a junk diet, but if you give your child fruit juice all day and nothing else, that's a junk diet, too.*
>
> Fima Lifshitz M.D.
> Maimonides Hospital
> Brooklyn, New York

energy needs of the infant leads to clear objectives for individual feedings. If the anorexia and disinterest are profound and skilled nursing not available, nasogastric tube feeding is required. An improvement in skin color, turgor, peripheral circulation and the affect of the child is evident after only a few hours of adequate feeding. Nurses in rehabilitation units in the third world comment that return of the child's smile is a strong sign of improvement. Tube feeding is continued until at least three consecutive days of weight gain have been observed. Dependence on tube feeding beyond this point is diagnostic of a severe feeding problem or more fundamental clinical disorder.

Behavioral problems are frequently prominent in the weaned or partially weaned infant with growth faltering. Here too, the surrogate mother is important. Attempts to neutralize adverse behavior requires the limiting of conflicting attractions through environmental control and the provision of background sights and sounds that do not distract from the feeding process. Increasing the "fun" of the feeding period is also therapeutic and can be carried out by varying the textures, colors, temperatures and shapes of foods, with playful rewards for compliance. Providing toys during the feeding period can be a useful adjunct.[26, 34]

A team approach to diagnosis and management is recommended.[20] Team members include nurses, social workers, dietitians, speech therapists, child developmentalists and pediatricians.[20] Consultation with the Children's Protective Agency is mandated if neglect is documented. Enrollment in the local and federal programs such as Well Child Clinic and WIC program ensures a continuity and comprehensiveness of care.

Therapeutic Objectives

Management should begin with a diet familiar to the infant and family. Management (Table 2) is divided into three phases:

- Introduction of adequate nutrient intake through stepwise "regrading" the diet over a 12-hour period;
- Restoration of nutritional deficits; and
- Catch-up growth.

In phase I, induction of adequate intake is usually begun with a cow milk formula. One half of the dietary volume of feed of the normal child of the same age is offered as a single feed. Depending on acceptance and tolerance, the quantity of formulas is advanced over 12 hours, so that in the following 24-hours a volume of formula sufficient to provide the energy needs of an average child of the same age is received. Care is taken to chart the clinical course between the extremes of continued starvation and a sudden increase in intake to full calories, by observation of gastrointestinal tolerance. Intolerance is characterized by vomiting and diarrhea of a significant nature. Spitting up and small volume starvation stools need to be differentiated from gastrointestinal intolerance. If dietary intolerance is detected, alternative feeding strategies for dietary intolerance as outlined above and in the chapter on Nutritional Care of the Chronically Ill should be followed. If phase one is uncomplicated, a diet appropriate for age is begun in phase two. The caloric level is advanced over the next two to four days to one and one-half times that required to provide adequate dietary energy for an average child of the same age. It is important to treat and prevent any specific nutritional deficiencies during phase two by providing vitamin and mineral supplementation. The diet and supplement should contain one and one-half times the daily requirement for intracellular electrolytes; zinc, potassium, magnesium and bone electrolytes; calcium; and phosphorus. Hematinics, including iron, folic acid, and B_{12}, are provided at three times the normal intake for age. As lean body mass develops very rapidly during phase two, the demand for intracellular electrolytes, bone electrolytes and the hematinics are increased compared with normal growth. Water shifts (Finkelstein's hydrolability) are associated with the restructuring of electrolyte balance and can make interpretation of daily weights perplexing. If there is no gastrointestinal disturbance and intake exceeds one and one-half

---

- **Phase 1 - Regrading**
  Quantity of the formula should be gradually increased at each feeding until 50% of expected energy intake for age is reached.
  Duration: 12 hours

- **Phase 2 - Restoring Nutritional Deficiencies**
  Child should receive 1 1/2 times the expected intake for age of calories and protein and 3 times the expected intake for age of micronutrients and hematinics.
  Duration: 3 to 5 days

- **Phase 3 - Catch-up Growth**
  Phase 2 diet should be continued and the child should be stimulated socially and physically. Work with the family to restore coping abilities and provide child-care training.
  Duration: 2 to 6 weeks (attained weight at time of discharge should be no more than 1 SD below the normal mean for age).

Table 2: Therapeutic objectives.

times the normal energy requirement for age, patience will be rewarded by a consistent weight gain after three or four days as normal new tissue is formed.

Phase three begins after two weeks of steady weight gain. A course must be charted between protective isolation of a malnourished child with impaired immune function and the need for social stimulation and physical activities in phase three. Discharge from rehabilitation care depends upon the nature of the family and the availability of support systems to assist them with their coping with the rehabilitation program at home.

Food aversion, vomiting, rumination and hostility are managed in a similar sequence, except that tube feeding is implemented to bypass these barriers to adequate food intake. The tube feeding extends into early phase three, when this mode feeding can be discontinued while oral bolus feedings are offered. It is important that the objectives for dietary intake are maintained during the transition from phase two and phase three and during the full extent of phase three. In many infants, feeding difficulties improve after recovery from malnutrition. The use of intravenous feedings is described in the chapter on Nutritional Care of the Chronically Ill.

Rules for Managing Growth Faltering

Clinical observations of infants with failure to thrive lead to the definition of rules to manage growth faltering

> • All growth faltering is an interactive child/family/societal problem, but even in severely aversive circumstances, growth faltering is rare.
> • The classification of organic and non-organic growth faltering is imprecise because all growth faltering falls within a spectrum between dietary deficiency and malnutrition due to other illnesses.
> • The morbidity and mortality of growth faltering are equally pernicious and regardless of classification. all cases require diagnostic and management attention.

Case Histories

Case #1: A two month-old white infant was hospitalized because of poor weight gain. Weight at 2-½ months was 4.10 kg compared with a birthweight of 3.25 kg. Behavioral assessment showed minimal backarching, but good eye contact and an easy social smile. The mother was 29 years old, married and had five other children, all under the age of seven years. Initially, the mother reported an intake of 35 to 40 ounces of formula a day or 170 calories/kg/day. The baby grew well in the hospital, but had not grown well at home. Following discharge, the mother kept a diet history which revealed that the infant was taking only four bottles a day for a total of 20 to 22 ounces or about 90 calories/kg/d. The visiting nurse also noted that the infant slept up to six hours, and did not demand feedings. The mother was so overworked with her other tasks that the infant's sleep was a welcome respite. The mother was instructed to awaken the infant to assure an adequate daily intake, and the baby subsequently thrived.[35]

Case #2: A Latino male who had failure to thrive since age 10 months underwent hospitalization and comprehensive evaluation at age 19 months. At this time, it was determined that he was allergic to milk and soy protein. His mother was given extensive instructions about which foods to avoid. After one week on a milk and soy-free diet, his weight had fallen off even further. In avoiding all the

prohibited foods, the mother was starving the child! With a change in the diet instructions (what to give rather than what to avoid) weight gain occurred.[35]

Case #3: Donna was referred at three months of age in the course of a hospitalization to clarify the causes of her failure to gain weight. Donna had gained weight in the hospital and the medical staff felt concerned about the mother's brief though frequent hospital visits and about the relative absence of holding and physical contact, which the staff interpreted as maternal rejection of Donna.

In a number of ways, Donna fit the classic non-organic growth faltering syndrome. At home, she was repeatedly ill with gastrointestinal disturbances and was unable to maintain or increase her weight, while during two hospitalizations she was able to gain weight adequately. Also, the nursing staff reported that Donna was a rewarding infant to work with, while her mother, Mrs. D., described her as an irritable and inconsolable baby who cried for hours and could not be soothed.

While no clear-cut organic cause for Donna's growth failure was ever found, a constellation of risk factors and the observations of the Infant-Parent Program worker assigned to the case strongly suggest that Donna was an unusually difficult baby. Donna was born at 37 weeks and was small for gestational age. Her head circumference was disproportionately small. Since her birth, she had several bouts of diarrhea, recurrent high fever, and a seizure of unexplained origin. Moreover, Donna was neurophysiologically immature and it required considerable persistent effort to console her when she was distressed. She was a weak sucker and easily distracted while feeding.

Home visits after Donna's discharge showed that Mrs. D. was capable of responding appropriately to Donna, and could successfully feed her and interact with her if she had emotional support and no external distractions. But there was a number of circumstances which precluded this from happening with any regularity. Mrs. D. was a single parent who worked full time to support her two young children. When she came home, she felt torn between her duties towards Donna and towards her 18-month old son, and she often gave precedence to the insistent demands of the older child, which were both easier to understand and easier to respond to than Donna's. In addition, the strain of the repeated illness, and, not least, the sense of blame Mrs. D. experienced from her contacts with the hospital staff, significantly contributed to this otherwise adequate mother's insecurity and uncertainty. These feelings fostered in turn a defensive stance of detachment toward her daughter and anger at the hospital staff for not finding an organic cause for Donna's illness. After sympathetic discussions of her predicament, and much support and help in identifying Donna's fleeting positive responses to their ministrations, Mrs. D. was able to do much better with her admittedly difficult infant, and the child's weight and medical condition stabilized. The improvements in the mother-child interaction and in the child's condition became even more marked after Mrs. D. married a man who provided financial support and who helped her with the two children.[35]

Case #4: Jamal was referred for non-organic growth faltering when he was 18 months old. This condition had been first identified by the pediatrician when Jamal was six months old and his weight had dropped from the 20th percentile at four months to below the third percentile at six months (height and head circumference had stayed at the 25th percentile and 10th percentile respectively). In the intervening year between diagnosis and referral, the pediatrician had conducted a comprehensive series of medical tests that ruled out organic causes for the condition. The pediatrician then reluctantly considered the possibility that Jamal's growth faltering was due to psychological factors. In making the referral, he expressed his misgivings about this possible diagnosis by emphasizing how loving Jamal's parents were and how attached Jamal was to them.

Our initial home visits confirmed the pediatrician's impression that there were reliable affective bonds between Jamal and his parents. Jamal seemed like an active and competent toddler and his parents were quite proud of him, complaining only that he was unresponsive to limit setting and that he sometimes wore them out with his constant activity. However, other factors began to emerge as our visits continued. Jamal's mother

> **We may not know how preterm babies who are growth restricted at birth got that way, but we certainly know how they stay that way - we don't feed them enough once they are born.**
>
> Bill Hay M.D.
> Department of Pediatrics
> University of Colorado
> School of Medicine

was an extremely passive, almost inert woman, with a thought disorder that was at first masked by her apparent reserve. Her favorite activity was to watch TV, she seldom took the initiative in interacting with Jamal or setting limits, and she often did not notice behaviors that required prompt intervention, such as Jamal's climbing on a stool to reach a favorite toy. The father was more actively involved with Jamal and tended to set appropriate limits, but he was often out of the house and his arrivals and departures were rather sudden and unexplained.

The home environment was an odd mixture of benignity and confusion. While Jamal appeared to be genuinely cherished by his parents, they themselves led highly unstructured, outwardly haphazard lifestyles in which the connection between intentions, actions and results were strikingly obscure. Such a lack of organization was clearly reflected in the attitude towards eating. Nobody in the family ate regular meals, and there was no consistent pattern for Jamal's feedings: the mother was usually vague when asked when and what Jamal had eaten. Also, while Jamal occasionally took things from the refrigerator, he was sometimes praised proudly for his initiative, sometimes scolded for taking the wrong thing or making a mess, and sometimes ignored. On the few occasions when, at our urging, Jamal was actually fed, things tended to go wrong: the oatmeal was too hot and Jamal burned himself, bringing the meal to a sad end; or he was given a huge slab of ham that was not cut for him and that he hardly managed to nibble on; or the mother started to reminisce about her life and forgot to finish her cooking. Jamal continually had a bottle available to him which might contain milk or Koolaid (a colored, sweetened drink) or nothing, but he was never observed to use it for nutritional purposes.

Jamal's parents were not worried about his failure to gain weight, and responded to the pediatrician's and our concerns with benign puzzlement. They pointed out that Jamal had so much energy he could not possibly be weak from lack of eating and were convinced that he would eventually catch up.

Our own view was that Jamal, an unusually active baby, had responded to his unstructured and unstructuring environment with precocious investment in motor activity to provide himself with more organized and manageable stimulation than his environment was able to offer him. Although he was well coordinated, this constant activity had a compulsive, preservative quality and a lack of goal-directedness that suggested a primitive form of self-stimulation. This inordinate investment in gross motor activity, which might have originated as a coping response to extreme absence of structure, seemed now to have become a partial determinant of Jamal's growth faltering because it interfered with his capacity to become aware of and respond to his hunger cues. In our view, Jamal's environment had not provided him at a crucial age with the reciprocal feeding exchanges necessary to help him develop adequate schemes of the relationship between hunger, feeding and the social interaction mediating these experiences of need and satiation. Jamal's response to this environmental failure had been two-fold: a loss of interest in food and quick decline in weight, which stabilized below the third percentile, and a concomitant turn to motor activity as a source of self-contingency and self-stimulation in the face of his mother's failure to serve as a responsive partner in the establishing reciprocal patterns of interaction.[35]

Historical Perspective...

The dietetic needs of
Marasmic Children
are fully met by

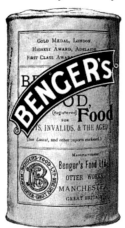

"Supplies every element necessary to healthy development."

"Retained when all other foods are rejected."

GOLD MEDAL, LONDON.
HIGHEST AWARD, ADELAIDE.
FIRST CLASS AWARD.

BENGER'S
FOOD,
(Registered)
FOR
INFANTS, INVALIDS, & THE AGED

Benger's Food Ltd.
OTTER WORKS
MANCHESTER
GREAT BRITAIN

"Incomparably superior to any"

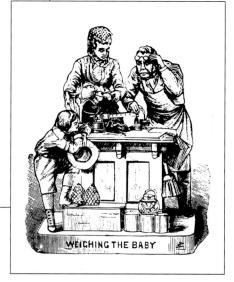

WEIGHING THE BABY

References

1. Parrot J. Etiologie de l'athrepsie. In: *Clinique Des Nouveau-Nes, L'Athrepsie.* Paris: G Masson; 1877:376-446.

2. Finkelstein H. *Lehrbuch Der Sauglingskrankheiten.* Berlin: Verlag Von Julius Springer; 1924:225.

3. Wilcox WD, Nieburg P, Miller DS. Failure to thrive. A continuing problem of definition. *Clin Pediatr.* 1989; 28:391-394.

4. Rathbun JM, Peterson KE. Nutrition in failure to thrive. In: Grand RJ, et al, eds. *Pediatric Nutrition Theory and Practice.* 1987:628.

5. Waterlow JC, Ashworth A, Griffiths M. Faltering in infant growth in less-developed countries. *Lancet.* 1980; 2:1176-1178.

6. Frank DA, Zeisel SH. Failure to thrive. *Pediatr Clin North Am.* 1988;35:1187-1206.

7. Peterson KE, Rathbun JM, Herrera MG. Growth data analysis in FTT treatment and research. In: Drotar D, ed. *New Directions in Failure to Thrive.* New York: Plenum Press; 1985:157-176.

8. Healy MJR, Yang M, Tanner JM, Zumrawi FY. The use of short-term increments in length to monitor growth in infancy. In: Waterlow JC, ed. *Linear Growth Retardation in Less Developed Countries.* New York: Raven Press; 1988:41-55.

9. Zumrawi FY, Min Y, Marshall T. The use of short-term increments in weight to monitor growth in infancy. *Ann Human Biol.* 1992;19:165-175.

10. Kusin JA, Kardjati S, de With C, Rengvist UH. When does growth faltering start? *Paediatr Indonesiana.* 1991; 31:26-40.

11. Albertsson-Wikland K, Karlberg J. Natural growth in children born small for gestational age with and without catch-up growth. *Acta Paediatr Suppl.* 1994;399:64-70.

12. Finkelstein H. *Lehrbuch Der Sauglingskrankheiten.* Berlin: Verlag Von Julius Springer; 1924:214.

13. Woolston J. Diagnostic classification: the current challenge in failure to thrive research. In: Drotar D, ed. *New Directions in Failure to Thrive.* New York: Plenum Press; 1985:225-233.

14. Kien CL. Failure to thrive. In: Walker WA, Watkins JB, ed. *Nutrition in Pediatrics.* Boston: Little Brown; 1985: 757-768.

15. Wilson EP. Failure to thrive. In: Schwartz MW, ed. *Principles and Practice of Clinical Pediatrics.* Year Book Med Publishers; 1987:389-393.

16. Bithoney WG, Rathbun JM. Failure to thrive. In: Levine MD, et al, eds. *Developmental-behavioral Pediatrics.* WB Saunders;, Philadelphia: 1983:557-571.

17. Garza C, Frongillo E, Dewey KG. Implications of growth patterns of breast-fed infants for growth references. *Acta Paediatr Suppl.* 1994;402:4-10.

18. Butte NF, Wong WW, Ferlic L, Smith EO, Klein PD, Garza C. Energy expenditure and deposition of breast-fed and formula-fed infants during early infancy. *Pediatr Res.* 1990;28:631-640.

19. Stuff JE, Nichols BL. Nutrient intake and growth performance of older infants fed human milk. *J Pediatr.* 1989;115:959-968.

20. Rathbun JM. Issues in the treatment of emotional and behavioral disturbances in failure to thrive. In: Drotar D, ed. *New Directions in Failure to Thrive.* New York: Plenum Press; 1985:311-314

21. Frank DB, Allen D, Brown JL. Primary prevention of failure to thrive: social policy implications. In: Drotar D, ed. *New Directions in Failure to Thrive.* New York: Plenum Press; 1985:337-357

22. Bithoney WG, Newberger EH. Child and family attributes of failure-to-thrive. *J Dev Behav Pediatr.* 1987;8:32-36.

23. Drotar D, Sturm L. Influences on the home environment of preschool children with early histories of nonorganic failure-to-thrive. *J Dev Behav Pediatr.* 1989;10:229-235.

24. Drotar D, Eckerle D. The family environment in nonorganic failure to thrive: A controlled study. *J Pediatr Psychol.* 1989;14:245-257.

25. Chatoor I, Egan J. Nonorganic failure to thrive and dwarfism due to food refusal: A separation disorder. *J Am Acad Child Psychiatr.* 1983;22:294-301.

26. Larson KL, Ayllon T, Barrett DH. A behavioral feeding program for failure-to-thrive infants. *Behav Res Ther.* 1987;25:39-47.

27. Finkelstein H. *Lehrbuch Der Sauglingskrankheiten.* Berlin: Verlag Von Julius Springer; 1924:215.

28. Goldson E. Neurological aspects of failure to thrive. *Dev Med Child Neurol.* 1989;31:816-826.

29. Mathisen B, Skuse D, Wolke D, Reilly S. Oral-motor dysfunction and failure to thrive among inner-city infants. *Dev Med Child Neurol.* 1989;31:293-302.

30. Walker-Smith JA. Cow's milk intolerance as a cause of postenteritis diarrhoea. *J Pediatr Gastroenterol Nutr.* 1982;1:163-173.

31. Walker-Smith JA. Cow milk-sensitive enteropathy:predisposing factors and treatment. *J Pediatr.* 1992;121:S111-S115.

32. Lifschitz CH, Hawkins HK, Guerra C, Byrd N. Anaphylactic shock due to cow's milk protein hypersensitivity in a breast-fed infant. *J Pediatr Gastroenterol Nutr.* 1988;2:141-144.

33. Shulman RJ, Lifschitz CH, Langston C, Gopalakrishna GS, Nichols BL. Human milk and the rate of small intestinal mucosal recovery in protracted diarrhea. *J Pediatr.* 1988;114:218-224.

34. Broughton D. Nonorganic failure to thrive. *Am Family Physician.* 1989;40:S63-S72.

35. Berkowitz C. Comprehensive pediatric management of failure to thrive: an interdisciplinary approach In: Drotar D, ed. *New Directions in Failure to Thrive.* New York: Plenum Press; 1995:193-210.

36. Lieberman AF, Burch M. The etiology of failure to thrive: an interactional approach. In: Drotar D, ed. *New Directions in Failure to Thrive.* New York: Plenum Press; 1985:259-277.

37. Klish WJ, Udall JN, Calvin RT, Nichols BL. The effects of intestinal solute load on water secretion in infants with acquired monosaccharide intolerance. *Pediatr Res.* 1980;14: 1343-1346.

Nutritional Care of the Chronically Ill
D.C. Wilson M.D. & P.B. Pencharz M.B., Ch.B., Ph.D.

Departments of Pediatrics and Nutritional Sciences,
University of Toronto,
Toronto, Canada

Reviewed by Buford L. Nichols M.D., Stanley H. Zlotkin M.D., Ph.D. and Mitchell B. Cohen M.D.

Introduction

Chronic illness in infancy and childhood is commonly associated with energy deficiency, and less commonly, with specific nutrient deficiencies. The vast majority of pediatric inpatients in any hospital in the world are under two years of age, so an understanding of nutritional care is mandatory for any pediatric resident, clinical dietician or family doctor. Undernutrition is commonly seen in healthy survivors of extremely premature birth, and is compounded by adverse sequelae of premature birth such as bronchopulmonary dysplasia (BPD). It is also common in neurodevelopmentally handicapped infants, and those with specific chronic illnesses such as cystic fibrosis, congenital heart disease, renal disease, liver disease and AIDS. In this chapter, we will consider the related factors that give rise to energy and nutritional imbalance, and then deal with the chronic illnesses mentioned above. Lastly, we will discuss the various management strategies that can be adopted.

Assessing of nutritional status is the first step in nutritional care, and should be part of the history and examination of any child. This has been covered in the chapter entitled "Diagnosing Nutritional Disorders" by S. Zlotkin. During growth measurement, it is useful to express weight as a percentage of ideal weight for height, age and gender.[1]

Practical Points

- *Undernutrition is common in chronically ill infants.*
- *Chronically ill infants make up a large proportion of inpatient and ambulatory pediatric practice.*
- *Nutritional status should be assessed in all infants.*
- *It is useful to express weight as % of ideal weight for height.*

Pathogenesis of Nutritional Imbalance

A variety of complex, related and unrelated factors will give rise to nutrient imbalance in the chronically ill child. As an example, we will consider energy imbalance. Figure 1 shows a model to explain the cause of energy deficit in patients with chronic illness. This model was first used for cystic fibrosis,[2] and later applied to bronchopulmonary dysplasia,[3] but it can be appropriately altered to suit any nutrient in any disease state. Using Figure 1 as a guideline, we will exemplify by considering energy imbalance in cystic fibrosis. The energy deficit in cystic fibrosis results from an imbalance between energy needs and intake (Table 1), and is determined by three factors: energy losses, energy expenditure and energy intake. Also, using Figure 1 as a guideline, we can explain any other nutrient deficiency, such as vitamin A deficiency in the preterm infant with BPD. Again, vitamin A deficiency will result from an imbalance between needs and intake, determined by increased losses, decreased intake and increased use. Preterm infants have a greater degree of fat malabsorption, and thus fat-soluble vitamin malabsorption, than term infants or adults, and this will cause increased intestinal loss. They may have reduced intake due to fat-free parenteral nutrition, fluid restriction for cor pulmonale or concomitant gastroesophageal reflux. Premature infants may have increased need in the body for repair of tracheobronchial epithelium damaged by barotrauma and hyperoxia.

Specific Chronic Illnesses

In this section, we will consider nutritional care in chronic illnesses such as cystic fibrosis, BPD, neurodevelopmental handicap, congenital heart disease,

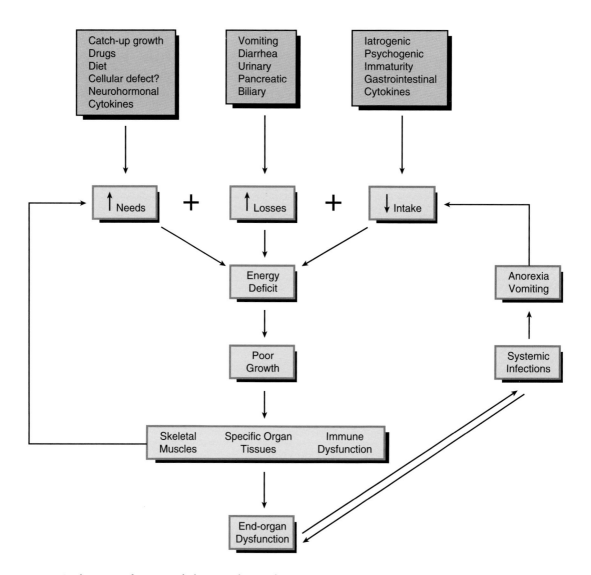

Figure 1: Pathogenesis of energy imbalance in chronic disease.

renal disease, hepatic disease and AIDS. However, any chronic disease could be considered using the approach described above. We will not consider inborn errors of metabolism, primary gastrointestinal diseases, chronic anemia and food allergy, which are discussed in later chapters of this book. General management issues are discussed in the final section of this chapter, but specific issues related to individual illnesses are considered in this section.

The Infant With Cystic Fibrosis

Cystic fibrosis (CF) is a common, inherited disorder of infancy, with an incidence of 1 in 2,500 newborns of

Northern European ancestry. There has been a marked increase in understanding the disease since the CF gene was identified in 1989.[4] About 10% of affected infants present in the neonatal period with bowel obstruction due to meconium ileus.[5] With more than 450 different mutations of the CF gene now described, we have gained considerable insight into genotype-phenotype relationships. Both from the clinical and the nutritional perspective, it is useful to divide mutations into those that cause pancreatic insufficiency (PI) and those that cause pancreatic sufficiency (PS).[6] PS patients have pancreatic disease, but have sufficient

Increased Losses	Decreased Intake	Increased Expenditure
Increased intestinal losses • Pancreatic insufficiency • Bile salt metabolism • Hepatobiliary disease • Gastroesophageal reflux Increased urinary losses • Diabetes mellitus	Reduced intake • Anorexia • Feeding disorders • Depression • Esophagitis • DIOS • Iatrogenic fat restriction	Pulmonary disease Primary defect

Table 1: Energy imbalance in cystic fibrosis. Adapted from Pencharz and Durie.[2]

exocrine function to permit normal nutrient digestion and absorption. They constitute about 15% of the CF population and have milder disease expression, with diagnosis at a later age, slower progression of lung disease, better nutritional status and a superior survival rate than PI patients. Therefore, infants who are diagnosed as having symptomatic CF have an overwhelming likelihood of having a PI phenotype, and thus require pancreatic enzyme supplementation.

Chronic undernutrition with weight retardation and linear growth failure has long been recognized as a problem in CF patient populations. In most CF centers, nutritional support is now seen as an integral part of the multidisciplinary care of CF patients, with aggressive programs instituted to prevent malnutrition. Growth retardation is seen as a consequence of energy imbalance. The importance of achieving normal nutritional status had been demonstrated by a comparative study of two closely similar CF clinics a decade ago (Boston & Toronto). Corey et al[7] found a marked difference in median age of survival, being 21 years in Boston and 30 in Toronto. The only difference in patient population or care was the approach to nutrition; a calorie-enriched diet was given in Toronto, with unrestricted dietary fat and additional enzyme supplements prescribed. It has been suggested that the goal of every CF center should be to support normal nutrition and growth for patients of all ages.[8]

The pathogenesis of the energy imbalance in CF is shown in Table 1, and will not be discussed further. Deficits of essential micronutrients can also occur. Deficiency of the fat soluble vitamins A, D, E and K

have been demonstrated at diagnosis of CF in infancy.[9] In infancy, particularly before diagnosis, clinical features of essential fatty acid deficiency can occur.

Nutritional support should be an integral part of the care of CF patients, with careful assessment at diagnosis, monitoring of growth rates and appropriate dietary counseling. Those infants who fail to grow at a normal rate deserve careful evaluation. Our diagnostic approach to nutrition evaluation and therapy is based on energy balance.[2] Key factors are energy intake, absorption and expenditure. Intake is determined by three-or five-day dietary record with absorption measured by a simultaneous three day stool collection. Energy expenditure is measured with indirect calorimetry.[10]

The majority of patients with CF are diagnosed in infancy because of neonatal screening programs, meconium ileus or nutritional disturbance. At the time of diagnosis, we work intensively with the patients to provide nutrition education and dietary counseling. We also institute appropriate therapeutic intervention, remembering that this is a time of rapid growth and high energy needs. There are three groups of infants who require particular attention at diagnosis. Some are profoundly anorexic and indifferent to food. Another group present with anemia, edema and hypoalbuminemia; these infants will have been fed on human milk or soy formula. The third group are those infants who have received surgical repair for meconium ileus. In these groups, a short course of parenteral nutrition with enteral tube feeding may be necessary. For most infants, there is rapid improvement from attention to caloric needs, vitamin needs and pancreatic enzyme supplementation; routine oral feeding with an appropriate

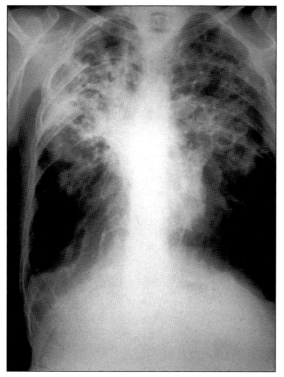

Figure 2: Chest X-ray of a child with severe cystic fibrosis.

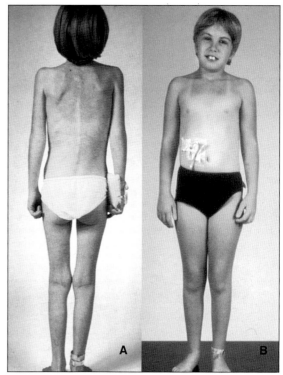

Figure 3: A. Eight-year old patient with cystic fibrosis and secondary malnutrition, before tube feeding, B. the same child after a period of g-tube feeds onto oral feeding only.

formula quickly becomes possible. Growth can also be maintained in breast-fed infants, provided calorie and sodium requirements are met. Some infants require a formula with higher energy density, but few require protein hydrolysates, medium chain triglyceride (MCT) or polysaccharide supplements. If so, these supplements usually need to be delivered by enteric tube.

Practical Points
- *CF may present with edema, anemia and hypoproteinemia in the first six months if breast-fed (borderline protein) or soy formula-fed (antitryptic effect).*
- *Sweat chloride may be falsely negative in the presence of edema and hypoalbuminemia.*
- *Nutritional care strongly affects survival.*
- *Infants with pancreatic sufficiency will not suffer nutritional problems.*
- *Normal nutrition and growth is possible in all children with CF.*

- *Both fat-soluble vitamin and essential fatty acid deficiency may be present at diagnosis.*
- *Routine oral feeding is possible in nearly all pancreatic insufficient infants, provided enzyme supplementation is given.*
- *A few infants will require aggressive nutritional intervention.*

The Infant with Bronchopulmonary Dysplasia

Preterm infants constitute 7% of all births, and those with birth weight <1,500 g make up 1%. Recent advances in neonatal intensive care, such as surfactant replacement therapy, have resulted in increasing survival of tiny preterm infants. However, these babies often require prolonged mechanical ventilation and prolonged duration of stay in the neonatal unit, and many survivors develop bronchopulmonary dysplasia (BPD). They have been shown to have prolonged periods of undernutrition due to difficulties with parenteral and enteral nutrition,[11] therefore fail to meet the recommended enteral energy intake of 120 kcal/kg/d.[12]

Undernutrition is very common in infants with BPD.[11] The problems with energy intake during the neonatal period have been described elsewhere;[11] as the infant becomes older, additional factors will also contribute.[3] Tachypnea, fatique, anorexia and gastrointestinal upset from drug use such as digoxin, and pain of esophagitis from gastroesophageal reflux are all factors. Energy needs are increased, due to raised energy expenditure, the use of drugs such as theophylline and salbutamol, and the need for catchup growth. Energy losses are increased, due to diuretic therapy, vomiting from drug-induced gastritis and gastroesophageal reflux (GER).

Nutritional care of babies with BPD includes recognizing potential problems early and starting an aggressive approach to parenteral and enteral feeding. High carbohydrate foods will increase carbon dioxide production. Use of balanced lipid-glucose-amino acid parenteral mixtures will lower metabolic rate, carbon dioxide production and glucose-derived lipogenesis, but will increase fat storage.[13] Use of glucose plus lipid in the newborn[14] has also been shown to increase the reutilization of amino acids for protein synthesis and increase energy storage for growth. The enteral diet of infants with BPD must be one with increased energy concentration because of the need for fluid restriction. A preterm milk fortifier can be added to human milk, and this milk, preterm formula and term formulas can have calorie supplements of glucose polymers, long chain triglycerides (LCT) or MCT. The delivery of nutrients can be orally, by naso-gastric tube or gastrostomy tube.

Vomiting due to gastroesophageal reflux is a common problem in babies with bronchopulmonary dysplasia. We recommend using food thickeners, positioning, correct dosage of the prokinetic cisapride and gastrojejunal tube feeding. If these fail, we recommend antireflux surgery. It should be noted, however, that chronic lung disease is the leading risk factor correlated with failure of pediatric antireflux surgery.[15]

Practical Points

- *Undernutrition is very common in infants with BPD.*
- *Early recognition of potential problems is important.*

- *An aggressive approach to nutritional management is needed.*
- *Both breast and formula milks need caloric supplements.*
- *GER is common and needs aggressive treatment.*

The Neurodevelopmentally Handicapped Infant

Both undernutrition and obesity are very real problems in infants with neurodevelopmental disability. Undernutrition is a frequent problem in children with severe cerebral palsy (spastic quadraplegia), who often have significant impairment of their eating and swallowing mechanisms.[16] Pseudobulbar palsy affects both swallowing and eating and thus results in both decreased feed intake and increased eating time. For many parents of handicapped children, feeding takes up to four to six hours per day, is punctuated by food spills, aspiration and regurgitation, and is the major difficulty in the daily management of their child.[17]

Nutritional needs of infants with severe neurological disability are poorly defined. Bandini et al[18] have shown that adolescents with cerebral palsy expend less energy than other adolescents. Children with spastic quadraplegia at age three to 20 years have reduced energy needs if fed exclusively by gastrostomy tube.[19] It is probable that the energy needs of non-ambulant children with neurodevelopmental handicap are lower than the recommended dietary allowance for age and gender.

Gastroesophageal reflux is a problem in the majority of neurologically disabled infants, and is thought to be due to a combination of delayed gastric emptying and intestinal dysmotility.[16] Reflux may limit energy intake, increase the risk of food aspiration and aspiration pneumonia and cause reflux esophagitis, with painful swallowing, anemia and stricture formation. We aim to treat reflux by medical therapy-appropriate positioning, food thickeners, antacids, the prokinetic agent cisapride and an H_2-blocker or proton pump inhibitor. Refeeding itself will improve GER in neurologically disabled children.[20] If reflux is still troublesome, we use a gastrojejunal tube. Anti-reflux surgery is used as a last option, due to the high complication rate and frequent need for revision operations in this

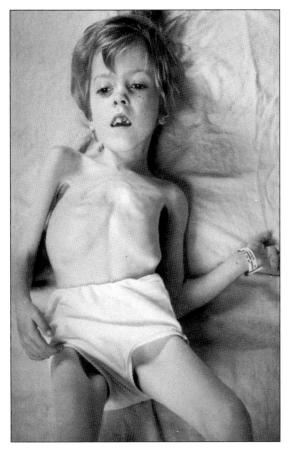

Figure 4: Two-year old child with spastic quadriplegia (and scoliosis) and an oro-motor feeding problem.

group of infants.[21] Fundoplication in children with spastic quadraplagia may be complicated by dumping syndrome, due to rapid gastric emptying, hyperglycemia and rebound hypoglycemia. Khoshoo et al[22] have shown that fundoplication-associated dumping syndrome can be managed simply and non-invasively by nutritional management alone, using a combination of a complex carbohydrates and a fat emulsion.

There is a growing recognition of the effect of undernutrition on brain growth and neurodevelopment. An infant who often chokes on or aspirates liquids or solids will be discomforted during feeding. Undernourished children generally feel miserable compared with well-nourished children. Time spent on feeding limits time for the caregiver to devote to other activities with the disabled infant, to siblings and to their own needs.

Assessing nutritional status by comparing weight and length with standard growth charts may be difficult, due to musculoskeletal deformities and muscle wasting due to atrophy. We consider skinfold measurements the most useful assessment when compared to population norms. Laboratory assessment is rarely helpful, except when GER leads to chronic intestinal blood loss.

The cause of the energy deficit in neurodevelopmentally handicapped infants can be summarized using Figure 1. Energy intake is decreased due to difficulties with eating and swallowing. Energy losses are increased due to gastroesophageal reflux. Energy needs are increased due to the need for catch-up growth.

Our approach to management is that of the Nutrition Committee of the Canadian Pediatric Society.[16] A multidisciplinary approach with clinical dietician, enterostomy nurse, feeding therapist, pediatric gastroenterologist/nutritionist, radiologist and possibly pediatric surgeon, dentist and neurologist is used. The first approach is to increase energy concentration of ingested food, provided that oral feeding is safe. This may be by adding fat to liquids and solids, or by high-energy liquid supplements. Supplemental tube feeding is often required; if more than a short-term measure is envisioned, a gastrostomy tube is preferable to a nasogastric tube. GER should be treated as discussed above. Jejunal feeding, when used, is given continuously via pump, rather than by bolus feeding. Restoration of oral feeding is sometimes possible, provided there is not progressive neurological deterioration (see later).

Obesity in the handicapped infant can become evident in the second year of life, setting a pattern that will lead to major problems in later childhood. Obesity not only leads to locomotor and cardiorespiratory compromise of the disabled child, but also is a significant problem for caregivers.[23]

Practical Points

- *Undernutrition is a major problem in neurodevelopmentally handicapped infants.*
- *Skinfold measurements are very useful in the non-ambulant child with muscle wasting.*
- *Oromotor feeding problems are common, resulting in undernutrition and/or chronic aspiration.*

- *Feeding of the infant may dominate the caregiver's life.*
- *GER is due to delayed gastric emptying and intestinal dysmotility, and requires aggressive medical therapy.*
- *Anti-reflux surgery is a last option.*
- *A multidisciplinary approach to management is required.*
- *If oral feeding is safe, increase the energy concentration of ingested food.*
- *Gastric or gastrojejunal tubes are the preferred type of tube feeding.*
- *If there is no feeding problem, obesity may begin to be a problem in the second year of life.*

Congenital Heart Disease

Undernutrition is common in infants with congenital heart disease (CHD). The related problems again include decreased energy intake, increased energy expenditure and increased energy losses (Figure 1). There is also an effect of the type of CHD. In the past, definitive surgical repairs were often delayed until middle or late childhood, with palliative surgical procedures performed in infancy. Nowadays, surgery is often performed in the neonatal period, such as the "switch" procedure for transposition of the great arteries. This has decreased long-term growth failure secondary to the effect of undernutrition during rapid growth in early life, and the high energy cost of catch-up growth.

The type of cardiac lesion has an effect on growth failure. A significant minority of cases of CHD are part of a malformation syndrome or chromosomal anomaly that itself has an associated growth problem – for example, coarctation of the aorta in Turner's syndrome or atrioventricular canal defect in Down's syndrome.

Decreased energy intake has a variety of causes. Anorexia is a major problem, due to drugs, hepatic congestion, congestive gastropathy, respiratory distress from congestive heart failure (CHF) and fatigue due to CHF. Eating or drinking is often prolonged, with frequent pauses, and sweating due to sympathetic overactivity. Early satiety may be a complication of some drugs. At a cellular level, anoxia and acidosis may alter metabolism to limit energy intake.[24]

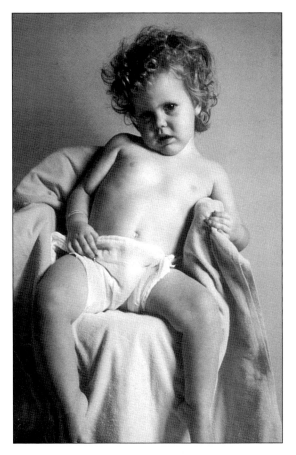

Figure 5: Same child pictured in Figure 4 after a period of g-tube feedings and gradation off tube feeding onto oral feeding only.

Energy needs are also high in infants with CHD. Increased metabolic rate is a common finding, especially if CHF is present.[25] Decreased energy intake and increased resting energy expenditure alone, therefore, should explain the commonly seen growth failure. However, there are confounding factors, such as the reduced energy expenditure from activity if an infant is chronically ill, and the reduced energy expenditure from decreased synthesis of new tissue in growth failure. A recent paper by Barton et al[26] is therefore very useful, because they measured total daily energy expenditure (energy expenditure due to resting energy expenditure plus the energy costs of growth and activity) in infants with severe CHD using the doubly labeled water method. Total daily energy expenditure was found to be raised, and significantly greater than that of healthy infants of a similar age.[26]

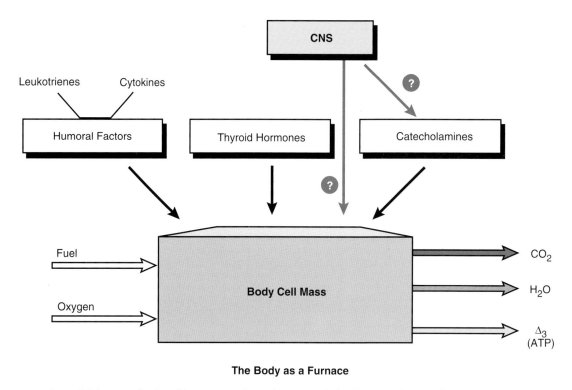

The Body as a Furnace

Figure 6: Model diagram developed by Azcue and Pencharz to include all known factors affecting energy expenditure in response to disease.

Increased energy losses may also be a feature. Gastroesophageal reflux is known to occur more frequently in infants with CHD. Vomiting may also occur secondary to drug-related gastritis. CHF, if severe, can lead to hepatic ischemia and fat malabsorption. CHF has also been suggested to cause edema and hypoxia of the gut with resultant malabsorption. Vaisman et al[27] studied seven infants with CHD who received regular diuretic treatment for CHF. Energy balance studies showed that these infants did not have a significant problem with malabsorption. Further, total body water and extracellular fluid were measured in the infants by deuterium dilution and corrected bromide space respectively, and the results suggested that normal weight gain will occur if the total body water is not overly expanded.[27]

Infants with significant CHD should be fed a high calorie diet, usually a milk with less water content and higher protein, carbohydrate and fat. Standard formulas (0.67 kcal/ml) are rarely appropriate because of the need for fluid restriction. Calorie requirement is at least 20% higher than standard (75-120 kcal/kg/d); most infants with major CHD need an energy intake of at least 140 kcal/kg/d to thrive.[24, 26, 28] Large fluid loads should be avoided, and sodium balance carefully adjusted. Unrestricted sodium may exacerbate CHF, but severe sodium restriction will not allow growth. Oral feeding is the route of choice, but many infants with established growth failure require tube feeding to achieve nutritional repletion.[28] Total parenteral nutrition (TPN) is rarely needed, except during the postoperative period or during a major illness where enteral feeding is not possible.

Practical Points
- *Undernutrition is common in infants with congenital heart disease.*
- *Decreased energy intake is related to anorexia, gastritis, increased respiratory effort and fatigue.*
- *Total daily energy expenditure is raised in infants with CHD.*

- *The need for fluid restriction should be compensated by increased energy concentration of foods.*
- *Most infants with major CHD need at least 140 kcal/kg/d to thrive.*
- *Some infants require tube feeding to reach caloric goals.*

Acquired Immunodeficiency Syndrome (AIDS)

During the first two years of life, infection of children with the human immunodeficiency virus (HIV) is a result of being born to HIV-infected mothers. These mothers are frequently of low socioeconomic status and are known to have poorer pregnancy outcomes, with low birthweights and more prematurity.[29] The study of Miller et al[29] is of particular interest since it compares the growth of children, born to HIV-infected mothers, who are either HIV-infected or who are not infected (have seroreverted). At birth there were no differences in size; however, over the first two years of life, the children with HIV-infection grew significantly more slowly in weight that the non-infected children. Growth failure in children[30] and depletion of body cell mass in adults[31] are adverse prognostic factors in patients with AIDS. It has therefore been reasoned that the maintenance of nutritional status, growth and body composition are of great importance in patients with HIV infection and AIDS.[32]

The known effects of AIDS on the nutrition of a patient are multiple and include both systemic infections, which result in anorexia and hypermetabolism,[32] and infections of the gut resulting in anorexia and malabsorption.[32-34] Thus, the adverse nutritional effects of AIDS are well represented by the model shown in Figure 1. The approach to management is to first identify and treat infections which may be bacterial, fungal, parasitic or viral. Frequently, particularly during disease exacerbations, the child is unable to ingest nutritional requirements for age. Further, their requirements may be increased, secondary to infection.[35] It has been shown that it is possible to successfully provide enteral tube nutrition support.[36] Since this need for nutritional support is ongoing, our view is that a percutaneous gastrostomy should be seriously considered. There are no clear data as to what type of

formula should be infused through the gastrostomy and the choice depends upon gut function. It is therefore appropriate to start with a lactose-free infant formula or pediatric polymeric feed. Use of a semi-elemental or elemental feed depends upon the absorptive function of the gut, which can be determined by a three-day fat balance. Only if it proves impossible to nourish with enteral nutrition would parenteral nutrition be used, as is the case with any other disease process. Other centers agree with this approach to nutritional support.[35, 37]

Our center's limited experience has been that it is possible to improve the nutritional status of a malnourished infant or child with HIV infection by enteral or parenteral nutritional support. What is not clear is how nutrition support affects the longer-term outcome. There is therefore an increasing emphasis being placed on careful growth and nutrition monitoring, with diet therapy and oral supplementation, in an effort to prevent malnutrition.[32]

Practical Points

- *Identify and treat any infections in the HIV-infected child – both gut and systemic infections will compromise nutritional care.*
- *A high index of suspicion for early undernutrition is required.*
- *Consider early use of a gastrostomy tube if growth begins to falter.*
- *Lactose-free infant formulas or pediatric polymeric formulas are the first line of feed type.*
- *TPN is used only if enteral nutrition has failed.*

Hepatic Diseases and Failure

A variety of diseases cause hepatic failure in young children.[38] The hepatic failure is usually associated with cholestasis, which significantly impairs fat digestion and absorption, thereby adversely affecting energy, fat-soluble vitamin[38-40] and essential fatty acid[41] status. The most common cause of end-stage liver disease in this group is extra-hepatic biliary atresia with secondary biliary cirrhosis. Patients with this condition have been shown to have increased resting energy expenditure.[42] Finally, many of these infants and children have anorexia[39, 43] due to mechanical issues (hepatomegaly and ascites compressing the stomach and bowel) and probably, to metabolic effects. The development of pediatric liver transplantation, and the recognition that nutritional status affects outcome, have resulted in an increased appreciation of the need for nutrition support.[39, 40, 43]

Nutritional management should include an assessment and monitoring of nutritional status. Weight/height measurements alone may result in a false impression of the energy status. Sokol and Stall[44] have pointed out the importance of measuring triceps skinfold thickness, since hepatomegaly and ascites can falsely increase weight. Experience has shown that the use of energy-dense feeds (usually 1 kcal/ml) are helpful. Replacement of some of the LCT with MCT has proven to help with the fat malabsorption. However, it is important to ensure that there is a generous intake of essential fatty acids or deficiency may occur. Kaufman et al[41] observed biochemical evidence of essential fatty acid deficiency in infants fed a very high MCT-containing formula (Portagen). Conversely, when the infants were switched to a lower MCT-containing formula with more essential fatty acids (Pregestimil) they noted an improvement in essential fatty acid status. Particular care must also be paid to the fat-soluble vitamins A, D, E and K because of the malabsorption. In addition, vitamin D is activated by 25-hydroxylation in the liver and this process may be compromised. Chin et al[40] observed low vitamin A and E levels in 69 and 62% of their patients and low 25-hydroxyvitamin D levels in 25% of the group. Clearly, blood vitamin concentrations need to be monitored and water soluble supplements given in high doses to normalize these levels.[39]

For many of the infants, diet therapy alone is not sufficient to maintain growth and nutritional status[39, 43]; supplemental tube feeds are required.[43, 45] Chin et al[43] demonstrated in a randomized crossover trial that the addition of a branched chain amino acid supplement (increasing branch chains from 25 to 38% of the protein) significantly improved growth and body composition. In our center, we have adopted the use of branch chain amino acid supplements to the base diet Pregestimil (a semi-elemental infant formula

with a casein hydrolysate protein source and 50% of the fat from MCT). Tube supplements, both naso-enteric and enterostomies, are used increasingly, with transpyloric placement of the tube if vomiting is a problem. From a practical point of view, an enterostomy is preferable to a naso-enteric tube, but the transplant surgeons are concerned that the enterostomy track may interfere with liver transplantation. So our current practice is to use a naso-enteric tube for a patient who is already on the transplant list and will therefore be transplanted in the next six months. Conversely, an infant who is severely malnourished and is therefore not a good candidate for transplantation will have an enterostomy inserted. Once nutritionally resuscitated, the patient will be listed for transplantation.

Practical Points

- *Cholestasis causes fat maldigestion and malabsorption, and adversely effects energy, fat-soluble vitamin and essential fatty acid status.*
- *Anorexia is common in infants with hepatic disease.*
- *Poor nutritional status has a negative effect on outcome of liver transplantation.*
- *Use of medium chain triglyceride supplements will increase energy absorption despite fat malabsorption.*
- *Adequate amounts of essential fatty acids must be supplied.*
- *Fat soluble vitamin status requires regular monitoring with alteration of amount of supplementation.*
- *Tube feeding is often necessary.*
- *Branched chain amino acid supplements should be used in end-stage liver disease.*

Renal Diseases and Failure

In the first two years of life, the two renal conditions that need to be considered from a nutritional standpoint are nephrotic syndrome and renal failure. Infants are generally too small to be managed with hemodialysis, but there is growing experience with the effect of peritoneal dialysis on nutritional status. Infants and young children with chronic renal failure often suffer from anorexia, which makes meeting their nutritional needs difficult.

Peritoneal dialysis only compounds the food intake problem. Thus, infants with renal failure tend to fail to thrive.[46-48]

As far as specific nutrients are concerned, the focus has been on protein, energy, phosphate, potassium and 1,25 dihydroxylcholecalciferol. In adults with chronic renal disease, it has been shown that protein restriction slows the progression of the renal disease and may therefore delay the need for dialysis and eventual transplantation. The situation in infants and children with chronic renal failure is more complex because protein restriction may impede linear growth.[49] Further, there are animal data that protein restriction may also impede kidney growth.[50] Finally, hepatic albumin synthesis is dependent upon an adequate protein intake.[51] Peritoneal dialysis is known to result in loss of amino acids, which increases protein needs to a degree. Currently, studies are ongoing to determine whether adding amino acids to peritoneal dialysate has any long-term benefit.[52] Our hospital practice is to feed infants at a protein level at, but not above, the requirement for age, at the same time trying to ensure an adequate non-protein energy intake. To achieve these goals, energy-dense formulas are used. These are usually based on a low-phosphate, low-electrolyte infant formula (Similac PM 60:40), to which is added non-protein energy sources such corn syrup solids (dextrins) and a vegetable oil. If the infant is consistently not able to ingest an adequate intake, then the possible use of supplemental enterostomy (gastrostomy or gastrojejunal) feeds are discussed with the family. Our philosophy is to try to minimize growth failure. Although there are limited data regarding the effects of chronic renal failure on energy expenditure,[46] our hospital experience with tube-feeding infants with renal disease and failure to thrive is that their energy requirements are not increased above those needed for recovery from undernutrition. Phosphate restriction is valuable in preventing hyperparathyroidism[53] and renal oseodystrophy. Currently, management consists of a restricted phosphate intake, plus oral phosphate binders if required. In addition, calcium metabolism is optimized by taking vitamin D supplements. Since 1-hydroxylation of vitamin D takes place in the kidney, supplemental 1,25 dihydroxycholecalciferol is given.

For infants with end-stage renal disease, the combination of peritoneal dialysis with aggressive nutritional support via nasogastric feeding minimizes growth failure.[48] With the introduction of percutaneous enterostomies at our hospital there has been increasing use of enterostomy feeding. When an infant is on peritoneal dialysis, peritoneal fluid has to be drained prior to enterostomy placement, but we have had only small technical problems in this situation.

Practical Points

- *Anorexia is common in infants with chronic renal disease.*
- *Provide infants with a protein intake equal to requirement for age and ensure good non-protein energy intake.*
- *Low-phosphate, low-electrolyte infant formulas are used.*
- *Formulas require increased energy concentration.*
- *Consider tube feeding if energy intake is consistently sub-optimal.*
- *Aggressive nutritional support is needed in end-stage renal disease.*
- *Enterostomy tubes can be placed in infants requiring peritoneal dialysis.*

Nutritional Management

Diet therapy, tube feeding, parenteral nutrition and the role of nutrition support teams will all be discussed. The nutritional management of every infant should be individualized, with attention paid to weight, postnatal age, degree of pre-existing malnutrition, type and severity of disease, presence of feeding incoordination, presence of GER and social circumstances.

Route of Feeding

Oral feeding is the route of choice in the chronically ill infant. However, oral feeding is often not safe, or voluntary oral intake is inadequate to allow appropriate growth. If safety is the concern, history alone may reveal that aspiration and choking are often associated

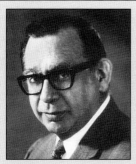

Harry Shwachman, M.D., (1910-1986) was a Hopkins graduate who trained in Pediatrics at the Children's Hospital, Boston. Shwachman spent an extra year in Pathology to study an unnamed disease now known as cystic fibrosis. This launched a career of benchmark contributions to pediatric clinical nutrition and gastroenterology. Shwachman was responsible for most of the clinical advances in CF care between 1941 and 1976. The highest recognition of the North American Society of Pediatric Gastroenterology and Nutrition is the Shwachman Award. Archives: CNRC (Photo courtesy of BCH)

with feeding. When in doubt, we recommend a feeding assessment by a trained occupational therapist; a radiological feeding study may be necessary. The safety of thin and thick liquids, thin and thick purees and solids are assessed.

If feeding incoordination or limited voluntary oral intake is present, involuntary enteral feeding is necessary. Nasogastric or nasojejunal feeding are effective if nutritional rehabilitation or supplementation will be brief – that is, no longer than six weeks. For longer periods, we recommend inserting a permanent feeding tube, such as a gastrostomy or gastro-jejunostomy tube. Gastro-esophageal reflux or aspiration of feeds that is unresponsive to diet and pharmacological maneuvers may require a tube placed past the ligament of Treitz in the jejunum.

Total parenteral nutrition is only used if intestinal failure, severe dysmotility or congenital anatomical or functional problems preclude the use of the gut. Partial parenteral nutrition, a combination of enteral and parenteral nutrition, may be necessary for variable periods in some patients.

Practical Points

- *Oral feeding is the route of choice, provided it is safe and allows normal growth.*
- *Feeding assessment by an occupational therapist is valuable.*

- *Naso-enteral feeding should not be used for long-term feeding.*
- *Gastrojejunostomy tubes are useful if GER and dysmotility are problematic.*
- *TPN is used only if enteral feeding fails.*

Formulas

All formulas fit into four basic categories: home-liquidized, polymeric, elemental and modular.[54] Only the first two may contain fiber. A detailed description of available formulas is provided in the appendix.

Home-liquidized formulas are table foods thinned with liquids and possibly with added vitamins and minerals. The only difference from normal food is the texture, so it is suitable for only a few infants with chronic illness, and never before one year of age. The constituents are whole proteins, long chain triglycerides and starch with di- and monosaccharides. One main advantage is their low cost.

Polymeric formulas contain protein, fat and carbohydrate in their non-hydrolysed forms (whole protein, mainly LCT, starch and glucose polymers) and are used in the absence of maldigestion and malabsorption. Although standard infant formulas contain lactose, few polymeric formulas do, due to the widespread presence of genetic or acquired lactase deficiency in the population requiring enteral feeding.[55] Polymeric formulas contain between 11 and 25% of total calories as whole proteins of high quality, and from 20 to 40% as fat. Fats include LCT and MCT; the former provide a calorie-dense energy source with essential fatty acids and fat soluble vitamins that also contribute to the formula's palatability. MCT are more easily digested and rapidly absorbed than LCT. Carbohydrate, which provides 46 to 66% of total calories, is primarily starch and partially hydrolysed starch (maltodextrins, oligo- and poly-saccharides).

Elemental formulas are used for infants with maldigestion or malabsorption, and are of no advantage in infants with a normal gastrointestinal tract.[55] The protein, carbohydrate and fat are more hydrolysed than those in polymeric formulas. They are fiber-free and may have high osmolality due to the presence of multiple small particles. Protein is supplied as amino acids or peptides up to tetrapeptides, hydrolysed from a high quality protein source. Fat is supplied mainly as the easily-absorbable MCT. Carbohydrate content may be higher than in polymeric formulas, with an increased amount of maltodextrins. They are more expensive than polymeric formulas, and their poor taste can lead to problems of acceptability in infants who have previously had breast milk or infant formulas.

Modular diets consist of individual nutrient components of fat, carbohydrate and protein, and can be used in combination or else to supplement other feeds.

There are some other formulas available. Supplements are often given to augment caloric intake in older children or in adults and are available as milk shakes, puddings or liquids. In infants, supplements are usually modules of fat or carbohydrate added to polymeric or elemental formulas. Specialty formulas that can be used in infancy include preterm formulas, low phosphate and protein formulas for renal disease and branched-chain amino acid-augmented formulas for liver disease.

Practical Points

- *Formula types are home-liquidized, polymeric, elemental and modular.*
- *Home-liquidized formulas are unsuitable for infants younger than one year.*
- *Polymeric formulas contain protein, fat and carbohydrate in non-hydrolysed forms.*
- *Elemental formulas are used if maldigestion or malabsorption are present, and nutrients are hydrolysed.*
- *Modular diets consist of individual nutrient components.*

Tube Feeding

Nasogastric or nasojejunal tubes are recommended for only short-term (<six weeks) feeding. Enterostomy

> *Much, if not most, malnutrition in the world today depends not only on the cataclysms of nature and man-made disasters such as war and civil disorder. It depends on failure to conserve, select, distribute and prepare food.*
>
> *Primary Health Care Pioneer*
> *The Selected Works of*
> *Dr. Cicely D. Williams*
> Naomi Baumslag, Editor
> World Federation of Public
> Health Associations
> and UNICEF

feeding tubes are used for longer-term feeding, even if this is supplemental and not total feeding. The surgically placed gastrostomy and jejunostomy tubes have now been augmented by percutaneous gastrostomy and percutaneous gastrojejunostomy tubes, both of which can be placed by an endoscopic or radiological technique.[54] The newer placement techniques and the increased availability of reliable replacement tubes and formula feeds has led to increased use of nutrition support teams. Currently, the Home Feeding Program at the Hospital for Sick Children, Toronto, has 250 patients on home overnight enteral feeds and 16 on home TPN.

Once the decision has been made to perform an enterostomy, the question becomes which technique will be used. Percutaneous enterostomies are only contraindicated if the liver or transverse colon is positioned directly over the proposed site. The two types of percutaneous enterostomy are endoscopic or radiological; the latter usually uses a retrograde rather than antegrade approach.[54] Retrograde percutaneous gastrostomy has been the method of choice at the Hospital for Sick Children since 1990. Surgically-placed tubes are usually used in the rare patients who require an anti-reflux surgical procedure as well as an enterostomy.

The decision to have a gastrostomy placed is often difficult for the infant's parents. Our Nutrition Support nursing team runs a pre-procedure clinic, with teaching and discussion of any concerns, and provides a teaching manual for parents. A gastrojejunal tube is inserted if there is a strong history of reflux or there is another indication for jejunal feeding. Infants are discharged three to five days after the procedure, and then seen at the gastrostomy tube clinic one week later. The initial catheter is changed to a balloon-type catheter at six weeks, and a skin level tube (button) at a minimum of three months later, when the tract is mature. Replacement tubes tend to be of the button type.

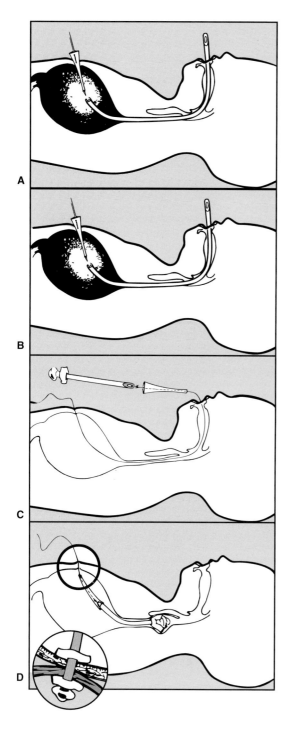

Figure 7: Four illustrations depicting the placement of a retrograde (radiologically) percutaneous gastrostomy.

The main indications for gastrojejunostomy or jejunostomy tube insertion include tracheal aspiration, GER that is unresponsive to medical therapy, gastroparesis, microgastria (congenital or post-surgical) and postoperative feeding after major surgical procedures. A standard polymeric formula is appropriate for most infants, and the isotonic strength is preferable to hyperosmolar elemental feeds.

Practical Points

- *Nasal tube feeding is used only for short periods.*
- *Enterostomy tubes may be placed surgically, endoscopically or radiologically.*
- *The only contraindication to percutaneous enterostomy is liver or colon lying over the proposed site.*
- *Retrograde percutaneous enterostomy is performed radiologically and has many advantages.*
- *Counseling of caregivers is required prior to enterostomy placement.*
- *Hyperosmolar feeds are unsuitable for patients fed directly into the jejunum.*

Reintroduction of Oral Feeding

Oral feeding is the goal for any chronically ill infant. For some, such as children with progressive neurological disease, oral feeding will never be safe. In other cases, resolving the medical problem or developmental improvement secondary to nutritional replenishment will allow the child to discontinue tube feeding. Our hospital experience is that lack of eating during a significant portion of infancy often leads to a behavioral eating problem when oral feeding is again possible. We suggest that assessment of oral-motor skills be repeated when developmental progress has occurred in the neurodevelopmentally handicapped infant or when the underlying medical condition has improved. In the former group, bulbar functional improvement is manifest by improved head control, disappearance of drooling, disappearance of stridor and the development of speech.[16] The aim of feeding assessment is again to answer the question of whether it is safe for the child to eat, and if so, which textures of food are safe. A child who aspirates liquids is often safe with pureed food. When it is safe for the child to eat, caregivers should be encouraged to give part of the daily intake by mouth. Overnight supplemental tube feeding by pump is a useful option to separate tube feeding from eating.[54] Even when safe, it may take months to wean the child from tube feeding. We have found the involvement of a trained infant psychiatrist to be of great help in successful behavioral modification.

Practical Points
- *Oral feeding can usually be reintroduced when medical problems have resolved and developmental progress has occurred.*
- *Reintroduction of oral feeding may be impossible in infants with progressive neurological disease.*
- *Behavioral problems are common when oral feeding is reintroduced.*
- *Simple clinical assessment provides clues that oral-motor skills have improved.*
- *Overnight supplemental feeding allows oral feeding by day.*
- *Involvement of an infant psychiatrist may be invaluable.*

Total Parenteral Nutrition
Total Parental Nutrition (TPN) is often needed as a sole or partial type of feeding when the infant with chronic illness requires hospitalization. However, it is uncommon for these infants to need TPN for home use. Indications for home TPN include short gut syndrome, chronic intestinal pseudo-obstruction, aganglionosis, hollow viscus myopathy and autoimmune enteropathy. Due to the success of the home overnight enteral feeding program, we average 12 patients and have never had more than 24 patients requiring home TPN at one time in the program at the Hospital for Sick Children, of whom about one-third are usually infants.

The parents or carers of an infant requiring home TPN require considerable teaching and back-up, which would be impossible without a nutrition support team. Complications of home TPN are significant, and include sepsis, catheter-related thrombosis[56] and hepatic dysfunction.[57] The latter is at its most

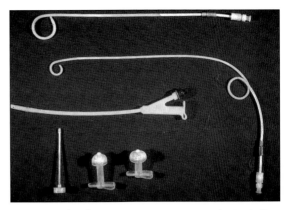

Figure 8: This shows various enterostomy tubes including from top to bottom: a Cope-loop g-tube; a GJ-tube; foley type g-tube; two sizes of a button g-tube with introducer.

severe in premature infants, in whom TPN-associated cholestasis may eventually necessitate liver or liver-small bowel transplantation.

Practical Points
- *TPN is often needed in hospital, but rarely at home.*
- *Home TPN is impossible in the absence of a nutrition support team.*
- *Home TPN may be complicated by sepsis, catheter-related thrombosis and hepatic dysfunction.*

Role of Nutrition Support Team
The establishment of a home feeding program, enteral or parenteral, requires a nutrition support team for optimal function. This is a multidisciplinary team, consisting of pediatric gastroenterologist/nutritionist, clinical dietician, nurse and possibly pharmacist. The team is involved in patient care, education and research, and has been shown to significantly improve care and provide cost-effective therapy.[55]

Case Histories
Case #1: A ten-week-old white male infant presented with poor weight gain, pallor and edema. He had been born at term weighing 3.1 kg to a primigravid mother after an uncomplicated pregnancy. He had been exclusively breast-fed until seven weeks of age, when supplementation with a formula milk was commenced for poor weight gain. He was referred to our service for

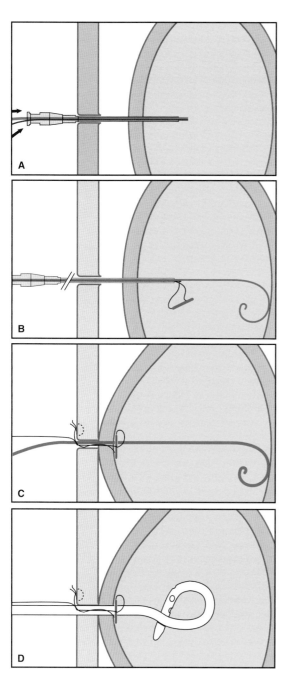

Figure 9: Four illustrations depicting the placement of a percutaneous endoscopy gastrostomy (PEG).

assessment of his poor weight gain and recently noted pallor and edema.

On admission, he was noted to be pale, edematous and a voracious feeder. His weight at 3.9 kg (<3rd centile) was 79% of ideal weight for height. The only other finding of note was a soft ejection systolic murmur.

Laboratory investigations included total protein of 41g/l, albumin of 24 g/l, hemoglobin of 73 g/l with normal indices and reticulocyte count of 9%. Due to clinical suspicion of cystic fibrosis, sudan stain of stool showed neutral fat, fecal fat loss was 21% of intake over 72 hours and sweat chloride was 57 mmol/l. The sweat chloride was considered a false negative.

His formula was changed to a casein hydrolysate with 50% MCT, and vitamin and pancreatic enzyme supplementation was begun, with dramatic response. Three weeks later, weight had risen to 5.8 kg, edema had resolved, and both hemoglobin and serum albumin levels were normal. Repeat sweat chloride was 94 mmol/l and CF genotype was determined to be homozygous for ΔF508.

Case #2: *A female infant aged 14 months was referred to our clinic with feeding difficulties. She had been born at 26 weeks gestation, weighing 746 g, and had required mechanical ventilation and surfactant replacement therapy for the respiratory distress syndrome. Her stormy neonatal course included multiple episodes of sepsis. She had intraventricular hemorrhage with ventricular dilatation. She was a postnatal age of five months at time of discharge home.*

Her parents took one to two hours per meal to feed her with a polymeric formula and small quantities of soft food. She vomited after meals, despite use of an H_2-blocker. She had had two episodes of possible aspiration pneumonia requiring hospital admission. Her weight at referral was 8.4 kg (<3rd centile) and triceps skinfold thickness was 4 mm (<5th centile).

A radiological feeding study with a trained occupational therapist showed oro-motor discoordination with minor reflux from above. Gastroesophageal reflux was also noted. A multidisciplinary approach to management included insertion of gastrostomy tube, use of calorie-supplemented formula and appropriate doses of cisapride and ranitidine.

Eight months later, her weight had risen to the 25th centile, oral feeding had been introduced and accounted for 50% of intake and there had been no more hospital admissions.

Historical Perspective...

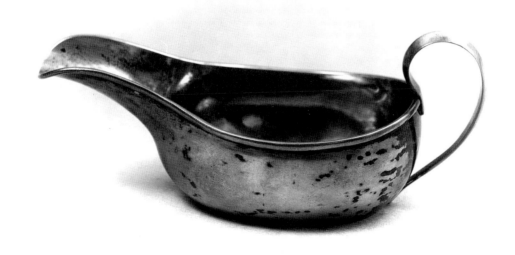

Pap boat, sterling silver, 1820.

References

1. Moore J, Durie PR, Forstner GG, Pencharz PB. The assessment of nutritional status in children. *Nutr Res.* 1985;5:797-799.

2. Pencharz PB, Durie PR. Nutritional management of cystic fibrosis. *Ann Rev Nutr.* 1993;13:111-136.

3. Grunow JE, Pencharz PB. Enteral nutrition in bronchopulmonary dysplasia. In: Baker S, Baker R, Davis A, eds. *Pediatric Enteral Nutrition.* New York: Chapman and Hall; 1994;238-250.

4. Kerem B-S, Rommens JM, Buchanan JA, et al. Identification of the cystic fibrosis gene: genetic analysis. *Science.* 1989;245:1073-1080.

5. Kerem E, Corey M, Kerem B-S, et al. Clinical and genetic comparisons of patients with cystic fibrosis, with or without meconeum ileus. *J Pediatr.* 1989;114:767-773.

6. Gaskin K, Gurwitz D, Durie P, et al. Improved respiratory prognosis in patients with cystic fibrosis with normal fat absorption. *J Pediatr.* 1982;100:857-862.

7. Corey M, McLaughlin FJ, Williams M, Levison H. A comparison of survival, growth and pulmonary function in patients with cystic fibrosis in Boston and Toronto. *J Clin Epidemiol.* 1988;41:583-591.

8. Ramsey BW, Farrell PM, Pencharz P, and the Consensus Committee. Nutritional assessment and management in cystic fibrosis: a consensus report. *Am J Clin Nutr.* 1992; 55:108-116.

9. Sokol RJ, Reardon MC, Accurso FJ, et al. Fat-soluble vitamin status during the first year of life in infants with cystic fibrosis identified by screening of newborns. *Am J Clin Nutr.* 1989;50:1064-1071.

10. Vaisman N, Pencharz PB, Corey M, Canny GJ, Hahn E. Energy expenditure of patients with cystic fibrosis. *J Pediatr.* 1987;111:496-500.

11. Wilson DC, McClure G, Halliday HL, Reid MMcC, Dodge JA. Nutrition and bronchopulmonary dysplasia. *Arch Dis Child.* 1991;66:37-38.

12. American Academy of Pediatrics Committee on Nutrition. Nutritional needs of low birthweight infants. *Pediatrics.* 1985;75:976-986.

13. Van Aerde JEE, Sauer PJJ, Pencharz PB, Smith JM, Swyer PR. Effect of replacing glucose with lipid on the energy metabolism of newborn infants. *Clin Sci.* 1989; 76:581-588.

14. Pencharz P, Beasley J, Sauer P, et al. Total body protein turnover in parenterally fed neonates: effects of energy source studied by using (15N) glycine and (1-13C) leucine. *Am J Clin Nutr.* 1989;50:1395-1400.

15. Taylor LA, Weiner T, Lacey SR, Azizkhan RG. Chronic lung disease is the leading risk factor correlating with the failure (wrap disruption) of antireflux procedures in children. *J Pediatr Surg.* 1994;29:161-166.

16. Nutrition Committee, Canadian Paediatric Society. Undernutrition in children with a neurodevelopmental disability. *Can Med Assoc J.* 1994;151:753-759.

17. Couriel JM, Bisset R, Miller R, Thomas A, Clarke M. Assessment of feeding problems in neurodevelopmental handicap: a team approach. *Arch Dis Child.* 1993;69: 609-613.

18. Bandini LG, Schoeller DA, Fukagawa NK, et al. Body composition and energy expenditure in adolescents with cerebral palsy or myelodysplasia. *Pediatr Res.* 1991;29:70-77.

19. Fried MD, Pencharz PB. Energy and nutrient intakes of children with spastic quadraplegia. *J Pediatr.* 1991;119: 947-949.

20. Lewis D, Khoshoo V, Pencharz PB, Goalladay ES. Impact of nutritional rehabilitation on gastroesophageal reflux in neurologically impaired children. *J Pediatr Surg.* 1994;29:167-170.

21. Spitz L, Roth K, Kiely EM, Brereton RJ, Drake DP, Milla PJ. Operation for gastro-oesophageal reflux associated with severe mental retardation. *Arch Dis Child.* 1993;68:347-351.

22. Khoshoo V, Roberts PL, Loe WA, Golladay ES, Pencharz PB. Nutritional management of dumping syndrome associated with antireflux surgery. *J Pediatr Surg.* 1994;29:1452-1454.

23. Bax M. Nutrition and disability. *Dev Med Child Neurol.* 1993;35:1035-1036.

24. Forchielli ML, McColl R, Walker WA, Lo C. Children with congenital heart disease: a nutrition challenge. *Nutr Rev.* 1994;52:348-353.

25. Menon G, Poskitt EME. Why does congenital heart disease cause failure to thrive? *Arch Dis Child.* 1985;60: 134-139.

26. Barton JS, Hindmarsh PC, Scrimgeour CM, Rennie MJ, Preece MA. Energy expenditure in congenital heart disease. *Arch Dis Child.* 1994;70:5-9.

27. Vaisman N, Leigh T, Voek H, Westerterp K, Abraham M, Duchan R. Malabsorption in infants with congenital heart disease under diuretic treatment. *Pediatr Res.* 1994; 36:545-549.

28. Schwarz SM, Gewitz MH, See CC, et al. Enteral nutrition in infants with congenital heart disease and growth failure. *Pediatrics.* 1990;86:368-373.

29. Miller TL, Evans SJ, Orav EJ, Morris V, McIntosh K. Growth and body composition in children infected with the human immunodeficiency virus. *Am J Clin Nutr.* 1993;57:588-592

30. Brettler DB, Fosberg A, Bolivar E, Brewster F, Sullivan J. Growth failure as a prognostic indicator for progression to acquired immunodeficiency syndrome in children with hemophilia. *J Pediatr.* 1990;117:584-588.

31. Kotler DP, Tierney AR, Wang J, Pierson RN. Magnitude of body cell mass depletion and the timing of death from wasting in AIDS. *Am J Clin Nutr.* 1989;50:444-447.

32. Hecker LM, Kotler DP. Malnutrition in patients with AIDS. *Nutr Rev.* 1990;48:393-401.

33. Anon. Is malabsorption an important cause of growth failure in HIV-infected children? *Nutr Rev.* 1991;49:341-343.

34. Powell KR. Approach to gastrointestinal manifestations in infants and children with HIV infection. *J Pediatr.* 1991;119:S34-S40.

35. Azcue MP, Pencharz P. Nutrition and AIDS (a selected summary). *J Pediatr Gastroenterol Nutr.* 1992;14:242-243.

36. Henderson RA, Saavedra JM, Perman JA, Huton N, Livingston RA, Yolken RH. Effect of enteral tube feeding on growth of children with symptomatic human immunodeficiency virus infection. *J Pediatr Gastroenterol Nutr.* 1994;18:429-434.

37. Simpser E. Nutritional support in children with HIV: Some answers, many questions. *J Pediatr Gastroenterol Nutr.* 1994;18:426-428.

38. Ramirez RO, Sokol RJ. Medical management of cholestasis. In: Suchy FJ, ed. *Liver disease in children.* St. Louis: Mosby; 1994:356-388.

39. Beath SV, Booth IW, Kelly DA. Nutritional support in liver disease. *Arch Dis Child.* 1993;69:545-549.

40. Chin SE, Shepherd RW, Thomas BJ, et al. The nature of malnutrition in children with end-stage liver disease awaiting orthotopic liver transplantation. *Am J Clin Nutr.* 1992;56:164-168.

41. Kaufman SS, Scrivner DJ, Murray ND, Vanderhoof JA, Hart MH, Antonson DL. Influence of Portagen and Pregestimil on essential fatty acid status in infantile liver disease. *Pediatrics.* 1992;89:151-154.

42. Pierro A, Koletzko B, Carnelli V, et al. Resting energy expenditure is increased in infants with extra hepatic biliary atresia and cirrhosis. *J Pediatr Surg.* 1989;24:534-538.

43. Chin SE, Shepherd RW, Thomas BJ, et al. Nutritional support in children with end-stage liver disease: a randomised crossover trial of a branched-chain amino acid supplement. *Am J Clin Nutr.* 1992;56:158-163.

44. Sokol RJ, Stall C. Anthropometric evaluation of children with chronic liver disease. *Am J Clin Nutr.* 1990;52:203-208.

45. Moreno LA, Gottrand F, Hoden S, Turk D, Loeuille GA, Farriaux J-P. Improvement of nutritional status in cholestatic children with supplemental nocturnal enteral nutrition. *J Pediatr Gastroenterol Nutr.* 1991;12:213-216.

46. Brocklebank JT, Wolfe S. Dietary treatment of renal insufficiency. *Arch Dis Child.* 1993;69:704-708.

47. Strife CF, Quinlan M, Mears K, Davey ML, Clardy C. Improved growth of three uremic children by nocturnal nasogastric feedings. *Am J Dis Child.* 1986;140:438-443.

48. Warady BA, Kriley M, Lovell H, Farrell SE, Hellerstein S. Growth and development of infants with end-stage renal disease receiving long-term peritoneal dialysis. *J Pediatr.* 1988;112:714-719.

49. Friedman AL, Pityer R. Benefit of moderate dietary protein restriction on growth in the young animal with experimental chronic renal insufficiency: importance of early growth. *Pediatr Res.* 1989;25:509-513.

50. Jakobsson B, Celsi G, Lindbland BS, Aperia A. Influence of differential protein intake on renal growth in young rats. *Acta Paediatr Scand.* 1987;76:293-299.

51. Kaysen GA, Jones H, Martin V, Hutchison FN. A low-protein diet restricts albumin synthesis in nephrotic rats. *J Clin Invest.* 1989;83:1623-1629.

52. Hanning RM, Balfe JW, Zlotkin SH. Effectiveness and nutritional consequences of amino acid-based vs glucose-based dialysis solutions in infants and children receiving CAPD. *Am J Clin Nutr.* 1987;46:22-30.

53. McCrory WW, Gertner JM, Burke FM, Pimental CT, Nemery RL. Effects of dietary phosphate restriction in

children with chronic renal failure. *J Pediatr.* 1987;111: 410-412.

54. Grunow JE, Chait P, Savoie S, Mullan C, Pencharz P. Gastrostomy feeding. In: David TJ, ed. *Recent Advances in Paediatrics 12*. Edinburgh: Churchill Livingstone; 1994;23-39.

55. Kirby DF, Delegge MH, Fleming CR. American Gastroenterological Association technical review on tube feeding for enteral nutrition. *Gastroenterology.*

1995;108:1282-1301.

56. Andrew M, Marzinotto V, Pencharz P, et al. A cross-sectional study of catheter-related thrombosis in children receiving total parenteral nutrition at home. *J Pediatr.* 1995;126:358-363.

57. Quigley EMM, Marsh MN, Shaffer JL, Markin RS. Hepatobiliary complications of total parenteral nutrition. *Gastroenterology.* 1993;104:286-301.

Meeting Energy Needs

Nancy F. Butte Ph.D.

USDA/ARS Children's Nutrition Research Center, Department of Pediatrics,
Baylor College of Medicine,
Houston, Texas

Reviewed by Berthold Koletzko M.D. and Jack Sinclair M.D.

"If the caloric intake is not sufficient to cover the energy output due to play and activity, the child will automatically restrict his activity so that the limited amount of food furnished will provide first for growth, primarily stature."

Frances G. Benedict

Practical Points

- *The contribution of the brain to basal metabolism is exceptionally high in the newborn period (70 %) and throughout the first years of life (60 to 65 %).*
- *The newly emerging data on total energy expenditure (TEE) of infants provide strong evidence that current recommendations for energy intake of infants are too high.*
- *The more rapid the weight gain, the higher the dietary protein:energy (P:E) ratio required.*
- *Mean energy intakes of breast-fed infants are lower than formula-fed infants after the first few months of life. Furthermore, energy intakes remain lower even after the introduction of solid foods.*
- *Total energy expenditure, sleeping energy expenditure, body temperature, and heart rates are lower in breast-fed infants than formula-fed infants.*
- *For each degree centigrade rise in body temperature, metabolic rate increases up to 13 %.*
- *The availability of fat is the major limiting factor in survival from infant malnutrition.*
- *If normal body composition is to be restored, the P:E ratio in the diet must be increased.*

- *In practice, the limiting factor in the diet is likely to be energy density, which can be increased by adding fat to the diet.*
- *Because restricting calories has deleterious effects on growth, resistance to infection and central nervous system development, specific caloric restriction is not recommended during infancy.*

Introduction

Energy requirements are fundamental to all other nutrient needs. Once energy requirements are fulfilled with a nutrient-balanced diet, the intake of other nutrients generally is ensured. Energy is required for all vital functions of the body at the cellular and organ level. At the cellular level, heat production is associated with the continuous catabolism and anabolism cycles of body tissue turnover, with transport systems, and with the regulation of body temperature. At the systemic level, energy is required to meet circulatory, respiratory, neurological and muscular demands. Energy requirements during infancy are higher than at any other time in life, because of the infant's higher basal metabolism and needs for growth.

Energy Metabolism
Components of Energy Utilization

Energy requirements during infancy may be partitioned into components of basal metabolism; thermic effect of feeding; thermoregulation at environmental temperatures above and below the zone of thermal neutrality; physical activity; and growth (Figure 1). Historically, direct calorimetry and respiratory gas exchange, also referred to as indirect calorimetry, have been used to measure the energy expenditure of

Gross Energy Intake

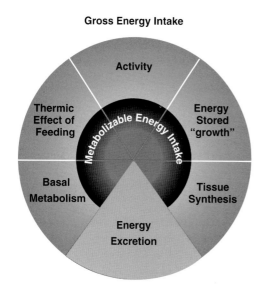

Figure 1: Partitioning of the energy requirements during infancy.

infants. A direct calorimeter measures the rate of heat lost through a layered series of circulating water pipes, heating elements and thermocouples. This apparatus is expensive to construct and technically difficult to operate. More commonly, heat production or energy expenditure is measured by respiratory gas exchange. Since energy is utilized in the body by means of chemical reactions, energy expenditure may be calculated using the energy equivalence of the oxygen consumed and carbon dioxide produced. The conventional unit for energy is calorie, defined as the amount of heat required to raise the temperature of one gram of water 1°C. One calorie is equivalent to 4.184 joules.

Basal Metabolism

Basal metabolic rate (BMR) is defined as that energy expended to maintain cellular and tissue processes fundamental to the organism. Specifically, it is the energy needed to maintain body temperature, support the minimal work of the heart and respiratory muscles, and to supply the energy requirements of tissues at rest. Some of the factors that affect basal metabolism are listed in Figure 2. Conventionally, BMR is measured under standard conditions where the individual is at rest in a thermoneutral environment after a 12- to 18-

hour fast. Heat production and heat loss are equal under thermoneutral conditions; body temperature is constant and maintained through control of skin circulation. The application of these criteria to infants would be impractical, so investigators have adopted various approaches to measure "basal metabolism" in sleeping infants. Some investigators have used sedatives to induce sleep;[1] others have opted to feed the infant.[2] Sleep and some sedatives will lower BMR, whereas feeding will augment it.

The basal metabolism of infants is accounted for primarily by the brain, liver, heart and kidney. Holliday et al.[3] analyzed BMR in relation to body weight and organ weight, and noted that oxygen consumption increased at a rate greater than that of organ weight or body weight during the intrauterine and postnatal periods. The increased oxygen consumption was attributed to increased enzymatic activity during the transition to extrauterine life. Thereafter, the metabolic activity of these vital organs was proportional to increases in organ weight. The contribution of the brain to basal metabolism was exceptionally high in the newborn period (70%) and throughout the first years of life (60 to 65%).

Basal metabolism of term infants has been investigated extensively.[1, 2] Reported BMR ranges from 43 to 60 kcal/kg/day. The high variability is attributable to biological differences in body composition, and technical differences in experimental conditions and methods. Nevertheless, it should be appreciated that standardized by body weight basal metabolism of infants is two to three times that of the adult.[4]

The BMR of healthy children under the age of three years may be predicted by the following equation derived by Schofield[4] from historical data:

Boys:
BMR(kcal/d) =
0.1673 Weight(kg) + 1517 Length(m) - 618

Girls:
BMR(kcal/d) =
16.25 Weight(kg) + 1023 Length(m) - 413

These equations may not apply to sick children whose metabolism and/or body composition might be altered. Basal metabolic rates of preterm infants are lower and increase at slower rates during the first month of extrauterine life than those of full-term infants. At thermoneutrality, metabolic rates did not exceed 40 kcal/kg/day in preterm infants weighing 1,000 to 2,000 gm at 2 to 31 days of age.[5] Oxygen consumption is higher in small for gestational age (SGA) infants than in appropriate for gestational age (AGA) preterms[6] due to their larger brain size and higher growth rates.

Thermic Effect of Feeding

The next component of energy production is the energy expended above basal metabolism in response to feeding. This is referred to as the thermic effect of feeding (TEF), or diet-induced thermogenesis (DIT). The TEF amounts to approximately 10% of the daily energy expenditure.[7] The major part of the rise in energy expenditure after a meal is due to the metabolic costs of transporting and converting the absorbed nutrients into their respective storage forms; this component has been referred to as "obligatory thermogenesis." Since infants normally are fed frequently and not subjected to prolonged fasting, the residual effect of feeding will exert a continual, albeit variable, influence on energy expenditure.

Flatt[8] has calculated the metabolic cost of substrate storage from stoichiometric equations. Expressed as a percentage of the glucose calories ingested, the conversion of glucose to glycogen dissipates 7% of the energy, whereas conversion of glucose to fat expends 26%. The TEF associated with fat is approximately 2 to 4%, depending on whether the absorbed fatty acids are oxidized or stored. With protein ingestion, approximately 25% of the energy is dissipated through peptide bond synthesis, gluconeogenesis, or ureagenesis.

The TEF in preterm infants[9] and in infants recovering from malnutrition[10] has been shown to be proportional to the rate of weight gain. These observations support the view that the increased energy expenditure is due to the metabolic costs of tissue synthesis.

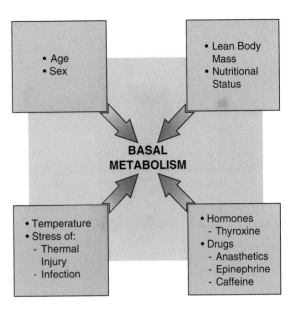

Figure 2: Factors that affect basal metabolism.

The measured TEF is greater than that would be expected from theoretical calculations. The difference between what is observed empirically and what is calculated theoretically has been referred to as facultative thermogenesis, whereby heat is produced but no work is performed.[7] Possible calorigenic mechanisms include sympathetic nervous stimulation of brown adipose tissue, accelerated sodium pump or activation of "futile cycles" of intermediate metabolism.

Thermoregulation

Thermoregulation constitutes an additional energy cost when infants are exposed to temperatures below and above their zone of thermoneutrality. The environmental temperature at which oxygen consumption and metabolic rate are at their lowest is described as the thermoneutral zone.[11] In the first 24 hours after birth, this temperature is 34 to 36°C for the naked infant and falls to 30 to 32° by seven to ten days of age. The amount of energy required to maintain normal body temperature is greater at lower than at higher temperatures. Basal oxygen consumption rates increase from 4.8 ml O_2/kg/min at zero to six hours postpartum to 7.0 ml O_2/kg/min at six to ten days of life, and remain fairly constant thereafter throughout the first

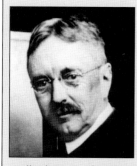

Graham Lusk Ph.D.

(1866-1932) An American, Lusk received his Ph.D. degree under Voit in Munich. He returned to teach Physiology at Yale and in 1898 moved to Bellevue Hospital and Cornell Medical Schools. He built a small calorimeter for studies of metabolism of small animals and babies. He collaborated with Howland in the first American studies of infant calorimetry. Lusk's book, *The Science of Nutrition*, went through four editions between 1906 and 1928. He was a lifelong friend of Rubner's. J Nutr. 41,1-12,1950 (Photo courtesy of NLM)

year of life.[12] At temperatures below the critical temperature, i.e., the lower end of the thermoneutral zone, energy expenditure increases proportionately to the drop in environmental temperature.

For preterm infants, neutral thermal environmental temperatures vary according to gestational age, postnatal age and body weight. Tables are available to adjust ambient temperatures.[13] Clothing and swaddling conserves body heat significantly. The energy expenditure of naked preterm infants maintained at 28 to 29°C exceeded that of swaddled infants maintained at 20 to 22°C (80 vs 58 kcal/kg/day).[5]

Facultative thermogenesis allows the infant to adapt to cold exposure. The neonate responds to cold exposure with an increase in metabolic rate which is thought to be mediated by increased sympathetic tone. This metabolic response is present in term infants and to a lesser extent in preterm infants. Neonatal heat production occurs mainly by nonshivering thermogenesis.[14] Oxidation of brown adipose tissue located between the scapulae, in the posterior triangle of the neck and around major vessels and organs of the mediastinum and abdomen is thought to make the most important contribution to nonshivering thermogenesis in infants.

Physical Activity

Activity represents an increasingly larger component of the total daily energy expenditure as the infant grows

and develops. The energy costs of the specific activities of infants can only be estimated from a very limited set of data. Using respiration calorimetry, 24-hour energy expenditure was measured in two full-term, breast-fed infants, three and six months of age.[15] Twenty-four hour energy expenditure rates, 74 and 70 kcal/kg/day, were only 20 to 30% above basal. Maximum muscular activity corresponded to an increase of 70% above basal. Early observations by Murlin[16] demonstrated that crying increased metabolism by 49% in newborns. Talbot suggested adding 15, 25 and 40% to basal metabolic rates to cover the activity needs of very quiet, normally active, and extremely active infants, respectively.[15]

Based on calorimetric studies of 70 healthy, full-term infants, Benedict and Talbot[2] estimated that activity may represent as much as 40% of total daily energy expenditure. The peak of energy expenditure for activity occurred at six months; thereafter, voluntary muscular control became more coordinated, and the energy expenditure more efficient.

From food intake and actometer records, Rose and Mayer[17] deduced that infants four to six months of age expended 27% of their energy intake on activity. Combining indirect calorimetry with heart rate monitoring, Spady[18] estimated that infants recovering from malnutrition expended 10 kcal/kg/day on activity; the average age of these children was 12.2 months.

Activity accounts for only a small proportion of the total heat production of low-birthweight infants. The contribution of activity to total energy expenditure in nongrowing, preterm infants was three kcal/kg/day, which was consistent with their sedentary state.[19] Growth was accompanied by a three-fold increase in energy expenditure.

Total Energy Expenditure

Total energy expenditure (TEE) of infants encompasses basal metabolism, thermoregulation, physical activity, and synthetic cost of growth. The doubly-labeled water method may be used to measure TEE. This method involves enriching the body water with deuterium and oxygen-18 (^{18}O), then determining the wash-out kinetics of both isotopes as their concentrations decline exponentially toward natural abundance levels. The concentra-

Reference	n	Age (mo)	TEE (kcal/d)	TEE (kcal/kg/d)	Comments
Lucas 1987[24]	12BF	0.9-1.4 2.3-2.8	306 (26)** 402 (19)	66.9 (24) 71.7 (8)	BF infants, Cambridge, UK
Prentice 1988[25]	15 12	12-24 24-36		83 (9) 81 (10)	Cambridge, UK
Roberts 1988[26]	18	3	408 (28)	72 (5)	MF infants, Cambridge, UK TEE/SMR=1.15
Vasquez-Velasquez 1987[27]	8 15 19 8	0-3 3-6 6-9 9-12	381 (88) 473 (106) 572 (121) 664 (133)	82 (23) 78 (21) 80 (16) 85 (12)	MF Gambian infants
Fjeld 1989[28]	22FF 19FF	16 16.3	629 (84) 692 (82)	90 (12) 84 (10)	FF infants, Lima, Peru Early recovery from malnutrition Late recovery from malnutrition
Butte 1990[29]	10BF 10FF	1	291 (48) 316 (42)	64 (7) 67 (8)	BF and FF infants, Houston, TX TEE/SMR=1.28, 1.26
	10BF 10FF	4	420 (49) 476 (58)	64 (8) 73 (9)	TEE/SMR=1.34, 1.36
Davies 1989, 1991[30, 31]	20BF 29FF	1.4 1.4	283 (80) 319 (97)	61.1 (17.8) 71.4 (19.1)	BF and FF infants, Cambridge, UK
	20BF 30FF	2.8 2.8	366 (73) 433 (118)	64.5 (12.6) 75.3 (19.6)	BF and FF infants, Cambridge, UK
	19BF 18FF	6.0 6.0	590 (119) 619 (78)	78.5 (13.7) 79.0 (11.2)	BF and FF infants, Cambridge, UK
	12BF 10FF	9.2 9.2	702 (124) 808 (184)	83.0 (14.8) 93.7 (21.2)	BF and FF infants, Cambridge, UK
Wells 1995[32]	18BF 20BF	1.5	454 (72) 464 (90)	74.1 (10.1) 78.5 (14.0)	BF and FF infants, Cambridge, UK
Butte 1993[33]	19BF 19BF	4 6	446 (97) 542 (83)	74.1 (13.9) 76.0 (6.9)	BF infants, Capulhuac, Mexico
Davies 1994[34]	23	18-30	1069 (254)		Cambridge, UK

* Abbreviations: Fx–isotope fractionation; RQ–respiratory quotient; TEE–total energy expenditure; BF–breast-fed; FF–formula-fed; MF–mixed-fed; SMR–sleeping metabolic rate
** Mean (SD)

Table 1: Total energy expenditure of infants by doubly-labeled water method.

tion of ^2H decreases as a result of body water being diluted by ingested unlabeled water and loss of labeled water through excretory pathways. The rate constant for ^2H is derived from the slope of the $\log_n$ ^2H enrichment against time and is a measure of the rate of water flux through the subject. The ^{18}O label is lost as water, but also as CO_2 because CO_2 in body fluids is in isotopic equilibrium with body water due to the action of carbonic anhydrase. The slope of the line representing ^{18}O is steeper than ^2H, and the difference between slopes repre-

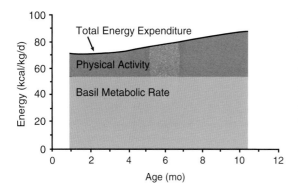

Figure 3: Total energy expenditure of infants, measured by the doubly-labeled water method, partitioned into basal metabolic rate[4] and physical activity.

sents CO_2 production. By knowing the chemical composition of the food- stuffs being oxidized, since this affects the energy equivalence of CO_2 produced, energy expenditure can be calculated from CO_2 production. The doubly-labeled water method has been validated in preterm infants and hospitalized term infants. In the validation studies, mean errors between the doubly-labeled water method and respiration calorimetry were 0.3±2.6%,[20] -0.9±6.2%,[21] -4.5±6%[22] and -0.4±11.5%.[23] Published data on the TEE of infants are summarized in Table 1. Standardized by weight, TEE ranged from 65 to 90 kcal/kg/d, increasing linearly with age. TEE of breast-fed infants was shown to be lower than formula-fed infants.[29, 30, 31] Energy expended on physical activity may be estimated from the difference between TEE and BMR; since most BMR measurements have been made in the fed state and because growth is thought to be a continuous process, the BMR includes the thermic effect of feeding and the energy cost of tissue synthesis. The energy expended on physical activity has been estimated for young infants: at one month infants expended 13 kcal/kg/d on activity, or 20% TEE, and at three to four month infants expended 16 to 18 kcal/kg/d, or 20 to 25% TEE.[32, 95, 29] As the infant approaches one year of age the activity component increases (Figure 3).

The newly emerging data on TEE of infants provide strong evidence that current recommendations for energy intake of infants are too high.[25] Current recommendations for dietary energy were derived from the observed intakes of healthy, thriving infants. Energy requirements preferably should be based on total energy expenditure, with an allowance made for growth. Revision of current recommendations, however, will require expansion of the available database on TEE of healthy infants, in terms of sample size, age range and geographic distribution across the entire age range of infancy.

Total energy expenditure of preterm infants has been measured over prolonged periods using respiration calorimetry and the doubly-labeled water method (Table 2). Mean 24-hour rates of energy expenditure ranged from 58 to 69 kcal/kg/d in stable preterm infants measured under thermoneutral conditions.[35, 36, 37, 20, 23]

Growth

Although the energy requirement for growth relative to maintenance is small, except for the first months of life, satisfactory growth is a sensitive indicator of whether energy needs are being met. The energy cost of growth may be divided into two components: the energy content of the tissues and the energy needed for synthetic processes. The total cost of growth from nutrient balance and growth studies approximates 4 to 6 kcal/gm of tissue gained, of which approximately 1.0 kcal/gm is oxidized for tissue synthesis.[18] The total cost of growth (kcal/g) varies with age, because the composition of the tissue synthesized changes with development (Figure 4).

The energy cost of growth may be computed from the separate costs of protein and fat deposition, since the components of weight gain change dramatically through the first year of life. In Table 3 the energy cost of growth has been estimated from rates of weight gain and components of weight gain, as described by Fomon[38] and standardized by median National Center for Health Statistics (NCHS) weights. The energetic efficiencies of synthesizing protein and fat were taken to be 42% (1 kcal deposited/2.38 kcal used) and 85% (1 kcal deposited/1.17 kcal used), respectively.[39] Energy equivalents for the fat and protein deposited were 9.25 kcal/g and 5.65 kcal/g, respectively. The energy cost of growth decreases appreciably during the first

Reference	No. Infants/ Measurements	Weight (g)	Age (d)	Energy Intake (kcal/kg/d)	TEE (kcal/kg/d)
Bell 1986[35]	5/9	1510	20	101	59.8 ± 9.5*
Schulze 1986[36]	5/12	1463	34	102-150	60.6 ± 3.4
Freymond 1986[37]	9	–	21	122	68.4 ± 4.4
Roberts 1986[20]	4	1635	23	–	58.2 ± 2.2 58.3 ± 1.3†
Jensen 1992[23]	12	1674	31	118	68.6 ± 5.8 68.3 ± 10.3†

* Mean ± SD, indirect calorimetry
† Mean ± SD, doubly-labeled water method

Table 2: Total energy expenditure (TEE) of preterm infants measured by indirect calorimetry and doubly-labeled water method.

years of life (Figure 5). Between birth and two months the energetic cost of fat and protein deposition is estimated at 29 to 42 kcal/kg/day. This value decreases to 10 kcal/kg/day at six months and to 2 kcal/kg/day at 18 to 24 months.

The energy requirement for maintenance takes precedence over protein synthesis. Protein synthesis is a high energy-requiring process, and the supply of energy influences the rate of whole body protein metabolism. Over the range of energy intake, 60 to 270 kcal/kg/day, energy intake and the rate of protein turnover are positively correlated.[40] When energy intake is below maintenance needs, growth will cease. The more rapid the weight gain, the higher the dietary protein:energy (P:E) ratio required. Growth rates of 10, 30 and 50 gm/day required P:E ratios of 5.6, 6.9 and 8.1%, respectively, in infants recovering from malnutrition.[41] Standard infant formulas and human milk have P:E ratios of about 12 and 8%, respectively.

Fetal and Neonatal Energy Metabolism
Glucose is the major energy substrate of the fetus, although fatty acids are transported to a limited extent.[42] Even though most of the glucose is oxidized, the fetus has an enhanced ability to utilize glucose anaerobically and therefore is somewhat resistant to hypoxia. Lipogenesis is active in fetal tissues. In the last two months of gestation, body fat content increases from 3.5 to 16% of body weight.[42]

In the immediate postpartum period, the infant mobilizes glucose from stored glycogen, until gluconeogenesis, fatty acid oxidation and exogenous food intake are established. The hepatic glycogen stores of the term infant may be depleted rapidly within the first 24 hours.[42]

Hypoglycemia may develop in infants with low glycogen stores. Preterm infants are particularly vulnerable because of low reserves and limited gluconeogenesis. Infants of diabetic mothers have sufficient stores, but glycogenolysis is inhibited by elevated serum concentrations of insulin and low serum concentrations of glucagon.[42]

There are major shifts in the pattern of fuel utilization in the neonatal period. The proportions of carbohydrate, fat, and protein oxidized by the body under resting conditions are determined primarily by the amount and composition of the food consumed. Approximately 10, 40 and 50% of the energy in human milk or formula are derived from protein, carbohydrate and fat, respectively. Since 50% of the calories in milk are derived from fat, fatty acid oxidation and ketone use emerge as major metabolic pathways in the neonatal period, and carbohydrate oxidation continues to be substantial. Plasma concentrations of cholesterol,

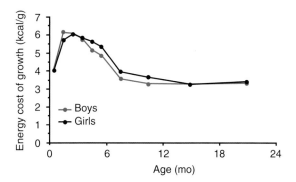

Figure 4: Total energy cost of growth (kcal/g) as a function of age.

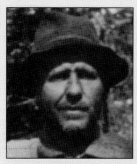

John Howland M. D.
(1873-1926) was a graduate of New York Medical School. He trained at Presbyterian Hospital with L. Emmett Holt, Sr., and was associated with Lusk at Cornell until 1910. Howland carried out the first studies of infant energy expenditure in Lusk's laboratory. In 1914, he joined Johns Hopkins Medical School as the first full-time Chairman of Pediatrics in the U.S. His insistence that chemical investigations were important to the investigation of childhood diseases lead to many nutritional discoveries. Howland's method of artificial infant feeding was based on that of Czerny, Heubner's successor in Berlin, and that of Holt. The highest recognition of the American Pediatric Society is the Howland Award. *Pediatric Profiles* (Photo courtesy of CNRC).

fatty acids, glycerol, and ketones rise after birth[43] and fall again at weaning, when dietary carbohydrate levels increase. Ketone body production and utilization are accelerated in the newborn even on a four-hour feeding schedule.[44] Ketone bodies can yield approximately 10 kcal/kg/day during the first days of life, which may be utilized by skeletal and cardiac muscle, the renal cortex, and the brain.

The preterm infant relies more on carbohydrate oxidation than the term infant, at least in the first weeks of life.[45] The contribution of carbohydrate oxidation to total energy expenditure declines from 80 to 65% by the sixth week of life, as fat oxidation increases from 14 to 30%.

Energy Requirements of Term Infants
Energy Balance

The energy balance of infants may be described simply as:
Gross energy intake=energy excreted+energy expended +energy stored.

Gross energy intake, measured by combustion in a bomb calorimeter, is greater than the energy available to the body when food is ingested, because most foods are not completely absorbed and protein is oxidized incompletely. Fats in particular are not completely absorbed. Fat absorption depends on the type of milk and age of the infant. Urea and other nitrogenous products are excreted in the urine. The gross energy values for milk (5.65 kcal/gm protein, 3.95 kcal/gm carbohydrate, and 9.25 kcal/gm fat) may be used to

estimate gross energy intake if a bomb calorimeter is not available.

Digestible energy refers to the energy absorbed by the individual, i.e., gross energy intake minus the heat of combustion of feces. Metabolizable energy is defined as digestible energy minus the heat of combustion of urine. Atwater's fuel values of 4 kcal/gm protein or carbohydrate and 9 kcal/gm fat have been used to convert the macronutrient composition of infant formulas to metabolizable energy. Application of the adult-derived Atwater's values to infant diets is satisfactory if the dietary fat is highly digestible and protein concentration modest. Because of higher excretory losses of nitrogenous substances and fat, metabolizable energy from high protein formulas and cow milk may be overestimated.

Energy balance data are limited in term infants (Figure 6).[46-48] Metabolizable energy ranged between 88 and 92% of intake. Energy storage was estimated at 26 to 27 kcal/kg/day in one study.[47]

Energy intakes of term infants have been documented by many investigators. There is growing concern that dietary methodologies are biased towards underestimation; however, the bias is not uniform

Boys	Weight	Weight Gain*	Fat Deposition		Protein Deposition		Fat Synthesis	Protein Synthesis	Total Energy Cost Growth		
(mo)	(kg)	(g/d)	(g/d)	(kcal/d)	(g/d)	(kcal/d)	(kcal/d)	(kcal/d)	(kcal/d)	(kcal/kg/d)	(kcal/g)
0-1	3.80	29	6	56	4	21	10	29	115	30	4.0
1-2	4.75	35	14	130	4	20	23	27	201	42	5.7
2-3	5.60	30	13	119	3	17	21	23	181	32	6.0
3-4	6.35	21	8	77	4	13	14	18	121	19	5.8
4-5	7.00	17	6	51	2	11	9	16	87	12	5.1
5-6	7.55	15	4	38	2	11	7	16	72	9	4.8
6-9	8.50	13	2	17	2	11	3	16	46	5	3.5
9-12	9.70	11	1	9	2	10	2	14	35	4	3.2
12-18	10.81	7	0.5	5	1	7	1	10	23	2	3.2
18-24	12.08	6	0.4	4	1	6	1	9	19	2	3.2
Girls (mo)											
0-1	3.60	26	6	52	3	19	9	26	105	29	4.0
1-2	4.35	29	13	118	3	16	21	22	177	41	6.1
2-3	5.05	24	10	93	3	15	16	20	145	29	6.0
3-4	5.70	19	7	68	2	12	12	16	108	19	5.7
4-5	6.35	16	6	55	2	11	10	15	90	14	5.6
5-6	6.95	15	5	45	2	11	8	15	79	11	5.3
6-9	7.97	11	2	16	2	10	3	14	43	5	3.9
9-12	9.05	10	1	11	2	10	2	13	36	4	3.6
12-18	9.98	9	0.9	8	2	8	2	11	29	3	3.2
18-24	11.34	6	0.5	5	1	6	1	8	20	2	3.3

* Monthly rates of weight gain[38]

Table 3: Energy cost of growth through infancy.

across all ages. Mean energy intakes of infants and toddlers have been shown to be accurate using the doubly-labeled water method.[34] Whitehead[49] compiled energy intakes of infants from literature predating 1940 through 1980. This large database revealed several findings. A highly significant curvilinear relation between energy intake per unit body weight and age was observed. The authors attributed the sharp fall in energy intake from zero to six months of age to the rapidly slowing of growth, the reduction in the rate of fat storage, and a decrease in energy needed for maintenance per unit body weight. The rise in energy intake from 6 to 12 months of age was attributed to the increase in physical activity as infants begin to crawl and then walk. A compilation of energy intakes of healthy infants reported after 1980 is presented in Table 4 and Figure 7. Overall mean intakes and the pattern of intake are similar before and after 1980. After the first months of life, the energy intakes of breast-fed infants were lower than formula-fed infants.

The discrepancy in energy intake between breast-fed and formula-fed infants, and its consequences, have been studied by a number of investigators. There is much confusion around the magnitude of the discrepancy, because of differences in study design, subject criteria and methods. Two technical problems arise in estimating energy intake from human milk. Breast-milk intakes measured by the test-weighing method require correction for insensible water loss (IWL) during the course of the measurement, but have been included in a few studies only.[68, 69] The systematic negative bias caused by not correcting for IWL is well recognized; the difficulty has been determining how much correction is necessary to fairly represent the ranges of metabolic rates, ambient temperatures, humidities and air circulation rates. IWL may cause approximately

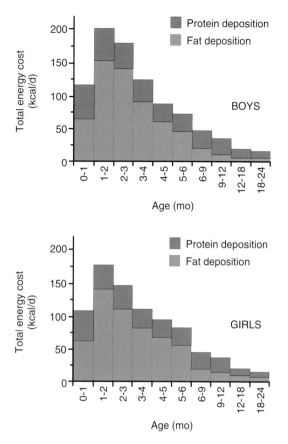

Figure 5: Total energy cost of protein and fat deposition (kcal/d) as a function of age.

3 to 6% underestimation of milk intake.[70, 71] Another source of confusion and error is the conversion of milk intake to energy intake. Milk sampling schemes varied across studies, affecting the fat and therefore the energy content of milk. Energy content of human milk was measured by bomb calorimetry in some studies; macronutrients were analyzed and converted to gross or metabolizable energy using Atwater factors in other studies; or a constant for the energy content of human milk was assumed. Consequently, mean energy content of human milk, measured or assumed, ranged from 0.65 to 0.76 kcal/g milk; this had a major impact on reported energy intakes.

Although the magnitude of the discrepancy is disputed, there is consensus that mean energy intakes of breast-fed infants are lower than formula-fed

infants after the first few months of life. Furthermore, energy intakes remain lower even after the introduction of solid foods.[62, 54, 68] These differences in energy intake are associated with distinct growth patterns. Weight gain is less rapid in breast-fed infants than in formula-fed infants.[72, 29] Differences in other physiological and behavioral outcomes also have been noted between feeding groups. Total energy expenditure,[29] sleeping energy expenditure,[29] body temperature and heart rates[73] were lower in breast-fed infants. A higher proportion of non-rapid eye movement (NREM) sleep was reported in breast-fed infants.[74] Importantly, no deleterious consequences of lower intakes have been observed in breast-fed infants, in terms of morbidity, activity, or behavioral development.[70]

Energy Requirements of Term Infants

The recommended dietary allowances (RDA) for infants are summarized in Table 5. These recommendations are based upon the median energy intakes of thriving, healthy infants. Appetite, activity and weight gain should be evaluated in determining an individual infant's energy requirement.

Historically, a factorial approach has been used to define energy requirements in older children and adults, which can be applied to infants. The infant's requirements for maintenance, thermic effect of feeding, physical activity and growth were summed to derive an estimate of total requirement (Figure 8). The prediction equations of Schofield were used for BMR (for infants at the NCHS 50th percentile weight for age). Because the measurements, for the most part, were made on fed infants, the thermic effect of feeding is included. Physical activity represented 20 to 35% of total energy expenditure. The components of weight gain described by Fomon[38] were applied. As seen in Figure 8, the current RDA for energy intake[76] exceeds this factorial estimation.

Application of the doubly-labeled water method to determine total energy expenditure provides an alternative means of estimating energy requirements. The total energy requirement of infants was estimated from total energy expenditure plus an allowance for

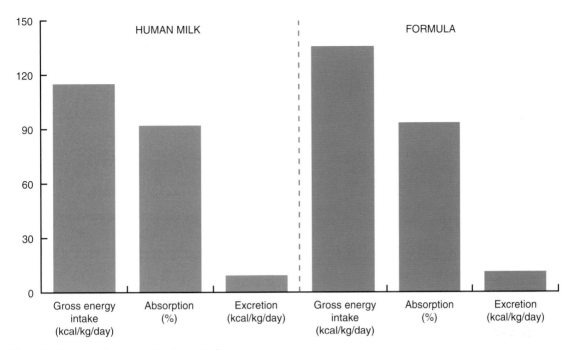

Figure 6: Energy balance studies of term infants.

energy deposition (Figure 9). These preliminary data provide strong evidence that current recommendations should be revised; however, confirmation of these observations will require expansion of the available database on total energy expenditure of healthy infants, in terms of sample size, age range and geographic distribution across the entire age range of infancy.

Altered Energy Requirements
Preterm Delivery

To achieve the remarkable growth potential of preterm infants, energy and nutrient intakes must be sufficient to support the intrauterine growth rate, or to exceed it if catch-up growth is needed. The amount of energy deposited for growth will depend on the weight gain composition. There is controversy over whether rates of fat deposition in the preterm infant should be similar to that of the fetus (14% of weight gain) or term infant (30 to 40% of weight gain).

Energy utilization of small for gestational age (SGA) and appropriate for gestational age (AGA) infants was compared using nutrient balance techniques and indi-

rect calorimetry.[82] SGA infants had lower absorption rates of fat and slightly higher metabolic rates. Somewhat surprisingly, the SGA infants tended to grow at rates higher than those of the AGA infants. However, the energy content of the newly formed tissues was less in the SGA infants, reflecting higher water and lower fat contents of the tissue gained.

In order to compensate for the preterm infant's intolerance of large intake volumes, the use of high-energy-density formulas (72 to 90 kcal/dl) was compared with standard formula (62 kcal/dl) in one study (Figure 10).[83] Although the percentage of energy absorption declined, net retention increased. However, growth rate during periods of feeding high-energy-density formula did not increase significantly. Apparently, greater amounts of adipose tissue were deposited. A further disadvantage of the high-energy-density formulas was that fasting and postprandial metabolic rates increased 10.4 and 12.8% respectively, offsetting the higher retention of energy. Absorption rates reported in this study were low compared with those of other investigations. The use of high-energy-density formulas cannot be recommended; metabolic rates were augmented, offsetting the increase in retention.

Reference	Country	Method	Age (mo)	No.	Energy Intake (kcal/kg/d)	Initial Feeding Mode
McKillop 1982[50]	Scotland	5-d weighed	3-6	71	97n	Formula
			6-12	91	96	Formula
			12-24	143	100	Formula
Hofvander 1982[51]	Sweden	1-d weighed	1	25	112	Breast Milk
				25	120	Formula
			2	25	108	Breast Milk
				25	107	Formula
			3	25	96	Breast Milk
				25	101	Formula
Dewey 1983[53]	U.S.A.	2-d weighed	1	17	113±19	Breast Milk
			2	20	105±25	Breast Milk
			3	19	93±26	Breast Milk
			4	19	93±19	Breast Milk
			5	17	85±20	Breast Milk
			6	18	89±24	Breast Milk
Butte 1984[53]	U.S.A.	1-d weighed	1	37	110±24	Breast Milk
			2	40	83±19	Breast Milk
			3	37	74±20	Breast Milk
			4	41	71±17	Breast Milk
Dewey 1984[54]	U.S.A.	2-d weighed	7	8	79±12	Breast Milk
			8	7	74±7	Breast Milk
			9	5	70±14	Breast Milk
			10	5	75±17	Breast Milk
			11	6	72±15	Breast Milk
			12	2	77±5	Breast Milk
Kohler 1984[55]	Sweden	2-d weighed	1.5	26	113	Breast Milk
				33	130	Formula
			3.5	21	96	Breast Milk
				32	116	Formula
			5.5	13	87	Breast Milk
				31	95	Formula
			6.5	12	83	Breast Milk
				30	90	Formula
Hitchcock 1984[56]	Australia	7-d record	12	125	88±18	
			18	142	102±20	
Forsum 1986[57]	Sweden	1-d weighed	1	22	114±19	Breast Milk
			2	22	97±16	Breast Milk
			2.5	22	92±15	Breast Milk
Hoffmans 1986[58]	The Netherlands	1-d weighed or recall	4	124	95±20	Breast Milk and Formula
			16	124	88±26	Breast Milk and Formula
			28	124	82±26	Breast Milk and Formula
Catassi 1988[60]	Italy	3-d weighed	12-15	12	91±22	
			15-18	10	83±13	
			18-24	18	82±18	
Wood 1988[61]	U.S.A.	1-d weighed	0.9	12	105±20	Breast Milk
			1.8	14	99±15	Breast Milk
			2.8	16	79±12	Breast Milk
			4.2	17	74±16	Breast Milk
			5.2	15	62±12	Breast Milk

Reference	Country	Method	Age (mo)	No.	Energy Intake (kcal/kg/d)	Initial Feeding Mode
Stuff 1989[62]	U.S.A.	5-d weighed	4	45	73±13	Breast Milk
			5	45	70±16	Breast Milk
			6	45	70±16	Breast Milk
			7	45	73±16	Breast Milk
			8	26	69±20	Breast Milk
			9	8	69±19	Breast Milk
Stuff 1990[63]	U.S.A.	5-d weighed	3n	40	104±17	Formula
			4	40	100±10	Formula
			5	40	95±11	Formula
			6	40	90±11	Formula
			7	23	86±11	Formula
			8	7	82±11	Formula
Butte 1990[64]	U.S.A.	3-d weighed	1	17	99±17	Breast Milk
				17	108±18	Formula
			4	15	74±12	Breast Milk
				16	101±9	Formula
Butte 1990[29]	U.S.A.	5-d weighed	1	10	101±16	Breast Milk
				10	118±17	Formula
			4	10	72±9	Breast Milk
				10	87±11	Formula
Paul 1990[65]	U.K.	7-d weighed	3	47	100±16	Breast Milk
			6	47	86±14	Breast Milk
			8	38	91±13	Breast Milk
			12	29	88±13	Breast Milk
			15	25	90±12	Breast Milk
			18	22	86±16	Breast Milk
Sauve 1991[66]	Canada	3-d record	4	29	110	Formula
			8	26	108	Formula
			12	31	130	Formula
Rasanen 1992[67]	Finland	3-d record	12-24	46	106±20	
Davies 1994[34]	U.K.	4-d weighed	18-30	23	78±12	
Heining 1993[68]	U.S.A.	4-d weighed	3	71	86±11	Breast Milk
				46	99±14	Formula
			6	56	80±13	Breast Milk
				42	95±15	Formula
			9	46	84±19	Breast Milk
				41	94±18	Formula
			12	40	90±18	Breast Milk
				40	98±21	Formula
Michaelsen 1994[69]	Denmark	1-d weighed	2	60	102±20	Breast Milk
			4	36	91±18	Breast Milk

Table 4: Energy intakes of infants during first two years of life.

Source	Age (months)	(kcal/kg)	(kJ/kg)
FAO/WHO/UNU, 1985[75]	0-3	116	485
	3-6	99	415
	6-9	95	100
	9-12	101	420
	12-24	boys 104, girls 108	boys 435, girls 452
United States, 1989[76]	0-6	108	452
	6-12	98	410
	12-36	102	427
United Kingdom, 1991[77]	1	115	480
	3	100	420
	6-36	95	400
Canada, 1992[78]	0-4	100	418
	5-12	100	418
	12	100	418
	24-36	93	389
Japan, 1991[79]	0	120	502
	2	110	460
	6	100	418
	12	88	368
	24	90-91	376-381
	36	92-93	385-389
Korea, 1989[80]	0-3	145	607
	4-6	107	448
	7-9	105	439
	10-12	106	444
	12-36	95	397
European Community[81]	1	115	480
	3	100	420
	6	96	400
	9	96	400
	12	96	400
	18	96	400
	24	96	400

Table 5: Recommendations for energy intakes of infants.

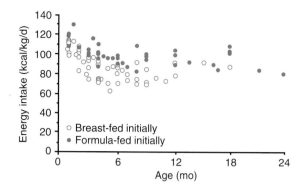

Figure 7: Energy intakes of healthy breast-fed and formula-fed infants reported after 1980.

The effect of varying protein and energy intakes on growth and metabolic parameters was examined in preterm infants.[85] A protein intake of 2.24 gm/kg/day was inadequate to support growth and normal plasma concentrations of albumin and prealbumin. Protein intakes of 3.5 to 3.6 gm/kg/day were well tolerated. Increasing energy from 115 to 150 kcal/kg/day did not improve protein utilization, but promoted greater fat accretion. The lower energy intake 115 kcal/kg/day was sufficient for complete utilization of 3.5 gm/kg/day of protein.

In general, when metabolizable energy exceeds 60 to 70 kcal/kg/day, energy storage will occur in preterm infants.[86] Further increases in metabolizable intake will result in increased excretion, expenditure and storage. Increasing energy intake alone may result in higher rates of expenditure and storage without changes in weight gain, due to a disproportionate accretion of fat. Higher rates of weight gain can be obtained with energy supplementation if protein and possibly minerals are supplemented as well. A total energy intake of 120 kcal/kg/d will support a weight gain of 18 to 20 g/kg/d, a protein retention of 2 g/kg/d, and a fat deposition of 20 to 25% of weight gain.[87] Energy requirements of preterm infants can be increased significantly by thermal stress, increased insensible water loss, respiratory distress and sepsis. The American Academy of Pediatrics states that 120 kcal/kg/d supports adequate growth of most preterm infants, but recog-

Energy balances of preterm infants fed formulas consisting of either a mixture of medium-chain triglycerides (MCT) and long-chain triglycerides (LCT) or predominantly LCT were compared.[84] The MCT afforded no advantage in terms of energy or nitrogen balance over the LCT. Moreover, gastrointestinal problems, ketonemia, increased urinary excretion of dihydroxy and ω–hydroxy fatty acids have been reported with MCT use.[84]

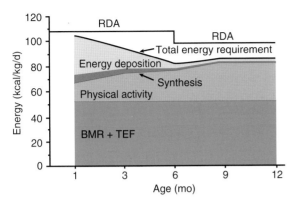

Figure 8: *Total energy requirements of infants estimated by the factorial approach.*

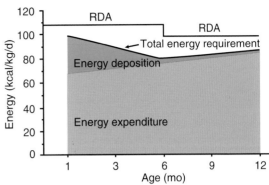

Figure 9: *Total energy requirements of infants estimated from energy expenditure and deposition.*

nizes that higher intakes may be required by sick or growth- retarded infants.[92]

Total Parenteral Nutrition

Total parenteral nutrition (TPN) is widely used to support the maintenance and growth needs of term and preterm infants who are unable to receive adequate nutrition enterally. The clinician must be knowledgeable about the choices of fuel sources and the appropriate caloric level to be administered.

Fuel Sources

Amino Acids. The amount of crystalline amino acids which may be administered is limited and the proportion oxidized will depend on the rate of protein synthesis and the total amount of energy infused.

Glucose. Glucose may function as a fuel source for all cells in the body, but it is essential for erythrocytes, the central nervous system, renal medulla, retina and a few other tissues. If glucose is not available, glucose-dependent cells can adapt by using ketone bodies as an energy source. There are several disadvantages of using glucose as the sole nonprotein fuel source: essential fatty acid deficiency; increased basal metabolism, increased secretion of insulin, catecholamines and cortisol; and

> *Solutions to health problems do not always lie in the medicine and bandages, but also in education and practical preventive measures.*
> *Primary Health Care Pioneer*
> *The Selected Works of Dr. Cicely D. Williams*
> Naomi Baumslag, Editor
> World Federation of Public Health Associations and
> UNICEF

lipid deposits in the liver.[88, 89] Glucose administration exceeding the resting metabolic rate will result in lipogenesis, with carbon dioxide production exceeding oxygen consumption. Carbon dioxide retention will stimulate ventilation and respiratory distress in patients with respiratory difficulties.[88] Under these circumstances, the respiratory quotient ($RQ=CO_2$ production/O_2 consumption) will rise.

Metabolic derangements of hyperglycemia and insulin resistance can be observed in post-traumatic conditions, depending on the clinical situation. Blood sugar concentrations may be normalized by decreasing the glucose concentrations in the TPN solution or by infusing insulin.

Fat. With use of fat emulsions, it is possible to prevent essential fatty acid deficiencies and to provide adequate calories via peripheral veins rather than by the central route. Prior to the advent of fat emulsions, it was not possible to deliver sufficient calories via peripheral veins. Alimentation solutions containing more than 12% glucose are associated with phlebitis and thrombosis.

Intralipid is most commonly used in the United States. It is an emulsion of soybean oil and egg yolk phospholipids, and consists of triglycerides of long-chain fatty acids.[88] Term infants tolerate and uti-

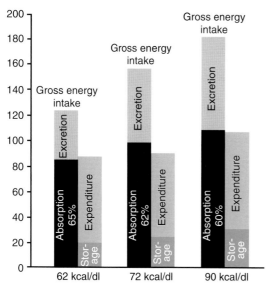

Figure 10: Energy balance in formula-fed preterm infants.

lize intravenous fat (IVF) well, but preterm infants metabolize it slowly and are prone to hyperlipidemia.[90] SGA infants use IVF slower than AGA infants. Reduced fat oxidation rates have been observed in preterms with septicemia.[88] Relative fat intolerance may be related to decreased lipoprotein lipase activity and lower stores of adipose tissue. The serum lipid concentrations of infected or respiratory-distressed infants receiving fat emulsions should be monitored to avoid hyperlipidemia, which has been associated with dysfunction of the reticuloendothelial system and alveolar gas exchange.[91] Lipid administration should be limited to 2 to 3 gm/kg/d. With caloric levels exceeding 80 kcal/kg/d, fat oxidation did not exceed 30% of total energy expenditure regardless of the fat level.[91]

Glucose Plus Fat. There is convincing evidence that the fuel source of choice is a combination of glucose and fat.[88] Most studies have demonstrated comparable nitrogen retention rates with glucose plus fat, or glucose alone.

Fat should provide 50% of the nonprotein calories when peripheral veins are used.[88] The ratio of glucose to fat may be increased if the central vein is utilized. In general, the amount of non-nitrogen energy should be derived from glucose and fat in equicaloric amounts.

Parenteral Energy Requirements

The parenteral energy requirement of term infants should be approximately 95 to 105 kcal/kg/day. The energy requirement of the VLBW infant is about 120 kcal/kg/day enterally and 110 to 120 kcal/kg/day parenterally.[92] Positive nitrogen balance was achieved with preterm infants infused with 60 kcal/kg/day but these infants were losing weight.[93] Growth requires a minimum of 70 kcal/kg/day in the VLBW infant.

Infection and Trauma

A characteristic response to infection and trauma is a rise in core body temperature and resting energy expenditure. Oxygen consumption was measured in adult patients with several febrile illnesses (tuberculosis, typhoid fever, malaria, bacterial pneumonia, and rheumatic fever).[94] These studies indicated that, for each degree centigrade rise in body temperature, the metabolic rate increased up to 13%.

During infection, fatty acids continue to be the major fuel source, but use of ketone bodies is decrease.[94] Uptake and utilization of branched-chain amino acids are accelerated in skeletal muscles to fuel gluconeogenesis in the liver and kidney.

When the energy cost of measles was estimated in Kenyan children 28 months of age,[95] a 75% fall was seen in energy intake and a slight decrease in absorption during acute illness. Basal metabolic rate was similar during measles and after recovery. The energy density of the diet tolerated during illness declined from 0.9 kcal/gm to 0.6 kcal/gm. Inadequate intake, not elevated expenditure, resulted in an energy deficit with this infectious disease.

The degree of hypermetabolism with trauma varies with the extent of the injury, the most extensive being in burn patients.[96] A 50% total body surface burn may double the metabolic rate. If the burn patient's body temperature is regulated at a high set point, the patient must be kept warm and heat losses minimized during the febrile state. If heat production exceeds thermoregulatory needs, physical and pharmacological measures should be employed to lower body temperature. In either case energy requirements should be determined and met with vigorous nutritional support.

Other Diseases

Bronchopulmonary dysplasia (BPD) typically is associated with slow growth. The impaired growth rate has been attributed to decreased nutritional intake during acute illness and to the increased work of respiration. Oxygen consumption was 25% higher in infants with BPD than in controls.[97] The increased energy requirements should be supported with aggressive nutritional therapy.

The metabolic rates of infants with congenital heart failure (CHF) are elevated in proportion to their degree of growth retardation and heart failure. The oxygen consumption of infants with CHF was 9.4 ml/kg/min, compared with 6.5 ml/kg/min in infants with cardiac heart disease (CHD) not in failure.[98] Infants with severe CHD who were markedly undergrown had abnormally high rates of oxygen consumption, whereas those with CHD whose growth was normal consumed oxygen at normal rates.[99]

Nutritional Marasmus

Nutritional marasmus is due to extreme underfeeding. Classical clinical signs include growth retardation, severe wasting of muscle and subcutaneous fat, occasionally mild hair changes and associated vitamin deficiencies.[100] Nonedematous protein energy malnutrition (PEM) or marasmus is primarily a deficiency of total calories. Unlike kwashiorkor (protein deficiency with variable reduction in energy), the marasmic child adapts to the insufficient intake. The edema, fatty liver and abnormal serum concentrations of lipase, amylase and cholesterol seen in kwashiorkor do not present in marasmus despite extreme emaciation.[101] Severe wasting does not preclude homeostasis; fat oxidation is intact despite depleted body fat. The availability of fat is the major limiting factor in survival from infant malnutrition.[102] Basal metabolic rates of marasmic infants were slightly elevated on admission (59.8 kcal/kg/day) and peaked during recovery (100.2 kcal/kg/day).[103]

There are many factors that cause marasmus: inadequate intake, increased energy requirements, reduced energy retention and increased excretory losses.[104] Inadequate intake can be a result of poverty, anorexia of illness, fasting imposed by hospital procedures and

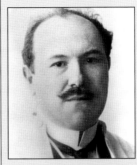

Leo Langstein Ph.D., M.D.

(1876-1933) studied chemistry under Emil Fischer, the Nobel laureate who named lactase. Langstein's pediatric training was under Heubner. He became the Director of the Kaiserin Auguste Victoria Children's Hospital (KAVH) in Berlin in 1911. Energy expenditure measurements were carried out at this hospital with Rubner's collaboration in 1915. Papers on childhood carbohydrate and protein digestion and on dietary requirement for iron appeared from the KAVH. Langstein's group first wrote about dietary lactose in 1906, first discovered glucose in diarrheal stools, and demonstrated a relationship between carbohydrate intake and acid balance. Langstein reviewed the Heubner and von Pirquet nutritional methods and felt that the von Pirquet nem system did not allow consideration of the needs of nutrients other than energy. *Pioniere der Kinderheilkunde* by J. Oehme (Photo courtesy of KAVH).

psychological stress. Energy requirements can be increased by infection, trauma, fever, neoplasm, hyperthyroidism and cardiorespiratory distress. Vomiting, diarrhea and malabsorption syndromes increase nutrient losses.

The prevalence of malnutrition among hospitalized pediatric patients has been reported to be 20 to 40%.[104] Risk factors for undernutrition include: weight less than 90% of standards, height less than 95% of standards, weight-for-height less than 90% of standards, rapid weight loss of 10% of usual weight, and no oral intake for greater than three days.

Protein energy malnutrition (marasmus) predisposes the infant to increased morbidity and mortality. Surgical outcome and postoperative complications are related to nutritional status, although this relationship has not been studied specifically in infants.[104] The effect of malnutrition on the immune response significantly impairs the malnourished infant's ability to resist infection.

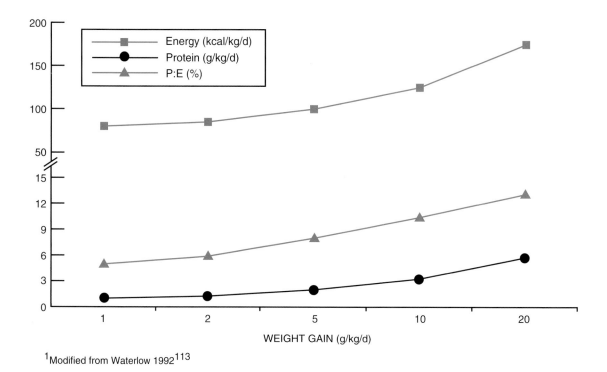

[1]Modified from Waterlow 1992[113]

Figure 11: Energy and protein requirements for "catch-up" growth of infants.[1]

The energy requirements of the marasmic infant are elevated during the recovery period. Growth depends as much on adequate energy as on protein and other essential nutrients. The malnourished child has lost adipose tissue and protein, primarily from muscle. Rates of "catch-up" growth vary widely, but maximum rates can be 10 to 20 times normal rates. Rapid rates of weight gain are accompanied by an increase in the TEF, presumably caused by increased protein synthesis.[105, 106] Waterlow[107] has estimated the energy and protein requirements for catch-up growth for an infant (Figure 11). If normal body composition is to be restored, the protein:energy ratio in the diet must be increased. In practice, the limiting factor in the diet is likely to be energy density, which can be increased by adding fat to the diet.

Obesity

Efforts to identify nutritionally-related infant diseases that persist later in life have focused much attention on

infant obesity. Data conflict in regard to the persistence of infant obesity into childhood, but there is strong evidence to support the persistence of childhood obesity into adult years.

A prospective study in Switzerland showed no relationship between skinfold thicknesses at one year and at puberty.[108] Tracking of body fatness from 12 months to five years was demonstrated in one prospective study, but a history of excess weight accounted for only 30% of the variance in body fat.[109] In contrast, Huenenmann[110] found that none of the children with high weight-height ratios at age three years had been categorized as such at six months. Rate of weight gain during infancy predicted subsequent obesity in some studies. Rapid weight gain during the first six months of life was related to excessive weight at school age.[110]

Suggested causes of infant obesity include genetic predisposition, excessive feeding, poor intake regulation, underactivity, maternal attitudes toward infant feeding and mother-child interactions. Inappropriate infant feeding practices may result in infant obesity. The decline in breast-feeding, excessive consumption of formula, and early introduction of solid foods have been suggested as possible causes. The neonate might not be fully able to regulate food intake. Initially, food consumption is controlled mainly by gastric filling and subsequently by additional regulatory mechanisms. Infants presented with two levels of formula density (67 or 133 kcal/dl) made some adjustment in total volume intakes, but only after 40 days of age were they able to make adjustments to control weight gain.[111] In one of the few studies relating infant activity levels to obesity, Rose and Mayer[17] showed heavier infants to be less active than lighter ones. In order to identify antecedents of obesity in infants, Kramer[112, 113] studied many clinical, socio-demographic and psychological factors (Figure 12). The main determinants of weight at 12 months were birthweight, sex, duration of breast-feeding and age at introduction of solid foods. However, most of the variance in weight and adiposity remained unexplained. Maternal and paternal obesity, beyond their effect on birthweight, did not predict infant size. At 24 months, the salient factors were birthweight, duration of breast-feeding, sex and relative maternal weight. Breast-feeding and later introduction of solid foods may offer a slight protective effect against obesity, but seem to be overshadowed by factors yet to be identified.

Because of the deleterious effects of caloric restriction on growth, resistance to infection and central nervous system development, specific caloric restriction is not recommended during infancy. Measures to guard against infant obesity can be implemented, however, by educating parents. Grossly inappropriate feeding practices should be corrected by pediatric health care providers.

Case Histories

Case #1: A one-month-old male infant was admitted to the hospital for failure to thrive. The infant was born prematurely at 34 weeks, birthweight 2.5 kg. The postnatal course was complicated by jaundice and treated with phototherapy. At one month the infant failed to demonstrate

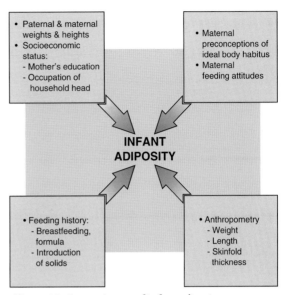

Figure 12: Determinants of infant adiposity.

appropriate growth: weight 2.70 kg, height 47.5 cm, head circumference 33.2 cm. The diet consisted of a standard cow milk-based formula for term infants providing 20 kcal/oz, three ounces every four hours. Despite failure to thrive, the infant had a voracious appetite. Physical examination revealed a wasted but otherwise normal infant. Laboratory data included: hemoglobin/hematocrit (Hgb/Hct) 8.6 gm/dl/25.0%; mean corpuscular hemoglobin/mean corpuscular volume (MCH/MCV) 33.5 pg/97.5 u³; White blood cell count 13200/mm³; urinalysis normal; serum aspartate transaminase/serum alanine transaminase (AST/ALT) 113/46 U/l; alkaline phosphatase 209 U/l; serum Ca/P 10.0/8.2 mg/dl; total protein/albumin (TP/AlB) 5.6/3.1 gm/dl; 72-hour stool fat 8.7 gm/d; stool weight 150 gm/d.

Diagnosis: Cystic fibrosis with malabsorption and anemia.
Treatment: A nutritionally complete dietary formulation with medium chain triglycerides such as Portagen (Mead Johnson & Co.) This is a formula consisting of maltodextrin, sodium caseinate, medium chain triglycerides, corn oil and lecithin and supplying 20 kcal per oz. Three ounces should be given every four hours; in addition, should be given a pancreatic enzyme supplement and a multivitamin mineral supplement plus additional iron.

Question: What was the suggestive evidence for diagnosis of cystic fibrosis?

Answer: Despite an intake of 133 kcal/kg/d, this infant was only growing at a rate of 6.7 gm/d. The excessive amount of fat in the stool represented 44% of the fat intake, or 22% of the total calories ingested. Poor growth associated with fat malabsorption suggested cystic fibrosis.

Question: What was the rationale for this diet prescription?

Answer: Medium-chain triglycerides are readily absorbed by the portal circulation. This diet formulation together with the pancreatic enzyme supplement should increase fat absorption in the child. A caloric intake of 200 kcal/kg/d should support sufficient catch-up growth.

Case #2: A three-week-old female was admitted to the hospital for failure to thrive. Pregnancy was complicated by maternal drug abuse. The infant was born at term; birthweight 2.1 kg, length 45 cm. Postnatal course was uneventful. The diet consisted of a cow milk-based formula for term infants supplying 20 kcal/oz, two ounces every four hours. On admission the infant weighed 2.4 kg and measured 48 cm in length. Physical examination revealed

no unusual findings. Laboratory data included Hgb/Hct 13/36, MCH/ MCV 29/83, WBC 11400, urinalysis normal, serum Ca/P 10.5/5.5, TP/Alb 6.0/4.0.

Diagnosis: Small for gestational age (SGA) infant with failure to thrive due to inadequate intake.

Treatment: Standard cow milk-based formula for term infants, supplying 20 kcal/oz, three ounces every three hours.

Follow-up: Weight at two months, 3.6 kg; length 52.5 cm.

Question: Describe the growth performance of this infant.

Answer: The child was below the 5th percentile in weight and height at birth and remained at this level after three weeks postpartum. The growth rate had been 14 gm/d during this interval. SGA infants usually have the potential for accelerated growth given a proper diet.

Question: What was the caloric intake of this infant at admission and what caloric intake was prescribed?

Answer: This child was receiving 100 kcal/kg/d on admission, which was probably inadequate for the relatively high energy requirement of SGA infants. The child was given the same formula at 200 kcal/kg/d after admission, and an appropriate growth rate of 34 gm/d was demonstrated on follow-up examination.

> *It is probable that many of these stunted babies survived their in utero milieu by utilizing all transferred calories for energy at the expense of growth. An interesting but unsubstantiated observation is that some of the most severely growth retarded in this group ingest (when they are not limited) volumes of milk much more appropriate to their gestational age than their actual weight.*
>
> Anthony Phillips M.D.
> University of Arizona Health
> Science Center
> Tucson, Arizona

Glossary

1. **Basal metabolic rate (BMR)** - the energy expended to maintain cellular and tissue processes fundamental to the organism, measured in the fasted state (12 to 18hr postprandially) while at rest in a thermoneutral environment.

2. **Thermic effect of feeding (TEF)** - the energy expended above basal metabolism in response to feeding, primarily attributed to the transport and conversion of absorbed nutrients into their respective storage forms; also referred to as diet-induced thermogenesis (DIT) or specific dynamic action of foods (SDA).

3. **Energy balance** - gross energy intake = energy excreted + energy expended + energy stored.

4. **Gross energy** - heat of combustion of food determined by bomb calorimetry.

5. **Digestible energy intake** - gross energy intake minus the heat of combustion of feces.

6. **Metabolizable intake** digestible energy intake minus the heat of combustion of urine.

7. **Calorie** - the amount of heat necessary to raise the temperature of one gram of water from 14.5 to 15.5°C.

8. **Joule** - the amount of energy expended when one kilogram weight is moved one meter's distance by one newton force. (1 cal = 4.184 joules).

9. **Indirect calorimetry** - the measurement of oxygen consumption and CO_2 production to determine energy expenditure.

10. **Total energy expenditure (TEE)** encompasses basal metabolism, thermogenesis, physical activity and synthetic cost of growth.

11. **Energy cost of growth** consists of the energy content of the tissues and the energy needed for synthetic processes.

Historical Perspective...

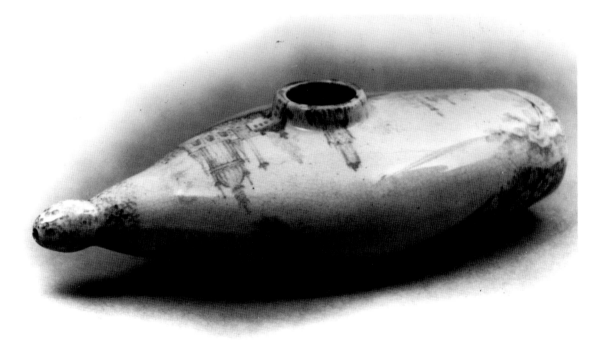

English, transfer-printed, pottery feeding bottle. Staffordshire, circa 1820.

References

1. Karlberg P. Determinations of standard energy metabolism (basal metabolism) in normal infants. *Acta Paediatr Scand.* 1952;41:Suppl 89.

2. Benedict FG, Talbot FB. Metabolism of growth from birth to puberty. Washington, DC. Carnegie Institute: 1921. Carnegie Institution of Washington publication 302;1-213.

3. Holliday M, Potter D, Jarrah A, Bearg S. Relation of metabolic rate to body weight and organ size. A review. *Pediatr Res.* 1967;1:185-195.

4. Schofield WN. Predicting basal metabolic rate, new standards and review of previous work. *Hum Nutr: Clin Nutr.* 1985;39C (Suppl 1):5-41.

5. Mestyan J, Jarai I, Fekete M. The total energy expenditure and its components in preterm infants maintained under different nursing and environmental conditions. *Pediatr Res.* 1968;2:161-171.

6. Sinclair JC, Silverman WA. Relative hypermetabolism in undergrown neonates. *Lancet.* 1964;2:49.

7. Danforth E. Diet and obesity. *Am J Clin Nutr.* 1985;41:1132-1145.

8. Flatt JP. The biochemistry of energy expenditure. In: Bray A, ed. *Recent Advances in Obesity Research II.* London: Newman Publishing Co; 1978:211-228.

9. Reichman BL, Chessex P, Putet G, et al. Partition of energy metabolism and energy cost of growth in the very low birth weight infant. *Pediatrics.* 1982;69:446-451.

10. Ashworth A. Metabolic rates during recovery from protein-calorie malnutrition: the need for a new concept of specific dynamic action. *Nature.* 1969;223:407-409.

11. Hill JR. The development of thermal stability in the newborn baby, In: Jonxis JHP, Visses HKA, Troelstra JA, eds. *The Adaptation of the Newborn to Extrauterine Life.* Leiden HE, Stenfert Kroese NV; 1964:223-228.

12. Widdowson EM. Nutrition. In: Davis JA, Dobbing J, eds. *Scientific Foundations of Pediatrics.* Philadelphia: WB Saunders Co; 1974:44-55.

13. Scopes J, Ahmed I. Range of critical temperatures in sick and preterm newborn babies. *Arch Dis Child.* 1966;41:417-419.

14. Penn D, Schmidt-Sommerfeld E. Lipids as an energy source for the fetus and newborn infant. In: Lebenthal E, ed. *Textbook of Gastroenterology and Nutrition in Infancy.*

15. Talbot FB. Twenty-four-hour metabolism of two normal infants with special references to the total energy requirements of infants. *Am J Dis Child.* 1917;14-25.

16. Murlin JR, Conklin MS, Marsh ME. Energy metabolism of normal new-born babies. With special reference to the influence of food and of crying. *Am J Dis Child.* 1925;29:128.

17. Rose HE, Mayer J. Activity, calorie intake, fat storage and the energy balance of infants. *Pediatrics.* 1968;41:18-29.

18. Spady DW, Payne PR, Picou D, Waterlow JC. Energy balance during recovery from malnutrition. *Am J Clin Nutr.* 1976;29:1073-1078.

19. Rubecz I, Mestyan J. The partition of maintenance energy expenditure and the pattern of substrate utilization in intrauterine malnourished newborn infants before and during recovery. *Acta Pediatr Acad Sci Hung.* 1975;16:335-350.

20. Roberts SB, Coward WA, Schlingenseipen K-H, Nohria V, Lucas A. Comparison of the doubly labeled water ($^2H_2^{18}O$) method with indirect calorimetry and a nutrient-balance study for simultaneous determination of energy expenditure, water intake, and metabolizable energy intake in preterm infants. *Am J Clin Nutr.* 1986; 44:315-322.

21. Jones PJH, Winthrop AL, Schoeller DA, Swyer PR, Smith J, Filler RM, Heim T. Validation of doubly labeled water for expenditure in infants. *Pediatr Res.* 1987; 21:242-246.

22. Westerterp KR, Lafeber HN, Sulkers EJ, Sauer PJJ. Comparison of short term indirect calorimetry and doubly labeled water method for the assessment of energy expenditure in preterm infants. *Biol Neonate.* 1991; 60:75-82.

23. Jensen CL, Butte NF, Wong WW, Moon JK. Determining energy expenditure in preterm infants: comparison of $^2H_2^{18}O$ method and indirect calorimetry. *Am Physiol Soc.* 1992;R685-R692.

24. Lucas A, Ewing G, Roberts SB, Coward WA. How much energy does the breast-fed infant consume and expend? *Br Med J.* 1987;295:75-77.

25. Prentice A, Lucas A, Vasquez-Velasquez L, Davies PSW, Whitehead RG. Are current dietary guidelines for young

Second Edition. New York: Raven Press; 1989:293-310.

children a prescription for overfeeding? *Lancet.* 1988;11: 1066-1069.

26. Roberts SB, Savage J, Coward WA, Chew B, Lucas A. Energy expenditure and intake in infants born to lean and overweight mothers. *N Engl J Med.* 1988;318:461-467.

27. Vasquez-Velasquez L. Energy metabolism in children. Ph.D thesis. University of Cambridge; 1987.

28. Fjeld CR, Schoeller DA, Brown KH. A new model for predicting energy requirements of children during catch-up growth developed using doubly labeled water. *Pediatr Res.* 1989;25:503-508.

29. Butte NF, Wong W, Garza C, Ferlic L, Smith EO, Klein PD. Energy expenditure and deposition of breast-fed and formula-fed infants during infancy. *Pediatr Res.* 1990; 28:631-640.

30. Davies PSW, Ewing G, Lucas A. Energy expenditure in early infancy. *Br J Nutr.* 1989;62:621-629.

31. Davies PSW, Day JME, Lucas A. Energy expenditure in early infancy and later body fatness. *Intl J Obesity.* 1991; 15:727-731.

32. Wells JCK, Davies PSW. Energy cost of physical activity in twelve week old infants. *Am J Hum Biol.* 1995;7:85-92.

33. Butte NF, Villalpando S, Wong WW, Flores-Huerta S, Hernandez-Beltran M, Smith EO. Higher total energy expenditure contributes to growth faltering in breast-fed infants living in rural Mexico. *J Nutr.* 1993;123:1028-1035.

34. Davies PSW, Coward WA. Total energy expenditure and energy intake in the pre-school child: a comparison. *British J Nutr.* 1994;72:13-20.

35. Bell EF, Rios FR, Wilmoth PK. Estimation of 24-hour energy expenditure from shorter measurement periods in premature infants. *Pediatr Res.* 1986;20:646-649.

36. Schulze KF, Stefanski M, Masterson J, et al. An analysis of the variability in estimates of bioenergetic variables in preterm infants. *Pediatr Res.* 1986;20:422-427.

37. Freymond D, Schutz Y, Decombaz J, Micheli JL, Jequier E. Energy balance, physical activity and thermogenic effect of feeding in premature infants. *Pediatr Res.* 1986; 20:638-645.

38. Fomon SJ, Haschke F, Ziegler EE, Nelson SE. Body composition of reference children from birth to age 10 years. *Am J Clin Nutr.* 1982;35:1169-1175.

39. Roberts SB, Young VR. Energy costs of fat and protein deposition in the human infant. *Am J Clin Nutr.* 1988;

48:951-955.

40. Golden M, Waterlow JC, Picou D. The relationship between dietary intake, weight change, nitrogen balance, and protein turnover in man. *Am J Clin Nutr.* 1977;30: 1345-1348

41. Young VR. Protein-energy interrelationships in the newborn: a brief consideration of some basic aspects. In: Lebenthal E, ed. *Textbook of Gastroenterology and Nutrition in Infancy.* New York: Raven Press; 1981:257-263.

42. Maniscalco WM, Warshaw JB. Cellular energy metabolism during fetal and perinatal development. In: Sinclair JC, ed. *Temperature Regulation and Energy Metabolism in the Newborn.* New York: Grune and Stratton; 1978:1-38.

43. Hahn P. Nutrition and metabolic development. *Can J Physiol Pharmacol.* 1985;63:525-526.

44. Bougneres PF, Lemmel C, Ferre P, Bier DM. Ketone body transport in the human neonate and infant. *J Clin Invest.* 1986;77:42-48.

45. Gudinchet F, Schutz Y, Micheli JL, Stettler E, Jecquier E. Metabolic cost of growth in the very low-birth weight infant. *Pediatr Res.* 1982;16:1025-1030.

46. Southgate DAT, Barrett IM. The intake and excretion of calorific constituents of milk by babies. *Br J Nutr.* 1966;20:363-372.

47. Fomon SJ, Filer LJ, Thomas LN, et al. Relationship between formula concentration and rate of growth of normal infants. *J Nutr.* 1969;98:241-254.

48. Meurling S, Arturson G, Zaar B, Eriksson G. Energy, fat, and nitrogen balance in healthy newborn infants during the first week after birth. *Acta Chir Scand.* 1981; 147:487-495.

49. Whitehead RG, Paul AA. Infant growth and human milk requirements. *Lancet.* 1981;2:161-3.

49. Whitehead RG, Paul AA, Cole TJ. A critical analysis of measured food energy intakes during infancy and early childhood in comparison with current international recommendations. *J Hum Nutr.* 1981;35:339-348.

50. McKillop FM, Durnin JVGA. The energy and nutrient intake of a random sample (305) of infants. *Hum Nutr: Appl Nutr.* 1982;36A:405-421.

51. Hofvander Y, Hagman U, Hillervik C, Sjölin S. The amount of milk consumed by 1-3 months old breast- or bottle-fed infants. *Acta Pædiatr Scand.* 1982;71:953-958.

52. Dewey KG, Lönnerdal B. Milk and nutrient intake of breast-fed infants from 1 to 6 months: relation to growth and fatness. *J Pediatr Gastroenterol Nutr.* 1983;2:497-506.

53. Butte NF, Garza C, Smith EO, Nichols BL. Human milk intake and growth in exclusively breast-fed infants. *J Pediatr.* 1984;104:187-195.

54. Dewey KG, Finley DA, Lönnerdal B. Breast milk volume and composition during late lactation (7-20 months). *J Pediatr Gastro Nutr.* 1984;3:713-720.

55. Köhler L, Meeuwisse G, Mortensson W. Food intake and growth of infants between six and twenty-six weeks of age on breast milk, cow's milk formula, or soy formula. *Acta Pædiatr Scand.* 1984;73:40-48.

56. Hitchcock NE, Owles EN, Gracey M, Gilmour A. Nutrition of healthy children in the second and third years of life. *J Fd Nutr.* 1984;41:13-16.

57. Forsum E, Sadurskis A. Growth, body composition and breast milk intake of Swedish infants during early life. *Early Hum Dev.* 1986;14:121-129.

58. Hoffmans MDAF, Obermann-de Boer GL, Florack EIM, Van Kampen-Donker M, Kromhout D. Energy, nutrient and food intake during infancy and early childhood: The Leiden Pre-School Children Study. *Hum Nutr: Appl.* 1986;40A:421-430.

58. Horst CH, Obermann-deBoer GL, Kromhout D. Type of milk feeding and nutrient intake during infancy: The Leiden Pre-School Children Study. *Acta Pædiatr Scand.* 1987;76:865-871.

60. Catassi C, Guerrieri A, Natalini G, Oggiano N, Coppa GV, Giorgi PL. Computerized dietary analysis in children aged 6-30 months. I. Method of the survey and energy intake. *Riv Ital Ped (IJP).* 1988;14:702-706.

61. Wood CS, Isaacs PC, Jensen M, Hilton HG. Exclusively breast-fed infants: growth and caloric intake. *Pediatr Nurs.* 1988;14:117-124.

62. Stuff JE, Nichols BL. Nutrient intake and growth performance of older infants fed human milk. *J Pediatr.* 1989;115:959-968.

63. Stuff JE, Montandon CM, Smith EO, Nichols BL. Between- and within-individual variation in formula intake of infants from 12 to 24 weeks of age. *Am J Clin Nutr.* 1991;51:525.

64. Butte NF, Smith EO, Garza C. Energy utilization of breast-fed and formula-fed infants. *Am J Clin Nutr.* 1990;51:350-358.

65. Paul AA, Whitehead RG, Black AE. Energy intakes and growth from two months to three years in initially breast-fed children. *J Hum Nutr Diet.* 1990;3:79-92.

66. Sauve RS, Geggie JH. Growth and dietary status of preterm and term infants during the first two years of life. *Can J Pub Health.* 1991;82:95-100.

67. Räsänen L, Ylonen K. Food consumption and nutrient intake of one- to two-year old Finnish children. *Acta Paediatr.* 1992;81:7-11.

68. Heinig MJ, Nommsen LA, Peerson JM, Lönnerdal B, Dewey KG. Energy and protein intakes of breast-fed and formula-fed infants during the first year of life and their association with growth velocity: The Darling Study. *Am J Clin Nutr.* 1993;58:152-161.

69. Michaelsen KF, Larsen PS, Thomsen BL, Samuelson G. The Copenhagen Cohort Study on Infant Nutrition and Growth: breast-milk intake, human milk macronutrient content, and influencing factors. *Am J Clin Nutr.* 1994;59:600-611.

70. Dewey KG, Heinig MJ, Nommsen LA, Lönnerdal B. Adequacy of energy intake among breast-fed infants in the Darling study: Relationships to growth velocity, morbidity, and activity levels. *J Pediatr.* 1991;119:538-547.

71. Butte NF, Wills C, Jean CA, Smith EO, Garza C. Feeding patterns of exclusively breast-fed infants during the first four months of life. *Ear Hum Devel.* 1985;12:291-300.

72. Dewey KG, Heinig MJ, Nommsen LA, Peerson JM, Lönnerdal B. Growth of breast-fed and formula-fed infants from 0 to 18 months: The Darling Study. *Pediatr.* 1992;89:1035-1041.

73. Butte NF, Smith EOB, Garza C. Heart rates of breast-fed and formula-fed infants. *J Pediatr Gastro Nutr.* 1991;13:391-396.

74. Butte NF, Jensen CL, Moon JK, Glaze DG, Frost JD, Jr. Sleep organization and energy expenditure of breast-fed and formula-fed infants. *Pediatr Res.* 1992;32:514-519.

75. FAO/WHO/UNU Expert Consultation. "Energy and protein requirements." Geneva: 1985. World Health Organization Technical Report Series 724.

76. Food and Nutrition Board. Commission on Life Sciences, National Research Council. *Recommended Dietary Allowances, 10th Edition.* Washington DC: National Academy Press; 1989.

77. Committee on Medical Aspects of Food Policy. *Dietary Reference Values for Food Energy and Nutrients for the United Kingdom.* London: HMSO; 1991.

78. Health and Welfare Canada. *Nutrition Recommendations. The Report of the Scientific Review Committee.* Ottawa, Canada: 1990. Supply and Services.

79. Health Promotion and Nutrition Division, Health Policy Bureau, Ministry of Health and Welfare. Tokyo, Japan: 1991.

80. Ministry of Health and Social Affairs. Kyonggi, Korea: 1989.

81. The Scientific Committee for Food, Aggett PJ, Arnal M, et al. *Reports of the Scientific Committee for Food* (Thirty-first series). Nutrient and energy intakes for the European Community. Luxembourg; Commission of the European Communities: 1993. Office for Official Publications of the European Communities; 1-248.

82. Chessex P, Reichman B, Verellen G, et al. Metabolic consequences of intrauterine growth retardation in very low birthweight infants. *Pediatr Res.* 1984;18:709-713.

83. Brooke OG. Energy balance and metabolic rate in preterm infants fed with standard and high energy formulas. *Br J Nutr.* 1980;44:13-23.

84. Whyte RK, Campbell D, Stanhope R, et al. Energy balance in low birth weight infants fed formula of high or low medium-chain triglyceride content. *J Pediatr.* 1986;108:964-971.

85. Kashyap S, Forsyth M, Zucker C, et al. Effects of varying protein and energy intakes on growth and metabolic response in low birth weight infants. *J Pediatr.* 1986;108: 955-963.

86. Whyte RK, Bayley HS, Sinclair JC. Energy intake and the nature of growth in low birth weight infants. *Can J Physiol Pharmacol.* 1985;63:565-570.

87. Putet G. Energy. In: Tsang RC, Lucas A, Uauy R, Zlotkin S, eds. *Nutritional Needs of the Preterm Infant.* Baltimore: Williams & Wilkins; 1993:15-28.

88. Ekman L, Wretlind A. Utilization of parenteral energy sources. In: Garrow JS, Halliday D, eds. *Substrate and Energy Metabolism.* London: John Libbey; 1985:222-231.

89. Shaw JCL. Parenteral nutrition in the management of sick low birthweight infants. *Pediatr Clin North Am.* 1973;20:333-358.

90. Sunshine P, Kerner JA. The use of intravenous fat emulsions in preterm infants. In: Kretchmer N, Minkowski A, eds. *Nutritional Adaptation of the Gastrointestinal Tract of the Newborn.* New York: Raven Press; 1983:163-175.

91. Committee on Nutrition, Academy of Pediatrics. Use of intravenous fat emulsions in pediatric patients. *Pediatrics.* 1981;68:738-743.

92. Committee on Nutrition, Academy of Pediatrics. Nutritional needs of low-birth-weight infants. *Pediatrics.* 1985;75:976-986.

93. Anderson TL, Muttart CR, Bieber MA, et al. A controlled trial of glucose versus glucose and amino acids in preterm infants. *J Pediatr.* 1979;94:947-951.

94. Beisel WR, Wannemacher RW, Neufeld HA. Relation of fever to energy expenditure. In: *Assessment of Energy Metabolism in Health and Disease.* Columbus, Ohio: Ross Laboratories; 1980:144-150.

95. Duggan MB, Milner RDG. Energy cost of measles infection. *Arch Dis Child.* 1986;61:436-439.

96. Aulick LH. Studies in heat transport and heat loss in thermally injured patients. In: *Assessment of Energy Metabolism in Health and Disease.* Columbus, Ohio: Ross Laboratories; 1980:141-144.

97. Weinstein MR, Oh W. Oxygen consumption in infants with bronchopulmonary dysplasia. *J Pediatr.* 1981;99: 958-961.

98. Krauss AN, Auld PAM. Metabolic rate of neonates with congenital heart disease. *Arch Dis Child.* 1975;50:539-541.

99. Lees MH, Bristow JD, Griswold HE, Olmstod RW. Relative hypermetabolism in infants with congenital heart disease and undernutrition. *Pediatrics.* 1965;36: 183-191.

100. Jelliffe DB. The assessment of the nutritional status of the community. Geneva: 1966. WHO; 187-189.

101. Hatch TF. Effects of protein-caloric malnutrition on the digestive and absorptive capacities of infants. In: Lebenthal E, ed. *Textbook of Gastroenterology and Nutrition in Infancy.* New York: Raven Press; 1981:767-776.

102. Kerr DS, Stevens CG, Robinson HM. Fasting metabolism in infants. 1. Effect of severe undernutrition on energy and protein utilization. *Metabolism.* 1978;27: 411-435.

103. Montgomery RD. Changes in the basal metabolic rate of the malnourished infant and their relationship to body composition. *J Clin Invest.* 1962;41:1653-1663.

104. Baker SS. Protein-energy metabolism in the hospitalized pediatric patient. In: Walker WA, Watkins JB, eds. *Nutrition in Pediatrics: Basic Science and Clinical Application.* Boston: Little Brown and Co; 1985:171-181.

105. Brooke OG, Ashworth A. The influence of malnutrition on the postprandial metabolic rate and respiratory quotient. *British J Nutr.* 1972;27:407-415.

106. Fjeld CR, Schoeller D, Brown KH. Body composition of children recovering from severe protein-energy malnutrition at two rates of catch-up growth. *Am J Clin Nutr.* 1989;50:1266-1275.

107. Waterlow JC. In: *Protein-energy Malnutrition.* London: Edward Arnold; 1992:253.

108. Hernesniemi I, Zachmann M, Prader A. Skinfold thickness in infancy and adolescence. A longitudinal correlation study in normal children. *Helv Pediatr Acta.* 1974;29:523-530.

109. Mellies M, Glueck C. Infant nutrition and the development of obesity. In: Lebenthal E, ed. *Textbook of Gastroenterology and Nutrition in Infancy.* New York: Raven Press; 1981:709-718.

110. Huenenmann RL. Environmental factors associated with preschool obesity. *J Am Diet Assoc.* 1974;64: 480-491.

111. Fomon SJ, Filer W, Thomas LN, et al. Relationship between formula concentration and rate of growth of normal infants. *J Nutr.* 1969;98:241-254.

112. Kramer MS, Barr RG, Leduc DG, et al. Determinants of weight and adiposity in the first year of life. *J Pediatr.* 1985;106:1014.

113. Kramer MS, Barr RG, Leduc DG, et al. Infant determinants of childhood weight and adiposity. *J Pediatr.* 1985;107:104-107.

Meeting Protein Needs

Kathleen J. Motil M.D., Ph.D.

USDA/ARS Children's Nutrition Research Center,
Department of Pediatrics,
Baylor College of Medicine,
Houston, Texas

Reviewed by Edward A. Liechty M.D.

Introduction

In 1784, in his book entitled A Treatise of the Diseases of Children, *Michael Underwood provided a comparative analysis of milk from women, cows, goats, asses, sheep and mares. He concluded that, "Cow's milk, while adequate for healthy, vigorous infants, is inferior to ass milk for the 'delicate' or 'sickly' infant." Although unknown to the physicians and midwives in the early 1900s, ass's milk is the only animal milk known to have a casein: whey content comparable to human milk.*

In spite of the notable advances in infant feedings made during the past half century, many nutritional problems contributing to infant morbidity and mortality remain unsolved. Protein and amino acid requirements in the infant remain controversial due to individual variability, nutrient interactions and the technical difficulties associated with precise determination of nutrient needs. Protein is essential for the structural components of the cells during the process of maturation, remodeling, and growth, as well as for the functional activity of synthetic and degradative enzymes and transport proteins of all body organs. Protein in the diet is important because it is the source of nitrogen and amino acids. Nitrogen is not stored by the body and must be replenished to avoid the irreversible consequences of protein deficiency. The body can synthesize and interconvert some amino acids, but nine (histidine, isoleucine, leucine, lysine, methionine, phenylalanine, threonine, tryptophan and valine) are considered essential and must be supplied by the diet. Objective criteria for determining the adequacy of dietary nutrients, particularly amino acids, are lacking. Some studies suggest that protein, rather than energy, is the most limiting nutrient in the young, and that the quality of protein, i.e., its amino acid composition, is the most important factor in the regulation and maturation of developmental processes.[1]

This chapter focuses on the physiology of protein and amino acid utilization, the determination of protein and amino acid needs in the infant, the deficiency and toxicity states associated with protein and amino acid metabolism, and a global perspective of the problems associated with dietary protein deficiency. Ultimately, a better understanding of these aspects of protein and amino acid metabolism will permit an improved approach to the nutritional management of infants in health and disease.

Physiology

The infant is born with a structurally underdeveloped body and organs that are functionally immature.[2] This immaturity lends itself to special consequences in relation to the digestion, absorption, utilization and excretion of dietary protein, and in determining protein and amino acid requirements during infancy.

John Clarke, in his writings of 1815, favored ass's milk if breast-feeding was impossible because cow's milk was "too rich, containing too much oil (fat) and cheesy (curd) matter." If ass's milk could not be found, skimmed cow's milk was mixed with barley, grits, rice or arrow root in a ratio of two-thirds to one-third. If this mixture did not agree with the child, a weak broth of mutton, chicken or beef was mixed with a "mucilaginous farinacous decoction" in a proportion of one to one.

Gastrointestinal Tract
Digestion and Absorption

Protein digestion begins in the stomach, where as much as 10% of ingested protein is denatured by hydrochloric acid (HCl) or acted upon by proteolytic enzymes such as pepsin. At the same time, peptide hor-

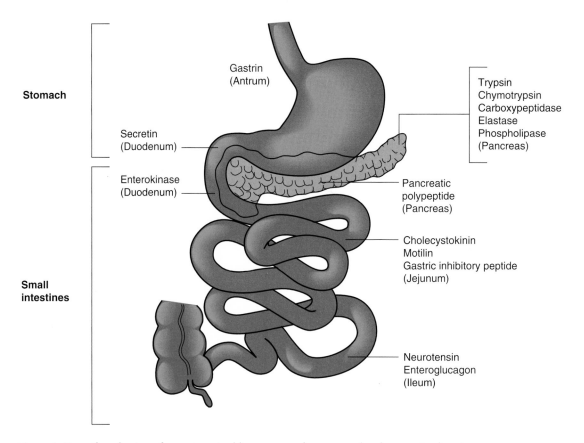

Figure 1: Sites of production of gastrointestinal hormones and enzymes related to protein digestion.

mones such as gastrin, and enterokinase, both of which are released by the gastrointestinal tract, facilitate the digestion of dietary proteins by enhancing gastric and intestinal motility and by stimulating the pancreas to release additional proteolytic enzymes (Fig. 1). Protein also is secreted into the intestinal lumen during digestion; as much as 30% of postprandial protein products may be of endogenous origin.

The majority of the peptides formed after luminal hydrolysis may be digested further; this takes place either at the surface of the cell, by peptidases located within the brush border of the enterocytes with subsequent transfer of amino acids across the mucosal cell membrane, or the peptides may be transported intact into the mucosal cell and hydrolyzed intracellularly in the soluble fraction of the cell. Amino acids and peptides are actively transported into the mucosal cells by carrier systems for dipeptides and for neutral,

basic and acidic amino acids. As the amino acids pass through the mucosal cells, they are transported to the liver via the portal vein, where they are metabolized further.

Digestion and Absorption in the Infant

The process of gastric and pancreatic digestion of protein is functionally immature in the infant.[3] The ability of the stomach to secrete HCl is established within 24 hours after birth, but does not attain adult capacity until the infant is two years of age. Despite the well-developed gastric parietal mass, HCl may be absent in the fasted state and may decrease postprandially, thereby reducing protein denaturation.[4] Gastric pepsins are also present in decreased amounts in infancy and do not attain adult levels until the infant is two years of age. Similarly, enterokinase is present at birth, but is only one-fifth as active in the infant as in the older child.[5] Pancreatic zymogen granules, which contain digestive enzymes, are present in adequate numbers in infants, but the activity of trypsin and chymotrypsin is less in infants than in older children.[5, 6] The functional immaturity of the stomach and pancreas is clinically relevant in situations where specific diseases such as cystic fibrosis remain undiagnosed, or during the course of enteric infections which result in significant villous atrophy. In this setting, reduced digestive capacity potentiates the problem of poor weight gain and may lead to protein malnutrition.

In contrast, the intestinal absorption of protein is functionally intact and relatively well-developed during infancy. Early in gestation, intestinal dipeptidase and tripeptidase activities have been detected in the brush border and cytoplasm of villous cells throughout the small bowel; these activities mature to adult levels by mid-gestation.[7] Carrier-mediated active transport systems for amino acids and dipeptides and tripeptides also are well-established in the fetal gut.[8] As a consequence, the infant has the ability to digest and absorb at least 80% of its protein intake.[9] Casein and whey proteins from human and cow milk are digested and absorbed equally well.

Macromolecular transport of intact protein in the human infant has not been clearly documented.[10] Studies suggest that the intestines of the infant may have a higher capacity for the absorption of macromolecules than the intestines of the adult.[11] Thus, the early introduction of specific foods of increased antigenic potential in the susceptible infant, such as one who sustains severe post-infectious villous injury, may put the infant at risk for protein sensitization.

Although the infant is able to digest and absorb protein, the development of the hormones and enzymes that regulate these processes in the gut is not well-characterized. Gastrin, enteroglucagon, vasoactive inhibitory polypeptide, gastric inhibitory polypeptide, neurotensin, motilin and pancreatic polypeptide are present at birth[12, 13] and rise significantly above adult values by 24 days of life. Plasma concentrations of these hormones also rise in response to a feeding, depending on the composition of the meal, i.e., carbohydrate alone vs. mixed protein and fat.[14] Although enteral feeding induces hormonal changes in the gastrointestinal tract of the infant, the functional significance of these observations is not understood clearly.

Rotch was the authority on infant feeding from 1890 until 1915. His concept of percentage feeding was based on the premises that cow milk protein was difficult to digest, while cow milk fat was harmless. In modifying the infant's feeding, a certain percentage of each food element was to be administered, rather than giving a certain amount of food. Based on the available information on the composition of human milk, Rotch developed the following formula: ¼ part cream, ⅛ part milk, one part water, one measure (3⅜ drams) of lactose, and 1/16 part lime water for each eight ounces.

Rotch believed that the tolerance to cow milk varied enormously according to age, and as little as 0.1% variation in a single food element could make the difference in digestibility. As a result, milk was prescribed with the same accuracy and precision as dangerous drugs. Although Rotch's percentage method was adopted universally in America, interest waned quickly because of the mathematical gymnastics necessary to feed infants.

Liver
Hepatic Protein Metabolism
Much less is known about the developmental aspects of protein metabolism in the infant's liver. As in the gut, hepatic protein synthesis, as measured by transport and acute phase reactant proteins, is functionally immature in infancy. All major plasma proteins derived from the liver are present at birth, although several, such as ceruloplasmin, low density lipoproteins and haptoglobin, are at concentrations below adult values. During the first postnatal week, lipoprotein levels rise abruptly in response to the increase in serum lipid concentrations; albumin and transferrin levels rise to adult concentrations after several months; and ceruloplasmin and complement factors rise to low normal adult levels by one year of age. Hepatic protein synthesis responds readily to altered dietary protein intake. Thus, in the clinical setting, a reduction of individual hepatic proteins confirms the presence of a protein deficiency state.

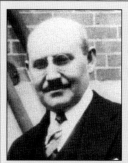

Lafayette B. Mendel Ph.D.
(1872-1935) received his degree under Chittenden at Yale. He taught at Yale for his entire career. Working with Thomas B. Osborne, they tested the quality of dietary proteins in rats. These studies demonstrated for the first time that some amino acids cannot be synthesized by the animal's body and are thus essential in the diet. A similar study with dietary lipids resulted in the discovery of vitamin A. Mendel published a book *Childhood and Growth* in 1906, in which he applied his studies on experimental animals to the child. J. Nutr. 60, 1-12, 1956 (Photo courtesy of CNRC)

Ureagenesis and Gluconeogenesis
The urea cycle provides the mechanism for the disposal of nitrogen from the catabolism of proteins and amino acids. Urea is made from the hydrolysis of the amino acid, arginine, when catalyzed by the enzyme arginase. The rate-limiting enzyme of the urea cycle is arginine synthetase. The activities of all the urea cycle enzymes are present at birth, but are reduced during infancy, presumably because of the need to conserve proteins and amino acids for tissue growth.[15] As a consequence, BUN concentrations are low because of the reduction in the proportion of body protein catabolized by the infant compared with that in the adult, averaging 4% in the former and 17% in the latter.

Gluconeogenesis is the metabolic process that results in the formation of glucose or glycogen from noncarbohydrate sources such as amino acids, lactate and glycerol. Skeletal muscle provides the principal gluconeogenic precursor, alanine, for glucose synthesis. The rate-limiting enzyme in gluconeogenesis is phosphoenolpyruvate carboxykinase. Gluconeogenesis becomes functionally important in the human only after birth.[16] The young infant is particularly susceptible to hypoglycemia because the large glucose requirement of the brain cannot be met when the infant is in the postabsorptive state. In general, glycogen stores are depleted rapidly. In addition, not all amino acids are gluconeogenic. Finally, the synthesis of glucose from pyruvate (derived from alanine) provides no additional new glucose.

Kidneys
In early infancy, the kidney has a minor role in the metabolism of proteins and amino acids because approximately 90% of the protein nitrogen ingested by the human infant is incorporated into newly synthesized body tissues and is not excreted as urea by the kidney. The functional capacity of the kidney to excrete urea nitrogen remains limited for the first two months of life. Renal tubular maturation can be induced by providing dietary protein.[17] Nevertheless, infants under four months of age have increased rates of urinary excretion, and lower net and percent tubular reabsorption of amino acids compared with older children.[18] Thus, the immaturity of kidney function also may contribute to increased protein and amino acid needs during infancy.

Protein and Amino Acid Needs
General Concepts
Although protein generally is not a limiting dietary nutrient during infancy, it is clear that dietary protein is essential for normal growth and development. Protein needs in the infant are determined primarily by the quantity of dietary nitrogen and amino acids required to maintain body composition, promote growth and support the functional aspects of body protein metabolism. From birth to four months of age, the average increase of body protein in the infant is 3.5 g/day (1.0 g·kg^{-1}·d^{-1}); thereafter, the infant accumulates protein in an amount that approximates 3.1 g/day (0.6 g·kg^{-1}·d^{-1}).[19, 20] This amounts to increases in body protein content from 11.4% at term to 17.5% at one year of age and represents an appreciable proportion of the protein requirement of the rapidly growing infant (Figure 2). However, the body is not 100% efficient in assimilating and using dietary nutrients for tissue deposition. Protein turnover studies using stable isotopes have demonstrated that the rate of protein synthesis in infants exceeds that of the adults by a factor of three- to fourfold. Although the discrepancy between protein synthesis and protein deposition appears to be

wasteful and inefficient, the recycling process of body protein metabolism readily permits remodeling of body tissues during periods of rapid growth.

The most significant achievement in the field of infant nutrition came from Arthur V. Meigs. His contribution was the accurate analysis of human and cow milk. In 1882, Meigs read a paper before the Philadelphia Medical Society that stated that human milk contained 0.7 to 1.2% casein and 7% sugar. In a second paper, in 1893, Meigs reiterated his findings and recommended a formula prepared as follows: 3 ounces of top milk (7% fat), 3 ounces of a 15% sugar solution, and 2 ounces of lime water. This mixture provided a nutrient content of casein, 1.1%; fat, 4.7%; sugar, 6.2%; and 21.7 kcal/oz. Meigs argued in favor of his formulation on the basis that this preparation was simple and that multiple formulations that could lead to errors were unnecessary as the infant advanced in age. Although Meigs's formula closely resembled human milk, it was not widely popularized in part because sweetened condensed milk (Gail Borden, 1856) had become available.

Protein quality, as well as quantity, must be considered in determining the nitrogen and amino acid needs of infants. Protein quality refers to the relative nutritional adequacy of the protein source in the infant's diet. The quality of a protein depends on its ability to supply sufficient essential amino acids to maintain body structure and function, and growth. A protein source is evaluated on the chemical analysis of its nitrogen and amino acid content; it also includes biologic tests such as nitrogen balance and the protein efficiency ratio, which assesses weight gain in relation to protein consumption.

The concept of the limiting amino acid is important to determine the nutritional quality of a protein on the basis of its constituent amino acids. In general, all amino acids must be provided simultaneously at the intracellular sites of protein synthesis. If deficits occur, rates of protein synthesis will be limited by the amino acid present in the least concentration relative to tissue needs. In this context, the amino acid profile for the ideal dietary protein for infants has been established by the Food and Agriculture Organization/World Health Organization and is based on the essential amino acid pattern of

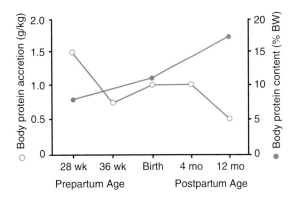

Figure 2: Body protein accretion in infancy.

human milk (Figure 3).[21] It is evident, however, that the amino acid content of food sources composed of high quality proteins, e.g., eggs, cow milk and beef, more than meet the amino acid needs of older infants.

Methods to Determine Nutrient Needs

Nitrogen and amino acid needs in the infant are determined two ways: by research methods, such as nitrogen balance and whole body protein turnover; or by clinical methods, such as correlating rates of growth with actual nutrient intakes and measuring individual proteins and amino acids, or their metabolites, in the body.

Research Methods and Concepts

Nitrogen balance determines how much dietary nitrogen is retained by the infant after obligatory urinary, fecal and other miscellaneous losses have been measured.[22] The protein content of food is estimated by chemical analysis for its nitrogen content, assuming that nitrogen accounts for 16% of protein by weight. The nitrogen balance technique has its limitations. In general, dietary intakes are overestimated and excretory losses are underestimated, leading to falsely elevated nitrogen balances. Furthermore, the variability of nitrogen balance among individuals averages 15%, and may lead to wide ranges in "requirement" values. Factors that contribute to the variability of nitrogen balance among individuals include alterations in the quality and quantity of dietary protein and energy sources; the nutritional status of the individual; the

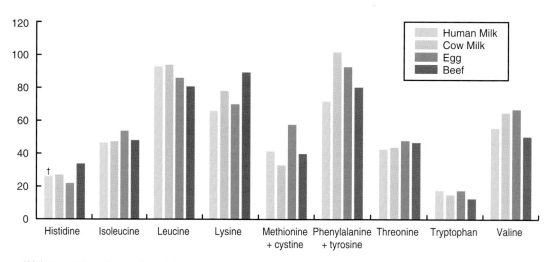

†Values expressed as mg/g protein

Figure 3: Amino acid profiles of high quality proteins. (Adapted from reference 21.)

variability in growth rates; hormonal factors such as insulin; growth hormone and insulin-like growth factors; and the presence or absence of disease.

More recently, protein needs of the infant have been estimated from whole body protein turnover studies using stable isotope techniques.[23, 24] In these studies, the ^{15}N or ^{13}C enrichments of amino acids, urinary urea or ammonia are measured during the oral or intravenous administration of ^{15}N or ^{13}C-labeled amino acids. Net protein retention can be calculated from the differences between the rates of body protein synthesis and breakdown estimated during the administration of the isotopically labeled amino acid. The kinetic isotope technique has limitations similar to those identified for nitrogen balance, as well as additional assumptions and errors inherent in the methods. Despite these problems, the kinetic isotope technique serves as an additional method to corroborate the findings of the nitrogen balance studies.

Clinical Measurements of Protein Adequacy

Growth rates of infants with measured amounts of formula consumption have been monitored to assess the adequacy of their dietary protein intakes in relation to their protein needs.[25-31] Although this technique permits a general assessment of dietary protein adequacy, it has several limitations. Growth studies require a large

number of individuals who can be followed for extended periods. Such studies assume that growth occurs at a constant rate, although variations in length and weight velocities are known to occur. Bias may be introduced because the participants are a generally healthy group of infants, rather than a group who is failing to thrive. With participant self-selection, correlations between linear growth rates or weight gains and dietary intakes may be difficult to ascertain due to the heterogeneity of the population studied. The measurement of formula consumption and dietary nutrient intakes provides an overestimate of "requirements," because the nutrients being consumed are not present in limiting amounts. If there is failure to thrive, identifying the limiting nutrient may be difficult because of the number of nutrients being monitored.

In the clinical setting, selected laboratory tests such as BUN and urinary nitrogen or urea excretion may be useful to determine dietary protein adequacy.[25-28] BUN concentrations serve as a useful predictor of how much dietary protein is taken in by the infant. Concentrations less than 1.2 mmol/L reflect a low intake of dietary nitrogen. Conversely, high BUN values greater than 7 mmol/L may be found in infants who receive feedings in which 20% or more of their energy content is derived from protein. However, high BUN values also may reflect dehydration in the presence of low dietary protein intakes or protein intakes of poor quality, thereby confounding the interpretation of the infant's dietary intake. Urinary nitrogen or urea excretion also correlates well with dietary nitrogen intake. Urinary urea accounts for 80% or more of the total nitrogen excreted by the well-fed infant. In individuals with low intakes of dietary protein, the proportion of urea nitrogen relative to total nitrogen may fall to 50%. However, the difficulties encountered in collecting timed urine samples from infants make this method impractical in the clinical setting and preclude its usefulness in assessing the adequacy of dietary protein intakes.

Serum concentrations of amino acids, or ratios among selected amino acids, may be used to assess the quality of the dietary protein source. Plasma amino acid patterns respond promptly to alterations in dietary protein intake. Low protein intakes are associated with an increased ratio of nonessential to essential amino acids. This is due to a fall in plasma lysine and branched-chain amino acids and a concomitant rise in glycine and serine levels.[32] However, using plasma amino acids to monitor dietary protein adequacy may be impractical because of the expense of these measurements. It has been suggested that preprandial plasma amino acid concentrations found in healthy, breast-fed infants serve as useful reference values to evaluate the adequacy of the infant's diet (Table 1).[33]

The hepatic transport proteins, albumin, transthyretin and retinol-binding protein, are used routinely to assess the protein status of infants and their response to nutritional intervention (Table 2).[34-37] Depressed serum albumin levels reflect longstanding dietary protein inadequacy; transthyretin and retinol-binding protein more accurately reflect the immediate response of visceral protein metabolism to protein intake because of their short half-lives (two days and 10 hours, respectively). However, other dietary factors such as energy intake and inflammation influence the serum concentrations of transthyretin and retinol-binding protein in infants (Figure 4).[38, 39] Nevertheless, these plasma proteins serve as useful indicators of the infant's response to nutritional rehabilitation during illnesses.

Amino Acid	Plasma Concentrations (µmol/L)		
	Mean	±SD	95% Confidence Interval
Threonine	133	30	70 - 210
Valine	155	31	90 - 220
Leucine	111	27	50 - 170
Isoleucine	58	15	30 - 90
Lysine	156	35	80 - 230
Methionine	36	7	20 - 50
Cystine	52	8	30 - 70
Histidine	76	20	30 - 190
Phenylalanine	46	11	20 - 70
Tyrosine	79	19	40 - 120
Tryptophan	60	19	20 - 100
Aspartic acid	28	11	0 - 50
Asparagine	48	15	20 - 80
Serine	159	78	0 - 330
Glutamic acid	134	51	20 - 240
Glutamine	496	166	140 - 850
Proline	201	56	80 - 320
Citrulline	14	4	10 - 20
Glycine	226	70	80 - 380
Alanine	386	123	120 - 650
Ornithine	77	37	0 - 160
Arginine	95	25	40 - 150
Cysteine/cystine	153	25	100 - 210
Taurine	84	39	0 - 170

Table 1: Protein amino acid concentrations in breast-fed term infants. (Adapted from reference 33.)

Historically, the role of protein in infant feeding was not an issue except for the presence of curd. Thomas Rotch pointed out that curds were difficult for the infant to digest, and Abraham Jacobi advocated the addition of cereals to milk to prevent the formation of large casein curds. Thomas S. Southworth and Oscar M. Schloss

Number of Infants	Gestational Age (wk)	Postpartum Age (wk)	Weight (kg)	Transthyretin (mg/dl)	Retinol Binding Protein (mg/dl)
50	Term	Birth	NA	12.8 ± 4.2	2.1 ± 0.6
31	37 - 40	Birth	NA	12.0 ± 3.9	2.3 ± 0.8
37	34 - 37	Birth	NA	8.8 ± 2.3	1.8 ± 0.5
10	AGA, 38 ± 4	4 ± 5	3.0 ± 0.8	9.1 ± 3.7	1.6 ± 0.5
15	SGA, 35 ± 4	5 ± 6	2.2 ± 0.5	8.3 ± 2.9	1.8 ± 0.6

Table 2: Serum transthyretin and retinol binding protein concentrations in infants. Values expressed as mean ± SD; NA = information not available. (Adapted from references 34-37.)

demonstrated that there were two types of curd: soft curds derived from fat and large hard curds derived from casein. Joseph G. Brennemann contended that the physical state of the casein curd was the important factor related to protein digestibility. This observation ultimately led to the process of homogenation.

Estimates of Protein and Amino Acid Needs in Infants
Enteral Protein Needs

Currently, human milk is considered to be the gold standard with respect to the protein and amino acid needs of infants. Human milk is the ideal food for the infant. However, the protein content of human milk is lower than that of cow milk and contains only 9 g/L of true protein and 2 g/L of protein equivalents from nonprotein nitrogen. Assuming an infant of average weight of 4 kg consumes 750 g/d of human milk, the true protein intake averages 1.7 $g \cdot kg^{-1} \cdot d^{-1}$ and the intake of protein equivalents from nonprotein nitrogen averages 0.4 $g \cdot kg^{-1} \cdot d^{-1}$. This low protein intake is offset by the high protein quality of human milk because of its unique protein and amino acid composition. Whey proteins, as opposed to casein proteins, are the major constituents of human milk. Human whey proteins are unique because of their high cystine content, their high cystine:methionine ratio, and their low aromatic amino acid content. Although concern has been raised about the low protein intake of breast-fed infants, human milk protein consumption satisfies the healthy infant's requirements for the maintenance, function and growth of body protein stores, without amino acid or solute excess and their associated metabolic complications.[40]

The estimates of protein needs during infancy have been derived by the factorial method, which takes into consideration nitrogen losses through urine, feces and miscellaneous tissues. The estimates of protein needs are thought to be 1.98 $g \cdot kg^{-1} \cdot d^{-1}$ during the first month of life; they then decrease rapidly to 1.18 $g \cdot kg^{-1} \cdot d^{-1}$ by four to five months of age and remain at this level until one year of age.[22] Although the protein intakes of breast-fed infants during the first two months of life approximate the values estimated by the factorial method, protein intakes between two and six months of age generally are less. These estimates also are lower than the current Recommended Dietary Allowances for protein, the latter averaging 2.2 $g \cdot kg^{-1} \cdot d^{-1}$ between birth and six months of age, 1.6 $g \cdot kg^{-1} \cdot d^{-1}$ between six months and one year of age, and 1.2 $g \cdot kg^{-1} \cdot d^{-1}$ between one and two years of age.[41]

In the last ten years, concerns have been raised that protein intakes of formula-fed infants are excessive, particularly at weaning.[25-31, 42-45] Dietary protein intakes of formula-fed infants are two- to three-fold higher than breast-fed infants of the same age. This high protein intake is thought to adversely affect the metabolic indices of protein utilization, including blood urea nitrogen and plasma amino acid concentrations.[46-48] The alterations in dietary protein utilization are the result of the quantity of protein consumed as opposed to qualitative differences in the casein and whey fractions of milk.[31] As a result, recommendations have been made to reduce the protein content of infant formulas. Nevertheless, one possible risk of lowering the total protein content of cow milk formulas is the inadequate intake of

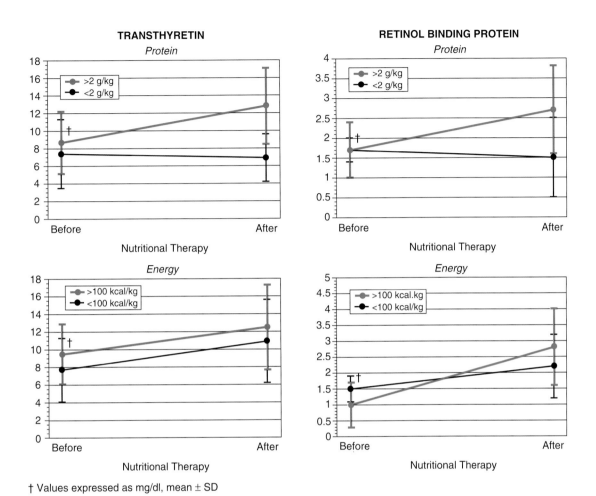

† Values expressed as mg/dl, mean ± SD

Figure 4: Influence of dietary protein and energy intakes on transthyretin and retinol-binding protein in infants. (Adapted from reference 38.)

tryptophan, the first limiting amino acid in cow milk.[30] Under these conditions, however, the addition of free tryptophan to cow milk preparations may result in a biochemical profile that more closely resembles that of the breast-fed infant.

Estimates of amino acid needs during infancy have been determined from studies in which variable levels of individual amino acids were administered to infants while monitoring nitrogen balance, growth rates, and biochemical measures of protein utilization. In addition, they have measured the amount of individual amino acids consumed by normally growing infants fed a variety of formulas.[21, 30, 41] When expressed per kilogram of body weight, the need for each essential amino acid declines progressively with increasing age. The requirements for essential amino acids decrease much more extensively than do those for total protein. In general, the proportion of total protein needs represented by essential amino acids decreases from 43% in infants to 36% in older children, and to 19% in adults. The nonessential nitrogen component of protein derived from nonessential amino acids is considered equally important. Supplementing protein-deficient diets with nonessential nitrogen restores positive nitrogen balance and promotes growth in infants.[49] Some nonessential amino acids such as glycine become "essential" to meet the needs of growth, especially in young infants.[50] Experts have proposed that the amino

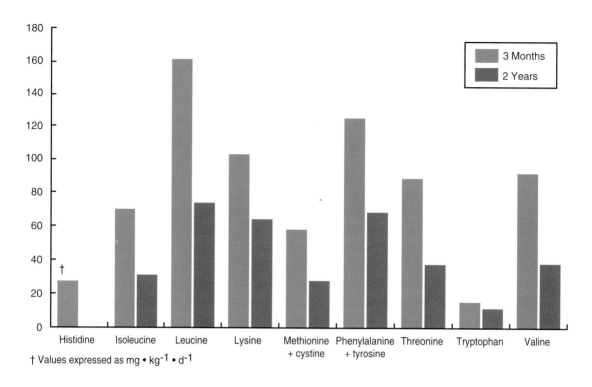

Figure 5: Estimates of amino acid requirements of infancy. (Adapted from reference 21.)

acid requirements for infants be met by amino acid consumption from a high-quality reference protein that is specific to the age group and that supports satisfactory growth (Figure 5).[21, 41]

Parenteral Protein Needs

Parenteral nutrition frequently is essential in the nutritional care of infants with intractible diarrhea, short bowel syndrome, congenital anomalies of the gastrointestinal tract, or severe malnutrition.[51] Infants with these disorders generally have specialized nutrient needs and greater nutrient requirements than older children and adults. For these reasons, parenteral nutrition in infants presents a number of challenges that are unique to this age group.

The use of parenteral nutrition in infants is determined by several factors, including the inability to meet nutrient needs of the infant by the enteral route and the duration of time before enteral refeeding can be established. If the infant's nutritional requirements cannot be met by the enteral route, then parenteral nutrition may be used to supplement or provide the sole source of nutrient intake. If adequate enteral nutrition cannot be established within three to four days, parenteral nutrition may be justified. Other factors include the infant's pre-existing nutritional status and underlying disease process. In general, the estimated survival time of healthy infants subjected to complete starvation is one and one-half months. If malnutrition and disease coexist, the rapid deterioration of the infant's nutritional status, when there is inadequate nutrient intake, can have profound effects on morbidity and mortality. Instituting parenteral nutritionas early as possible, if clinically warranted, may provide substantial benefit.

Meeting the protein needs of infants who receive parenteral nutrition is a major challenge. Protein requirements peak in the young, growing infant and decline with age. Protein precursors are needed for both tissue formation and the synthesis of enzymes, hormones, neurotransmitters and bile salts. Although most of the information pertaining to protein requirements in pediatric parenteral nutrition have been obtained from studies of preterm infants, the same principles are believed to apply to older infants.

The nitrogen source in parenteral solutions is derived from synthetically-manufactured crystalline amino acids. Although the amount of nitrogen retained generally is related to the level of nitrogen intake, an amino acid intake of 2 to 3 g·kg⁻¹·d⁻¹ results in nitrogen retention comparable to that observed in enterally-fed infants. The efficient use of protein can be best achieved when 150 to 200 nonprotein kilocalories per gram of nitrogen are administered concomitantly. The current use of crystalline amino acid solutions has solved the problem of poor nitrogen utilization and hyperammonemia associated with the administration of protein hydrolysates. Furthermore, the use of basic salts of histidine and substituting acetate for chloride in the lysine salts have eliminated the problem of hyperchloremic metabolic acidosis. However, metabolic complications associated with amino acids, including azotemia, hyperammonemia and acidosis, may occur with intravenous intakes of more than 4 g·kg⁻¹·d⁻¹.

The optimal quantity of each amino acid needed to meet the nutritional requirements of growing infants has yet to be determined. Certain amino acids considered to be nonessential in adults currently are regarded as semi-essential for infants. For example, cysteine, histidine and tyrosine are considered to be important additions for pediatric parenteral solutions.[51] Arginine is being considered as semi-essential for infants. Taurine is thought to help prevent nutrition-associated cholestasis.[52]

Currently, the composition of recommended amino acid solutions is based on the amino acid profiles of breast-fed infants and human milk.[33] Whether this combination of amino acids is best for the healthy or ill infant is unknown. One amino acid solution (Trophamine, Kendall McGaw, Irvine, CA) is thought to be most suitable for use in infants because it supplies essential and nonessential amino acids in sufficient quantities to maintain normal plasma amino acid profiles, promote superior weight gain and optimize nitrogen retention.[54] It also contains taurine to reduce the risk of parenteral nutrition-associated cholestasis. Furthermore, the addition of cysteine hydrochloride to this solution lowers the pH of the solution and allows the addition of extra calcium and

phosphorus without the risk of precipitation.[54] This feature is important because of the increased mineral needs of the rapidly growing infant.

Deficiency

Kwashiorkor is the clinical syndrome that results from dietary protein deficiency. Kwashiorkor develops in infants fed a low-protein, high-carbohydrate diet for prolonged periods, or may be precipitated by acute episodes of infections during periods of chronic protein-energy malnutrition (marasmus). Infants less than one year of age are at increased risk for developing malnutrition secondary to protein deficiency. Although typically found in developing countries, this type of malnutrition is encountered frequently in hospitals in developed countries. The prevalence of kwashiorkor in hospitalized, nutritionally-at-risk infants may be as high as 33%.[55] Kwashiorkor in the hospitalized infant most often results from gastrointestinal disorders such as infectious gastroenteritis or cystic fibrosis. However, primary protein deficiency may result from inappropriate feeding practices such as overdiluting formulas, feeding homemade formulas with inappropriate composition, feeding milk-free diets low in protein, prolonged breast-feeding without adequate supplementation, or parental neglect.

The classic features of kwashiorkor include irritability, edema, ascites, hypoproteinemia, hypoalbuminemia; it can also cause skin abnormalities such as hyperpigmentation, hyperkeratosis, desquamation and ulcerated lesions. The hair becomes sparse, depigmented and is plucked easily from the scalp. The cheeks become prominent, leading to a "moon-face" appearance. Hepatomegaly due to fatty infiltrates of the liver is evident. Intestinal fat malabsorption may be severe and prolonged. Carbohydrate malabsorption is variable, although lactose intolerance is commonplace. Anthropometric measurements such as weight may not reflect nutritional deficits due to subcutaneous fat stores and the presence of peripheral edema.

Serum albumin concentrations are the most frequently monitored laboratory values to make the diagnosis of kwashiorkor. Serum albumin is a sensitive indicator of the protein status of the body.

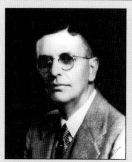

William C. Rose Ph.D.

(1887-1985) took his degree at Yale under Mendel. Rose discovered the essential amino acid threonine and was the first to determine the amino acid requirements of normal adults. He served as Chairman of Biochemistry at the University of Illinois from 1922-1954 and trained 58 Ph.D. candidates. J. Nutr. 111, 1311-1320, 1981 (Photo courtesy of NLM)

Depressed albumin levels can result in an increased risk of infection, prolonged hospital stay, increased morbidity particularly after surgery and increased mortality. Serum transthyretin and retinol-binding protein levels also are depressed in the acutely malnourished state; however, their measurements are more useful when used to assess the adequacy of the diet during refeeding (Figure 4).[56] Other laboratory findings of protein deficiency include reduced hemoglobin and hematocrit levels indicating anemia; depressed lymphocyte counts, particularly the T-cell subclass; and altered serum electrolytes including hyponatremia, hypokalemia and a reduction of serum bicarbonate.

The treatment of kwashiorkor includes first managing the dehydration and acute infection, followed by providing an adequate dietary intake and treating or correcting the underlying problem. The goal of nutritional therapy in kwashiorkor is to achieve maximal weight gain within the shortest time in a safe manner. In general, establishing adequate dietary intake by the oral route is the safest method to refeed the infant. However, in younger and more severely affected infants, voluntary refeeding is difficult to accomplish. In this setting, the infant with kwashiorkor can be refed enterally by a nasogastric tube that permits gradual but steady increases in nutrient intakes. Continuous milk feedings are useful because the volume or concentration of nutrients in the formula does not exceed the limited digestive and absorptive capacity of the intestinal tract. Bolus feedings can be instituted once adequate weight gain is in progress.

The choice of macronutrients in the diet should reflect the alterations in gut function. Whole protein of high quality may be used, which provides approximately 8 to 13% of the total energy intake; in most settings, a protein hydrolysate is chosen because of the combination of nutrients in commercial preparations that meet the functional needs of the gut. A mixture of long and medium chain triglycerides will reduce the likelihood of steatorrhea. Lactose intolerance should be assumed and a lactose-free feeding that provides complex polymers of glucose should be given.

Initial dietary intakes should be low, unless gastrointestinal tolerance has been established. In the setting of severe kwashiorkor, fluids cannot provide sufficient nutrients because volumes greater than 100 to 120 cc·kg^{-1}·d^{-1} compromise the clinical status of the child. Under these conditions, the concentration of individual nutrients such as energy may be increased in a step-wise fashion from 0.67 to 1.0 kcal/cc to optimize nutrient intake while restricting fluid load.

Most infants with kwashiorkor will require inordinately high nutrient intakes to achieve catch-up growth in weight and length. Maximal rates of weight gain have been seen in infants receiving protein and energy intakes of 4 to 5 g·kg^{-1}·d^{-1} and 200 kcal·kg^{-1}·d^{-1}, although average weight gains of 60 g/d can be accomplished with energy intakes of 150 to 175 kcal·kg^{-1}·d^{-1}. The formula most frequently used to calculate daily protein and energy needs for catch-up growth is the following:

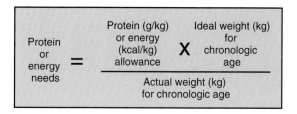

The infant's ideal weight is determined from the weight identified at the fiftieth percentile for chronologic age on the NCHS growth chart. Alternatively, higher or lower percentile values for weight may be used if the premorbid growth curve of the infant is known. Actual intakes are derived from the Recommended Dietary Allowances for infants less than two years of age and average 1.8 to 2.0 g·kg⁻¹·d⁻¹ for protein and 100 to 110 kcal·kg⁻¹·d⁻¹ for energy.

Tolerance to feeds is determined by monitoring fecal patterns. Increased stool output with refeeding is commonplace, but does not warrant a change in therapy unless the stools are persistently positive for glucose and organic acids. Occult bleeding is consistent with a degree of protein sensitization, but resolves rapidly. Wet stool weights between 150 and 200 g/d generally are acceptable in most infants. Stool number is of no value.

Careful attention must be given to the mineral status of the infant during refeeding. Hypokalemia and hypophosphatemia frequently complicate the refeeding process and may result in life-threatening consequences unless the deficiencies are corrected. Zinc supplementation (2 to 9 mg·kg⁻¹·d⁻¹) also may speed recovery by enhancing the rate of weight gain.

The clinical outcome of the infant with kwashiorkor is determined by the course and successful treatment of the underlying cause of the disorder. Although mortality may be high in kwashiorkor, once the initial fluid and electrolyte imbalances and infections are resolved, mortality should be lower than one percent.

Toxicity

Milk-Protein Allergy

Allergy to cow milk is the most common "toxic" response to dietary protein, but occurs in less than 8% of infants.[57] Approximately 30% of those infants with cow milk protein allergy also have sensitivity to soy proteins. A family history of atopy may be found in 60% of infants with milk protein sensitivity. The pathogenesis of this syndrome has not been explained, although an immunologic mechanism is suspected.

> *Biochemistry, research, and surveys are not sufficient if nutrition and health care are to reach the grassroots - the individual in the home - where it is needed.*
> *Primary Health Care Pioneer*
> *The Selected Works of*
> *Cicely D. Williams*
> Naomi Baumslag, Editor
> World Federation of Public
> Health Associations and
> UNICEF

Cow milk protein allergy is apparent usually before six months of age with 75% of all infants having symptoms within the first two months of life. The clinical features include vomiting, diarrhea, colic, abdominal pain, failure to thrive, atopic dermatitis, bronchial wheezing and shock. Some infants may develop a malabsorptive syndrome characterized by diarrhea, fat and carbohydrate malabsorption and failure to thrive. A more subtle manifestation of milk protein allergy is the presence of occult intestinal bleeding with or without diarrhea, constipation, iron deficiency anemia, hypoproteinemia and hypoalbuminemia.[58, 59] Frank intestinal bleeding from sensitization to milk proteins is observed most commonly after severe bouts of acute infectious gastroenteritis or in infants with a family history of atopy.[60]

Although there are no laboratory tests that diagnose cow milk or soy protein allergy, a peripheral eosino-philia, depressed serum albumin and elevated IgE concentrations and positive stool guaiac are consistent with the allergy. Small bowel biopsies may show an intestinal lesion with shortening of villous height, lengthening of the crypts and increased intraepithelial lymphocytes. Colonic biopsies may demonstrate inflammation with eosinophilic infiltrates of the mucosa.

The diagnosis of milk protein allergy can be made when symptoms disappear after milk products are withdrawn from the diet, then recur when the milk product is reintroduced. Human milk serves as a preventive measure, although potential allergens may be transferred through maternal milk, thereby sensitizing the infant.[61] Soy formulas are preferred as an initial treatment choice because of their low cost, availability and palatability, although in severely sensitized infants, casein or whey protein hydrolysate formulas, meat-based formulas or amino acid preparations may be necessary. In general, milk challenges should be

Type	Defect	Dietary Treatment
Hyperphenylalaninemias Phenylketonuria Hyperphenylalaninemias Dihydropteridin Hereditary tyrosinemia Transient neonatal tyrosinemia	Phenylalanine hydroxylase Phenylalanine hydroxylase, tyrosine enzymes Cofactor Several enzymes of tyrosine metabolism p-OH-phenylpyruvate oxidase	↓ Phenylalanine ↓ Phenylalanine ↓ Phenylalanine; 5-OH-tryptophan supplement ↓ Tyrosine ↓ Phenylalanine, tyrosine; vitamin C supplement
Histidinemia	?	? Histidine
Maple syrup urine disease	Branched-chain ketoacid dehydrogenase complex	↓ Leucine, isoleucine, valine
Urea cycle defects Hereditary urea cycle defects Transient hyperammonemia of infancy	Ornithine transcarbamylase argininosuccinate synthetase, argininosuccinate lyase, arginase Several urea cycle enzymes	↓ Protein; ketoanalogues of essential amino acids, arginine supplements ↓ Protein; ketoanalogues of essential amino acids, arginine supplements

Table 3: Common inborn errors of amino acid and protein metabolism.

delayed until the infant is at least one year old and has not received milk for at least six months. However, infants with a mild reaction to cow milk protein may be rechallenged every four to six months to see if symptoms persist. Challenges should be performed in the office setting under appropriate observation by medical personnel. Appropriate equipment should be available to deal with the possibility that an immediate hypersensitivity reaction such as anaphylaxis or shock may occur. Tolerance to cow milk usually develops between one and three years of age.

Infantile Colic

Infantile colic is a syndrome in which an otherwise healthy and well-fed infant has paroxysms of irritability, fussing, or crying lasting for a total of more than three hours per day and occurring on more than three days in any one week. Spontaneous recovery often is observed at three to four months of age. The prevalence of infantile colic is estimated to range between 10 and 30%.

Although the etiology of colic is unknown, one of the theories is that milk protein sensitivity causes this disorder. Studies that support this argument demonstrate that a large proportion of formula-fed infants have symptomatic improvement with the removal of cow milk protein from the diet.[62] Others have shown in some breast-fed infants a relationship between the prevalence of colic and the mother's consumption of cow milk protein.[63] Nevertheless, epidemiologic studies document that the frequency of colic is similar among infants who are breast-fed, formula-fed or who receive a combination of both milk sources.[64] Furthermore, counciling parents has been shown to improve colic, even more so than the removal of dietary cow milk protein, suggesting that inappropriate parent-infant interactions may lead to symptoms most commonly associated with infantile colic.[65] At the present time, the consensus is that hypersensitivity to cow's

Age (months)	Phenylketonuria	Tyrosinemia		Maple syrup urine disease			Urea cycle defects		
	PHE	TYR	MET	LEU	ISO	VAL	PRO	CIT	ARG
0-2	65	70	40	75	80	85	1050	180	550
2-6	50	70	40	75	80	85	—	—	—
6-12	40	40	20	—	—	—	—	—	—

Values expressed as mg·kg^{-1}·d^{-1}; PHE=phenylalanine, TYR=tyrosine, MET=methionine, LEU=leucine, ISO=isoleucine, VAL=valine, PRO=protein, CIT=citrulline, ARG=arginine

Table 4: Recommended amino acid and protein intakes in some inborn errors of metabolism of infancy. (Adapted from reference 66.)

milk protein is not the cause of colic in most healthy infants, although a clinical trial of a milk protein-free diet may be warranted in some infants.

Inborn Errors of Amino Acid Metabolism

Toxicity to individual amino acids is manifested as inborn errors of metabolism. The most common inborn errors include phenylketonuria and the hyperphenylalaninemias, histidinemia, disorders of branched-chain amino acids and disorders of urea cycle enzymes (Table 3). Most inborn errors of metabolism are associated with severe clinical manifestations. Mental retardation, seizures and other neurologic and behavioral manifestations such as irritability, hyperkinesis, hypertonicity, tremors and microcephaly are seen in the untreated patient. Many of the inborn errors of metabolism are fatal when metabolic complications such as hypoglycemia and hyperammonemia develop.

Nutritional therapy provides the mainstay for the treatment of children with inborn errors of metabolism.[66] (See Chapter 14, "Inborn Errors of Metabolism - Challange for the Twenty-First Century", Berry/Leslie). Specialized formulas are readily available for selected inborn errors of amino acid metabolism (see Appendix). For example, phenylketonuria can be treated by administering a formula that is phenylalanine-depleted and supplementing it with a standard infant formula and low-protein foods. The formula must be provided in amounts that maintain plasma phenylalanine concentrations within 3 to 9 mg/dL to optimize neurologic performance. In contrast, treatment of the urea cycle

disorder is accomplished by providing a limited amount of dietary protein with or without essential amino acid supplementation. Additional supplementation with citrulline or arginine may be necessary because of a relative insufficiency of these amino acids. Protein-free supplements also may be required to meet basic energy and micronutrient needs. Maple syrup urine disease, when unresponsive to pharmacologic doses of thiamine, is managed with a milk substitute free of branched-chain amino acids. Small amounts of branched-chain amino acids are required to achieve a near-normal concentration of all plasma amino acids and to avoid amino acid imbalances, which of themselves lead to potentially fatal outcomes. Protein and amino acid requirements have been estimated for selected inborn errors of metabolism (Table 4).

Global Perspectives of Protein Deficiency

Protein-energy malnutrition is a major nutritional problem in populations characterized by limited availability of food, poor environmental conditions favoring infections, ignorance of optimal feeding practices of childhood, and unstable socioeconomic and political circumstances. Although infants in such settings are capable of adapting to dietary deprivation, infections commonly precipitate kwashiorkor, further aggravating their protein deficiency. The mechanisms that account for this adverse outcome are not clear. Several explanations have been proposed, including: 1) the diversion of hepatic protein synthesis from synthesizing albumin and other transport proteins to producing

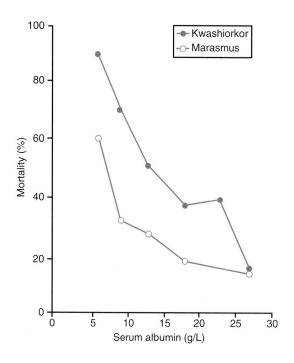

Figure 6: Relationship between mortality and serum albumin concentrations in children with protein-energy malnutrition. (Adapted from reference 69.)

acute phase reactants; 2) the acceleration of muscle protein catabolism associated with stress-mediated hormonal changes, i.e., increased cortisol and epinephrine levels; and 3) the enhancement of gluconeogenesis from amino acids to support the energy needs of the body.[67, 68] As a result of the infectious process, rapid protein loss ensues, amounting to as much as 2% of muscle protein per day during severe infections. The result is an increased mortality rate, an outcome that can be illustrated by the relationship between plasma albumin levels and rates of death in malnourished children (Figure 6).[69]

Although infections may precipitate protein deficiency, dietary protein insufficiency also predisposes the child to infections by altering the child's immune responsiveness. Dietary protein restriction has been shown to affect cell-mediated immunity by reducing the number of lymphocytes entering mitosis, and prolonging their cell cycle. The diminished production of

the cytokine, interleukin-1, by mononuclear cells also has been associated specifically with dietary protein deficiency. These defects in immune function can be reversed with adequate nutritional rehabilitation.

Breast-feeding has been advocated universally as the method of feeding infants from disadvantaged environments, regardless of the level of economic and social development of the country. Breast-feeding has a protective effect for the infant against a number of gastrointestinal and respiratory infections, including gastroenteritis, pneumonia, otitis media, bacteremia and meningitis.[70] Human milk contains a number of specific proteins, including lactoferrin, lysozyme and secretory IgA, that serve to protect the infant against infections; these indirectly influence the growth and development of the infant. Despite the lower concentration of protein in human milk, the amino acid composition of human milk proteins is thought to be optimal for normal infant growth and development.

Case Histories

Case #1: The patient is a four-week-old preterm infant born at 28 weeks' gestational age. His hospital course was complicated by hyaline membrane disease requiring prolonged ventilatory support and high concentrations of oxygen. Fluid intakes were limited to 90 ml·kg⁻¹·d⁻¹. The infant also had sepsis, but was on day six of appropriate antibiotic therapy. In order to maintain his nutritional status, the infant was given total parenteral nutrition by a "central" venous line. Protein intake by this route was estimated to be 2.5 g·kg⁻¹·d⁻¹. Energy intake (20% dextrose and 10% Intralipid) averaged 75 kcal·kg⁻¹·d⁻¹. Routine laboratory monitoring of this patient revealed a blood urea nitrogen (BUN) of 18.5 mmol/L (normal 7) and a triglyceride level of 3.50 mmol/L (normal 1.69). You have been consulted to explain these abnormalities and to recommend an appropriate treatment regimen.

Question: *What are protein and energy "requirements" versus "allowances" in the newborn infant and in children in general?*

Answer: *"Requirements" represent absolute values of nutrients that meet the metabolic need of the individuals. "Allowances" are estimates of nutrient needs of the body based on obligatory losses and the amount of the nutrient required to keep the individual in metabolic equilibrium. Absolute* nutrient requirements are difficult to ascertain. Recommended daily allowances for protein and energy in bottle-fed infants less than one year of age are 1.5 to 2.0 g·kg⁻¹·d⁻¹ and 98 to 108 kcal·kg⁻¹·d⁻¹.

Question: *Why are the BUN and triglyceride concentrations elevated? What metabolic pathways may be involved?*

Answer: *BUN and triglycerides are elevated because of an inadequate supply of nonprotein energy source. Excess protein is catabolized via gluconeogenesis and utilized for glucose formation. Nitrogen from endogenous protein breakdown is converted to urea because nitrogen is toxic; however, urea cannot be excreted quickly by the infant's immature kidney. Serum triglycerides are not metabolized in the face of inadequate dietary protein and energy intakes due to inadequate synthesis of the enzyme lipoprotein lipase.*

Question: *What role does the theory of the limiting nutrient have in this case?*

Answer: *Energy is a limiting nutrient for protein metabolism.*

Question: *What treatment program would you institute?*

Answer: *Liberalize intravenous fluids and supply additional nonprotein energy as glucose. These changes result in resolution of the metabolic disturbances.*

Case #2: A three-month-old infant was admitted for evaluation of failure to thrive. On admission, the infant's weight was 4.08 kg. Poor weight gain was noted since one month of age. The infant was breast-fed for the first two months of life, then supplemented with a soy protein formula. On physical examination the infant appeared proportionate in size, despite poor weight gain. Laboratory screening revealed a blood hemoglobin of 80 g/L (normal 110) and serum albumin of 30 g/L (normal 35). A sweat test was consistent with the diagnosis of cystic fibrosis. You have been consulted to explain the apparent discrepancy between the clinical appearance of this child and the laboratory findings, and to provide recommendations for therapeutic management.

Question: *What is the nutritional diagnosis in this infant? What other physical findings help to make this diagnosis?*

Answer: *The nutritional diagnosis is kwashiorkor. The etiology is due to a protein deficiency rather than energy.*

Clinical findings include edema, hypoproteinemia, hypoalbuminemia, and skin rashes; these are in contrast to general wasting seen in marasmus.

Question: *Why do you think this child failed to gain weight while receiving human milk and a soy formula? What is the relationship between these milk sources and protein quantity and quality?*

Answer: *Human milk contains 9 mg/L of protein nitrogen and may have been limited in quantity rather than overall quality. The quality of a protein is assessed by its amino acid composition. Soy formulas have trypsin inhibitors. In an infant who has limited trypsin due to pancreatic insufficiency, these formulas often do not support growth.*

Question: *What would happen if you treated this child's anemia with oral iron therapy?*

Answer: *Anemia would not resolve with iron therapy alone in a protein-deficient patient because hemoglobin must be synthesized from proteins to carry iron.*

Question: *What therapeutic approach would you take with this child and what laboratory measurements would you obtain to monitor the infant's progress?*

Answer: *Change the infant's formula to a casein- or whey-based preparation and provide pancreatic enzyme replacement. Albumin can be measured to monitor the infant's progress, but the turnover time is ten days. More rapidly turning-over proteins such as transthyretin or retinol-binding protein may reflect recovery earlier.*

Case #3: A nine-month-old infant was admitted because of recurrent vomiting, diarrhea, pallor, and weight loss. The infant was breast-fed for the first six months of life, then weaned to whole cow milk. On physical examination the infant was irritable and pale; minimal weight loss was apparent. Laboratory examination revealed a blood hemoglobin of 100 g/L (normal 110), a serum albumin of 30 g/L (normal 35) and guaiac-positive stools. An upper gastrointestinal x-ray evaluation was negative for gastroesophageal reflux and pyloric outlet obstruction. Serum electrolytes failed to demonstrate a metabolic disorder. While in the hospital, the infant was noted to have projectile vomiting and worsening diarrhea. As an afterthought, the infant's mother commented that she was fed goat milk as an infant.

Question: What is the nutritional diagnosis in this child? What etiologic factor is thought to cause this problem?

Answer: The diagnosis is cow milk protein allergy. The etiologic factor is thought to be due to the presence of β-lactoglobulin, a protein present in cow milk but not in human milk.

Question: How does this clinical problem relate to lactose intolerance? In what other situations might you see this problem and lactose intolerance combined?

Answer: Cow milk protein allergy is a clinical syndrome thought to be IgE-mediated. Carbohydrate intolerance is a clinical syndrome related to altered intestinal absorptive

capacity or the genetic background of the individual. The latter is not IgE-mediated and is not an "allergy." Both of these entities may be seen in severe diarrheal disease caused by rotavirus.

Question: What is the relationship between cow milk, soy formula, and goat milk in this clinical entity?

Answer: There may be cross-reactivity among cow, soy and goat milk proteins, insofar as 30% of children with cow milk sensitivity will be "allergic" to soy protein.

Question: How would you treat this infant?

Answer: Change the infant's formula to a protein hydrolysate preparation or provide human milk. In severely sensitized infants, an amino acid/dipeptide preparation may be necessary.

Historical Perspective...

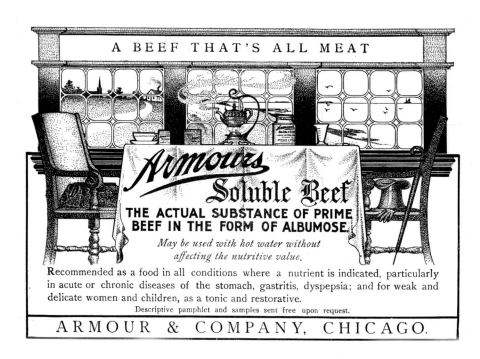

References

1. Miller SA. Nutrition in the neonatal development of protein metabolism. *Fed Proc.* 1970;29:1497-1502.

2. Motil KJ. Development of the gastrointestinal tract. In: Wyllie R, Hyams J, eds. *Pediatric Gastrointestinal Disease. Pathophysiology, Diagnosis, Management.* Philadelphia: WB Saunders Co; 1993:3-16.

3. Grand RJ, Watkins JB, Torti FM. Development of the human gastrointestinal tract. A review. *Gastroenterology.* 1976;70:790-810.

4. Euler AR, Byrne WJ, Cousins LM, Ament ME, Walsh JH. Increased serum gastrin concentrations and gastric acid hyposecretion in the immediate newborn period. *Gastroenterology.* 1977;72:1271-1273.

5. Antonowicz I, Lebenthal E. Developmental patterns of small intestine enterokinase and disaccharidase activities in the human fetus. *Gastroenterology.* 1977;72:1299-1303.

6. Hadorn B, Zoppi G, Shmerling DH, Prader A, McIntyre I, Anderson CM. Quantitative assessment of exocrine pancreatic function in infants and children. *J Pediatr.* 1968;73:39-50.

7. Heringova A, Koldovsky O, Jirsova V, Uher J, Noack R, Friedrich M, Schenk G. Proteolytic and peptidase activities of the small intestine of human fetuses. *Gastroenterology.* 1966;51:1023-1027.

8. Levin RJ, Koldovsky O, Hoskova J, Jirsova V, Uher J. Electrical activity across human foetal small intestine associated with absorption processes. *Gut.* 1968;9:206-213.

9. Fomon SJ. *Nutrition of normal infants.* St. Louis: Mosby; 1993:121-139.

10. Walker WA, Isselbacher KJ. Uptake and transport of macromolecules by the intestine. Possible role in clinical disorders. *Gastroenterology.* 1974;67:531-550.

11. Axelsson I, Jacobsson I, Lindberg T, Polberger S, Bendediktsson B, Räihä NC. Macromolecular absorption in preterm and term infants. *Acta Paediatr Scand.* 1989; 78:532-537.

12. Aynsley-Green A. Hormones and postnatal adaptation to enteral nutrition. *J Pediatr Gastroenterol Nutr.* 1983;2: 418-427.

13. Lucas A, Aynsley-Green A, Bloom SR. Gut hormones and the first meals. *Clin Sci.* 1981;60:349-353.

14. Lucas A, Bloom SR, Aynsley-Green A. Gut hormones and "minimal enteral feeding." *Acta Paediatr Scand.* 1986;75:719-723.

15. Räihä NC, Suihkonen J. Development of urea-synthesizing enzymes in human liver. *Acta Pediatr Scand.* 1968;57:121-124.

16. Räihä NC, Lindros KO. Development of some enzymes involved in gluconeogenesis in human liver. *Ann Med Exp Biol Fenn.* 1969;47:146-150.

17. Edelmann CM Jr, Wolfish NM. Dietary influence on renal maturation in premature infants. *Pediatr Res.* 1968; 2:421-422.

18. Brodehl J, Gellissen K. Endogenous renal transport of free amino acids in infancy and childhood. *Pediatrics.* 1968;42:395-404.

19. Widdowson EM. Growth and composition of the fetus and newborn. In: Assali NS, ed. *Biology of Gestation,* Vol II. New York: Academic Press Inc; 1968:23.

20. Widdowson EM, Southgate DAT, Hey EN. Body composition of the fetus and infant. In: Visser HKA, ed. *Nutrition and Metabolism of the Fetus and Infant.* The Hague Martinus Nijhoff Publishers; 1979:169-174.

21. *Energy and Protein Requirements. Food and Agriculture Organization/World Health Organization.* Geneva, World Health Organization: 1985. WHO Tech. Rpt. No. 724.:121.

22. Fomon SJ. Requirements and recommended dietary intakes of protein during infancy. *Pediatr Res.* 1991;30: 391-395.

23. Pencharz PB, Steffee WP, Cochran W, Scrimshaw NS, Rand WM, Young VR. Protein metabolism in human neonates: nitrogen-balance studies, estimated obligatory loss of nitrogen and whole-body turnover nitrogen. *Clin Sci Mol Med.* 1977;52:485-498.

24. Pencharz PB, Masson M, Desgranges F, Papageorgiou A. Total-body protein turnover in human premature neonates: effects of birthweight, intra-uterine nutritional status and diet. *Clin Sci.* 1981;61:207-215.

25. Lönnerdal B, Chen C-L. Effects of formula protein level and ratio on infant growth, plasma amino acids, and serum trace elements. I. Cow's milk formula. *Acta Paediatr Scand.* 1990;79:257-265.

26. Lönnerdal B, Chen C-L. Effects of formula protein level and ratio on infant growth, plasma amino acids, and serum trace elements. II. Follow-up formula. *Acta Paediatr Scand.* 1990;79:266-273.

27. Axelsson IE, Jacobsson I, Räihä NC. Formula with reduced protein content: Effects on growth and protein metabolism during weaning. *Pediatr Res.* 1988;24:297-301.

28. Räihä N, Minoli I, Moro G. Milk protein intake in the term infant. *Acta Paediatr Scand.* 1986;75:881-886.

29. Janas LM, Picciano MF, Hatch T. Indices of protein metabolism in term infants fed human milk, whey-predominant formula, or cow's milk formula. *Pediatrics.* 1985;75:775-784.

30. Hanning RM, Paes B, Atkinson SA. Protein metabolism and growth of term infants in response to a reduced-protein, 40:60 whey:casein formula with added tryptophan. *Am J Clin Nutr.* 1992;56:1004-1011.

31. Janas LM, Picciano MF, Hatch T. Indices of protein metabolism in term infants fed either human milk or formulas with reduced protein concentration and various whey/casein ratios. *J Pediatr.* 1987;110:838-848.

32. Alleyne GA, Hey RW, Picou DL. *Protein-energy malnutrition.* London: Edward Arnold Ltd; 1977:154.

33. Wu PY, Edwards N, Storm MC. Plasma amino acid patterns in normal term breast-fed infants. *J Pediatr.* 1986;109:347-349.

34. Giacoia GP, Watson S, West K. Rapid turnover transport proteins, plasma albumin, and growth in low birth weight infants. *J Parent Ent Nutr.* 1984;8:367-370.

35. Sasanow SR, Spitzer AR, Pereira GR, Heaf L, Watkins JB. Effect of gestational age upon prealbumin and retinol binding protein in preterm and term infants. *J Pediatr Gastroenterol Nutr.* 1986;5:111-115.

36. Vahlquist A, Rask L, Peterson A, Berg T. The concentration of retinol binding protein, prealbumin, and transferrin in the sera of newly delivered mothers and children of various ages. *Scand J Clin Lab Invest.* 1975;35:569-575.

37. Polberger SK, Fex GA, Axelsson IE, Räihä NC. Eleven plasma proteins as indicators of protein nutritional status in very low birth weight infants. *Pediatrics.* 1990; 86:916-921.

38. Helms RA, Dickerson RN, Ebbert ML. Retinol-binding protein and prealbumin: Useful measures of protein repletion in critically ill, malnourished infants. *J Pediatr Gastroenterol Nutr.* 1986;5:586-592.

39. Fleck A. Clinical and nutritional aspects of changes in acute-phase proteins during inflammation. *Proc Nutr Soc.* 1989;48:347-354.

40. Räihä NC. Milk protein quantity and quality and protein requirements during development. *Adv Pediatr.* 1989;36:347-368.

41. *Food and Nutrition Board/National Research Council Recommended Dietary Allowances,* 10th ed. Washington DC: National Academy of Sciences: 1989:66.

42. Lönnerdal B, Zetterstöm R. Protein content of infant formula—how much and from what age? *Acta Paediatr Scand.* 1988;77:321-325.

43. Beaton GH, Chery A. Protein requirements of infants: a re-examination of concepts and approaches. *Am J Clin Nutr.* 1988;48:1403-1412.

44. Axelsson IE, Räihä NC. Protein and energy during weaning. *Adv Pediatr.* 1992;39:405-440.

45. Fomon SJ, Sanders KD, Ziegler EE. Formulas for older infants. *J Pediatr.* 1990;116:690-696.

46. Axelsson I, Borulf S, Righand L, Räihä NC. Protein and energy intake during weaning. I. Effects on growth. *Acta Paediatr Scand.* 1987;76:321-327.

47. Axelsson I, Borulf S, Räihä NC. Protein and energy intake during weaning. II. Metabolic responses. *Acta Paediatr Scand.* 1987;76:457-462.

48. Axelsson I, Borulf S, Abildskov K, Heird W, Räihä NC. Protein and energy intake during weaning. III. Effects on plasma amino acids. *Acta Paediatr Scand.* 1988;77: 42-48.

49. Snyderman SE, Holt LE Jr, Dancis J, Roitman E, Boyer A, Balis ME. "Unessential" nitrogen: a limiting factor for human growth. *J Nutr.* 1962;78:57-72.

50. Jackson AA, Shaw JCL, Barber A, Golden MH. Nitrogen metabolism in preterm infants fed human donor breast milk: the possible essentiality of glycine. *Pediatr Res.* 1981;15:1454-1461.

51. Heird WC. Amino acid and energy needs of pediatric patients receiving parenteral nutrition. *Pediatr Clin N Am.* 1995;42:765-789.

52. Van Goudoever JB, Sulkers EJ, Timmerman M, Huijmans JG, Langer K, Carnielli VP, Sauer PJ. Amino acid solutions for premature infants during the first week of life: The role of N-acetyl-L-cysteine and N-acetyl-L-tyrosine. *JPEN.* 1994;18:404-409.

53. Howard D, Thompson DF. Taurine: an essential amino acid to prevent cholestasis in neonates? *Ann Pharmacother.* 1992;26:1390-1392.

54. Heird WC, Dell RB, Helms RA, Greene HL, Ament ME, Karna P, Storm MC. Amino acid mixture designed to maintain normal plasma amino acid patterns in infants and children requiring parenteral nutrition. *Pediatrics.* 1987;80:401-408.

55. Baker S. Protein-energy malnutrition in the hospitalized pediatric patient. In: Walker WA, Watkins JB, eds. *Nutrition in Pediatrics Basic Science and Clinical Application.* Boston: Little Brown and Co; 1985:171-181.

56. Georgieff MK, Sasanow SR. Nutritional assessment of the neonate. *Clin Perinatol.* 1986;13:73-89.

57. Halpern SR, Sellars WA, Johnson RB. Development of childhood allergy in infants fed breast, soy, or cow milk. *J Allergy Clin Immunol.* 1973;51:139-151.

58. Iacono G, Carroccio A, Cavataio F, Montalto G, Cantarero MD, Notarbartolo A. Chronic constipation as a symptom of cow milk allergy. *J Pediatr.* 1995;126: 34-39.

59. Wilson JF, Lahey ME, Heiner DC. Studies on iron metabolism. V. Further observations on cow's milk-induced gastrointestinal bleeding in infants with iron deficiency anemia. *J Pediatr.* 1974;84:335-344.

60. Ziegler EE, Fomon SJ, Nelson SE, Rebouche CJ, Edwards BB, Rogers RR, Lehman LJ. Cow milk feeding in infancy: further observations on blood loss from the gastrointestinal tract. *J Pediatr.* 1990;116:11-18.

61. Lake AM, Whitington PF, Hamilton SR. Dietary protein-induced colitis in breast-fed infants. *J Pediatr.* 1982;101:906-910.

62. Lothe L, Lindberg T, Jakobsson I. Cow's milk formula as a cause of infantile colic: a double brand study. *Pediatrics.* 1982;70:7-10.

63. Jakobsson I, Lindberg T. Cow's milk proteins cause infantile colic in breast-fed infants: a double blind crossover study. *Pediatrics.* 1983;71:268-271.

64. Thomas DW, McGilligan K, Eisenberg LD, Lieberman HM, Rissman EM. Infantile colic and type of milk feeding. *Am J Dis Child.* 1987;141:451-453.

65. Taubman B. Parental counseling compared with elimination of cow's milk or soy milk protein for the treatment of infant colic syndrome. A randomized trial. *Pediatrics.* 1958;81:756-761.

66. Caballero B. Dietary management of inborn errors of amino acid metabolism. *Clin Nutr.* 1985;4:85-94.

67. Beisel WR. Magnitude of the host nutritional responses to infection. *Am J Clin Nutr.* 1977;30:1236-1247.

68. Powanda MC. Changes in body balances of nitrogen and other key nutrients: description and underlying mechanisms. *Am J Clin Nutr.* 1977;30:1254-1268.

69. Waterlow JC. Protein-energy malnutrition. Challenges and controversies. *Proc Nutr Soc.* 1991;37:59-86.

70. Beaudry M, DuFour R, Marcoux S. Relation between infant feeding and infections during the first six months of life. *J Pediatr.* 1995;126:191-197.

Managing Dietary Carbohydrate Intolerance

Buford L. Nichols M.D.

Children's Nutrition Research Center,
Baylor College of Medicine, Department of Pediatrics,
Houston, Texas

Reviewed by James W. Hansen M.D., Ph.D., A. Wesley Burks M.D. and C. Lawrence Kien M.D., Ph.D.

Historical

Hans Helge, Chairman of Pediatrics, the Free University of Berlin and Chief of Pediatrics at the Kaiserin Victoria Children's Hospital: "In Germany, at the turn of the century, we had many infant patients with intestinal decomposition who had a death rate of approximately 20%. One of the leading German pediatricians who had to take care of these malnourished children was Heinrich Finkelstein. He was the first to recognize food intolerances in infants and found much opposition to his claim that carbohydrate intolerance existed in these patients and that the existing choices of carbohydrates for feeding these infants was very poor. From 1901 to 1918, Finkelstein was the head of The Infant Asylum and City Orphanage in Berlin. Under his leadership the mortality decreased from 50 to 10% in two years. In 1918, he became the Director at the Kaiser and Kaiserin Frederich Children's Hospital in Berlin, which still is affiliated with the University of Berlin. Finklestein had to leave Germany after 1933. He immigrated to Chile where he was the guest of his former students. He died from typhoid fever in 1942, at the age of 77. In the 1920s and 1930s, Finklestein's textbook was thought to be the "Bible of Pediatrics." He described many cases of young infants with "intestinal decomposition," all artificially fed from birth, who became progressively malnourished from chronic diarrhea. Finkelstein demonstrated that these patients could not tolerate 5% lactose in their feedings. He managed them by substituting 5% glucose oligosaccharides (partially malted starches) for lactose and many infants stopped having diarrhea and gained weight. Although the caloric intake was constant, weight loss occurred each time lactose was fed and weight was gained when glucose oligosaccharides were substituted. Another Berlin Chairman of Pediatrics (Adalbert Czerny, 1863-1941), believed that the diarrhea of the malnourished infant was the consequence of excess dietary fat. Using carefully designed feeding trials, Finklestein, working with L.F. Meyer (later Director of Pediatrics at Hadassah Municipal Hospital in Tel Aviv, Israel), was able to document that infants with intestinal decomposition gain weight on a fat-containing diet only if fed a glucose oligomer-containing formula.

Finklestein and Meyer also are recognized for their introduction of protein milk (German; Eiweissmilch). This, the first modular formula, was prepared by precipitating casein from skimmed cow's milk and washing the curds until free from lactose. With the modular formula feedings Finkelstein was able to stop "fermentative diarrhea," now called carbohydrate intolerance. Because the lactose was lost during preparation of protein milk, other carbohydrates could be added. Glucose oligosaccharide-containing modular formulas were well tolerated and diarrhea disappeared in one to three days, and most infants gained weight on these protein milk/glucose oligomer feedings. Approximately 10% of the infants with intestinal decomposition failed to tolerate protein milk, so Finkelstein fed them whole human milk. Finkelstein thought that cow's milk formula should be given to these children after four to six weeks on the protein milk/glucose oligomer diet. He thus appears to have first described the transient carbohydrate intolerance of malnourished infants" (from *Grand Rounds at Department of Pediatrics,* Baylor College of Medicine, January 19, 1983).

The Fate of Carbohydrates in the Diet

(L: carbo, pertaining to carbon-named because the elements are in a proportion to yield water (CHO)n) The major carbohydrates in the infant diet are few and simple in structure when compared to dietary lipids and proteins (Table 1).

Substrate Classifications:		
Chemical	Dietary	Enzyme
Lactose	milk sugar	Lactase-phlorizin
Sucrose	table sugar	Sucrase-isomaltase
Isomaltrose	dextrins	Sucrase-isomaltase
Maltrose	malt sugar	Maltase-glucoamaylase
Amylose	starch sugar	α Amylose
Amylopectin	starch sugar	β Amylose

Table 1: Metabolizable carbohydrates in infant diets.

Milk Sugar

Lactose *(L: saccharum lactis from Gr:, pertaining to milk)* or milk sugar is a disaccharide which, after hydrolysis, yields glucose *(Gr: sweet)* and galactose *(Gr:, pertaining to milk)* (Figure 1). In the small intestine, enzymatic *(Gr: leaven)* hydrolysis is carried out by a brush border lactase-phlorizin hydrolase, which is anchored to the luminal surface of the enterocyte. The associated phlorizin hydrolase, product of the same gene, serves to hydrolyze carbohydrates from membrane lipids. The two catalytic domains are homologous to each other and to similar glycosidase enzymes *(Gr: of yeast)* and bacteria.[1, 2, 3]

Table Sugar

Sucrose *(Gr:, a sweet juice from vegetable origin)*, or table sugar, is the most common disaccharide in the diet of the mature human. On hydrolysis it yields glucose and fructose *(L:, fruit)* (Figure 1). In the small intestine, enzymatic hydrolysis is carried out by a brush border sucrase-isomaltase hydrolase which is anchored to the luminal surface of the enterocyte. There is internal homology between the two parts of the enzyme and with a lysosomal hydrolase, which share the same active site.[1, 2, 3]

Starches

Sucrose and the starches are the most common carbohydrates in the post-weaning human diet (Figure 2). The starches are a mixture of two structurally different polysaccharides, amylose *(Gr:, starch)*, linear α-1-4-gluco-glucose polymers of about 300 units and amylopectin *(amylo+Gr:, congealed)*, with additional α-1-6-gluco-glucose links (about 4% of total) which result in a branched configuration of polymers of a thousand or more glucose units (Figure 1). The dietary starches have a mixture of approximately 25% amylose with amylopectin. The distinction is of nutritional significance because of the nature of the enzymatic hydrolysis.[1, 2, 4]

There are two families of amylase enzymes, but only α amylase is found in human salivary and pancreatic secretions. α amylase acts by hydrolysis of the internal 1-4 linkages of amylose and amylopectin. The enzyme bypasses the 1-6 linkages and produces linear dextrins *(L:, a mixture of products from the hydrolysis of starch which are dexterorotary in polarized light)* and branched isomaltose of about six glucose units. These products are not fermentable *(L:, leaven)* without additional enzymatic processing by β-amylase which hydrolyses the internal 1-4 and 1-6 linkages. The combined α and β-amylases produce di- and tri-saccharides (oligosaccharides) such as maltose *(Ger: malz sugar produced from starch by the action of malt)* and isomaltose *(Gr; , equal + maltose)* which are hydrolyzed to fermentable monosaccharides.

In mammals, this latter step is carried out by sucrase-isomaltase and maltase-glucoamylase. Sucrase makes up about 10% of the brush border membrane protein and accounts for 80% of the maltase activity. It splits both 1-4 (maltose) and 1-6 (isomaltose) glucosidic bonds. Maltase-glucoamylase makes up about 2% of the brush border membrane protein and accounts for the remaining maltase activity. It splits only the 1-4 oligosaccharide bonds. Glucoamylase enzyme substrate specificity is not fully documented, but is thought to be for glucose oligosaccharides produced by the amylase digestion (malting) of starches.[1, 3] Malted starches were first introduced into infant feeding formulas by Liebig[5] in 1866. These smaller glucose oligosaccharides, known as the dextrins, are of importance to contemporary infant feeding because they are added to formulas to bypass limited lactose digestibility and to reduce the luminal osmolar *(Gr; pushing)* load produced by smaller disaccharides.[6, 7]

There are carbohydrates in the diet that are poorly digested by the adult upper intestine. These are struc-

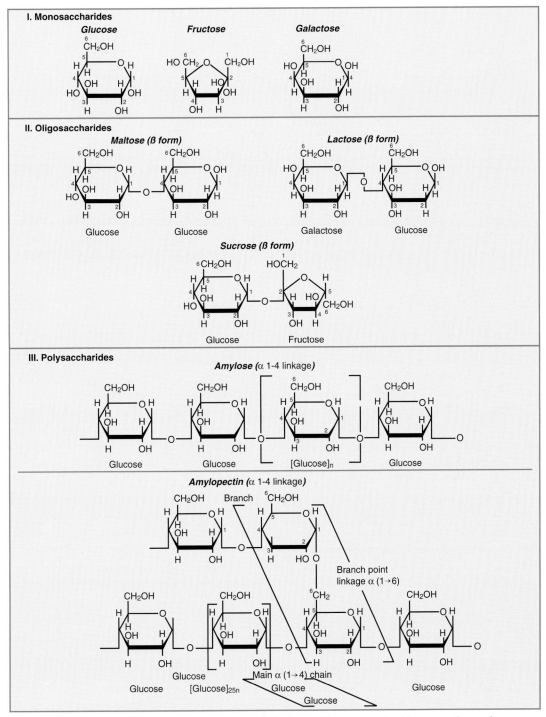

Figure 1: Chemical structure of the principal dietary carbohydrates. The monosaccharides are made up of pyranose rings and furanose rings with six and five members, respectively. The linkages in the oligosaccharides and polysaccharides are in an alpha or beta configuration. These are illustrated by maltose and lactose. Among the polysaccharides, amylose and amylopectin have alpha linkages and cellulose has a beta linkage similar to that found in lactose. Alpha-amylase cleaves amylose at the internal alpha linkages. Beta-amylase cleaves the reducing glucose sequentially. The reducing glucose is shown at the right of these diagrams.

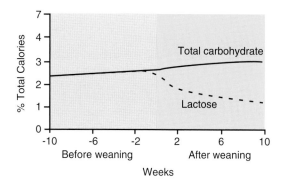

Figure 2: Contribution of carbohydrates to energy intake in breast-fed infants at weaning. Diet was changed to semi-solid foods and formula at weaning (0 weeks). (n = 40) Data courtesy of Janice Stuff, Children's Nutrition Research Center, Houston, Texas.

tural oligosaccharides and polysaccharides of the plant cell wall. These become significant components of the infant's diet at weaning when cereals, fruits and vegetables are added. Beyond sucrose, raffinose *(Fr: to refine)* is the most common oligosaccharide in plants. It is an α-galactose-α-glucose-β-fructose. It also exists with additional galactose as a tetrasaccharide stachyose *(Gr: nettle plants)* and pentasaccharise verbascose *(L: the mullen plant)*. None of these oligosaccharides are hydrolyzed in the small intestine, but all are fermented by the normal anaerobic flora of the colon. They produce hydrogen during colonic fermentation.[8]

Dietary fibers are a group of plant polysaccharides that contribute to intestinal function by binding water and maintaining fecal bulk. The pectins are a mixture of soluble polysaccharides. They are partially esterified linear polymers of galactose interspersed with rhamnose *(Gr: the buckthorn plant, used as a purgative)* decorated with side chains of glucose and galactose. Between 15 and 55% of pectins are digested in the adult small intestine but only 5% appears in feces. Bacterial enzymes account for the colonic salvage of carbon from pectin not absorbed in the small intestine.[9] Hemicelluloses *(L: half+a store-room)* are branched polymers of pentose and hexose sugars, which include xylose *(Gr: wood, thus wood sugar)*, arabinose, mannose *(Heb. manna)*, galactose and uronic *(Gr: urine)* acids. Digestion appears to be similar to the pectins; less than 30% of the dietary hemicelluloses appear in the adult

stool. Cellulose is a linear β-1-4 glucose polymer found in wood and similar plant tissues. The molecular structure is stabilized into structural ribbons by hydrogen bonding. About 95% of dietary cellulose appears unchanged in adult human feces.

Soon after birth, the colonic flora of the normal infant has a wide repertoire of hydrolase enzyme activities that function to digest carbohydrate and ferment sugars into metabolizable volatile fatty acids: acetate, butyrate and propionate. This function of colonic bacterial flora is analogous to that of the function of rumenal flora in herbivores. Glucose and galactose fermentation by specific bacterial strains in the colon is associated with release of hydrogen gas and is the basis for the clinical test used to detect proximal carbohydrate malabsorption by measurement of H_2 appearing in breath.[4, 10] Many of the carbohydrates malabsorbed from a mixed diet in the upper intestine are recovered by this "scavenging" pathway. An overview of carbohydrate digestion and absorption is presented in Figure 3.

Disaccharide Digestion

The disaccharidase enzyme activities are sensitive to developmental and dietary factors. In the rat and rabbit, lactase activities are high at birth and decline when weaned to the adult diet. The activities of sucrase are virtually absent until weaning occurs. Glucoamylase activity is present from birth, but increases on the adult diet. In adult animals, sucrase, maltase and glucoamylase activities increase when a high carbohydrate diet is fed, but lactase activity is independent of dietary levels of lactose.[3] In the pig and human, a modified pattern of enzyme activities is observed in which lactase is more sustained after weaning. Many humans lose lactase enzyme activity after about four years of age. This is a selective loss of lactase gene expression. In the pig and human, sucrase and glucoamylase activities are present from birth. In the pig, sucrase and glucoamylase activities increase on high carbohydrate diets.[3] All of the brush border disaccharidase activities increase in severely malnourished rats and pigs.[11, 12] This may be due to the developmental arrest imposed by experimental malnutrition. In malnourished infants all of the disaccharidase activities are reduced, but lactase activity is less than maltase<sucrase<glucoamylase.

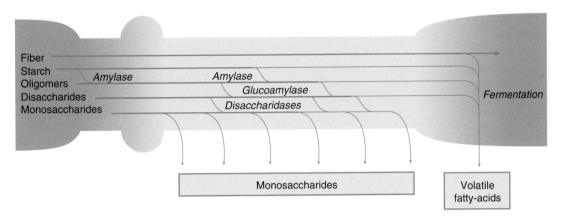

Figure 3: Carbohydrate digestion and absorption in adult humans. The digestive processes are indicated by vertical twin circles. Assimilation from the intestine is shown at the right of the diagram. The level of digestion and absorption is shown on the vertical axes. The complexity of the carbohydrates is greater on the left of the diagram and diminishes on the right. Note that absorption is limited to glucose, fructose, galactose, lactate and volatile fatty acids. The relative digestibility of the energy present in the different forms of dietary carbohydrates is indicated along the bottom of the diagram. Clinical disorders in children are indicated in a similar format in Table 2.

The paradoxical difference between the enzyme alterations in malnourished animals and children appears to be a consequence of the associated chronic mucosal inflammation of malnourished infants living under adverse sanitary conditions.

The primary structure of human lactase was reported in 1988.[13] It is synthesized as the 1927 amino acid precursor (pro lactase) and subsequently modified in size and glycosylation to mature lactase. Studies carried out on biopsies from adults with lactose intolerance found a spectrum of changes. The mature form was reduced to 15% of total lactase protein. The lactase gene has been studied in two adult hypolactasia subjects, and it was concluded that these subjects can code for lactase synthesis as well as controls. In larger studies there was good correlation between loss of lactase mRNA and reduction in enzyme activity. These two studies have not excluded a genetic mutation in some patients with the adult type of hypolactasia.

The primary structure of human sucrase has been known since 1992.[14] There are 1,827 amino acids in the precursor molecule (pre-sucrase-isomaltase), which is subsequently split into two subunits in the intestinal lumen. There are internal homologies between sucrase and isomaltase subunit domains. Human sucrase deficiency has been investigated in biopsy samples. A spectrum of alterations have been observed. In one group there was a failure to cleave the precursor to the two mature subunits; another had no defect in proteolysis but an accumulation in the cytoplasmic compartments. A third group had normal synthesis and processing, but appeared to have a mutation blocking the active site.[15, 16]

The primary structure of maltase-glucoamylase is unknown. It is synthesized as a 255,000 Da protein which is converted to the mature 335,000 D glycosylated form. It is not proteolytically processed as are lactase and sucrase.[16] Studies of maltase-glucoamylase-enzyme activity after partial proteolysis indicate that the maltase region is associated with the anchor end and the glucoamylase on the free terminus.[3,17] The glucoamylase portion is more highly glycosylated, consistent with the structure of yeast glucoamylases.[18] α-amylase activities in salivary and pancreatic secretions are absent in the premature infant and in the first six months of postnatal life, and become depressed or absent in older, malnourished infants.[4, 19, 20] α-amylase is not present in the mucosa of the small intestine, but is produced by colonic bacteria and yeast flora. It is believed that small intestinal glucoamylase is able to substitute for α-amylase by splitting the one to four

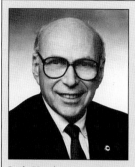

Norman Kretchmer Ph.D., M.D.

(1923-1995) received his degrees from U. of Minnesota and State U. of New York College of Medicine and trained in pediatrics at Cornell/New York Hospital where he was associated with S. Z. Levine, a student of Lusk. Kretchmer was Chairman of Pediatrics at Stanford U. from 1959-1978. His group discovered the developmental regulation of lactase and opened the way to contemporary understanding of lactose intolerance in infants with diarrhea. Kretchmer also pioneered in the study of ethnic lactose malabsorption. He served as Director of The National Institute of Child Health & Human Development from 1974 to 1981. From 1981 to 1994, Kretchmer was Professor of Nutritional Sciences at U. of California. Kretchmer, N. *Memorial lecture: lactose and lactase - a historical perspective.* Gastro. 61, 805-813,1971. (Photo courtesy of Mrs. Kretchmer)

dextrins arising from salivary and pancreatic-amylase hydrolysis or when fed as malted starches. In addition, glucose oligosaccharides or malted starches are frequently added to infant formulas to serve as emulsifiers and reduce intestinal luminal osmolar load.[21]

Monosaccharide Absorption

Only monosaccharides are normally absorbed into the body. Of the three major dietary monosaccharides, glucose and galactose are transported actively. The glucose/galactose transporter has a size of 72,000 D. It penetrates the luminal membrane. In the presence of luminal sodium the carrier has a high affinity site for luminal glucose. A carbonyl group on the transporter shifts from the lumenal to the intracellular membrane surface, and the glucose molecule and two sodium ions are internalized. The intracellular shift in the binding site releases the sodium ions and reduces the affinity of the transporter for the glucose, which is released into the cytoplasm of the enterocyte. The sodium ions are removed from the cytoplasm by the Na,K-ATPase at the basolateral membrane.[11, 12] As the mucosal absorption of sodium is linked to the active transport of glucose, both sodium and water absorption are stimulated by the presence of luminal glucose or galactose.

The mechanism of fructose absorption, that also requires a specific carrier, is independent of sodium transport and is not blocked by drugs which inhibit glucose and galactose absorption. The efficiency of glucose and galactose absorption is approximately 98%.[22] Studies in normal adult humans indicate that the transport rate of monosaccharides is limited by the overall process of starch and sucrose digestion, and not absorption. In contrast, hydrolysis of lactose is slower than the absorption of an equivalent mixture of glucose and galactose. Lactose digestion is the slowest of all the small bowel carbohydrate digestive-absorptive processes.[23]

In addition to the dietary carbohydrates and endogenous mucins *(Sanscr.: snivel from the nose)* that are not digested or absorbed in the adult upper small bowel, immaturity or acquired defects in small bowel carbohydrate digestion or absorption increase the delivery of unabsorbed carbohydrates to the colon. Most normal breast-fed infants rely on colonic fermentation to complete the digestion of the large lactose load (7%) in human milk. The mechanisms of normal colonic salvage of proximally unabsorbed carbohydrate are poorly determined. The colonic digestion of starches proceeds more slowly by β-amylase digestion. The practical consequence of β-amylase digestion is that the hydrolysis of the starch becomes a limiting step for colonic salvage.

Colonic Bacterial Fermentation

The biochemistry of bacterial fermentation *(L: yeast leaven)* in the colon is complex. Microorganisms make up approximately 50% of fecal dry solids. The extracellular products of normal fermentation are the volatile fatty acids: acetic, propionic and butyric. The volatile fatty acids produced by fermentation are absorbed rapidly from the lumen of the normal colon. Under conditions of disturbed colonic bacterial metabolism, intermediary compounds, e.g., lactate, pyruvate, and succinate, are found in the stool. The presence of these three abnormal acids in the stool accounts for the fall in fecal pH seen in failure of colonic salvaging. In normal adults, more than 70% of the energy available from the original carbohydrate entering the colon is thus absorbed from the lumen;[24] however, this is less efficient than the nearly total small bowel absorption of monosaccharides. Mucus is the endogenous carbohydrate source for colonic microbial fermentation during fasting. It has been estimated that 20 to 40 g of proximally unabsorbed carbohydrate and endogenously produced mucus are fermented daily by the colon of the normal adult.[24] Langstein was the first to report in 1906 that some children with diarrhea have unabsorbed glucose in the stool. He also discovered that the normal colonic flora converts glucose into lactic acid. It has now become clear that disturbances of colonic fermentation account for the clinical symptoms of carbohydrate malabsorption, but the mechanisms of controling normal colonic fermentation are still not understood.[25] Human milk regulates the nature and function of colonic flora within narrow limits, favoring the bacterial hydrolysis and fermentation of lactose. The smaller molecular weight carbohydrates and their products, the volatile acids, are the principal dietary source of proximally malabsorbed osmolar forces in the lumen of the intestine; they increase the volume of luminal contents and account for an osmolar diarrhea in clinical carbohydrate intolerance.

We have the baby weighed today
The nursing time is set,
At last we find we are so wise
We can begin to standardize
No baby now need fret;
In spite of this the baby grows
But why it does God only knows.

"Infant Feeding"
(Lines suggested by papers
on infant feeding)
Dr. John Rurah
Pediatrics of the Past
John Ruhrah, M.D., Editor
Paul B. Hoeber, Inc,
New York, NY

Carbohydrate Intolerance

Small intestine carbohydrate malabsorption becomes clinical intolerance only in unusual circumstances. When the colonic capacity to ferment carbohydrate is exceeded by the unabsorbed dietary load, symptoms of intolerance (e.g., diarrhea) occur. The presence of diarrhea, which improves when dietary carbohydrates are reduced or eliminated from the diet, characterizes clinical carbohydrate intolerance. The major osmotic forces in fluid entering the colon are derived from oligosaccharides, lactose, sucrose or glucose, which displace electrolytes. Normally, the electrolytes in ileal fluid and any unabsorbed carbohydrates are fermented to volatile fatty acids, are rapidly absorbed by the normal colonic epithelium. This absorption results in a reduction of luminal osmolality and facilitates the colonic absorption of water.

Inadequate colonic salvage results in diarrhea when the amount of ileal effluent is too large for the normal colon and its flora to manage, or when disorders in the colonic mucosa prevent the salvage of the ileal load. During secretory diarrhea, due to enterotoxins (e.g., from cholera or enterotoxigenic Escherichia coli), large volumes of ileal fluid enter the colon and pass relatively unchanged into the stool. This ileal secretion has a high sodium concentration (>100 mM) that persists even during prolonged fasting. The sodium concentrations in the stools of patients with carbohydrate intolerance are reduced (usually less than 60 mM) because of the presence of organic, osmotically-active components resulting from imperfect colonic salvage of unabsorbed carbohydrates in the small intestine. The passage of very large amounts of unabsorbed carbohydrates into the normal colon can alter the capacity of the colonic microflora for salvage. This involves a quantitative and qualitative failure of fermentation and transport, with accumulation of luminal organic acids causing a reduction in pH to levels of 4 to 5.5, and the presence of undigested carbohydrate and unabsorbed organic acids (>80 mOsm) in the stool.

Disorders of Carbohydrate Digestion and Absorption

There are three types of carbohydrate malabsorption in young children (Table 2):

1. The ontogenic forms related to the normal immaturity of the digestive functions during intrauterine and extrauterine development.
2. The genetic forms are congenital conditions which are inherited (inborn errors of metabolism).
3. The acquired forms are more difficult to classify because of the variability in their severity.

Developmental Forms of Carbohydrate Maldigestion and Malabsorption

Primary Lactase Deficiency

Although very small premature infants have low mucosal lactase activity, they tolerate lactose feedings.[38]

Classification	Colonic Bacterial Metabolism	Exocrine Amylase	Brush-Border Hydrolase	Monosaccharide Transport
1) Ontogenic	3 days of postnatal age	4 months of postnatal age	Sucrase: 20 weeks of gestation Lactase: 30 weeks of gestation; After 24 months of age[a]	15 weeks of gestation
2) Genetic		Cyctis Fibrosis Shwachman-Diamond Syndrome	Sucrase-isomaltase deficiency[a] Lactase deficiency[a] Postgastroenteritis[ab]	Glucose-galactose malabsorption
3) Acquired	Antibiotic therapy	Protein-energy malnutrition Chronic pancreatitis	Postintestinal surgery[ab] Celiac disease[ab] Milk protein hypersensitivity[ab] Protein-energy malnutrition[ab] Cytotoxic agents[ab]	Postgastroenteritis[ab] Postintestinal surgery[ab]

[a]Symptomatic intolerance
[b]Abnormal mycosal histology

Table 2: Types of carbohydrate malabsorption in infants.

It has been shown that lactose digestion in full-term infants is completed by colonic hydrolysis and fermentation of the proximally malabsorbed carbohydrate.[26, 27]

Genetic Forms of Carbohydrate Maldigestion and Malabsorption

Genetic Sucrase-Isomaltase Deficiency

This is a rare recessive disease. The symptoms do not occur unless sucrose, dextrin or starch is fed. Although diarrhea occurs in infants, older children and adults tolerate usual quantities of these carbohydrates. The mucosa is normal by light and electron microscopy. The enzymes sucrase and isomaltase are deficient in the small intestinal mucosal tissue. Management consists of eliminating sucrose and limiting the quantity of starch in the diet.

Genetic Lactase Deficiency

Genetic lactase deficiency of the newborn is an excessively rare disease. These infants usually have diet-induced diarrhea following the first feeding of lactose-containing milk, including human milk. The intestinal mucosa is normal by light and electron microscopy. There is a selective reduction of lactase enzyme activity in jejunal mucosal biopsy samples. The disease is thought to be inherited as an autosomal recessive trait. Management consists of eliminating lactose from the diet.

The adult form of lactase deficiency has its onset after four years of age. In some ethnic groups, up to 100% of adults have low small intestinal lactase enzyme activities. This form of hypolactasia only rarely causes gastrointestinal symptoms. The diagnosis of genetic hypolactasia requires the presence of normal sucrase enzyme activity and mucosal histology. There have been recent insights into the nature of adult forms of hypolactasia. When lactase immunoisolates are separated according to their sizes, three isoforms of 260-, 200- and 160-kDa are found.[24] It has been determined that the 200,000 Da form is the first to be synthesized. This pro-lactase is processed in the endoplasmic reticulum and Golgi apparatus to a complex glycosylated form which is proteolytically cleaved into the mature 160,000 D form found in the brush border membrane. Two types of adult subjects with low lactase SA and normal mucosal morphology have been recognized.[24, 28-30] In phenotype I, no lactase mRNA or synthesis can be detected. In phenotype II, lactase mRNA is present and synthesis occurs, but is associated with defective processing from the precursor to the mature, active luminal enzyme. Additional phenotypes may exist.[31] In phenotype II subjects, accumulation of lactase has been observed by immunoprecipitation and within the Golgi region by immunoelectron microscopy.[24] Diarrhea is rarely observed in the hypolactasic adult, presumably due to reduced milk intake and normal colonic salvage.

Genetic Glucose-Galactose Malabsorption

This rare disorder is a form of diet-induced diarrhea which is present from birth. It is characterized by intolerance when glucose, galactose or disaccharides are fed, and responds to the withdrawal of these carbohydrates. Glucose-galactose malabsorption is inherited in an autosomal recessive fashion. The mucosa are normal on histologic examination. Mucosal uptake of glucose and galactose is absent, while amino acid transport is normal. The defect appears to be a specific absence of the mucosal glucose and galactose transport mechanisms, but the genetic abnormalities cover a wide spectrum. The transport of fructose is normal and the infants respond to a fructose-containing diet with relief of diarrhea and normal growth. With age, these children eventually tolerate moderate amounts of starch and milk, presumably through colonic compensatory mechanisms.

> We need to remember that sucrose, fructose and starch are entirely unnatural for suckling mammals.
>
> Susan Henning Ph.D.
> Department of Pediatrics
> Baylor College of Medicine
> Houston, Texas

Acquired Forms of Carbohydrate Maldigestion and Malabsorption

Nutritional Inadequacies

In children, chronic dietary protein inadequacy or energy deficiency can alter parotid and pancreas production and secretion of α-amylase. Knowledge of the mechanisms of these adaptive responses is incomplete.[32]

The feeding of increased sucrose, lactose or starch can increase the sucrase, lactase and amylase activities in adult humans.[22] In the human malnourished child, reductions of jejunal lactase activities are very common.[33] Animals with similar degrees of malnutrition have elevations of lactase activities. The paradoxical human response may occur because of associated villus atrophy and inflammatory reactions in the mucosa of malnourished children dwelling in unsanitary environments and suffering

from acute and chronic intestinal infections. The lactase isoform patterns and reduced mRNA levels observed in severely malnourished infants (personal unpublished data) are consistent with a transcriptional and post-translational suppression similar to the phenotype II hypolactasic adults in Italy. Older infants with severe degrees of malnutrition and hypolactasia seldom have clinical intolerance. It has recently been demonstrated that young malnourished infants with hypolactasia and clinical intolerance also have an acquired defect in the colonic salvage of the malabsorbed carbohydrate.[34]

Acute Diarrhea

Infections that affect the small intestine can alter digestive functions, although the mechanisms behind many of these reductions are unknown. Rotavirus infections preferentially invade and cause shedding of the enterocytes at the tip of the villi. This results in an associated reduction in lactase activity and transport of glucose. The recovery of disaccharidase and monosaccharide digestive and absorptive mechanisms requires 7 to 14 days.[31, 35] By mechanisms similar to those contributing to the loss of lactase activity observed in chronic mucosal inflammatory diseases such as active celiac and graft vs. host diseases, acute inflammatory disorders of the intestine may directly cause acquired hypolactasia. Only rarely will a well-nourished infant have a recurrence of transient diarrhea when rehydrated with an oral rehydrating solution; but about 10% of malnourished infants will have recurrent intolerance of rehydrating solutions containing 5% glucose. Recurrence of carbohydrate-induced intolerance is much less common with the contemporary 3% than with older 5% glucose oral electrolyte solutions. The 3% glucose solutions were designed and promoted because of the discovery that in cholera, water losses were reduced by dietary glucose. The mechanism of water secretion in cholera is well documented and the response to dietary glucose is mediated by the improved absorption of luminal sodium by the glucose transporter. It is likely that the number of glucose trans-

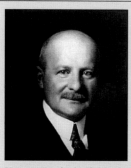

Heinrich Finkelstein Ph.D., M.D.

(1865-1942) received a geology degree before entering the study of medicine. He was an assistant of Heubner's for seven years. From 1918 until 1933, Finkelstein served as Director of Kaiser and Kaiserin Friedrich Children's Hospital in Berlin. With Heubner, reforms in infant stimulation, sanitation and diet were instituted, which reduced failure to thrive from 80 to 10% among children hospitalized in the infants' ward. Finkelstein studied the effect of individual food components on intestinal function and growth of malnourished infants and first demonstrated clinical lactose intolerance. *Pediatric Profiles* editor B. S. Veeder, Mosby St. Louis, 1957, 104-108. (Photo courtesy of NLM)

porters is reduced in viral diarrheas like rotavirus which cause a shedding of enterocytes, and that the higher unabsorbed glucose concentrations cause an osmolar pooling of fluid in the lumen of the bowel.

Acquired Carbohydrate Intolerance

In 1962, a syndrome was described in a small group of young infants who failed to recover formula tolerance after having been treated for dehydration from acute diarrhea.[36-38] This disorder was referred to as *intractable diarrhea, protracted diarrhea, post-gastroenteritis syndrome, acquired or temporary monosaccharide and disaccharide intolerance, cow milk intolerance, sugar-induced diarrhea and diarrhea grave rebelle.* Whether these clinical descriptions are synonymous is unclear. All, however, fulfill the earlier criteria of Brenneman[39] for a syndrome called "intestinal decomposition" (gut rot):

1. Complete relief of the intestinal symptoms when food is withdrawn.
2. Recurrence of diarrhea when an excess of the offending food (or the offending carbohydrate in the food) is given.
3. Absence of gross pathological lesions in the intestinal mucosa.
4. Malnutrition with increased susceptibility to infections.

Because of the difficulty in nomenclature and lack of uniformity in diagnostic criteria and therapeutic management, we will present our personal experience as a guide to the health worker responsible for the care of infants with similar symptoms.[38,40-43]

Clinical Presentation

In our experience, "decomposition" is suspected during the refeeding of infants with diarrhea admitted to hospital. Certain clinical features at admission suggest that the recovery will be complex and prolonged. The average infant with decomposition is about 30 days of age and always less than 270 days old. Weight gain since birth is less than 12 gm/day and the body weight is frequently less than birth. Many have a previous history of feeding difficulty or diarrhea before the onset of the current illness. The severity and frequency of the diarrhea does not distinguish these infants from others with a benign course; however, the duration of diarrhea before hospital admission is slightly longer, and the degree of dehydration at the time of admission is more severe, than in infants with uncomplicated acute diarrhea. Family history and infectious vectors do not differentiate the infant who will develop decomposition. Feeding history also does not set apart those infants who will develop decomposition; however, we have never seen this disorder occur in an exclusively breast-fed infant.[36, 41]

Physical examination reveals a moderately to severely marasmic infant. Wasting of subcutaneous and muscle tissue is apparent, and the abdomen is usually distended. Other than the presence of atrophy of the papillae over the dorsum of the tongue, no signs of specific nutrient deficiencies are evident. The body weight is usually less than birth weight and the weight/length index, skinfold measurement and arm/head circumference ratio all confirm the presence of moderate to severe malnutrition. The hydration state of the infants is difficult to assess at admission; however, the weight gain after rehydration averages 5% of initial body weight.[43, 44] Mucosal biopsies of jejunal tissue reveal moderate to severe villous atrophy.

Diagnostic Criteria

The diagnosis becomes evident during oral refeeding. In the first hours after admission, the priority is restitution of circulatory adequacy through vigorous rehydra-

Fluid Intake

A. Record volume and exact nature of each feeding.
B. Note acceptance, regurgitation and duration of feeding.

Fluid Losses

A. Preweigh all diapers to nearest gram and record weight of diaper. Reweigh soiled diapers and record change in diaper weight and time of evaluation. Note size of stool (small, medium, normal, large, extra large); consistency of stool (formed, "mushy", "runny", liquid); color (green, brown, yellow, white) and any other observations (blood, parasites, pH).
B. If it is not possible to weigh stools, mark each diaper with date and time; fold and store in plastic bag under bed to allow inspection by physician. Discard after daily rounds.

Body Weight

A. Weigh every 8 hours until stable; record weight to nearest gram.
B. Check calibration of each scale with standard weights.

Loose Stools

A. Avoid urine contamination when possible; record when not possible. Use indicator paper to measure pH, report to nearest 0.5 units.
B. Use urine dipstix to measure glucose, read 1000 = 100 = 1+, 2000 = 2+, etc. Immerse the dipstix in fresh stool and read color reaction as indicated in directions. Note: sucrose is not a reducing sugar but bacterial hydrolases result in presence of increased glucose in the stools.

Table 3: Quantitative observations required for refeeding young infants recovering from diarrhea.

tion. Our practice is to withhold all formula feeding for a maximum of 12 hours during rehydration. Before oral feedings are begun, the stooling must have improved and urine output must be adequate. If preliminary intravenous rehydration is required, oral feedings are begun with an oral electrolyte solution (3% glucose in a balanced salt solution). Once the infant is stabilized, a stepwise program of refeeding is instituted (Fig. 2). Key observations are made during this critical period (Table 3).

The basic features of these observations are frequent evaluations of hydration as reflected in weight gain and urine output, careful recording of the characteristics of all stools, and full documentation concerning the type, volume, and time of each feeding. These observations should be available in any clinical setting. In our approach, refeeding formulas are divided into two classes, those of fixed composition, and formulas made with modules of carbohydrate, protein and lipid that can be tailored according to the patient's specific tolerance and nutritional needs (Table 4). The use of modular formulas is generally restricted to hospitalized patients because of the increased risks of formula contamination in the home.

The findings used to identify carbohydrate intolerance are listed in Table 3. A recurrence of diarrhea during refeeding is a major sign of intolerance. If diarrhea resolves with fasting and then recurs after refeeding the same or a lower glucose level, decomposition is confirmed. The presence of reduced pH and the presence of glucose in the stool are diagnostic under these circumstances. Only rarely are these fecal changes observed in infants who have a rapid recovery to a full diet for age. These diagnostic signs and the therapeutic step-by-step refeeding schedule help to identify the nature of the intolerance (Fig.2). Nutritional rehabilitation is required if intolerance to 3% glucose in the formula, and severe mucosal atrophy on small bowel biopsy are present. A second failure when refeeding is attempted is an indication for short-term complementary peripheral intravenous nutrition during the continued testing of formula tolerance. Peripheral nutrition should be limited to those infants who require intravenous supplementation for less than 48 hours.

Before total intravenous therapy (TPN) is implemented, nasogastric infusions of modular formulas are always tried; such infusions, however, are not effective

Formula	Carbohydrate	Protein	Fat	Indication
Complete				
Cow milk	Lactose	Cow's casein and whey	Vegetable and animal	Normal digestive function
Soy	Sucrose, glucose oligosaccharides	Soy	Soy	Lactose intolerance Cow milk protein hypersensitivity
Hydrolyed protein	Sucrose, glucose oligosaccharides	Hydrolyed casein or whey	Medium-chain triglycerides (MCT)	Cow milk and soy protein hypersensitivity Pancreatic insufficiency
Modular				
Casein based	0-7%	Casein	0-3%	Sucrose and glucose intolerance
Soy based	0-7%	Soy	Soy	Sucrose and glucose intolerance
Hydrolyzed casein based	0-7%	Hydrolyzed casein	MCT	Cow's milk protein hypersensitivity
Hospital produced modular				
Cow milk based	0-7%	Washed casein	0-3%	Sucrose and glucose intolerance
Chicken puree based	0-7%	Blended chicken	Animal (trace)	Cow's milk protein hypersensitivity

Table 4: Formulas for the management of refeeding of young infants recovering from diarrhea.

when the infant does not tolerate formulas containing 3% or less glucose. Steps must be taken to support the nutritional rehabilitation during the period of the modular formula testing; these infants are malnourished and cannot tolerate continued hypocaloric feedings for prolonged periods. Signs of impending nutritional crisis are hypothermia, bradycardia and progressive anorexia. These clinical signs call for aggressive nutritional support. Hydration must be maintained independently of nutritional management. Only hydrated infants are candidates for the modular approach to refeeding.

Glucose is the first sugar tested during the refeeding program because neither the sucrose nor the glucose polymers in the original refeeding formula is tolerated. Some physicians begin refeeding with lactose-containing formulas. However, we abandoned this practice in the very young infant. Tolerance to sucrose, lactose, glucose polymers and glucose can be tested by giving a load of these sugars of 2 g/kg by

mouth and following blood glucose concentrations at 15-minute intervals over a one-hour period. Infants with decomposition fail to demonstrate a normal rise in blood glucose in this absorption test. Theoretically, proximal carbohydrate malabsorption could be detected if a rise in breath hydrogen levels occurs following colonic salvage of the carbohydrate from a test load of formula. In our experience, the infants with decomposition have defective colonic salvaging and do not demonstrate breath hydrogen responses to proximal malabsorption of carbohydrates. As a rule, those infants who excrete glucose in the stools do not produce elevations in breath hydrogen after an oral carbohydrate challenge.

When infants have difficulties tolerating a 4 to 5% glucose feeding, they are fed by nasogastric infusions using the same carbohydrate source and quantity. In many cases, these feedings are tolerated more readily than intermittent bolus feedings. The substitution of 1 or 2% of glucose polymers for an equivalent amount of

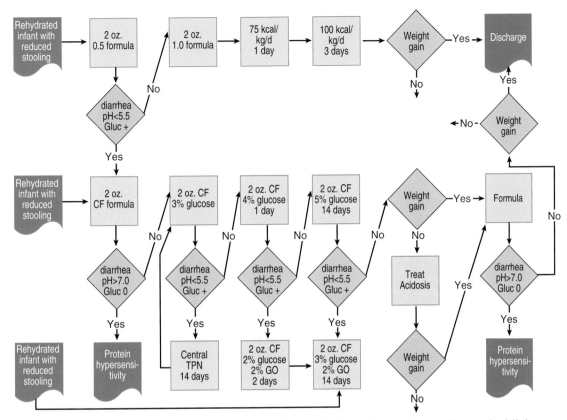

Figure 4: Algorithm outlining the diagnosis and therapy of clinical carbohydrate intolerance. See text for full discussion. Formula: Any previously tolerated complete formula (0.5 is half strength and 1.0 is full strength). CF, carbohydrate-free modular formula; GO, Glucose oligosaccharides; TPN, total parenteral nutrition; Gluc, Glucose; grey diamond, decision point; orange, starting or finishing positions; yellow boxes, therapy. This sequence of feeding trials was pioneered by Finkelstein in the early 20th century.

the glucose in the formula is another variation that is frequently tolerated.[42]

Differential Diagnosis

The genetic disorders of carbohydrate digestion, except for glucose-galactose malabsorption, will respond to the management approach given in Figure 4. In the case of glucose-galactose malabsorption, fructose can be substituted for glucose in the modular formula. However, we have not found fructose to be useful in managing decomposition, presumably because its absorption is also impaired.

Systemic disorders can lead to a decomposition syndrome. Several infants with severe combined immunodeficiency have presented with this syndrome, and we have found that clinical carbohydrate intolerance is rare in hypolactasic malnourished children who have mature immunoglobulin A transport to the intestinal lumen (unpublished data). The large amount of IgA, lactoferrin and other factors in mother's milk may contribute to the preservation of colonic salvage pathways in breast-fed infants. Specific hypersensitivity syndromes are known to produce diarrhea; therefore, we test each infant with the carbohydrate-free dietary module to identify the most clearly manifested hypersensitivity. Less clear-cut immunological disturbances may exist in infants who successfully pass this challenge; however, we believe that our success with manipulating the carbohydrate in the diet has rendered milk protein hypersensitivity a moot question. We have found that septicemia, chronic urinary tract infection and abscess delay the recovery of infants with

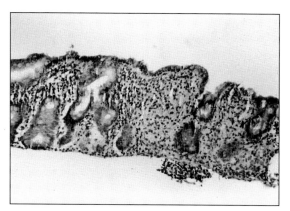

Figure 5: Mucosal biopsy of Jose F. (case 1). Note that the mucosa lacks long finger-like villus structures and that the crypts are short and have few mitotic figures. The number of lymphocytes are increased in the epithelium and lamina propria.

decomposition, and can precipitate the onset of the syndrome in other infants with poor nutritional status. Epidemics of rotavirus infection in the infant unit frequently precipitate this complication. A decomposition syndrome was observed in very young infants after intestinal surgery. The frequency of this complication has declined with the successful implementation of routine total intravenous nutrition during the post-operative period.

The identification of the various secretory diarrheas of infancy is based upon the infant's failure to respond to fasting[23], and the high sodium concentration (70 mEq/L) in his stools.[45] Confusion with tropical enteropathy, cystic fibrosis and celiac disease is not a problem because of the very young age of the decomposition subjects, the marked malabsorption of fat in infants with cystic fibrosis, and the history of gluten intake in infants with celiac disease.[36]

Case Histories

Case #1: Jose F. was admitted to the Ben Taub Hospital Pediatric Service in Houston at 36 days of age. Three days before, he had developed vomiting and diarrhea. He had been started on the breast but was discharged on a cow milk formula. On admission he weighed less than birth weight and was severely malnourished as well as dehydrated. The arm/FOC ratio was 0.24 (< 0.28 = severe malnutrition). Examination of stools were positive for shigella and rotavirus.

After initial rehydration, Jose was offered a 5% glucose oral electrolyte solution which was well tolerated. He was started on half-strength soy formula containing glucose oligosaccharides. This was advanced to full-strength formula which was well tolerated, but weight gain was poor.

After 11 days of adequate intake and poor weight gain he began to have an increased number of green, mucus-filled stools that were positive for glucose. When Jose was fasted, he had a remission of his diarrhea and glucose spillage. We attempted to refeed with a modular soy formula that was tolerated with 4% but not 5% glucose. He was changed to a modular casein formula, but had a recurrence of glucose + diarrhea with 1% glucose. Jose was then fed the 5% glucose oral electrolyte solution and became acutely dehydrated. He next received total intravenous nutrition for 36 days and was successfully weaned to a hydrolyzed casein and glucose formula, on which he continued to thrive.

A mucosal biopsy was obtained at the time that intravenous feeding was begun (Figure 5). The biopsy revealed almost total villar atrophy. There was an increase in the number of epithelial and lamina propria lymphocytes. There were no goblet cells visualized and only rare mitotic figures in the crypt areas. On electron microscopy there were reduced numbers of microvilli on the luminal surface. The mucosa was much improved, but still abnormal by light and electron microscopy, when a repeat biopsy was obtained at the end of the period of intravenous nutrition. It appears that the loss of villi and microvilli resulted in reduced mucosal absorption of luminal glucose.[42]

Case 2: Lucas A.B.C. was admitted to the Children's Institute at the University of Sao Paulo at 213 days of age. He had onset of acute diarrhea at about 180 days, which responded to outpatient oral rehydration. The diarrhea persisted intermittently until he was suddenly admitted to the in-patient service with acute dehydration. On the previous day he had vomiting and fever and had passed 10 mucus-filled, green stools. A thorough search for pathogenic agents was unrewarding. Lucas required intravenous fluid therapy for seven days.

He was first fed a diluted whole milk formula. He had a relapse of diarrhea on this feeding associated with pH < 5.5 and presence of 2+ glucose in the stools. The diarrhea stopped and fecal pH and glucose became normal when he was changed to a lactose-free sucrose/casein formula.

Before illness, his diet had been human milk until two months of age. This had been followed by introducing *whole milk diluted ⅓ with 5% table sugar. Fruit and fruit juices were introduced at two months; cereal, egg yolks and prepared dinners at three months.*

At admission his z score ht/age was -3.37; wt/age -3.36 and wt/ht -1.09. The arm/head circumference was .27 (Normal =.32). He appeared severely malnourished and dehydrated. After admission, a mucosal biopsy was done. It revealed deep crypts and short villi (Figure 6). There was patchy necrosis of the epithelial layer and patchy hemorrhage and edema in the lamina propria. The enterocytes were columnar. The brush border appeared mostly intact but had some irregularities, goblet cells were depleted and the basement membrane was prominent. There were rare mitotic figures in the crypt . One crypt abscess was present. The biopsy was assayed for lactase enzyme SA; 4.7 U/gm (normal > 10 U/gm). No enzyme activity could be detected by mucosal histochemistry; however, a strong mucosal staining for lactase was present by immunohistology. Western blotting demonstrated that the mature form of mucosal lactase was decreased from a normal value of 77 to 43% of the total immunoprecipitable enzyme. This reduction in mature lactase form and discrepancy between weak enzyme activity and strong immuno histology staining suggested a

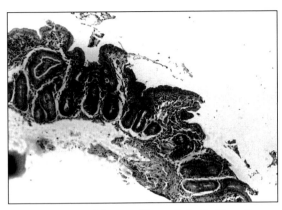

Figure 6: Mucosal biopsy of Lucas A. B. C. (Case 2). Note the shortened villi and deep crypts. There was patchy loss of the epithelial layer by light and EM examination. There are increased epithelial and lamina propria lymphocytes. Only rare mitotic figures appear in the crypt epithelium. A crypt abscess is present.

defect in the maturation of lactase,[23] perhaps the consequence of primary malnutrition. The patient was discharged on a lactose-free diet and did well on follow up in the outpatient department. (Courtesy of Dr. Francisco Carrazza, Children's Institute at the University of Sao Paulo).

Historical Perspective...

References

1. Hassid WZ, Ball CE. Oligosaccharides. In: Pigman W, ed. *The Carbohydrates. Chemistry, Biochemistry, Physiology.* New York, NY: Academic Press Inc; 1957:492-506.

2. Whistler RL, Corbett WM. Polysaccharides. In: Pigman W, ed. *The Carbohydrates. Chemistry, Biochemistry, Physiology.* New York, NY: Academic Press Inc; 1957: 644-647 and 672-683.

3. Semenza G, Auricchio S. Small-intestinal disaccharidases. In: Scriver CR, Beaudet AL, Sly WS, Valle D, eds. *The Metabolic Basis of Inherited Disease.* New York, NY: McGraw-Hill; 1989:2975-2997.

4. Shulman RD, Wong WW, Irving CS, Nichols BL, Klein PD. Utilization of Dietary Cereals by Young Infants. *J Pediatr.* 1983;103:23-28.

5. Liebig J. *Suppe fur Sauglinge.* Braunschweig: Friedrich Biemeg und Sohn; 1866:5-11.

6. Svensson B. Regional distant sequence homology between amylases, æ-glucosidases and trans-glucanosylases. *FEBS Lett.* 1988;230:72-76.

7. Hong SH, Marmur J. Primary structure of the maltase gene of the MAL6 locus of Saccharomyces carlsbergensis. *Gene.* 1986;41:75-84.

8. Cristofaro E, Mottu F, Wuhrmann JJ. Involvement of the raffinose family of oligosaccharides in flatulence. In: Sipple HL, McNutt KW, eds. *Sugars in Nutrition.* New York: Academic Press; 1974:313-336.

9. Eastwood MA, Passmore R. Dietary fibre. *Lancet.* 1983; 2:202-206.

10. Lifschitz CH, Irving CS, Gopalkrishna GS, Evans K, Nichols BL. Carbohydrate malabsorption in infants studied with the breath hydrogen test. *J Pediatr.* 102: 371-375.

11. Galluser M, Belkhou R, Freund J-N, Duluc I, Torp N, Danielsen M, Raul F. Adaption of intestinal hydrolases to starvation in rats: effect of thyroid function. *J Comp Physiol. B.* 1991;161:357-361.

12. Pond WG, Heath J, Dudley MA, Burrin D, Krook L. Changes in Body Composition and in visceral organs in response to severe protein deficiency in genetically lean and obese infant pigs. 1993. (In Press)

13. Mantei N, Villa M, Enzler T, Wacker H, Boll W, James P, Hunziker W, Semenza G. Complete primary structure of human and rabbit lactase-phlorizin hydrolase: implications for biosynthesis, membrane anchoring and evolution of the enzyme. *EMBO J.* 1988;7:2,705-2,713.

14. Chantret I, Lacasa M, Chevalier G, Ruf J, Islam I, Mantei N, Edwards Y, Swallow D, Rousset M. Sequence of the complete cDNA and the 5' structure of the human sucrase-isomaltase gene. *Biochem J.* 1992;285: 915-923.

15. Naim HY, Roth J, Sterchi EE, Lentze MJ, Milla P, Schmitz J, Hauri H-P. Sucrase-isomaltase deficiency in humans. *J Clin Invest.* 1988;82:667-679.

16. Naim HY, Sterchi EE, Lentze MJ. Structure, biosynthesis, and glycosylation of human small intestinal maltase glucoamylase. *J Biol Chem.* 1988;263:19709-19717.

17. Lee L, Fostner G. High molecular weight soluble neutral maltase-glucoamylases in the intestine of the suckling rat. *Biochem Cell Biol.* 1990;68:1103-1111.

18. Jespersen HM, Macgregor EA, Sierks MR, Svensson B. Comparison of the domain-level organization of starch hydrolases and related enzymes. *Biochem J.* 1991;280:51-55.

19. Rossiter MA, Barrowman JA, Dand A, Wharton BA. Amylase content of mixed saliva in children. *Acta Paediatr Scand.* 1974;63:389-392.

20. Danus O, Urbina AM, Valenzuela I, Solimano G. The effect of refeeding on pancreatic exocrine function in marasmic infants. *J Pediatr.* 1970;77:334-337.

21. Shulman RJ, Kerzner B, Sloane HR, Boutton TW, Wong WW, Nichols BL, Klein PD. Absorption and oxidation glucose polymers of different lengths in young infants. *Pediatr Res.* 1986;20:740-743.

22. Herman RH. Hydrolysis and absorption of carbohydrates, and adaptive responses of the jejunum. In: Sipple HL, McNutt KW, eds. *Sugars in Nutrition.* New York: Academic Press; 1974:145-172.

23. Gray GM. Carbohydrate digestion and absorption. *Gastroenterology.* 1970;58:96-107.

24. Cummings JH. Fermentation in the human large intestine: Evidence and implications for health. *Lancet.* 1983;2:1206-1209.

25. Lifschitz CH, Carrazza FR, Feste AS, Klein D. *In vivo* study of colonic fermentation of carbohydrate in infants. *J Pediatr Gastroenterol Nutr.* 1995;20:59-64.

26. Maclean WC, Fink BB, Schoeller DA, Wong W, Klein PD. Lactose assimilation by full-term infants: relation of (13C) and H2 breath tests with fecal (13C) excretion. *Pediatr Res.* 17:629-633.

27. Lifschitz CH, Smith EO, Garza C. Delayed complete functional lactase sufficinecy in breast-fed infants. *J Pediatr Gastroenterol Nutr.* 1983;2:478-482.

28. DeCurtis M, Senterre J, Rigo J, Putet G. Carbohydrates derived energy and gross energy absorption in preterm infants fed human milk or formula. *Arch Dis Child.* 1986;61:867-870.

29. Harvey CB, Wang Y, Hughes LA, Swallow DM, Thurrell WP, Sams VR, Barton R, Lanzon-Miller S, Sarner M. Studies on the expression of intestinal lactase in different individuals. *Gut.* 1995;28-33

30. Naim HY, Lacey SW, Sambrook JF, Gething M-JH. Expression of a full-length cDNA coding for human intestinal lactase-phlorizin hydrolase reveals an uncleaved, enzymatically active, and transport-competent protein. *J Biol Chem.* 1991;266:12313-12320.

31. Barnes GL, Townley RRW. Duodenal mucosal damage in 31 infants with gastroenteritis. *Arch Dis Child.* 48: 343-349.

32. Desnuelle P, Figarella C. Biochemistry. In: Howat HT, Sarles H, eds. *The Exocrine Pancreas.* London: WB Saunders; 1979:86-125.

33. Prinsloo JG, Wittmann W, Kruger H, Freier E. Lactose absorption and mucosal disaccharidases in convalescent pellagra and kwashiorkor children. *Arch Dis Child.* 1971; 46:474-478.

34. Tolboom JJM, Ralitapole-Maruping AP, Mothebe M, Kabir H, Molatsell P, Fernandes J. Carbohydrate malabsorption in children with severe protein energy malnutrition. *Trop Geogr Med.* 1984;36:5-365.

35. Sack DA, Rhoads M, Molla A, Molla AM, Wahed MA. Carbohydrate malabsorption in infants with rotavirus diarrhea. *Am J Clin Nutr.* 1982;36:1112-1118.

36. Anderson CM, Gracey M. Disorders of carbohydrate digestion and absorption. In: Anderson CM, Burke V, Gracey M, eds. *Paediatric Gastroenterology.* 2nd ed. Oxford: Blackwell Scientific Publications; 1987:353-374.

37. Laplane R, Polonovski C, Etienne M, Debray P, Lods JC, Pissaro B. L'intolerance aux sucres a transfert intestinal actif. *Arch Fr Pediatr.* 1962;19:895-944.

38. Klish WJ, Udall JN, Rodriguez JT, Singer DB, Nichols BL. Intestinal surface area in infants with acquired monosaccharide intolerance. *J Pediatr.* 1978;92:566-571.

39. Brenneman J. *Notes on Infant Feeding, Maternal and Artificial.* Butler, Indiana: Harry R Farnham; 1919:3-77.

40. Nichols BL. Pathogenesis of glucose malabsorption in acquired monosaccharide intolerance. In: Lifschitz F, ed. *Carbohydrate Intolerance in Infancy.* New York: Marcel Dekker; 1982:105-119.

41. Calvin RT, Klish WJ, Nichols BL. Disaccharidase activites, jejunal morphology and carbohydrate tolerance in children with chronic diarrhea. *J Pediatr Gastroenterol Nutr.* 1985;4:949-953.

42. Klish WJ, Udall JN, Calvin RT, Nichols BLT. The effect of intestinal solute load on water secretion in infants with acquired monosaccharide intolerance. *Pediatr Res.* 1980;14:1343-1346.

43. Nichols VN. Epidemiology of acquired monosaccharide intolerance. In: Lifschitz F, ed. *Carbohydrate Intolerance in Infancy.* New York: Marcel Dekker; 1982:21-29.

44. Jalili F, Smith EO, Nichols VN, Mintz AA, Nichols BL. A comparison of acquired monosaccharide intolerance and acute diarrheal syndrome. *J Pediatr Gastroenterol Nutr.* 1982;1:81-89.

45. Dahlqvist A. Enzyme deficiency and malabsorption of carbohydrates. In: Sipple HL, McNutt KW, eds. *Sugars in Nutrition.* New York: Academic Press; 1974:187-214.

Importance of Dietary Lipids
Berthold Koletzko, M.D.

Professor of Paediatrics
Kinderpoliklinik, Ludwig-Maximilians-University of Munich
Pettenkoferstr. 8a, D-80336 München, Germany

Reviewed by Nancy F. Butte Ph.D., Frank R. Greer M.D., Richardo Uauy M.D., Ph.D.
and Margit Hamosh Ph.D.

Introduction

> *"In fact we can conclude that dietary fat (in its chemical meaning), even in infants, can be completely substituted by sugar."*
>
> Franz von Groer, Vienna (1919)[1]

For a long time, dietary fats for infants and children were only considered a largely exchangeable source of energy. Compared with other nutrients such as protein, relatively little attention had been given to the amount and composition of dietary fat supplied to young children. This attitude has changed completely. Today, we know that the quality of dietary lipid supply in early childhood is of major importance for growth, body composition, infant development, and long-term health.[2-5] Thus, the choices made about dietary lipid supply during the first years of life are of great practical importance.

Practical Points

Lipids have a number of different physiological functions:

- *Lipids are the predominant dietary energy source for infants and young children, providing some 40 to 55% of the energy in human milk, and a similar proportion in many infant formulas. In contrast to proteins and carbohydrates, lipids can store energy in the body in almost unlimited amounts.*
- *The palatability of foods is greatly influenced by their lipid components, which are important for texture, flavor and aroma.*
- *Dietary lipids slow gastric emptying and intestinal motility, thereby may modulate the satiety value of food.*
- *Dietary lipids provide essential polyunsaturated fatty acids and lipid soluble vitamins.*
- *In the body, lipids are the major means of energy storage, with a much higher energy deposition per g of tissue than with glycogen or protein.*
- *Lipids serve as structural components of all tissues, particularly as indispensable parts of all cell and plasma membrane systems. The composition of structural lipids affects cell membrane functions, such as membrane fluidity, activity of membrane-bound enzymes and receptors, metabolite exchange and signal transduction. The brain and other neural tissues are particularly rich in structural lipids, and lipid supply and metabolism have been shown to affect neural functions.*
- *Some long-chain polyunsaturated fatty acids are precursors for bioactive lipid mediators, including prostaglandins, thromboxanes, and leukotrienes. These eicosanoids are powerful regulators of numerous cell and tissue functions (e.g. thrombocyte aggregation, inflammatory reactions and leukocyte functions, vasoconstriction, and the closure of the ductus arteriosus Botalli).*
- *Dietary lipid intake and cholesterol metabolism, even at a young age, may modulate the development of vascular lipid deposition and occurrence of early arterial lesions.*

The importance of lipid metabolism for infant growth becomes apparent if one considers that 35% of

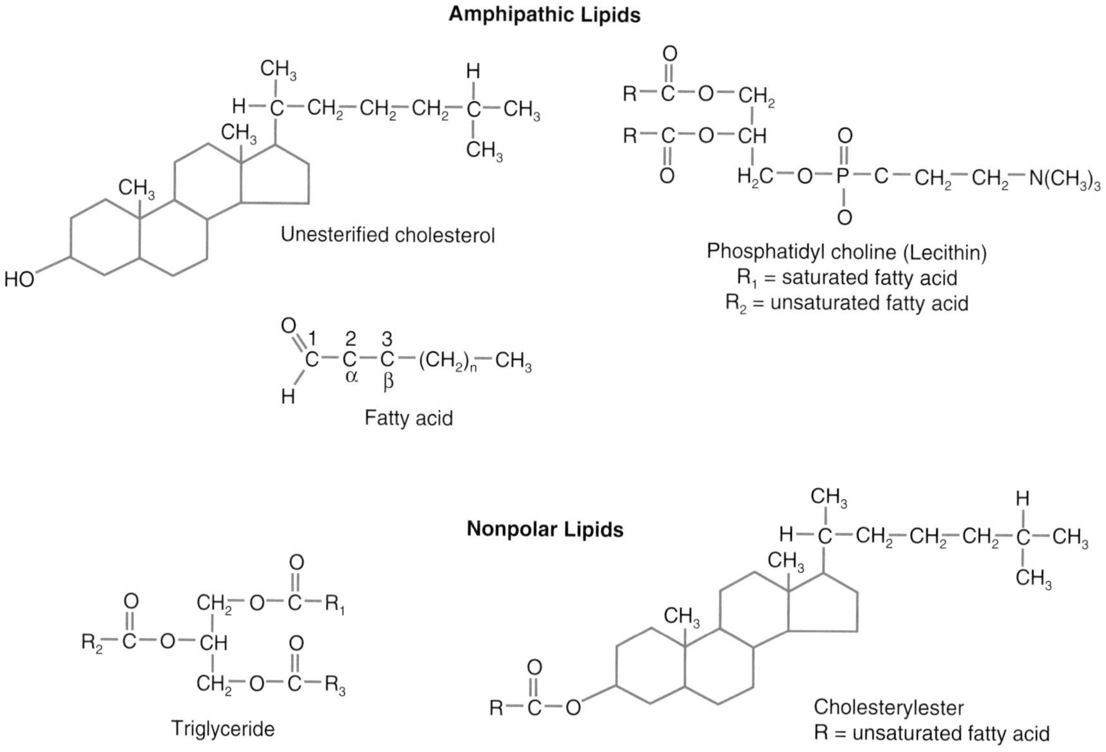

Figure 1: Structure of triglycerides and cholesterol esters (nonpolar lipids) and of mono- and diglycerides, phospholipids and cholesterol (amphipathic lipids with some affinity to water).

an infant's weight gain in the first six months of life is contributed by body fat, which equals about 90% of the energy stored in growing tissues during this period.[6] The purpose of this chapter is to review physiological properties of lipids and their roles in foods for infants and young children.

Physiology
Characteristics of Lipids

Lipids can be generally defined as substances that have no or very limited solubility in water, but are soluble in organic solvents (e.g., chloroform, hexane). Most of our dietary fats are triglycerides formed by three fatty acids esterified to a glycerol backbone (Figure 1). Vegetable oils, for example, consist almost entirely of triglycerides. Physicochemical properties of triglycerides (e.g., the melting point of a fat) are determined by the composition of its fatty acids. Watery foods may contain triglycerides either as a separate lipid layer or as an emulsion (such as milk). Emulsification can be achieved by amphipathic lipids that contain both hydrophobic parts, which associate with neutral lipids, as well as hydrophilic components, which interact with polar molecules such as water. Amphipathic lipids include phospholipids, monoglycerides and unesterified cholesterol and plant sterols (Figure 1). In contrast, cholesterol esters (esterified with a long-chain fatty acid) are non-polar.

In the body, triglycerides serve as the main form of storage and transport of fatty acids. Phospholipids and cholesterol, due to their amphipathic nature, are indispensable components of the lipid bilayer in all cell membranes (Figure 2). The amount of different phospholipids and cholesterol in membranes as well as the fatty acid pattern of incorporated phospholipids modulate membrane fluidity, permeability for metabolite exchange and degranulation of vesicles, activity of membrane bound enzymes and receptors, and signal transduction. Phospholipids and cholesterol are also incorporated into the surface of lipoproteins to allow the transport of non-polar (oily) lipids in the watery plasma. In addition, cholesterol is required in considerable amounts as the precursor for the synthesis of steroid hormones and bile acids. While dietary cholesterol contributes to the cholesterol pool in plasma and tissues, the major portion is derived from endogenous synthesis primarily in the liver, the activity of which is modulated by the diet.[8-11] An inborn defect of this endogenous cholesterol synthesis is associated with severe mental retardation in children with the Smith Lemli Opitz-syndrome.[12, 13]

The characteristics of esterified lipids depend largely on the nature of their fatty acids. The chain length of a fatty acid is the major determinant of its melting point; solubility in different media; energy content, efficacy of absorption; chain length also determines metabolic properties such as degree of deposition or oxidative degradation and effect on cholesterol metabolism. Conventionally, fatty acids are classified by chain length into four groups:

Fatty acids are either saturated, monounsaturated (contain one double bond) or polyunsaturated (two or more double bonds) (Figure 3). Double bonds occur in two isomeric forms, *cis* and *trans* (Figure 4). Plant and mammalian metabolism introduce almost entirely *cis*-configurated double bonds into fatty acids, in which both parts of the adjoining carbon chain point to the same direction of the double bond and, therefore, the molecule is bent becoming more flexible and fluid (Figure 4). *Trans*-isomeric fatty acids are formed primarily by rumen bacteria (in the forestomach of cows, goats and sheep) and by technical fat hydrogenation. *Trans*-fatty acids have a straight carbon chain, with a tertiary structure similar to saturated fatty acids (Figure 4). *Trans*-fatty acids have lower melting points and are less fluid than their respective *cis*-isomers.

In biochemistry, the position of double bonds within a fatty acid is conventionally described by distance to the terminal methyl group (the omega end of the fatty acid), because this part of the molecule is usually unchanged in human metabolism. Since fatty acids are activated by reacting with coenzyme A at the

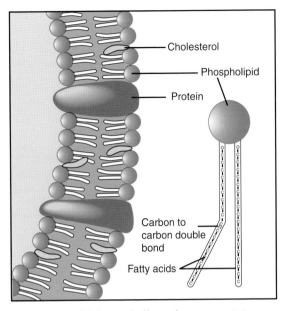

Figure 2: Lipid bilayer of cell membranes containing phospholipids and cholesterol.

carboxyl end, enzymatic biochemical alterations such as chain elongation, chain shortening by β-oxidation or introduction of double bonds occur at this part of the molecule. In contrast, the methyl or omega end of a fatty acid is little changed in intermediary metabolism. Therefore, omega-6 (ω-6 or n-6) or ω-3 fatty acids (with their terminal double bonds located 6 or 3 carbon atoms, respectively, from the terminal end of the molecule) remain ω-6 or ω-3 fatty acids in human metabolism, unless they are oxidized. Polyunsaturated fatty acids with their terminal double bonds in ω-6 (e. g., linoleic acid) or ω-3 positions (α-linolenic acid) are essential nutrients because man and higher animals cannot introduce double bonds in the ω-6 or ω-3 positions.[14]

Short formulas are used to describe fatty acids, which indicate the number of carbon atoms and double bonds as well the position of the terminal double bond. The saturated palmitic acid with 16 carbons and no double bonds is abbreviated as 16:0, the monounsaturated oleic acid with 18 carbons and 1 double bond in ω-9 position as 18:1ω-9, and the ω-6 polyunsaturated linoleic acid as 18:2ω-6 (cf. Table 1). The typical fatty acid composition of selected fats and oils is shown in Table 2.

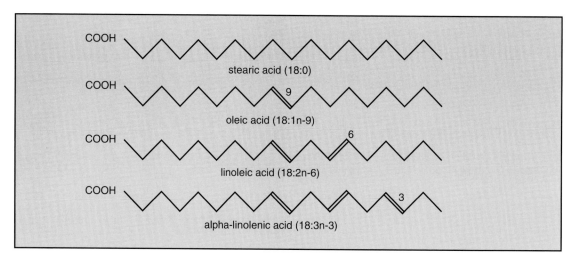

Figure 3: Long-chain saturated (stearic acid, 18:0), cis-monounsaturated (oleic acid, 18:1ω-9), and ω-6 (linoleic acid, 18:2ω-6) and ω-3 (a-linolenic acid, 18:3ω-3) polyunsaturated fatty acids.

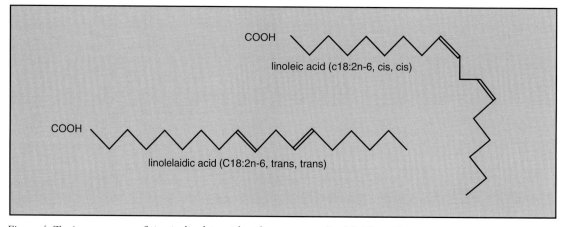

Figure 4: Tertiary structure of cis, cis, linoleic acid and trans, trans, linolelaidic acid.

Lipids in Human Milk

Human milk contains about 4% lipids, but the variation of fat content is large. Mammary alveolar cells synthesize milk fat, and this synthesis is stimulated by emptying of the breast through nursing and by prolactin secreted from the anterior lobe of the pituary gland (Figure 5). The major proportion of milk fat is formed from circulating lipids derived from the mother's diet and body stores. In addition, part of the milk fat can be synthesized *de novo* in the mammary gland from glucose, which results primarily in the formation of saturated fatty acids with 10 to 14 carbon atoms.[15] The proportion of these endogenously synthesized fatty acids with medium and intermediate chain length increases when breast-feeding women consume diets with a low fat and a high carbohydrate content.[16] The alveolar cells package and secrete the lipids into the lumen in the form of milk fat globuli (Figure 6). Milk fat globuli have a hydrophobic core consisting of triglycerides, and a hydrophilic membrane formed from phospholipids, cholesterol and proteins, which allows their dispersion in the watery environment of milk. Some 97 to 99% of the total milk fat is made up of triglycerides, whereas only relatively small proportions are contributed by diglycerides (0.7%), monoglycerides

Trivial Name	Systematic Name	Chain Length (C-atoms)	Number of Double Bonds	Position of Terminal Double Bond	Short Formula	Essential Fatty Acid
Short-chain saturated fatty acids						
acetic		2	0		C2:0	
propionic		3	0		C3:0	
butyric		4	0		C4:0	
caproic	hexanoic	6	0		C6:0	
Medium-chain saturated fatty acids						
caprylic	octanoic	8	0		C8:0	
capric	decanoic	10	0		C10:0	
Intermediate-chain saturated fatty acids						
lauric	dodecanoic	12	0		C12:0	
myristic	tetradecanoic	14	0		C16:0	
	pentadecanoic	15	0		C15:0	
Long-chain saturated fatty acids						
palmitic	hexadecanoic	16	0		C16:0	
margaric	heptadecanoic	17	0		C17:0	
stearic	octadecanoic	18	0		C18:0	
arachidic	eicosanoic	20	0		C20:0	
behenic	docosanoic	22	0		C22:0	
lignoceric	tetracasanoic	24	0		C24:0	
***Cis*-monounsaturated fatty acids**						
palmitoleic	cis-hexadecenoic	16	1	ω-7	C16:1ω-7	
oleic	cis-octadecenoic	18	1	ω-9	C18:1ω-9	
vaccenic	cis-octadecenoic	18	1	ω-7	C18:1ω-7	
***Trans*-monounsaturated fatty acids**						
elaidic	*trans*-octadecenoic	18	1 (*trans*)	ω-9	C18:1ω-9t	
trans-vaccenic	*trans*-octadecenoic	18	1 (*trans*)	ω-7	C18:1ω-7t	
***Cis*-polyunsaturated fatty acids**						
linoleic	octadecadienoic	18	2	ω-6	C18:2ω-6	✔
α-linolenic	octadecatrienoic	18	3	ω-3	C18:3ω-3	✔
γ-linolenic	octadecatrienoic	18	3	ω-6	C18:3ω-6	✔
dihomo-γ-linolenic	eicosatrienoic	20	3	ω-6	C20:3ω-6	✔
Mead	eicosatrienoic	20	3	ω-9	C20:3ω-9	
arachidonic	eicosatetraenoic	20	4	ω-6	C20:4ω-6	✔
	eicosapentaenoic	20	5	ω-3	C20:5ω-3	✔
cervonic	docosahexaenoic	22	6	ω-3	C22:6ω-3	✔
***Trans*-polyunsaturated fatty acids**						
linolelaidic	*trans*-octadecadienoic	18	2 (*trans*)	ω-6	C18:2ω-6t	

Although a large number (>250) of different fatty acids are found in the human body, the major portion is comprised by straight chain fatty acids with an even number of 10 to 24 carbon atoms. Fatty acids can be saturated or unsaturated (containing *cis*- or *trans*-configured double bonds.)

Table 1: Some physiologically important fatty acids.

Fatty acid	Corn	Saf-flower	Sun-flower	Soybean	Olive	Low erucic rapeseed	Evening primrose	Black currant	Shark oil	Coconut	MCT	Butter	Human milk
8:0										7.6	65-75	1.1	
10:0										5.7	25-35	2.5	0.7
12:0										45.0	1-2	2.8	4.4
14:0	1.4								6.1	17.2		10.0	6.7
16:0	10.0	5.7	6.2	9.5	10.8	3.8	9	7.4	27.8	8.6		26.2	21.8
16:1	0.5		0.5	0.5	1.5	0.5			5.9			2.3	2.7
18:0	2.4	2.4	4.8	3.4	2.4	1.4	1	0.8	4.2	2.4		12.1	8.2
18:1	31.1	11.4	21.9	20.1	71.7	60.1	7	10.4	16.2	6.7		25.1	34.3
18:2ω6	50.0	74.0	60.2	53.4	8.0	19.1	71	48.1	0.3	1.4		2.3	10.8
18:3ω3	0.9	0.5	0.5	7.6	0.95	8.6		12.7				1.4	0.8
18:3ω6							10	17.1					0.2
20:4ω6									5.1				0.4
20:5ω3									3.5				n.d.
22:1						0.5							0.1
22:6ω3									16.4				0.2

Table 2: Fatty acid composition (% wt/wt) of selected oils and fats. (Adapted from 79, 160.)

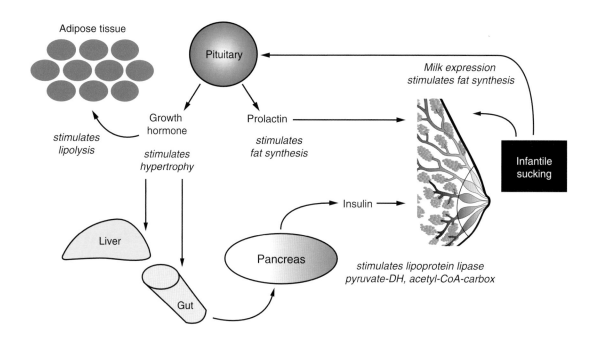

Figure 5: Regulation of human milk fat synthesis.

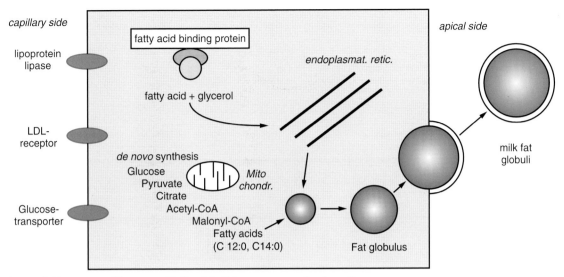

Figure 6: Formation of human milk fat globuli in mammary alveolar cells.

(traces), free fatty acids (0.4%), phospholipids (0.3%) and cholesterol (0.25%).[17, 18]

The fat content of human milk increases during the first four weeks (Figure 7) of lactation, which is accompanied by a rising average size of the milk fat globules and, therefore, a decreasing ratio of phospholipids and cholesterol (membrane lipids) to triglycerides (core lipids).[17, 18] Also, human milk fat increases, and the ratio of phospholipids and cholesterol to triglycerides decreases, during each nursing. This physiological phenomenon has been utilized clinically in poorly thriving preterm infants fed their mothers' expressed breast milk, where preferential feeding of the last two-thirds of milk obtained during expression (hindmilk) led to significantly improved weight gain.[19]

The diet of lactating women influences, to some extent, the fatty acid composition of human milk lipids. For example, the contents of trans fatty acids in milk reflect the maternal dietary intake of trans fatty acids and are higher in North America and Europe than in rural Africa, where little hydrogenated fat is consumed.[16, 20] However, the degree of variation of milk fatty acids is buffered to a certain extent by metabolic regulation,[21] such as the extensive utilization of endogenous lipid stores for human milk fat synthesis even in well-nourished breast-feeding women. Human milk fat usually is rich in monounsaturated fatty acids and provides the essential fatty acids linoleic and a-

linolenic acids, as well as their long-chain polyunsaturated metabolites such as arachidonic and docosahexaenoic acids. Since milk phospholipids are an important source of long-chain polyunsaturated fatty acids, the decrease of milk phospholipid content during the first month after birth is accompanied by a decrease of milk arachidonic and docosahexaenoic acids.[17, 7] The milk of mothers who delivered premature babies tends to have slightly higher amounts of endogenously synthesized fatty acids with 10 to 14 carbon atoms, but there is no consistent difference in the essential fatty acid content throughout the first month of lactation.[7] The contents of long-chain polyunsaturated fatty acids in mature human milk are relatively stable and rather similar in different geographic regions with different dietary compositions (Table 3). Even women consuming predominantly vegetarian diets with little dietary intake of preformed arachidonic acid maintain high milk contents of arachidonic acid,[16, 22] which again demonstrates the important effect of maternal metabolism, in addition to diet, on human milk lipid composition.

Lipid Digestion, Absorption and Transport

The digestion of dietary lipids is initiated in the stomach by the action of lingual and gastric lipases, which hydrolyze primarily triglycerides.[23, 24] After entering the duodenum, lipids are solubilized in mixed micelles

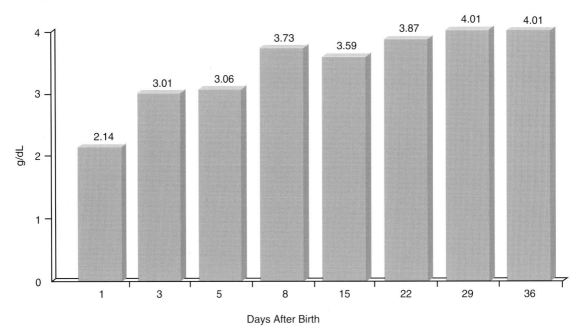

Figure 7: Increase of milk fat content with duration of lactation (mean milk triglyceride content of British & German women, day 1-36 of lactation. Hibberd et al, Arch Dis Child 1982).

	Africa (10 studies)	Europe (14 studies)
linoleic acid	12.0 (3.3)	11.0 (1.6)
arachidonic acid	0.6 (0.2)	0.5 (0.2)
total ω-6 LC-PUFA	1.5 (0.3)	1.5 (0.3)
α-linolenic acid	0.8 (0.4)	0.6 (0.2)
docosahexaenoic acid	0.3 (0.3)	0.3 (0.1)
total ω-3 LC-PUFA	0.6 (0.5)	0.6 (0.5)

Table 3: Essential fatty acids (% wt/wt, median and inter quartile range) in studies on mature human milk from Africa and Europe. (Adapted from 20.)

formed with conjugated bile acids. Hydrolysis is achieved by the concerted action of the pancreatic enzymes lipase, colipase, cholesterol ester lipase (which was shown to be identical to bile salt-stimulated human milk lipase), phospholipase A_2 and intestinal lipase. Liberated fatty acids and monoglycerides are absorbed by the intestinal mucosa and, in the case of short and medium chain fatty acids, also the gastric mucosa.[25] The

solubility and efficacy of absorption is greater for unsaturated than for saturated fatty acids, and it decreases with increasing chain length.[26] The absorption of long-chain saturated fatty acids is enhanced if they are esterified in the β- or sn-2-position of the triglyceride molecule. While saturated fatty acids are esterified in more or less random order within triglycerides of vegetable fats, the major portion of the saturated palmitic acid (16:0) in human milk triglycerides is in the sn-2-position.[17] Lipolytic hydrolysis will cleave the fatty acids in sn-1- and sn-3-positions, and palmitic acid from human milk will appear primarily in the remaining monoglyceride. Thereby, absorption is facilitated because palmitic acid monoglyceride is more polar and has a higher water-solubility than free palmitic acid (Figure 8). Clinical trials in formula-fed infants confirmed a better absorption of palmitic acid from triglycerides with preferential esterification in the sn-2 position compared to randomly esterified palmitic acid.[27] Calcium absorption is also improved, because there is less formation of insoluble calcium soaps with the saturated palmitic acid. However, healthy infants fed either human milk or current infant formulas (without structured triglycerides or bile salt-stimulated lipase) achieve a very efficient fat absorption, usually >90 to 95% of intake.

Following absorption of fatty acids and monoglycerides, triglycerides are resynthesized in the intestinal mucosa and packed together with phospholipids, cholesterol, cholesterol esters, lipid soluble vitamins and apoproteins B48 and E into chylomicrons, which are secreted via the lymphatic system into the circulation. Most of their triglyceride content is hydrolyzed by lipoprotein lipase bound to endothelial cells, and the liberated fatty acids are taken up by peripheral tissues (e.g., muscle, adipose tissue) (Figure 9). The activity of lipoprotein lipase is enhanced by apoprotein CII and in most tissues by insulin, while it is inhibited by apoprotein CIII.[28] The production of apoprotein CIII is regulated by nuclear receptors acting as gene transcription factors, such as apoprotein AI regulatory protein.[29]

The type of dietary fat consumed modulates the metabolism of chylomicrons. Consumption of unsaturated fatty acids results in larger chylomicrons that are cleared more effectively by lipoprotein lipase, because it has a higher affinity to unsaturated fatty acids. Hence, diets rich in ω-6 and ω-3 polyunsaturated fatty acids can reduce postprandial chylomicron levels by half.[30-33] After triglyceride removal, the remaining chylomicron remnant is taken up primarily in the liver by LDL receptors (apoprotein B/E receptors) or by apoprotein E mediated chylomicron remnant receptors.[34]

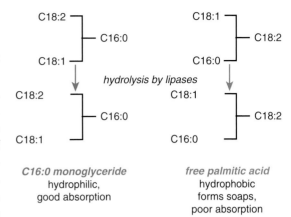

Figure 8: Predominant esterification of palmitic acid in the sn-2 position of human milk triglycerides facilitates absorption.

Triglyceride-rich Very Low Density Lipoproteins (VLDL) containing apoproteins B100 and E are synthesized by the liver and catabolized by endothelial lipoprotein lipase (Figure 9). Hepatic triglyceride synthesis depends primarily on the balance between fatty acid uptake and oxidation, because there appears to be only limited *de novo* synthesis of fatty acids. A diet high in saturated fatty acids effectively increases plasma VLDL, whereas VLDL are reduced by unsaturated fatty acids and particularly by long-chain ω-3 polyunsaturated fatty acids (fish oils) that not only enhance the rate of lipolysis but also decrease hepatic VLDL synthesis.[35, 36] Although VLDL content of cholesterol is to some extent modulated by dietary cholesterol intake, hepatic cholesterol synthesis usually exceeds dietary intake by far.[37, 38]

Hydrolytic clearance of VLDL triglycerides transforms these particles to Intermediary Density Lipoproteins (IDL), which can be taken up by the liver or converted further in the circulation to Low Density Lipoproteins (LDL), again influenced by the type of dietary fat. Mediated by binding of apoprotein B100 to the LDL receptor, LDL is taken up by the liver and peripheral tissues. The major regulator of LDL receptor synthesis, and hence of LDL uptake, is the intracellular cholesterol pool.[39] In addition, dietary saturated fatty acids suppress LDL receptor activity and LDL removal.[40-42] LDL may be modified by peroxidation, which is enhanced by proxidants (e.g., unbound iron

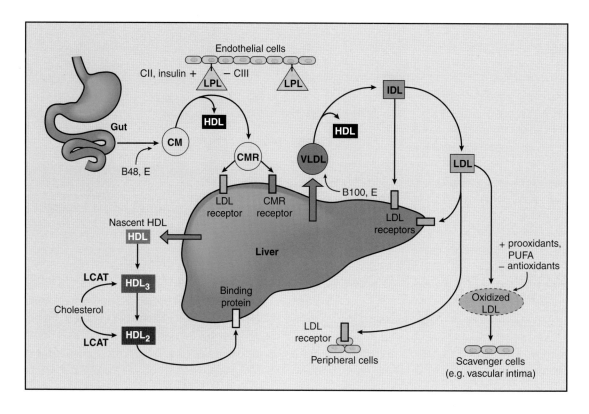

Figure 9: Schematic depiction of lipoprotein metabolism.

and copper) and polyunsaturated fatty acids but inhibited by antioxidants (e.g., α-tocopherol and β-carotene). Modified (oxidized) LDL is rapidly removed from the plasma by scavenger cells in various tissues, including the vascular intima. Thus, vascular lipid deposition is enhanced by high plasma concentrations of LDL (increased by dietary saturated fat, particularly by the saturated fatty acids lauric, myristic and palmitic acids with 12 to 16 carbons atoms, by *trans*-monounsaturated fatty acids), and by peroxidative LDL modification (enhanced by an excess of proxidants and polyunsaturates and a poor dietary intake of antioxidants).[43]

Disc-shaped nascent High Density Lipoproteins (HDL) contain apoproteins AI and AII and are secreted by the liver and the gut, or they are formed in the circulation during lipolysis of triglyceride-rich lipoproteins (chylomicrons and VLDL). Cholesterol from peripheral tissues is taken up by HDL, esterified by the action of Lecithin Cholesterol Acyl Transferase (LCAT), and thereby transformed from nascent HDL to HDL_3 and

HDL_2, which can be taken up in the liver by specific binding proteins.[44] High HDL levels have a strong protective effect against vascular cholesterol deposition and development of atherosclerosis.[45] Diet affects HDL levels. Polyunsaturated fatty acids both of the ω-6 and the ω-3 series reduce LCAT activity:[46, 47] therefore, high dietary intakes have the untoward effect of lowering protective HDL.[48-51] Diet also modulates the activity of Cholesterol Ester Transfer Protein (CETP), which mediates redistribution of newly formed cholesterol esters from HDL to VLDL and LDL.[52] Dietary cholesterol, saturated fats and *trans*-monounsaturated fats increase plasma CETP and LDL.[47, 53, 54] Table 4 shows a summary of the effects of dietary lipid intake on plasma LDL and HDL cholesterol levels.

Lipids and Energy Balance

The biological energy value of dietary long-chain triglycerides (around 9 kcal/g) is about 2.25 fold higher than that of carbohydrates and protein. The biological

Effects of dietary lipid intake on plasma lipoprotein cholesterol		
	LDL Cholesterol	**HDL Cholesterol**
Saturated fatty acids (12:0, 14:0, 16:0)	↑↑↑	↑
***Trans*-monosaturated fatty acids**	↑↑	↓
***Cis*-monosaturated fatty acids**	↓↓	↑
ω-6 polyunsaturated fatty acids	↓↓	↓
ω-3 polyunsaturated fatty acids	↑	≈
Cholesterol	↑	≈

Table 4: Effects of dietary lipid intake on plasma lipid protein cholesterol.

energy value of lipids for growing infants and young children, as reflected in the capacity to generate adenosine triphosphate (ATP) and deposit tissue during growth, appears to differ even more from non-lipid calories. During the first half year of life of a healthy full-term infant, lipids contribute about 35% of his weight gain or about 90% of the energy retained in his newly formed tissue.[6] Although the infant can synthesize lipids for tissue deposition *de novo* from carbohydrates or proteins, the capacity of this endogenous synthesis appears rather limited,[55] and it would result only in non-essential fatty acids with an unfavorable tissue composition. Moreover, endogenous lipid synthesis also requires an increased energy intake, because a substantial amount of the energy from dietary carbohydrates and proteins would be lost in energetically futile use of ATP for the synthesis of molecules for storage as metabolic fuel or tissue components.[56] For example, the synthesis of fat from glucose requires about 25% of the glucose energy invested for the cost of synthesis, whereas the synthesis of fat from fat requires only about 1 to 4% of the energy invested.[57] The extent of energy loss *in vivo* is difficult to determine, but a higher thermogenic effect of dietary carbohydrates and proteins as compared to long-chain lipids is well known.[58, 59] Studies supplying isoenergetic diets with different fat contents actually found a higher body

> *Fats for fun: From high fat to low fat with age: First to increase intelligence then to increase lifespan.*
>
> Kurt Widhalm M.D.
> Vienna, Austria

weight and fat gain and a lower energy expenditure on the higher fat diets.[59-61]

It is important to note that dietary medium-chain triglycerides (MCT) do not provide the same energy balance as long-chain triglycerides (LCT). MCT contain primarily saturated fatty acids with eight and ten carbon atoms and are effectively used for the treatment of fat malabsorption, because they have a high water solubility and are rapidly cleaved by lipases.[62] Due to the shorter chain length of their fatty acids, their energy content (per g fat) is about 15% lower than that of LCT. Moreover, MCT are rapidly oxidized and have a high thermogenic effect, because they can reach the liver directly without prior incorporation into chylomicrons and quickly enter the mitochondrion for β-oxidation, for a large part without the need for binding to coenzyme A and for carnitine-mediated transport into the mitochondria.[62, 63] When greater amounts of MCT are supplied in the diet, they are metabolized in several tissues by carnitine-dependent mechanisms and may indeed increase the need for carnitine.[64, 65] Even if about one-half of the medium-chain fatty acids supplied are not oxidized, they are also not deposited to any appreciable extent in human tissues as such but first need to be chain elongated, again an energy-consuming process.[66, 67] In fact, some studies evaluating the use of dietary MCT found that they induce a

Recommending body	Age range (months):			
	0-4 (-6)	6-12	12-24	24-36
Am. Acad. Pediatr., Comm. on Nutr., 1986 (160)				30-40
Am. Acad. Pediatr., Comm. on Nutr., 1992 (161)				30
Canadian Soc. Pediatr., 1993 (162)	no restriction of fat intake			
European Union 1995 (163)	≥40-58.5	(≥32-58.5*)		
European Soc. f. Peadiatr. Gastro. & Nutr. (ESPGAN), Comm. on Nutr., 1991 & 1994 (42, 89)	≥40-58.5	(≥32-58.5*)		30-35
World Health Organization/Food & Agriculture Organization 1994 (105)	50-60		30-40	30-40

*recommendation for follow-on formulae only, but not for total diet

Table 5: Some recommendations on the dietary intake of fat (in%) for infants and young children.

greater thermogenic effect[68] but have no advantage with respect to energy balance or weight gain.[69, 70]

Compared with the theoretical considerations regarding energy balance on low- or high-fat diets, the practical advantages of diets with relatively high contents of long-chain lipids for covering the high energy needs of young children may be even greater. The high palatability and caloric density of high-fat diets usually also results in a higher total energy intake. Thus, it is not surprising that obese individuals tend to have a greater weight gain on high-fat diets.[59, 71-73] On the contrary, failure to thrive has been observed in school age children given very low-fat diets with lipid contents <25% of energy intake (en%).[74] For healthy infants in the first half year of life, a high dietary lipid intake similar to the amount found in human milk (about 40 to 55% of energy content) appears desirable (Table 5).

Essential Fatty Acid Metabolism

Vegetable oils contain the parent essential fatty acids linoleic acid (18:2ω-6) and in most cases also α-linolenic acid (18:3ω-3). These two fatty acids have specific biological functions, for example, linoleic acid

is an indispensable structural component of certain dermal lipids with importance for the epidermal water barrier.[75] Moreover, linoleic and α-linolenic acids serve as precursors for the synthesis of physiologically important long-chain polyunsaturated fatty acids (LC-PUFA) with 20 and 22 carbon atoms, such as dihomo-γ-linolenic (20:3ω-6), arachidonic (20:4ω-6), eicosapentaenoic (20:5ω-3) and docosahexaenoic (22:6ω-3) acids (Figure 10). Human milk lipids contain preformed LC-PUFA in considerable amounts (Table 3), whereas vegetable oils and conventional infant formulas based on vegetable oils do not.[76, 77] LC-PUFA are essential components of all membrane systems and are incorporated in relatively large amounts in membrane-rich tissues, such as the brain, during early growth.[4, 78] Some LC-PUFA, namely dihomo-γ-linolenic (20:3ω-6), arachidonic (20:4ω-6) and eicosapentaenoic (20:5ω-3) acids, also serve as precursors for the formation of prostaglandins, prostacyclin, thromboxanes, leukotrienes and other lipid mediators that are powerful regulators of various cell and tissue processes (such as thrombocyte aggregation, inflammation, leukocyte functions, vasoregulation and the closure of the ductus arteriosus Botalli).

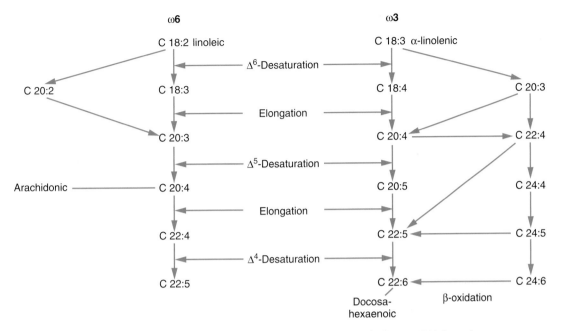

Figure 10: Pathways for biosynthesis of long-chain polyunsaturated fatty acids (LC-PUFA) from the precursors linolenic and α–linolenic acids. The presence of a direct Δ⁴-Desaturation has recently been questioned.

It has previously been assumed that a dietary supply of linoleic and α-linolenic acids would suffice to meet all human requirements of essential fatty acids, because the organism would synthesize sufficient amounts of LC-PUFA endogenously at all times. LC-PUFA are formed from the precursors by consecutive desaturation and chain elongation steps and, in the case of docosahexaenoic acid synthesis, it also involves indirect steps via 24-carbon fatty acids (Figure 10). The fetus *in utero* and the fully breast-fed infant do not depend on active endogenous synthesis, because the placenta and human milk lipids supply preformed LC-PUFA in amounts considered to meet the need for deposition in membrane-rich tissues.[5, 16, 79, 80] In contrast, premature infants fed vegetable oil-based formulae without LC-PUFA develop rapid LC-PUFA depletion of plasma lipids and red blood cell membranes, which indicates a limited activity of endogenous LC-PUFA synthesis.[81, 82] In premature infants, ω-6 LC-PUFA depletion has been associated with reduced growth;[83-86] ω-3 LC-PUFA depletion-induced alterations of electroretinogram responses and reduced visual acuity during the first months of life;[86-88] and an apparent disadvantage of cognitive development at a corrected age of one

year,[89] which could be corrected by LC-PUFA supplementation in the form of fish oil. Therefore, it is recommended in Europe that formulas for low birthweight infants (LBWI) should provide LC-PUFA.[90] Several products have become available, which differ in concentrations, relative contributions of the various essential fatty acid metabolites and lipid sources used.[91] There are still questions about the optimal dosage and composition of fatty acids in formulas[5] and the safety of supplementation, since some forms of LC-PUFA enrichment of LBWI formula may disturb infant growth and increase vitamin E requirements.[92, 93] Further research is required in this area.

These considerations on lipid supply for premature infants cannot be directly extended to healthy, full-term infants, because compared with low birthweight infants, they have larger body stores of lipids and LC-PUFA at birth, while their LC-PUFA requirements per kg bodyweight are lower because of their slower growth rate. The extent to which healthy infants synthesize LC-PUFA endogenously can be estimated today *in vivo* with stable isotope methods.[94] With this technique, we estimated linoleic acid conversion in healthy, full-term infants aged 18±4 days (mean±SD)

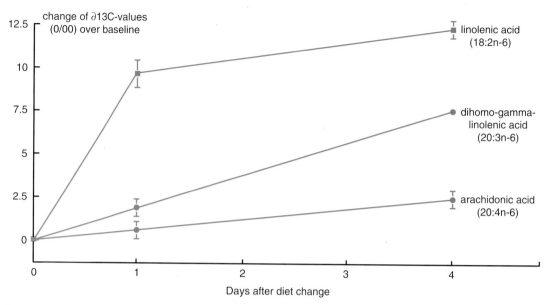

Figure 11: ^{13}C-enrichment (change of $\delta^{13}C$ ovr baseline) of plasma fatty acids in term infants fed a diet with increased ^{13}C-enrichment of linoleic acid. The increase of ^{13}C-contents in the linoleic acid metabolites dihomo-γ-linolenic acid and arachidonic acid indicates endogenous synthesis of LC-PUFA. (Modified from Demmelmair et al, 1995.)

given a diet providing linoleic acid with an increased content of the stable isotope ^{13}C.[94] ^{13}C-contents in different ω-6 fatty acids in infant plasma were measured and revealed a clear increase of ^{13}C-content, not only in the precursor linoleic acid, but also in its long-chain metabolites after the diet change (Figure 11). These data prove an active endogenous linoleic acid conversion, but the rate of conversion is slow. Using a simplified isotope balance equation, we estimate that the contribution of arachidonic acid synthesis to the total plasma arachidonic acid pool is only in the order of about 6% per day.[95] In agreement with these results, feeding studies indicate that healthy, full-term infants fed formula without LC-PUFA cannot match the LC-PUFA status of breast-fed infants for at least two months after birth (Figure 12).[96] The resulting depletion of ω-3 LC-PUFA in formula-fed term infants also extends to structural brain lipids, as was shown in babies who had died from sudden infant death syndrome.[97, 98] Similar to the cited findings in low birthweight infants, ω-3 LC-PUFA depletion in term infants has been associated with reduced visual acuity in the first half year of life.[99-102] In view of these observations, the possibility of LC-PUFA enrichment of infant formula (for healthy, full-term infants) is presently being evaluated.[103] Some investigators have reported beneficial effects from LC-PUFA enrichment of infant formula on visual and cognitive development in term infants;[101, 102, 104] another study reported in abstract form found no advantage, and a delay in speech development.[105] Some manufacturers of infant formulas for healthy term infants offer products with added LC-PUFA,[91] as it has been recommended by some expert groups.[106, 107] However, further research is required to study in more detail metabolic effects, functional outcome and safety related to the various forms of LC-PUFA supply for infants.

Needs of Term Infants
Total Lipids

Public health efforts in adult populations often emphasize the importance of limiting the dietary intake of saturated and total fats to prevent cardiovascular disease, obesity, type II diabetes and certain forms of cancer. This has also led to a reduction of total lipid intakes in many young childhood populations, reaching average values as low as 28 to 30% of energy at 6 to 12 months of age in different studies;[108-111] some 10% of the infants in these

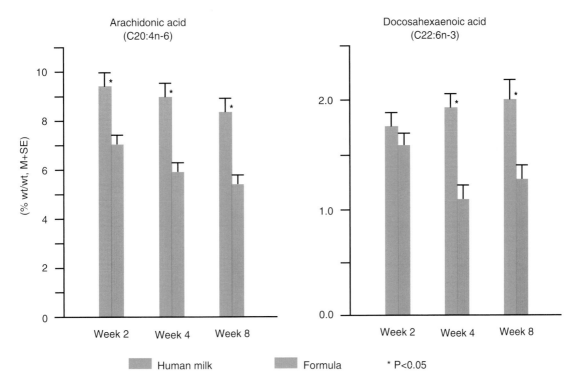

Figure 12: Contribution of the major LC-PUFA arachidonic acid (20:4ω6) and docosahexaenoic acid (20:6ω3) to plasma phospholipids of healthy term infants fed human milk or vegetable based infant formula at 2, 4 and 8 weeks of life. The lower values in formula fed infants indicate that at least up to the age of 2 months, their capacity for endogenous LC-PUFA synthesis from dietary precursors is not sufficient to match the essential fatty acid status of breast fed infants. (Modified from 95).

studies are at lipid intakes below about 22% of energy intakes.[111] In contrast, fully breast-fed infants have dietary lipid intakes of about 50% of energy intakes, which is considered beneficial for energy balance and growth (cf. above). Adverse effects of low-fat diets on weight gain and longitudinal growth in young children have been documented.[74, 111, 112] As a further adverse effect, it has been proposed that chronic non-specific diarrhea (toddlers diarrhea, "pea and carrot diarrhea") may be a complication of low-fat diets.[113] Since chronic, non-specific diarrhea is considered a motility disorder, it may improve after an increase of fat intake which slows gastric emptying and small intestinal motility.

The main argument put forward for a restricted total lipid intake in young children is that it may be beneficial for prevention of cardiovascular disease at a later age. However, preventive effects are expected only from a reduction of saturated and *trans*-monounsatu-

rated fats, not of total lipids[114] (Table 4). In fact, epidemiological studies in a population born in the 1920s raised the possibility that poor growth during the first year of life, which is associated with a low dietary energy density, may even increase the risk of cardiovascular mortality later in life.[115] There is no firm basis to favor low total fat intakes in children with normal body weight during the first two to three years of life.

Although there is a certain degree of variability between recommendations of different authorities on dietary total fat intakes in early childhood (Table 5), most bodies do not advise low-fat diets at an early age. During the period of rapid growth in the first four to six months of life, the contribution of total fat to energy intake should be similar to full breast-feeding, above about 40% of energy. With increasing age, a stepwise reduction to about 30 to 35% of energy at the age of two to three years appears reasonable (Table 6), because this

Heart healthy childhood diet	
• saturated fatty acids	• ≤ about 8-12 en%
• *trans*-fatty acids	• low intake
• polyunsaturated fatty acids	• about 6-10 en%
• monounsaturated fatty acids	• no limitation
• cholesterol	• ≤ about 300 mg/day
• antioxidative vitamins	• generous intake desirable
• sodium chloride	• low intake desirable
• complex carbohydrates	• generous intake desirable
• total fat intake	• about 30-35 en% (as one practical way to achieve a limited intake of saturated and *trans*-fatty acids)

Table 6: Childhood diet and prevention of coronary heart disease in later life. Recommended diet for children from the age of two to three years onwards and for adolescents.[42]

is one way to achieve the desirable limited intake of saturated and *trans*-unsaturated fatty acids (Table 6).

Polyunsaturated Fatty Acids

The exact essential fatty acid requirements of healthy infants and young children are not known, which explains a certain variability between recommendations on dietary intake (Table 7). The factorial approach and balance studies conventionally used to define requirements of many nutrients is of limited value for essential fatty acids because of their large and multiple body pools. Moreover, one must expect considerable inter- and intraindividual variability of dietary requirements, which may vary with prenatal nutrient supply, body weight, postnatal and postconceptional age, growth rate, metabolic and endocrine

factors, other dietary components and many other variables.[116] Clinical deficiency symptoms with impaired weight gain and skin changes may occur at PUFA intakes below 1% of energy, and abnormal patterns of serum fatty acids in infants at PUFA intakes below about 2 to 4.5% of energy.[116-118]

The minimal intake of linoleic acid (18:2ω-6) recommended for young infants is in the range of 2.7 to 4.5% of energy (Table 7). In Europe, a maximum level of 10.8% of energy was set[90, 119] because of concerns over potential adverse effects of very high intakes, including enhanced lipid peroxidation and α-tocopherol requirements, inhibition of arachidonic acid and prostaglandin formation, and immunosuppression.[115, 119] The European reference intakes for linoleic acid for children in the second year of life were set lower (3% of energy intake, cf. Table 7) than in the first year (4.5% of energy intake) in consideration of the lower growth rate and higher body stores after the first year.[121]

It is generally acknowledged that the infant also needs ω-3 fatty acids. In Europe, an α-linolenic acid (18:3ω-3) intake of 0.5 % of energy has been set as the minimum level of intake with infant formulas[119] and also as the reference intake throughout the second year of life[121] (Table 7). Moreover, the ratio between dietary linoleic and α-linolenic acids has been considered a variable of potential importance, because both fatty acids compete for the same enzyme system for conversion into LC-PUFA (Figure 10). There are indications that variations of the dietary linoleic/α-linolenic acid ratio modulate the relative contents of the metabolites arachidonic and docosahexaenoic acids in infantile cell membrane lipids.[122] For European infant formulas, the range of acceptable of linoleic/α-linolenic acid ratios was set as 5-15.[90, 119]

No unanimous agreement has been reached so far on dietary provision of preformed LC-PUFA. The ESPGHAN (European Society for Paediatric Gastroenterology, Hepatology and Nutrition) Committee on Nutrition concluded in 1991 that LC-PUFA "supplementation to infant formulas, i.e. for infants born at term, might be of advantage, but further data on this question are required prior to a definite recommendation".[90] In contrast, the British Nutrition foun-

Recommending body	Age range (months):			
	0-4 (-6)	6-12	12-24	24-36
Am. Acad. Pediatr., Comm. on Nutr., 1976 (164)	≥2.7 LA			
Brit. Nutr. Found. 1992 (121)	4 LA, 0.2 AA, 0.4 ALA, 0.2 DHA			
European Soc. f. Paediatr. Gastro. & Nutr. (ESPGAN), Comm. on Nutr., 1991 (89)	4.5-10.8 LA 0.3-2.2 ALA	(4.5-10.8 LA*) (0.3-2.2 ALA*)		
European Union 1991 & 1995 (131, 163) requirements for infant formulae & follow-on formulae	2.7-10.8 LA 0.5-2.2 ALA *(LC-PUFA optional: ω-6 ≤2%, ω-3 ≤1% of fatty acids)*	(≥2.7 LA*)		
European Union population reference intakes, 1993 (119)		4.5 ω-6 0.5 ω-3	3 ω-6 0.5 ω-3	3 ω-6 0.5 ω-3
World Health Organization/Food & Agriculture Organization 1994 (105)	600 mg/kg LA 50 mg/kg ALA 40 mg/kg AA 20 mg/kg DHA			

Abbreviations: LA=linoleic acid, AA=arachidonic acid, ALA=α-linolenic acid, DHA=docosahexaenoic acid; LC-PUFA=long-chain polyunsaturated fatty acids
*recommendation for follow-on formulae only, but not for total diet

Table 7: Some recommendations on the dietary intake of polyunsaturated fatty acids (% of energy intake) for infants and young children.

dation advises that all infant formula should contain 0.2% of energy each of arachidonic and docosahexaenoic acids.[123] Also, the International Society for the Study of Fatty Acids and Lipids (ISSFAL)[124] and an expert committee of the World Health Organization and the Food and Agriculture Organization of the UN[107] recommended adding preformed LC-PUFA to infant formula. Current revisions of regulations on infant formula in the European Union permit the optional addition of ω-6 LC-PUFA up to 2% and ω-3 LC-PUFA up to 1% of fatty acids,[119] but no minimal level of intake has been set. However, there is no indication of a requirement or benefit of a supply of preformed LC-PUFA after the first months of life.

Deficiency

Franz von Goer in 1919[1] described the first cases of essential fatty acid deficiency in great detail, but due to the limited understanding of the physiological bases, misinterpreted his observations (cf. introduction). Two infants with low-birthweight (2,400 and 1,900 g) were fed from birth with skim milk and added sugar. After three and six months, respectively, body weight gain came to a standstill, and the infants showed recurrent vomiting, anorexia and infections. After a diet change, with some delay the infants started to thrive again.

In the late 1920s, linoleic acid deficiency was rediscovered in rats raised from birth on fat-free diets; they failed to thrive after two to three months and developed

	Plasma sterolesters of 29 premature infants (day 4 of life) (133)		Plasma phospholipids of 53 healthy children (age 1-15 years, mean 7.5 years) (134)	
	18:1-trans	Total trans	18:1-trans	Total trans
Linoleic acid (18:2ω-6)	r=-0.14 (n.s.)	r=0.01 (n.s.)	r=-0.02 (n.s.)	r=-0.04 (n.s.)
Arachidonic acid (20:4ω-6)	r=-0.45 (P<0.05)	r=-0.38 (P<0.03)	r=-0.33 (P=0.015)	r=-0.32 (P=0.018)
Ratio arachidonic/ linoleic acid	r=-0.46 (P<0.05)	r=-0.36 (P<0.05)	r=-0.28 (P=0.045)	r=-0.26 (P=0.062)

Table 8: Trans octadecenoic acid (18:1-trans) and total trans fatty acids in plasma lipids of premature infants and of healthy children do not correlate with the major dietary essential fatty acid linoleic acid, but show significant inverse relations to the desaturation product arachidonic acid as well as the product substrate ratio of ω-6 essential fatty acid conversion, which is compatible with trans fatty acid induced inhibition of essential fatty acid conversion. (Adapted from 166.)

scaly skin lesions.[125] In human infants, systematic feeding studies on infants in an orphanage later confirmed the occurrence of essential fatty acid deficiency after one to three months of feeding a low-fat diet, with failure to thrive and dry, leathery, desquamative dermatitis (Figure 13).[126] These skin lesions could be corrected with supplying about 1% of energy as linoleic acid. Since then, numerous cases on human essential fatty acid deficiency have been reported on low-fat diets, chronic fat malabsorption or fat-free parenteral nutrition.[127, 128] Deficiency of ω-3 fatty acids has been associated with neurological symptoms in a child[129] and with skin changes in old people,[130] and from these observations the minimal requirement of ω-3 fatty acids has been estimated as about 0.2 to 0.5% of energy.

Potential Adverse Effects of Dietary Lipids

Some dietary lipids may induce untoward effects in infants and young children. Unsaponifiable ingredients in sesame seed oil were reported to cause allergic reactions,[131] and cyclopropenoids in cotton seed oil were found to impair essential fatty acid desaturation;[132] therefore, the use of both oils for infant formula has been banned in Europe.[90, 119, 133]

Trans fatty acids impair the conversion of linoleic acid to its long-chain metabolites *in vivo* in animals and *in vitro* in animal cells and human fibroblasts, apparently caused by competitive inhibition of desaturating enzymes.[134] Inverse correlations between *trans* fatty acids and LC-PUFA were found in human premature infants and in healthy children (Table 8).[135, 136] These findings are compatible with impairment of LC-PUFA synthesis in man, a potentially serious side effect of *trans* fatty acids in view of the importance of LC-PUFA availability for infant growth and development.[14, 83] Furthermore, a reduction of pre- and postnatal growth was observed in animals exposed to high levels of *trans* fatty acids.[134] Similarly, an inverse correlation between *trans* fatty acid values in plasma lipids and birthweight was observed in premature infants.[135] Since there is no advantage in the use of oils with high contents of *trans* fatty acids for the production of foods for infants and young children, the European Union set an upper limit of 4% of total fat for the *trans* fatty acid content of infant formula and follow-on formula.[119]

Erucic acid is a long-chain monounsaturated fatty acid (22:1ω9) found in high amounts in some types of rapeseed oil (high erucic acid rapeseed oil). Absorbed erucic acid is oxidized slowly; it may accumulate in myocardium and cause structural and functional abnormalities in myocardial mitochondria as well as

Author/year	Age at follow up (years)	Serum cholesterol (mg/dl)		P
		Breast-fed	Formula-fed	
Friedman et al 1975	1.5-2	155±6	155±5	n.s.
Wart et al 1980	2.5	152±17	141±12	<0.05
Huttunen et al 1983	5	189±4	182±4	n.s.
Crawford et al 1981	6	188±26	195±27	n.s.
Fomon et al 1984	8	163±27	164±29	n.s.
Hodgson et al 1978	7-12	172±27	157±29	<0.02

Table 9: Results of follow-up studies on the effect of infant feeding on serum cholesterol values in later life. There is no indication for a consistent long-term effect. (Adapted from Rey & Bresson, 1995 (167).)

myocardial lipidosis.[137, 138] Such side effects were observed at high but not at low (< 1 % of dietary fatty acids) levels of intake.[138] In contrast to Canada, rapeseed oils with low erucic acid contents may not be used for infant formula production in the USA.[139] In Europe, an upper limit of erucic acid contents of 1% of fatty acids was set for infant formula and follow-on formula;[119] thus low erucic acid rapeseed and borrage oils may be used for formula production there.

Oils with high contents of saturated fatty acids with intermediate chain length (lauric acid, 12:0, and myristic acid, 14:0) such as coconut and palm kernel oil have been used in relatively high proportions to produce some types of infant formula, because fatty acids of intermediate chain length are well absorbed and, in contrast to long-chain fatty acids, tend not to bind to and reduce absorption of calcium and magnesium.[140] Human milk has relatively low contents of lauric (around 5 to 7%) and myristic acids (around 6 to 8%). There is concern about high dietary intakes of lauric and myristic acids, because of all fats these are the two fatty acids with the strongest cholesterol-raising effect.[141, 142] Although conclusive data on the phyiological effects in infants are not available, untoward effects on lipoprotein metabolism and vascular lesions cannot be excluded. Therefore, the lauric and myristic acid contents in European infant formula and follow-on formula were restricted to a maximum of 15% each.[119, 133]

Human milk contains considerable amounts of cholesterol (about 200 mg/l),[17] while contents in infant for-mula based on vegetable oil are negligible. Consequently, breast-fed infants tend to have higher serum cholesterol values and a lower endogenous cholesterol synthesis than infants fed formula.[10] Experimental studies in rats found that postnatal feeding of milk with a higher cholesterol content led to lower serum cholesterol in adulthood, which raised the hypothesis that postnatal cholesterol exposure could program a favorable metabolic cholesterol handling in later life. However, follow-up studies of human infants fed human milk or formula do not provide any basis to assume a beneficial long-term effect on human serum cholesterol values (Table 9). On the contrary, follow-up studies of newborn baboons randomly assigned to postnatal feeding with breast milk or commercial infant formula revealed higher serum cholesterol values and more extensive arterial lipid deposition in those primates previously breast-fed. It remains unclear whether this difference is causally related to postnatal cholesterol intake or to other differences between breast milk and the formula used.

Lipids in Infant Formula

The fat content of most regular infant formula is in the range of about 3.5 to 4 g/100 ml, similar to human milk.[5, 18, 77, 143] The choice of fats used in infant formula should allow for efficient absorption and provide a balanced supply of metabolic substrates, in particular of essential polyunsaturated fatty acids and lipid soluble vitamins, in the absence of adverse effects. Blends of different fats, for the major part different vegetable

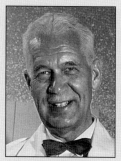

Arild E. Hansen M.D., Ph.D. (1899-1962) took his graduate degrees at the University of Minnesota. Hansen's pioneering work with eczema-prone infants soon found in 1937 that their serum fatty acids were low in polyunsaturated fatty acids, and that the eczema improved in response to diet supplementation with essential fatty acids (EFA). While Chairman of Pediatrics at University of Texas Medical Branch in 1958, Hansen discovered that evaporated cow milk diluted with sugar (Marriott's bottle feeding formula) lead to eczema and EFA deficiency in children and thus proved the importance of EFA in the human diet. Holman R. T: George O. Burr and the Discovery of Essential Fatty Acids. J Nutr.118, 535-540, 1988 and J. Pediatr. 63, 1179-1181, 1963 (Photo courtesy of A. Goldman)

oils, are used for formula to achieve a suitable triglyceride fatty acid composition. These triglycerides are emulsified with added phospholipids, such as soybean and egg lecithins, and monoglycerides. Compared with human milk, many current infant formulas tend to have somewhat lower contents of monounsaturated fatty acids and higher levels of saturated fatty acids. Since long-chain saturated fatty acids are not very well absorbed by the infant, oils providing medium and intermediate-chain fatty acids, such as coconut oil and medium chain triglycerides (Table 2), are often used as part of the fat body in regular infant formula. This is the case particularly in low-birthweight infant formulae and in special dietary products (cf. appendix: Hansen, composition of infant formulae) intended for use in infants with fat malabsorption caused by cholestasis, pancreatic disorders or other diseases. Infantile fat absorption is improved by the use of oils rich in monounsaturated fatty acids, such as high oleic acid sunflower seed oil and low erucic acid rapeseed oil, and to a limited extent also by the use of structured lipids with esterification of long-chain saturated fatty acids in the sn-2 position; this is however limited by their relatively high costs.

All infant formula and special dietary products for use in infants need to provide essential fatty acids both of the ω-6 and the ω-3 series. Most infant formulas

contain linoleic and α-linolenic acids in amounts similar to or greater than typical human milk contents (Table 3). More recently, some low birthweight infant formulas and a few term infant formulae with added metabolites of linoleic and α-linolenic acids have become available in some countries.[91] Different sources for enriching of formulas with such metabolites are available; fish oils, which provide docosahexaenoic and eicospentanoic acids in varying proportions, oils that contain the linoleic acid metabolite γ-linolenic acid (evening primrose oil, borrage oil or black currant seed oil), some special fish oils and egg phospholipid fractions that provide arachidonic acid, and biotechnologically-produced microbial oils from microalgae and fungi that can provide docosahexaenoic and arachidonic acids (686, 685, 683). It remains to be determined whether some of these sources have advantages over others for the infant.

Parenteral Lipid Emulsons

Full parenteral feeding of infants requires using lipid emulsions and to supply fatty acids to meet their high energy needs for maintenance and growth, which cannot be covered with the use of glucose and amino acids alone. Lipid emulsions consist of different oils (Table 10) emulsified with egg yolk phospholipids, to which glycerol is added to achieve isoosmolarity. The fat particles in the emulsions resemble endogenously-produced chylomicrons in size, physicochemical properties and metabolism.[144-146] The enzyme lipoprotein lipase plays the central role in clearing infused fat particles by hydrolysing the tryglyceride-rich core and liberating fatty acids and gylcerol for tissue uptake and utilization. Hepatic lipase contributes to removal of the triglyceride-depleted remnant particles.[145, 146] Lipolysis of infused triglycerides usually is very efficient in mature neonates, even after surgery.[147] In contrast, infused phospholipids from the infusion tend to accumulate in the infant's plasma. In addition to the phospholipids in the coating of triglyceride rich particles, the emulsions contain significant amounts of excess phospholipid in the form of vesicles, that after infusion take up cholesterol from cell membranes until reaching equimolar saturation.[148, 149] The extent of the resulting hyperphospholipidemia and hypercholes-

Oil Base	Soybean	Soybean/ MCT	Soybean/ Borrage	Olive/ Soybean	Soybean/ Fish
Product name (manufacturer)	Intralipid (Pharmacia), Ivelip (Clintec), Lipofundin (Braun), Lipovenös (Fresenius), Liposyn III (Abbott)	Lipofundin MCT (Braun)	PFE 4501 (Pharmacia) (167)	ClinOleic (Clintec)	Lipovenös + Omegavenös, 9+1 parts mix (Fresenius) (168)
triglycerides (%)	10, 20 &30%	20%	20%	20%	10%
ratio phospholipids/ triglycerides (mg/g)	120, 60 & 40	60	60	60	66
glycerol (%)	2.5	2.5	2.25	2.25	2.5
kcal/ml	1.1-2.0	1.9	2.0	2.0	1.1
Fatty acid composition (% wt/wt)					
medium chain (8:0+10:0)	n.d.	50	n.d.	n.d.	n.d.
palmitic (16:0)	9-11.2	5	11.2	13.5	10.8
stearic (18:0)	4-4.2	2	6.1	2.9	3.7
oleic (18:1ω9)	20.4-26	12	20.9	59.5	19.9
linoleic (18:2ω6)	52.4-54.5	27	55	18.5	49.7
α-linolenic (18:3ω3)	8-8.5	4	7.0	2	6.5
γ-linolenic (18:3ω6)			3.5		
arachidonic (20:4ω6)	n.d.-0.2	n.d.		0.2	0.2
eicosapentaenoic (20:5ω3)	n.d.	n.d.		n.d.	2.4
docosahexaenoic (22:6ω3)	n.d.-0.1	n.d.		0.1	2.3

Table 10: Composition of some intravenous lipid emulsions. (Based on manufacturers data and 168, 169.)

terolemia in the infant depends on the amount of excess phospholipid infused;[150] therefore, emulsions with a low phospholipid/triglyceride ratio (such as the usual 20% emulsions) are preferred for use in infants and young children.

An important advantage of lipid emulsions over glucose solutions is their high energy density in an isoosmolar solution, which is also well tolerated in peripheral vein infusions. The survival of peripheral vein catheters in infants can be significantly prolonged when the same dosage of nitrogen and calories is infused, but with a higher lipid/glucose ratio and hence a lower osmolarity of the infusate. Moreover, the additional infusion of lipids, compared to glucose and amino acids only, significantly reduces infantile energy expenditure, presumably because the infant can avoid the high energetic cost of glucose conversion to fatty acids. Since the respiratory quotient of lipids (about 0.7) is markedly lower than that of glucose (1.0), lipid infusion at the same level of energy intake will also reduce infantile CO_2-production, which may ease weaning from the respirator in some patients.

Prospective[151] and retrospective[152] studies in very low-birthweight neonates have associated very early lipid infusion during the first days of life with a poor outcome, such as increased rates of chronic lung dis-

	Patient	Reference values (median and interquartile range), (169)
Linoleic acid (18:2ω6)	6.2	14.7 [4.0]
Arachidonic acid (20:4ω6)	3.8	7.9 [3.3]
α-linolenic acid (18:3ω3)	n.d.	0.1 [0.04]
Docosahexaenoic acid (22:6ω3)	1.1	2.3 [1.0]
Mead acid (20:3ω9)	1.7	n.d.

Table 11: Fatty acid composition of plasma phospholipids on day eight of life in a term infant with essential fatty acid deficiency due to fat free parenteral feeding (n.d.=not detectable).

ease and retinopathy of prematurity; other observations do not confirm such an association.[153] The limited data available from clinical studies point to a possible risk of early lipid infusion for very immature and sick infants with extremely low birthweight, but this questions needs to be evaluated further. At this time, there is no indication of similar risks associated with parenteral feeding of mature infants. One hypothesis is that infusion of highly unsaturated fats to sick and very immature infants during the first days of life might expose them to enhanced oxidative stress, which might contribute to adverse outcomes.[154-156] Although this hypothesis remains to be tested, it appears prudent to provide infants receiving lipid emulsions with an adequate supply of antioxidants such as vitamin E.

Of the different emulsions available (Table 10), those based on soybean oil have been most extensively evaluated, and are most widely used in infants. Soybean oil emulsions provide both precursor essential fatty acids of the ω-6 and the ω-3 series. In contrast, previously used safflower oil emulsions did not contain appreciable amounts of ω-3 fatty acids, therefore, they are inadequate for feeding infants for more than a few days. An emulsion containing a mixture of soybean oil providing long-chain fatty acids and MCT oil was reported to have advantages in adult intensive care patients, but experience with this emulsion in infants is still limited.[157] The established lipid emulsions are rich in precursor-essential fatty acids, but contain only small amounts of LC-PUFA from the phospholipid emulsifier. Therefore, new products with metabolites of the classical essential fatty acids, such as γ-linolenic acid and long-chain ω-3 fatty acids, have been developed to improve the fatty acid supply to the infant (Table 10). Also, emulsions with a reduced content of the precursor-essential fatty acids achieved by mixing soybean oil with MCT or olive oil (Table 10) might have beneficial effects on infantile essential fatty acid metabolism. Further results on the clinical evaluation of these different emulsions in infants are awaited with great interest.

Today, the standard choice for use in infants is a soybean oil emulsion with a low phospholipid/triglyceride ratio, which should be infused continuously over 20 to 24 hours/day. The daily dose can be increased stepwise from 1 g/kg bodyweight to 2 to 3 g/kg. Dosages above 3 g/kg should only be used in selected cases with repeated monitoring of serum triglyceride concentrations. Dosage reduction is recommended if serum triglycerides exceed 150 mg/100 ml.

The coinfusion of lipid emulsions, heparin and high concentrations of calcium may lead to aggregation of the lipid particles (creaming of the emulsion) and should be avoided.[157] Similarly, serum of children with high concentrations of C-reactive protein (CRP) mixed *ex vivo* with lipid emulsion induces creaming.[159,160] Since the *in vivo* effects are not known, we tend to lower the dose of infused lipids to about 0.5 g triglyceride/kg bodyweight & day in patients with a transient rise of CRP to >2 mg/100 ml.

Case History

Case #1: *This infant was born as the first child of healthy parents after 39 weeks of an uneventful pregnancy with a weight of 3420 g. At first breast-feeding, the infant coughed severely and became dyspneic. X-ray of the thorax revealed aspiration in the right upper pulmonary lobe, and a contrast esophagogram indicated esophageal atresia with tracheoesophageal fistula. The infant was fed parenterally with amino acids and glucose, and surgery was performed on day two of life. Postoperatively, the child could not be weaned from the respirator, aspiration pneumonia was diagnosed and treated with antibiotics. The baby received nothing per os and was fed by a central venous catheter with amino acids, increased stepwise to a daily dose of 2.5 g/kg day, and glucose, increased stepwise to a daily dose of 14.5 g/kg day, but no lipids. The pulmonary infiltration did not show satisfactory improvement, and wound healing was poor. From day eight of life onwards, the skin was noted to be extraordinarily dry and scaly, particularly at forehead, hands (Figure 13) and feet. Plasma zinc levels and alkaline phosphatase were normal. Analysis of plasma phospholipid fatty acids revealed reduced levels of essential fatty acids and increased Mead acid (Table 11).*

Diagnosis: *Essential fatty acid deficiency*

Treatment: *The infant received a soybean oil emulsion intravenously (initial dose 1 g triglycerides/kg daily, dosage increased to 2 g/kg), and the skin symptoms cleared within a few days.*

Comment: *In enterally-fed infants with severe fat malabsorption, e.g., due to severe cholestasis, it may take several months before essential fatty acid deficiency becomes manifest. However, because parenteral feeding with a high continuous glucose supply stimulates insulin secretion and*

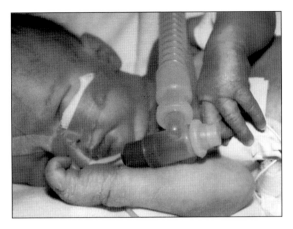

Figure 13: Scaly, dry dermatitis in an eight-day old newborn infant with confirmed essential fatty acid deficiency. The infant suffered from tracheoesophageal fistula treated surgically on day two of life, and from aspiration pneumonia, and received fat free parenteral nutrition. See detail in color atlas (page 240).

blocks lipolysis, endogenous essential fatty acid stores cannot be utilized and clinical signs of essential fatty acid deficiency may occur within about a week. Biochemical markers of essential fatty acid deficiency are:

a) subnormal values of essential fatty acids in plasma lipids, and

b) increased plasma values of Mead acid (ω9 eicosatrienoic acid, 20:3ω9). Mead acid is a metabolite of the non-essential oleic acid (18:1ω9). Usually there is no appreciable Mead acid synthesis because the binding of the precursor oleic acid to the desaturating enzyme is competitively inhibited by linoleic and α-linolenic acids, both of which have a higher binding affinity. Thus, the occurrence of increased plasma levels of Mead acid indicates low intracellular linoleic and α-linolenic acid levels.

Historical Perspective...

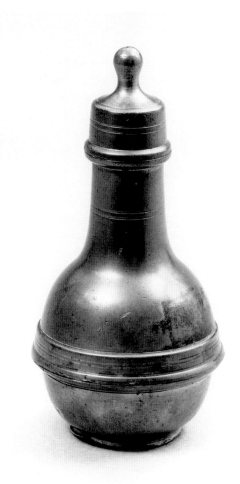

English, circa 1780 - This pewter feeder is a type common to England,
France and Holland from 1600 to 1800

References

1. von Gröer F. Zur Frage der praktischen Bedeutung des Nährwertbegriffes nebst einigen Bemerkungen über das Fettminimum des menschlichen Säuglings. *Biochem Z.* 1919;97:311-329.

2. Hamosh M. Fat needs for term and preterm infants. In: Tsang R, ed. *Nutrition During Infancy.* Raven; 1990.

3. Innis SM. Reviewed by: Gross SJ, Hamosh M, Koletzko B, Uauy R. Fat. In: Tsang RC, Lucas A, Uauy R, Zlotkin S, eds. *Nutritional Needs of the Preterm Infant.* Baltimore: Williams & Wilkins; 1993:65-86.

4. Koletzko B. Fats for brains. *Eur J Clin Nutr.* 1992;46: S51-S62.

5. Koletzko B, Thiel I, Springer S. Lipids in human milk: a model for infant formulae? *Eur J Clin Nutr.* 1992;46: S45-S55.

6. Fomon SJ, Haschke F, Ziegler EE, Nelson SE. Body composition of reference children from birth to age 10 years. *Am J Clin Nutr.* 1982;1169-1175.

7. Genzel-Boroviczény O, Wahle J, Koletzko B. Fatty acid composition of human milk during the first month after preterm and preterm delivery. *Eur J Pediatr.* 1997; 156:142-147.

8. Russell DW. Cholesterol biosynthesis and metabolism. *Cardiovasc Drugs Ther.* 1992;6:103-110.

9. Rudney H, Panini SR. Cholesterol biosynthesis. *Curr Opinion Lipidol.* 1993;4:230-237.

10. Wong WW, Hachey DL, Insull W, Opekun AR, Klein PD. Effect of dietary cholesterol on cholesterol synthesis in breast-fed and formula-fed infants. *J Lipid Res.* 1993; 34:1403-1411.

11. Wong WW, Hachey DL, Clarke LL, Zhang S. Cholesterol synthesis and absorption by 2H2O and 18O-cholesterol and hypocholesterolemic effect of soy protein. *J Nutr.* 1995;125:S612-S618.

12. Tint GS, Salen G, Batta AK, et al. Correlation of severity and outcome with plasma sterol levels in variants of the Smith-Lemli-Opitz syndrome. *J Pediatr.* 1995;127:82-87.

13. Abuelo DN, Tint GS, Kelley R, Batta AK, Shefer S, Salen G. Prenatal detection of the cholesterol biosynthetic defect in the Smith-Lemli-Opitz syndrome by the analysis of amniotic fluid sterols. *Am J Med Genet.* 1995; 56:281-285.

14. Decsi T, Koletzko B. Polyunsaturated fatty acids and infant nutrition. *Acta Paed Suppl.* 1994;395:1-7.

15. Thompson BJ, Smith S. Biosynthesis of fatty acids by lactating human breast epithelial cells: an evaluation of the contribution to the overall composition of human milk fat. *Pediatr Res.* 1985;19:139-143.

16. Koletzko B, Thiel I, Abiodun PO. Fatty acid composition of mature human milk in Nigeria. *Z Ernährungwiss.* 1991;30:289-297.

17. Jensen RG. *The Lipids of Human Milk.* Boca Raton: CRC Press; 1989.

18. Jensen RG. *Handbook of Milk Composition.* San Diego: Academic Press; 1995.

19. Valentine CJ, Hurst NM, Schanler RJ. Hindmilk improves weight gain in low-birth-weight infants fed human milk. *J Pediatr Gastroenterol Nutr.* 1994;18:474-477.

20. Koletzko B. Zufuhr, Stoffwechsel und biologische Wirkungen trans-isomerer Fettsäuren bei Säuglingen. *Die Nahrung.* 1991;35:229-283.

21. Koletzko B, Thiel I, Abiodun PO. The fatty acid composition of human milk in Europe and Africa. *J Pediatr.* 1992;120:S62-S70.

22. Sanders TAB, Reddy S. The influence of a vegetarian diet on the fatty acid composition of human milk and the essential fatty acid status of the infant. *J Pediatr.* 1992;120:S71-S77.

23. Hamosh M. *Lingual and gastric lipases: their role in fat digestion.* Boca Raton, FL: CRC Press; 1988.

24. Bernback S, Blackberg L, Hernell O. The complete digestion of human milk triacylglycerol in vitro requires gastric lipase, pancreatic co-lipase-dependent lipase, and bile salt stimulated lipase. *J Clin Invest.* 1990;85:1221-1226.

25. Hamosh M, Bitman J, Liao TH, et al. Gastric lipolysis and fat absorption in preterm infants: effects of medium-chain triglyceride or long-chain triglyceride-containing formulas. *Pediatrics.* 1989;83:86-92.

26. Chappell JE, Clandinin MT, Kearney-Volpe C, Reichmann B, Swyer PW. Fatty acid balance studies in premature infants fed human milk or formula: effect of calcium supplementation. *J Pediatr.* 1986;108:439-447.

27. Filer LJ, Mattson FH, Fomon SJ. Triglyceride configuration and fat absorption in the human infant. *J Nutr.* 1969;99:293-298.

28. Olivecrona T, Bengtsson-Olivecrona G. Lipoprotein lipase and hepatic lipase. *Curr Opin Lipidol.* 1990;1:222-230.

29. Ladias JAA, Karathanasis SK. Regulation of the apolipoprotein AI gene by ARP-1, a novel member of the steroid receptor superfamily. *Science.* 1991;251: 561-565.

30. Quarfordt SH, Goodman DWS. Heterogeneity in the rate of plasma clearance of chylomicrons of different size. *Biochem Biophys Acta.* 1966;116:382-385.

31. Ockner RK, Hughes FB, Isselbacher KJ. Very low density lipoproteins in intestinal lymph: role in triglyceride and cholesterol transport during fat absorption. *J Clin Invest.* 1969;48:2367-2373.

32. Ockner RK, Jones AL. An electron microscopic and functional study of very low density lipoproteins in intestinal lymph. *J Lipid Res.* 1970;11:284-292.

33. Weintraub MS, Zechner R, Brown A, Eisenberg S, Breslow JL. Dietary polyunsaturated fats of the ω-6 and ω-3 series reduce postprandial lipoprotein levels. Chronic and acute effects of fat saturation on postprandial lipoprotein metaabolism. *J Clin Invest.* 1988;82:1884-1893.

34. Brown MS, Herz J, Kowal RC, Goldstein JL. The low-density receptor-related protein: double agent or decoy? *Curr Opin Lipidol.* 1991;2:65-72.

35. Rustan AC, Nossen JO, Christiansen EN, Drevon CA. Eicosapentaenoic acid reduces hepatic synthesis and secretion of triacylglycerol by decreasing the activity of acyl-CoA:1,2-diacylglycerol acyltransferase. *J Lipid Res.* 1988;29:1417-1426.

36. Singer P, Wirth M, Berger I. A possible contribution of decrease in free fatty acids to low serum triglyceride levels after diets supplemented with n-6 and n-3 polyunsaturated fatty acids. *Atherosclerosis.* 1990;83: 167-175.

37. Spady DK, Woollett LA, Dietschy JM. Regulation of plasma LDL-cholesterol levels by dietary cholesterol and fatty acids. *Ann Rev Nutr.* 1993;13:355-381.

38. Hegsted DM, Ausman LM, Johnson JA, Dallal GE. Dietary fat and serum lipids: an evaluation of the experimental data. *Am J Clin Nutr.* 1993;57:875-883.

39. Dawson PA, Hofmann SL, van der Westhuyzen DR, Sudhof TC, Brown MS, Goldstein JL. Sterol-dependent repression of low density lipoprotein receptor promotor mediated by 16-base pair sequence adjacent to binding site for transcription factor Sp 1. *J Biol Chem.* 1988;263: 3372-3379.

40. Shepherd J, Packard CJ, Grundy SM, Yeshurun D, Gotto AM, Taunton OD. Effects of saturated and polyunsaturated fat diets on the chemical composition and metabolism of low density lipoproteins in man. *J Lipid Res.* 1980;21:91-99.

41. Fox JC, McGill HC, Carey KD, Getz GS. *In vivo* regulation of hepatic LDL receptor mRNA in the baboon. Differential effects of saturated and unsaturated fat. *J Biol Chem.* 1987;262:7014-7020.

42. Spady DK, Woollett LA. Interaction of dietary saturated and polyunsaturated triglycerides in regulating the processes that determine plasma low density lipoprotein concentrations in the rat. *J Lipid Res.* 1990;31:1809-1819.

43. ESPGAN Committee on Nutrition. Committee Report: childhood diet and prevention of coronary heart disease. *J Pediatr Gastro Nutr.* 1994;19:261-269.

44. Tozuka M, Fidge N. Purification and characterization of two high-density-lipoprotein-binding proteins from rat and human liver. *Biochem J.* 1989;261:239-244.

45. Stampfer MJ, Sacks FM, Salvini S, Willett WC, Hennekens CH. A prospective study of cholesterol, apolipoproteins, and the risk of myocardial infarction. *N Engl J Med.* 1991;325:373-381.

46. Gjone E, Nordoy A, Blomhoff JP, Wiencke I. The effects of unsaturated and saturated dietary fats on plasma cholesterol, phospholipids and lecithin:cholesterol acyltransferase activity. *Acta Med Scand.* 1972;191:481-484.

47. Abbey M, Clifton PM, McMurchie EJ, McIntosh GH, Nestel PJ. Effect of a high fat/cholesterol diet with or without eicosapentaenoic acid on plasma lipids, lipoproteins and lipid transfer protein activity in the marmoset. *Atherosclerosis.* 1990;81:163-174.

48. Weisweiler P, Janetschek P, Schwandt P. Influence of polyunsaturated fats and fat restriction on serum lipoproteins in humans. *Metabolism.* 1985;34:83-87.

49. Ginsberg HN, Barr SL, Gilbert A, et al. Reduction of plasma cholesterol level in normal men on an American Heart Association step 1 diet or a step 1 diet with added monounsaturated fat. *N Engl J Med.* 1990;322:574-579.

50. Mata P, Alvares-Sala LA, Rubio MJ, Nuno J, de Oya M. Effects of long-term monounsaturated- vs. ployunsaturated-enriched diets on lipoproteins in healthy men and women. *Am J Clin Nutr.* 1992;55:846-850.

51. Mensink RP, Katan M. Effect of dietary fatty acids on

serum lipids and lipoproteins. A meta-analysis of 27 trials. *Arterioscler Thromb.* 1992;12:911-919.

52. Tall AR. Plasma lipid transfer proteins. *J Lipid Res.* 1986;27:361-367.

53. Stein Y, Dabach Y, Hollander G, Stein O. Cholesteryl ester transfer activity in hamster plasma: increase by fat and cholesterol rich diets. *Biochem Biophys Acta.* 1990; 1042:138-141.

54. Quinet EM, Agellon LB, Kroon PA, et al. Atherogenic diet increases cholesteryl ester transfer protein messenger RNA levels in rabbit liver. *J Clin Invest.* 1990;85:357-363.

55. Flatt JP. The difference in the storage capacities for carbohydrate and for fat, and its implications in the regulation of body weight. *Ann NY Acad Sci.* 1987;499: 104-123.

56. Newsholme EA. Substrate cycles: their metabolic, energetic and thermic consequences in man. *Biochem Soc Symp.* 1978;43:183-205.

57. Flatt JP, Ravussin E, Acheson KJ, Jéquier E. Effects of dietary fat on postprandial substrate oxidation and on carbohydrate and fat balances. *J Clin Invest.* 1985;76: 1019-1024.

58. Dauncey MJ, Bingham SA. Dependence of 24 hour energy expenditure in man on the composition of nutrient intake. *Br J Nutr.* 1983;50:1-13.

59. Lean MEJ, James PT. Metabolic effects of isoenergetic nutrient exchange over 24 hours in relation to obesity in women. *Int J Obes.* 1988;12:15-27.

60. Wood JD, Reid JT. The influence of dietary fat on fat metabolism and body fat deposition in meal-feeding and nibbling rats. *Br J Nutr.* 1975;34:15-24.

61. van Aerde JE, Sauer PJ, Pencharz PB, Smith JM, Heim T, Swyer PR. Metabolic consequences of increasing energy intake by adding lipid to parenteral nutrition in full term infants. *Am J Clin Nutr.* 1994;59:659-662.

62. Bach AC, Babayan V. Medium-chain triglycerides: an update. *Am J Clin Nutr.* 1982;36:950-962.

63. Baba N, Bracco EF, Hashim SA. Enhanced thermogenesis and diminished deposition of fat in response to overfeeding with diet containing medium chain triglyceride. *Am J Clin Nutr.* 1982;35:678-682.

64. Borum PR. Medium-chain triglycerides in formula for preterm neonates: Implications for hepatic and extrahepatic metabolism. *J Pediatr.* 1992;120:S139-S145.

65. Rebouche CJ, Panagides DD, Nelson SE. Role of carnitine in utilization of dietary medium-chain triglycerides by term infants. *Am J Clin Nutr.* 1990;52: 820-824.

66. Sarda P, Lepage G, Roy CC, Chessex P. Storage of medium-chain triglycerides in adipose tissue of orally fed infants. *Am J Clin Nutr.* 1987;45:399-405.

67. Carnielli V, Sulkers EJ, Moretti C, et al. Conversion of octanoic acid into long-chain saturated fatty acids in premature infants fed a formula containing medium-chain triglycerides. *Metabolism.* 1994;43:1287-1292.

68. Seaton TB, Welle SL, Warenko MK, Campbell RG. Thermic effect of medium-chain and long-chain triglycerides in man. *Am J Clin Nutr.* 1986;44:630-634.

69. Brooke OG. Energy balance and metabolic rate in preterm infants fed standard and high-energy formulas. *Br J Nutr.* 1980;44:13-23.

70. Whyte RK, Campbell D, Stanhope R, Bayley HS, Sinclair JC. Energy balance in low birth weight infants fed formula of high or low medium-chain triglyceride content. *J Pediatr.* 1986;108:964-971.

71. Kendall A, Levitsky DA, Strupp BJ, Lissner L. Weight loss on a low-fat diet: consequence of the imprecision of the control of food intake in humans. *Am J Clin Nutr.* 1991;53:1124-1129.

72. Tremblay A, Plourde G, Despres JP, Bouchard C. Impact of dietary fat content and fat oxidation on energy intake in humans. *Am J Clin Nutr.* 1989;49:799-805.

73. Astrup A, Buemann B, Christensen NJ, Toubro S. Failure to increase lipid oxidation in response to increasing dietary fat content in formely obese women. *Am J Physiol.* 1994;266:592-599.

74. Lifshitz F, Moses N. Growth failure. A complication of dietary treatment of hypercholesterolemia. *Am J Dis Child.* 1989;143:537-542.

75. Elias PM. Epidermal lipids, barrier function, and desquamation. *J Invest Derm.* 1983;80:44-49.

76. Koletzko B, Bremer HJ. Fat content and fatty acid composition of infant formulae. *Acta Paediatr Scand.* 1989;78:513-521.

77. Decsi T, Behrendt E, Koletzko B. Fatty acid composition of Hungarian infant formulae revisited. *Acta Paediatr Hung.* 1994;34:107-116.

78. Decsi T, Koletzko B. Polyunsaturated fatty acids in infant nutrition. *Acta Paediatr.* Suppl. 1994;395:31-37.

79. Koletzko B, Müller L. *Cis-* and *trans*-isomeric fatty acids in plasma lipids of newborn infants and their mothers. *Biol Neonate.* 1990;57:172-178.

80. Koletzko B, Mrotzek M, Bremer HJ. Fatty acid composition of mature human milk in Germany. *Am J Clin Nutr.* 1988;47:954-959.

81. Koletzko B, Schmidt E, Bremer HJ, Haug M, Harzer G. Effects of dietary long-chain polyunsaturated fatty acids on the essential fatty acid status of premature infants. *Eur J Pediatr.* 1989;148:669-675.

82. Koletzko B, Edenhofer S, Lipowsky G, Reinhardt D. Effects of a low birthweight infant formula containing docosahexaenoic and arachidonic acids at human milk levels. *J Pediatr Gastro Nutr.* 1995;21:200-208.

83. Koletzko B, Braun M. Arachidonic acid and early human growth: is there a relation? *Ann Nutr Metab.* 1991;35:128-131.

84. Carlson SE, Cooke RJ, Werkman SH, Tolley EA. First year growth of preterm infants fed standard compared to marine oil n-3 supplemented formula. *Lipids.* 1992;27:901-907.

85. Leaf AA, Leighfield MJ, Costeloe KL, Crawford MA. Long chain polyunsaturated fatty acids and fetal growth. *Early Hum Dev.* 1992;30:183-191.

86. Carlson SE, Werkman SH, Tolley EA. Effect of long-chain n-3 fatty acid supplementation on visual acuity and growth in preterm infants with and without bronhcopulmonary dysplasia. *Am J Clin Nutr.* 1996 (in press).

87. Uauy R, Birch DG, Birch EE, Tyson JE, Hoffman DR. Effect of dietary omega-3 fatty acids on retinal function of very-low-birth-weight neonates. *Pediatr Res.* 1990;28:485-492.

88. Carlson SE, Werkman SH, Rhodes PG, Tolley EA. Visual-acuity development in healthy preterm infants: effect of marine-oil supplementation. *Am J Clin Nutr.* 1993;58:35-42.

89. Carlson SE, Wilson WW. Docosahaenoic acid (DHA) supplementation of preterm (PT) infants: effect on the 12-month Bayley mental developmental index (MDI). *Pediatr Res.* 1994;35:20A[Abstract].

90. ESPGAN Committee on Nutrition. Committee report. Comment on the content and composition of lipids in infant formulas. *Acta Paediatr Scand.* 1991;80:887-896.

91. Koletzko B. Lipid supply for infants with special needs. *Eur J Med Res.* 1997;2:69-73.

92. Carlson SE, Werkman SH, Peeples JM, Wilson WM. Growth and development of premature infants in relation to n-3 and n-6 fatty acid status. In: Galli C, Simopoulos AP, Tremoli E, eds. *Fatty acids and lipids: biological aspects.* Basel: S Karger AG; 1994:63-69.

93. Koletzko B, Decsi T, Sawatzki G. Vitamin E status of low birthweight infants fed formula enriched with long-chain polyunsaturated fatty acids. *Int J Vit Nutr Res.* 1995;65:101-104.

94. Demmelmair H, Sauerwald T, Richter T, Koletzko B. New insights into lipid and fatty acid metabolism via stable isotopes. *Eur J Pediatr.* In Press.

95. Demmelmair H, von Schenck U, Behrendt E, Sauerwald T, Koletzko B. Estimation of arachidonic acid synthesis in fullterm neonates using natural variation of 13C-abundance. *J Pediatr Gastro Nutr.* 1995;36:31-36.

96. Decsi T, Thiel I, Koletzko B. Essential fatty acid status in full term infants fed breast milk or formula. *Arch Dis Child.* 1995;72:F23-F28.

97. Farquharson J, Cockburn F, Patrick WA, Jamieson EC, Logan RW. Infant cerebral cortex phospholipid fatty-acid composition and diet. *Lancet.* 1992;340:810-813.

98. Makrides M, Neumann MA, Byard RW, Simmer K, Gibson RA. Fatty acid composition of brain, retina, and erythrocytes in breast- and formula-fed infants. *Am J Clin Nutr.* 1994;60:189-194.

99. Makrides M, Simmer K, Goggin M, Gibson RA. Erythrocyte docosahexaenoic acid correlates with the visual response of healthy, term infants. *Pediatr Res.* 1993;34:425-427.

100. Jorgensen MH, Jonsbo F, Holmer G, Hernell O, Michaelsen KF. Breast-fed (BF) term infants have a better visual acuity than formula fed (FF) infants at the age of 2 and 4 mo. *FASEB J.* 1994;8:460[Abstract].

101. Makrides M, Neumann M, Simmer K, Pater J, Gibson R. Are long chain polyunsaturated fatty acids essential nutrients in infancy? *Lancet.* 1995;345:1463-1468.

102. Carlson SE, Ford AJ, Werkman SH, Peeples JM, Koo WK. Visual acuity and fatty acid status of term infants fed human milk and formulas with and without docosahexaenoate and arachidonate from egg yolk lecithin. *Pediatr Res.* 1996 (in press).

103. Decsi T, Koletzko B. Growth, fatty acid composition of plasma lipid classes, and plasma retinol and tocopherol concentrations in fullterm infants fed formula enriched with long-chain polyunsaturated fatty acids. *Acta Paediatr.* 1995;84:725-732.

104. Agostoni C, Trojan S, Bellu R, Riva E, Giovannini M. Neurodevelopmental quotient of healthy term infants at 4 months and feeding practice: the role of long-chain polyunsaturated fatty acids. *Ped Res.* 1995;38:262-266.

105. Janowsky JS, Scott DT, Wheeler RE, Auestad N. Fatty acids affect early language development. *Ped Res.* 1995; 37:110A[Abstract].

106. The British Nutrition Foundation. *Unsaturated fatty acids. Nutritonal and physiological significance. The report of the British Nutrition Foundation's Task Force.* London: Chapman & Hall; 1992:1-211.

107. WHO-FAO. Fats and oils in human nutrition. Report of a joint expert consultation. Rome: Food and Agriculture Organization of the UN: 1994.

108. Persson LA, Johansson E, Samuelson G. Dietary intake of weaned infants in a Swedish community. *Hum Nutr App Nutr.* 1984;38:247-254.

109. Martinez GA, Ryan AS, Malec DJ. Nutrient intakes of American infants and children fed cow`s milk or infant formula. *Am J Dis Child.* 1985;139:1010-1018.

110. Lapinleimu H, Viikari J, Jokinen E, et al. Prospective randomised trial in 1062 infants of diet low in saturated fat and cholesterol. *Lancet.* 1995;345:471-476.

111. Michaelsen KF, Jorgensen MH. Dietary fat content and energy density during infancy and childhood; the effect on energy intake and growth. *Eur J Clin Nutr.* 1995. (in press).

112. Hansen D, Michaelsen KF, Skovby F. Growth during treatment of familial hypercholesterolemia. *Acta Paediatr.* 1992;81:1023-1025.

113. Cohen SA, Hendricks KM, Eastham EJ, Mathis RK, Walker WA. Chronic nonspecific diarrhea. A complication of dietary fat restriction. *Am J Dis Child.* 1979;133: 490-492.

114. ESPGAN Committee on Nutrition. Committee report: comment on childhood diet and prevention of coronary heart disease. *J Pediatr Gastroenterol Nutr.* 1994;19: 261-269.

115. Barker DJP. *Fetal and Infant Origins of Adult Disease.* London: BMJ Publishing group; 1992.

116. Koletzko B. Minimal, optimal, maximal essential fatty acid requirements during infancy: term infants. In: Ghisolfi G, Putet G, eds. *Essential Fatty Acids and Infant Nutrition.* Paris: John Libbey Eurotext; 1992:147-156.

117. Naismith DJ, Deeprose SP, Supramaniam G, Williams MJH. Reappraisal of linoleic acid requirement of the young infants, with particular regard to use of modified cow`s milk formulae. *Arch Dis Child.* 1978;53:845-849.

118. Crawford MA, Hassam AG, Rivers JPW. Essential fatty acid requirements in infancy. *Am J Clin Nutr.* 1978;31: 2181-2185.

119. Scientific Committee for Food. Report of the Scientific Committee for Food on the essential requirements for infant formulae and follow-on formulae. 1993[Abstract].

120. Caroll KK. Upper limits of nutrients in infant formulas: polyunsaturated fatty acids and trans fatty acids. *J Nutr.* 1989;119:1810-1813.

121. Nutrient and energy intakes for the European Community. *Reports of the Scientific Committtee for Food.* Thirty-first series. Luxembourg; Commission of the European Communities: 1993. Office for Official Publications of the European Communities. 1-248.

122. Clark KJ, Makrides M, Neumann MA, Gibson RA. Determination of the optimal ratio of linoleic to alpha-linolenic acid in infant formulas. *J Pediatr.* 1992;120: S151-S158.

123. British Nutrition Foundation. *Unsaturated fatty acids: nutritional and physiological significance.* The report of the British Nutrition Foundation`s task force. London: Chapman & Hall; 1992.

124. ISSFAL Board Statement. Recommendations for the essential fatty acid requirement for infant formulas. *ISSFAL Newsletter.* 1994;1:4-5.

125. Burr GO, Burr MM. A new deficiency disease produced by the rigid exclusion of fat from the diet. *J Biol Chem.* 1929;82:345-367.

126. Wiese HF, Hansen AE, Adam DJD. Essential fatty acids in infant nutrition. I. Linoleic acid requirement in terms of serum di-, tri- and tetraenoic acid levels. *J Nutr.* 1958;66:345

127. Yamanaka WK, Clemans GW, Hutchinson ML. Essential fatty acids deficiency in humans. *Prog Lipid Res.* 1981;19: 187-215.

128. Koletzko B. Essentielle Fettsäuren: Bedeutung für Medizin und Ernährung. *Akt Endokr Stoffw.* 1986;7:18-27.

129. Holman RT, Johnson SB, Hatch TF. A case of human linolenic acid deficiency involving neurological abnormalities. *Am J Clin Nutr.* 1982;35:617-623.

130. Bjerve KS, Mostad IL, Thoresen L. Alpha-linolenic acid deficiency in patients on long-term gastric tube feeding: estimation of linolenic and long-chain unsaturated n-3 fatty acid requirement in man. *Am J Clin Nutr.* 1987;45: 66-77.

131. Hayakawa R, Matsunaga K, Suzuki M. Is sesamol present in sesame oil? *Contact Dermatitis.* 1987;17:133-135.

132. Phelps RA, Shenstone FS, Kemmerer AR, Evans RJ. A review of cyclopropenoid compounds: biological effects of some derivates. *Poult Sci.* 1965;44:358-394.

133. Commission of the European Communities. Commission directive of 14 May 1991 on infant formulae and follow-on formulae. *Official J of the European Communities.* 1991.

134. Koletzko B. Zufuhr, Stoffwechsel und biologische Wirkungen *trans*-isomerer Fettsäuren bei Säuglingen. *Die Nahrung - Food.* 1991;35:229-283.

135. Koletzko B. Trans fatty acids may impair biosynthesis of long-chain polyunsaturates and growth in man. *Acta Paediatr Scand.* 1992;81:302-306.

136. Decsi T, Koletzko B. Do trans fatty acids impair linoleic acid metabolism in healthy children? *Ann Nutr Metab.* 1995;39:36-41.

137. Dupont J, White PJ, Johnston KM, et al. Food safety and health effects of canola oil. *J Am Coll Nutr.* 1989;8: 360-375.

138. Kramer JG, Farnworth ER, Johnston KM, Wolynetz MS, Modler HW, Sauer FD. Myocardial changes in newborn piglets fed sow milk or milk replacer diets containing different levels of erucic acid. *Lipids.* 1990;11: 729-737.

139. Food and Drug Administration. Direct food substances affirmed as generally recognized as safe: low erucic acid rapeseed oil. *Fed Register.* 1985;50:3745-3755.

140. Koletzko B, Tangermann R, von Kries R, et al. Intestinal milkbolus-obstruction in formula fed premature infants given high doses of calcium. *J Pediatr Gastro Nutr.* 1988; 7:548-553.

141. Grundy SM, Vega GL. Plasma cholesterol responsiveness to saturated fatty acids. *Am J Clin Nutr.* 1988;47:822-824.

142. Hayes KC, Pronczuk A, Diersen-Schade D. Dietary saturated fatty acids (12:0, 14:0, 16:0) differ in their impact on plasma cholesterol and lipoproteins in non-human primates. *Am J Clin Nutr.* 1991;53:491-498.

143. Koletzko B, Bremer HJ. Fat content and fatty acid composition of infant formulas. *Acta Pediatr Scand.* 1989;78:513-521.

144. Carpentier Y. Intravascular metabolism of fat emulsions. *Clin Nutr.* 1989;8:115-125.

145. Koletzko B. Die Bedeutung der Fettapplikation in der Ernährungstherapie von Säuglingen und Kleinkindern. In: Grünert A, Reinauer H, eds. *Fettemulsionen. Betrachtungen zur Pathophysiologie, Toxikologie und Klinischen Anwendung.* München: Zuckschwerdt Verlag; 1993:116-121.

146. Hamosh M, Hamosh P. Lipoprotein lipase, hepatic lipase, and their role in lipid clearing during total parenteral nutrition. In: Lebenthal E, ed. *Total Parenteral nutrition: indications, utilisation, complications, and pathophysiological considerations.* New York: Raven Press; 1986:29-58.

147. Koletzko B. Stoffwechsel einer Lipidemulsion bei parenteral ernährten Neugeborenen: Analyse der Plasma-Lipoproteine. In: Grünert A, Reinauer H, eds. *Fettemulsionen. Betrachtungen zur Pathophysiologie, Toxikologie und Klinischen Anwendung.* München: Zuckschwerdt Verlag; 1993:122-128.

148. Messing B, Peynet J, Poupon J, et al. Effect of fat-emulsion phospholipids on serum lipoprotein profile during 1 mo of cyclic total parenteral nutrition. *Am J Clin Nutr.* 1990;52:1094-1100.

149. Griffin E, Breckenridge WC, Kuksis A, Bryan MH, Angel A. Appearance and characterization of lipoprotein X during continuous Intralipid infusion in the neonate. *J Clin Invest.* 1979;64:1703-1712.

150. Haumont D, Deckelbaum RJ, Richelle M, et al. Plasma lipid and plasma lipoprotein concentrations in low birth weight infnats given parenteral nutrition with twenty or ten percent lipid emulsion. *J Pediatr.* 1989;115: 787-793.

151. Hammerman C, Aramburo MJ. Decreased lipid intake reduces morbidity in sick premature neonates. *J Pediatr.* 1988;113:1083-1088.

152. Cooke RWI. Factors associated with chronic lung disease in preterm infants. *Arch Dis Child.* 1991;66:776-779.

153. Gilbertson N, Kovar IZ, Cox DJ, Crowe L, Palmer NT. Introduction of intravenous lipid administration on the first day of life in the very low birth weight neonate. *J Pediatr.* 1991;119:615-623.

154. Pitkänen O, Hallman M, Andersson S. Generation of free radicals in lipid emulsion used in parenteral nutrition. *Ped Res.* 1990;29:56-59.

155. Tomsits E, Rischak K, Szollar L. Long-term effects of unsaturated fatty acid dominance on the release of free radicals in the rat. *Ped Res.* 1994;36:278-282.

156. Neuzil J, Darlow BA, Inder TE, Sluis KB, Winterbourn CC, Stocker R. Oxidation of parenteral lipid emulsion by ambient and phototherapy lights: potential toxicity of routine parenteral feeding. *J Pediatr.* 1995;126:785-790.

157. Rubin M, Harell D, Naor N, et al. Lipid infusion with different triglyceride cores (long-chain vs. medium-chain/long-chain tirglycerides): effect on plasma lipids and bilirubin binding in premature infants. *J Parent Ent Nutr.* 1991;15:642-646.

158. Raupp P, von Kries R, Schmidt E, Pfahl HG, Günther O. Incompatibility between fat emulsion and calcium plus heparin in parenteral nutrition of premature babies. *Lancet.* 1988;1:700.

159. Hulman G, Fraser I, Pearson HJ, Bell PRF. Agglutination of Intralipid by sera of acutely ill patients. *Lancet.* 1982; 2:1426-1427.

160. Lindh A, Johansson B, Lindholm M, Rössner S. Agglutinate formation in serum samples mixed with intravenous fat emulsions. *Crit Care Med.* 1985;13:151-154.

161. Souci SW, Fachmann W, Kraut H. *Die Zusammensetzung der Lebensmittel. Nährwert Tabellen 1989/90.* 4th ed. Stuttgart: Wissenschaftliche Verlagsgesellschaft; 1989: 1-1028.

162. American Academy of Pediatrics.Committee on Nutrition. Prudent life-style for children: dietary fat and cholesterol. *Pediatrics.* 1986;78:521-525.

163. Jialal I, Grundy SM. Effect of dietary supplementation with alpha-tocopherol on the oxidative modification of low density lipoprotein. *J Lipid Res.* 1992;33:899-906.

164. Working group of the Canadian Pediatric Society and Health Canada. Nutrition recommendations update; dietary fat and children. Ottawa; Health Canada: 1993.

165. Commission of the European Communities. Commission Directive amending Directive 91/321/EEC on infant formulae and follow on formulae (draft). Eur Comm: 1995. Document III/5769-EN. (in press).

166. American Academy of Pediatrics C. Commentary on breast-feeding and infant formulas, including proposed standards for formulas. *Pediatrics.* 1976;57:278-285.

167. Koletzko B, Decsi T. Adipose tissue trans fatty acids and coronary heart disease. *Lancet.* 1995;345:1107-1108.

168. Rey J, Bresson JL. Langfristige Auswirkungen der Ernährung im Säuglingsalter. In: *Die Ernährung des Jungen Kindes.* New York: Raven Press; 1996.

169. Rubin M, Moser A, Naor N, Merlob P, Pakula R, Sirota L. Effect of three intravenously administered fat emulsions containing different concentrations of fatty acids on the plasma fatty acid composition of premature infants. *J Pediatr.* 1994;125:596-602.

170. Simoens CH, Richelle M, Rössle C, Derluyn M, Deckelbaum R, Crapentier Y. Manipulation of tissue fatty acid profile by intevenous lipids in dogs. *Clin Nutr.* 1995;14:177-185.

171. Decsi T, Koletzko B. Fatty acid composition of plasma lipid classes in healthy subjects from birth to young adulthood. *Eur J Pediatr.* 1994;153:520-525.

Nutritional Aspects of Gastrointestinal Disorders of Infancy
Kathleen J. Motil M.D., Ph.D.

USDA/ARS Children's Nutrition Research Center,
Department of Pediatrics,
Baylor College of Medicine,
Houston, Texas

Reviewed by Reginald C. Tsang M.B.B.S.

Introduction

The nutritional abnormalities associated with gastrointestinal diseases generally are the result of defects in digestion and absorption. Problems such as fat malabsorption, carbohydrate intolerance, protein-losing enteropathy and specific vitamin and mineral deficiencies frequently complicate the course of gastrointestinal diseases such as cystic fibrosis, celiac disease, inflammatory bowel disease and short gut syndrome. Defects in digestion and absorption result in increased enteric losses of nutrients which, if untreated, lead to frank malnutrition and growth failure. Although individual laboratory tests provide qualitative or quantitative assessments of specific abnormalities of digestion and absorption, the severity of these defects can be assessed over the long-term by their impact on the global nutritional status of the child. Strategies that compensate for the specific defects of digestion and absorption will reverse the adverse nutritional consequences associated with these disorders. In this chapter, we will consider the gastrointestinal factors that lead to the inadequate digestion and absorption of dietary nutrients. We will then consider the role of these factors in specific gastrointestinal disorders such as celiac disease, short bowel syndrome and inflammatory bowel disease. Finally, we will present nutritional strategies that help to overcome the adverse nutritional consequences of maldigestion and malabsorption.

Practical Point

• *Nutritional deficits associated with common gastrointestinal disorders are the result of defects in digestion and absorption.*

Pathogenesis of Nutritional Deficits in Gastrointestinal Disorders

The digestion of all macronutrients within the gastrointestinal tract is accomplished by intraluminal and mucosal factors.[1, 2] The intraluminal factors include hydrochloric acid, biliary and pancreatic secretions, bacterial fermentation, and mucosal enzymes. Thus, gastrointestinal disorders that disrupt any one of these digestive components will result in increased enteric nutrient losses and lead to progressive malnutrition as a consequence of reduced nutrient availability. The absorption of all nutrients is dependent on the total absorptive surface of the gut, both its absolute length and relative surface area, as well as on specific transport mechanisms, which facilitate the transfer of nutrients across the intestinal mucosa for use by the body. Thus, gastrointestinal diseases that result in a shortened bowel length or some degree of villous atrophy also result in increased enteric losses, and consequently, malnutrition. Malnutrition itself is associated with pancreatic insufficiency, villous atrophy and small bowel bacterial overgrowth, all of which further aggravate intestinal protein loss, carbohydrate and fat malabsorption, and vitamin and mineral deficiencies.

Cystic fibrosis is the classic entity in which primary pancreatic insufficiency leads to profound fat malabsorption, thereby reducing the availability of dietary fat as an energy source. Enteric losses of dietary energy set the stage for nutrient imbalances that result in poor utilization of other dietary nutrients. Adverse clinical outcomes of energy deficits include hypoproteinemia; generalized edema; a "leaky" gut associated with bowel wall edema; and subsequently, a protein-losing enteropathy. Pancreatic enzyme replacement reverses the malabsorptive process and leads to improved nutritional status. Achlorhydria associated with histamine H_2 receptor therapy further enhances the therapeutic effect of pancreatic enzyme replacement.

Practical Points

- *Intraluminal factors that facilitate digestion include hydrochloric acid, biliary and pancreatic secretions, bacterial fermentation and mucosal enzymes.*
- *Mucosal factors that facilitate absorption include total bowel length and surface area, as well as specific transport systems.*
- *Maldigestion and malabsorption increase enteric nutrient losses and result in malnutrition; if these problems remain untreated, malnutrition further aggravates intestinal dysfunction.*

Specific Gastrointestinal Disorders

The most common pediatric gastrointestinal disorders that have significant adverse nutritional consequences include cystic fibrosis, celiac disease, inflammatory bowel disease and short gut syndrome, the latter generally being associated with the post-surgical complications of necrotizing enterocolitis and other gastrointestinal anomalies. Cystic fibrosis has been discussed elsewhere in this book; thus, this chapter will focus on the latter three entities. The approach to managing the nutritional aspects of these specific gastrointestinal disorders will be presented in each section, while general aspects of nutritional management will be found in the final section of this chapter.

Celiac Disease

Celiac disease, also known as gluten-sensitive enteropathy, is a genetic disorder in which the intestinal tract is permanently intolerant of dietary gliadin and related proteins and results in a flat villous lesion.[3] Gliadin is one of four classes of proteins found primarily in wheat, but also in other grains including rye, barley and oats. Feeding practices other than gluten consumption may influence celiac disease.[4] For example, breast-feeding can protect against its onset.[5] In addition, the type and

> *If you learn your "nutrition" from a biochemist, you are not likely to learn how essential it is to blow the baby's nose before expecting him to suck. Or to realize when it is that a child needs cuddling just as much as calories.*
>
> Primary Health Care Pioneer
> The Selected Works of
> Dr. Cicely D. Williams
> Naomi Baumslag, Editor
> World Federation of Public
> Health Associations
> and UNICEF

amount of cereal introduced into the infant's diet may affect the clinical features of this disease.[6]

The pathogenesis of celiac disease shows features of cell-mediated intestinal damage characterized by a lymphocytic infiltrate of the villi, followed by crypt hyperplasia, and subsequent villous atrophy. The clinical features of celiac disease vary widely, depending on the age of presentation. In infancy, celiac disease presents with symptoms of chronic diarrhea, abdominal distention, vomiting, irritability and failure to thrive.[7] In adolescence, the disorder may manifest itself primarily with extraintestinal symptoms such as short stature,[8] delayed puberty, anemia, arthritis and minor abdominal complaints.[9] Other diseases such as dermatitis herpetiformis, thyroiditis, sarcoidosis, insulin-dependent diabetes mellitus, IgA nephropathy, IgA deficiency and cystic fibrosis are found with greater frequency than expected in celiac disease.[10-12]

The nutritional complications of celiac disease are the consequences of inadequate dietary nutrient intake relative to metabolic need because of intestinal malabsorption and increased enteric losses. Individual nutrient deficiencies of protein, vitamins and minerals are commonplace in celiac disease. Fat and carbohydrate malabsorption, the latter in the form of lactose intolerance, is also a common feature of this disorder. A quantitative fat study, which measures the amount of fecal fat excreted over 72 hours relative to the amount of dietary fat consumed during the same time interval, is the best method to confirm fat malabsorption. A lactose hydrogen breath test is useful to demonstrate the presence of lactose intolerance; the one-hour xylose absorption test is a nonspecific indicator of generalized malabsorption associated with a flat villous lesion. Fat-soluble vitamin deficiencies often parallel fat malabsorption. Depressed serum vitamin A and E concentrations, low 25-hydroxyvitamin D_3 concentrations and prolonged prothrombin time are useful tests to detect vitamin A, E, D and K deficiencies, respectively. A protein-losing enteropathy frequently accompanies celiac disease when chronic diarrhea occurs. Serum albumin concentrations may be precipitously low and fecal α_1-antitrypsin concentrations may be strikingly high when this nutritional complication is present.[13] Increased fecal losses of calcium, magnesium, phosphorus and zinc, as well as iron deficiency anemia,[14] also occur in the presence of chronic diarrhea. Hemoglobin levels,[15] individual serum mineral concentrations and alkaline phosphatase levels help to identify these deficiencies.

Global malnutrition, failure to thrive and linear growth failure can result from individual nutrient deficiencies that persist for a prolonged period of time. In this setting, muscle wasting, loss of subcutaneous fat tissue, linear stunting and bone demineralization are clinically apparent. Other features of malnutrition such as hepatomegaly, edema, dermatoses and sparse, brittle hair become readily apparent. Growth measurements, including height and weight, as well as triceps skinfold thickness and mid-arm muscle circumference,[16] are essential to determine the severity of the nutritional insult.

A strict, gluten-free diet is the cornerstone of the management of children with celiac disease. The diet should exclude wheat, rye, barley and oats. Rice, corn and potato are used as wheat substitutes. A gluten-free diet is recommended indefinitely for both symptomatic and asymptomatic children because of the long-term association between celiac disease and malignancy. Normalization of the intestinal mucosa occurs after approximately six months of a gluten-free diet in compliant patients.[17, 18] A low-fat, lactose-free diet may be necessary for a brief, two- to four-week period of time to reduce symptoms associated with malabsorption. Although a gluten-free diet alone will improve the complications of celiac disease such as hypocalcemia and osteoporosis,[19-21] specific vitamin, mineral and trace element deficiencies should be corrected individually. Replacement therapy generally can be discontinued once clinical and histologic recovery on a gluten-free diet has been documented, feeding patterns have normalized and catch-up growth has been accomplished.[22] A nutritional specialist is an essential part of the clinical team. The dietitian should instruct parents on the details of a gluten-free diet to enhance patient compliance.[23] Parental education is important for compliance because many commercial food preparations contain "hidden" gluten products that may not be readily apparent. Local family support groups often are helpful in exchanging information about new food products that are gluten-free.

Practical Points

- *Celiac disease is a disorder in which the gastrointestinal tract is permanently intolerant of dietary gliadin, a protein found primarily in wheat, but also in other grains including rye, barley and oats.*
- *The nutritional complications of celiac disease may include fat malabsorption, lactose intolerance, a protein-losing enteropathy, iron deficiency anemia, fat-soluble vitamin and mineral deficiencies, malnutrition and growth failure.*
- *A strict, gluten-free diet administered indefinitely is the cornerstone of the management of celiac disease.*
- *A low-fat, low-lactose diet supplemented with multivitamins and minerals is indicated for the child newly diagnosed with celiac disease.*
- *Parental education is important because many commercial food preparations contain "hidden" gluten products.*

Short Bowel Syndrome

Short bowel syndrome is a gastrointestinal disorder in which malabsorption, fluid and electrolyte losses and malnutrition occur after massive small bowel resection. This resection is usually used for abdominal crises associated with necrotizing enterocolitis and other gastrointestinal anomalies.[24, 25] As much as 90% of the small intestine may be resected without significant long-term problems in sustaining nutrition, provided that the distal ileum and ileocecal valve remain intact. However, severe diarrhea may be present even though less than 25% of the small bowel has been resected if the distal ileum and ileocecal valve have been removed. This discouraging outcome may be offset by the fact that the small bowel of the infant has the ability to adapt and the capacity for significant growth and development, provided that adequate nutritional support is forthcoming.[26]

The most common causes of short bowel syndrome are jejunoileal atresia (32% of cases), volvulus (29% of cases), necrotizing enterocolitis (19% of cases), gastroschisis (12% of cases) and less frequently, total colonic aganglionosis (Hirschsprung's disease) with proximal extension into the terminal ileum.[27-32] The pathogenesis of the short bowel syndrome results from the loss of intestinal surface area for absorption of fluid, salts and all nutrients, coupled with altered intestinal motility, all of which lead to rapid transit of luminal contents and diminished digestive and absorptive capacity. The digestive and absorptive capacity of the residual small bowel depends on six factors: 1) the length of the remaining small bowel; 2) whether the remaining small bowel is proximal (jejunal) or distal (ileal); 3) the presence or absence of the ileocecal valve; 4) the presence or absence of the colon; 5) the degree of intestinal adaptation over time; and 6) the presence or absence of residual bowel disease or surgical complications. Thus, the shorter the residual segment, the worse the digestive and absorptive activity of the small bowel. Resection of the duodenum will lead to iron and calcium deficiencies and result in anemia and osteopenia, while extensive resection of the jejunum will lead to lactose intolerance and small bowel bacterial overgrowth. Resection of the terminal ileum and ascending colon results in bile salt and vitamin B_{12} deficiencies and a reduction in sodium and chloride absorption. Resection of the ileocecal valve permits colonic reflux and subsequent proliferation of colonic bacteria in the residual small bowel, further aggravating bile salt and vitamin B_{12} deficiency. Partial or total colectomy enhances the likelihood that severe dehydration, hypovolemia, hypokalemia, hypomagnesemia and hyponatremia will occur.

The complications arising from small bowel resection, including gastric and intestinal motility disturbances; profound malabsorption of minerals, trace elements and vitamins; gastric hyperacidity; small bowel bacterial overgrowth; cholelithiasis; nephrolithiasis; and rarely, lactic acidosis, adversely affect the nutritional status of the infant. The rate of gastric emptying and intestinal transit is inversely proportional to the length of the remaining small bowel and increases in the absence of the ileocecal valve and colon. Deficiencies of calcium, magnesium, iron and zinc are further aggravated by intestinal resection and may be associated with symptoms of tetany, osteopenia, spontaneous fractures and iron deficiency anemia. Fat-soluble vitamin (A, D, E, K) deficiencies worsen with profound steatorrhea. Vitamin B_{12} deficiency is invariably present when ileal resection is extensive. Small bowel bacterial overgrowth further aggravates the functional capacity of the remaining ileum to absorb vitamin B_{12} and may interfere with folate absorption throughout the small bowel. Gastric hyperacidity, a transient complication of small bowel resection, interferes with intraluminal digestion because hydrochloric acid inactivates pancreatic enzyme activity. Nephrolithiasis may occur in the presence of malabsorption because intraluminal calcium binds with unabsorbed fatty acids instead of other dietary products such as oxalate. Gallstones may form because of the interruption of the enterohepatic pathway and subsequent bile stasis within the biliary tract. Lactic acidosis may occur when the dietary intake of carbohydrates has been liberalized in the presence of small bowel bacterial overgrowth, resulting in the fermentation of sugar and the formation of D-lactate, a disaccharide associated with neurologic symptoms.

Nutritional support is the mainstay of therapy for short bowel syndrome because it allows intestinal adaptation to occur, thereby improving the prospects for long-term survival, normal growth and the resumption of enteral feeding in children with this disorder. Although parenteral alimentation permits intestinal growth to occur, it alone is insufficient to stimulate intestinal hyperplasia. Providing intraluminal nutrients is essential for the hyperplastic response of the intestinal cell mass, emphasizing the need to supplement enterally as soon as possible.[33, 34] The major nutrients responsible for the adaptive response of the gut mucosa include long-chain fatty acids,[35] disaccharides,[36] whole proteins and free amino acids,[37, 38] and possibly glutamine[39, 40] or nucleotides.[41, 42] Small feedings of these nutrients enhance mucosal adaptation because direct exposure of the gut to nutrients stimulates the functional activity of mucosal surface transport systems and the release of intestinal and extraintestinal hormones such as enteroglucagon,[43] secretin and cholecystokinin,[44] as well as pancreatic secretions and growth factors,[45] all of which are essential to maintain adequate absorptive function. Nevertheless, enteral feedings increase the number of episodes of sepsis in infants with short bowel syndrome because of bacterial translocation from the gut into the blood stream.[46]

Managing short bowel syndrome relies on the nutritional knowledge of the team of individuals required to care for infants and children with this disorder. The management of short bowel syndrome should focus on: 1) Stabilizing fluid and electrolyte needs to prevent dehydration and electrolyte imbalances; 2) instituting parenteral nutrition to provide nutrients essential to maintain tissue structure and function and for growth; 3) using pharmacologic agents judiciously to minimize gastric hypersecretion and diarrheal losses; 4) introducing oral hydration solutions and enteral formulas to stimulate small bowel adaptation; 5) watching for complications of parenteral nutrition including mechanical obstruction of catheters,[47] central line-related sepsis,[48] nutrient imbalances, cholestatic liver disease and cholelithiasis; 6) restoring normal linear and ponderal growth; and 7) reversing food aversion and loss of oromotor skills.

The first priority in the nutritional management of short bowel syndrome is placing a multilumen central venous line to deliver parenteral nutrition. The goals of parenteral nutrition are to replace fluid, electrolyte and mineral losses and to provide adequate amino acids and non-nitrogen energy sources to support normal growth and development of the infant. Excessive fluid and electrolyte losses from stools or an ileostomy should be estimated by measuring the differences between dry and wet diaper or ostomy bag weights, and by analyzing the liquid portion of the stool for its sodium, potassium and chloride concentrations. Fecal or ostomy losses are likely to be greater in newly created than in well-established anastomoses and ostomies. A solution of 0.45% sodium chloride administered via a second catheter lumen should be used to replace fluid losses on a volume-per-volume basis. Deficits in serum sodium and potassium concentrations should be corrected by adding the appropriate amount of sodium and potassium to the replacement solution to reverse the blood abnormalities. When fluid and electrolyte losses are more predictable, replacement solutions can be added directly to the parenteral nutrition solution. Furthermore, in the presence of high-output ostomies or prolonged use of total parenteral nutrition, supplemental trace elements, including zinc, copper, chromium, manganese, selenium and molybdenum may be required to avoid deficiencies of these nutrients.[49]

The second priority in the nutritional management of short bowel syndrome is placing a gastrostomy button for the provision of enteral feedings. Although the gastric button serves as the major access site for the enteral administration of rehydration solutions and milk-based formulas, all infants should be encouraged promptly to take oral feedings to stimulate the suck reflex and to reduce the likelihood of oral food aversions. A continuous infusion, rather than intermittent bolus, of all gastrostomy feedings is

> *By this name I mean to designate a disease, called in Philadelphia, the "vomiting and purging of children." From the regularity of its appearance in the summer months, it is likewise known by the name of "the disease of the season." It prevails in most of the large towns in the United States. It is distinguished in Charleston, in South Carolina, by the name of "the April and May disease", from making its first appearance in those two months. It seldom appears in Philadelphia til the middle of June, or the beginning of July, and it generally continues til near the middle of September. Its frequency and danger are always in proportion to the heat of the weather.*
>
> Benjamin Rush
> "An Inquiry Into the Cause and Cure of the Cholera Infantum,"
> *Pediatrics of the Past,*
> An anthology compiled and edited by
> John Ruhräh M.D., 1925
> Paul B. Hoeber, Inc. Publishers,
> New York, NY

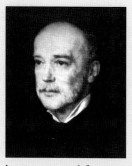

Samuel Gee M.D. (1839-1911) described the Celiac Affection in 1888. Gee was an English scholar of the classical literature and couched his report with quotations from the fourth century. Gee reported, "The celiac disease is commonest in patients between one and five years old: it often begins during the second year of life. Signs of the disease are yielded by the feces; being loose but not watery, more bulky than the food taken. Add emaciation and cachexia, and we have a complete picture of the disease." Coeliac Disease: 100 years edited by P. J. Kumar and J. A. Walker-Smith. Univ. of Leeds, Leeds, 1988 (Photo courtesy of J. Walker-Smith)

preferable because of enhanced nutrient absorption and better weight gain using this method.[50, 51] Combined glucose and electrolyte solutions should be the first type of enteral feeding administered to assess the intestinal response to individual nutrients. Once tolerance has been established, an elemental or polymeric formula may be initiated, although a milk-based preparation composed of a protein hydrolysate, glucose polymer and mixed medium- and long-chain fat source generally is the formula of choice. Enteral feedings should be given initially in amounts that approximate 10% or less of the total daily fluid requirements. At the same time, additional sodium or potassium acetate will need to be added to the parenteral nutrition solution, or sodium citrate will need to be provided orally, to compensate for the acid production and bicarbonate consumption associated with feeding. Stool volume, pH and glucose content should be monitored frequently for evidence of excessive fluid loss, acid production or carbohydrate malabsorption that would mitigate against too rapid advancement of enteral feedings. Advances in formula volume and nutrient concentrations should be made slowly to insure successful adaptation of the intestine. Parenteral nutrition should be reduced concurrently without compromising nutrient intake. A combination of cyclic parenteral nutrition and gastrostomy feedings may reduce the cholestatic complications of intra-

venous alimentation and simultaneously permit a more normal lifestyle. Regardless of the pattern of parenteral and enteral nutrition in infants with short gut syndrome, careful, routine monitoring of serum proteins, glucose, electrolytes, minerals and trace elements is mandatory to avoid the clinical consequences of nutrient imbalances or deficiencies.

The transition from parenteral nutrition and enteral ostomy feedings to oral bolus feedings generally is gradual and requires months or years to accomplish. The rapidity of this process depends on the length of the remaining small bowel and the degree of intestinal hyperplasia. Carbohydrate malabsorption typically is a persistent problem of short bowel syndrome.[52, 53] Lactose generally is tolerated poorly by most infants, although the inclusion of yogurt and milk in the diet has been recommended.[54] Use of dietary carbohydrate may be enhanced by adding complex polysaccharide (starch) or nonstarch fermentable fiber, although these dietary manipulations have not been well studied in infants.[39, 55] Although a high-carbohydrate, low-fat diet traditionally has been recommended,[56, 57] recent evidence suggests that a high-fat, low-carbohydrate diet may be a better choice for these infants. A high-fat (long-chain triglyceride) diet does not aggravate ostomy fluid, electrolyte or mineral losses, and may improve total energy intake despite increased fecal fat losses[58, 59] because the proportion of dietary fat absorbed remains constant.[60] Nevertheless, malabsorption of fat-soluble vitamins, vitamin B_{12} and minerals (calcium, magnesium, zinc) is common during oral refeeding and warrants supplementation. Drug-nutrient interactions, e.g., cholestyramine, also may aggravate fat-soluble vitamin and folate deficiencies. Small bowel bacterial overgrowth may be associated with inflammation and subsequent iron deficiency anemia because of intestinal blood loss. Periodic screening of these vitamin and mineral levels is mandatory. Oral administration of most vitamin and mineral supplements generally is sufficient, although parenteral administration of vitamins D and K and magnesium may be required. Subcutaneous administration of vitamin B_{12} may be necessary if a significant amount of terminal ileum has been resected. Finally, a low-oxalate diet that excludes chocolate, tea, colas, spinach and carrots is indicated when hyperoxaluria (greater than 50 mg/d) is detected to prevent nephrocalcinosis.

Practical Points

- *Short bowel syndrome is a disorder in which malabsorption, fluid and electrolyte losses and malnutrition occur after massive small bowel resection.*
- *The nutritional complications of short bowel syndrome are more likely to occur when a long segment of bowel has been resected and when the ileocecal valve and colon have been removed.*
- *The nutritional complications of short bowel syndrome may include deficiencies of all fat-soluble vitamins, folate and vitamin B_{12}, all minerals and two trace minerals, iron and zinc; lactose intolerance; carbohydrate and fat malabsorption; protein-losing enteropathy; malnutrition; and growth failure.*
- *Parenteral nutrition (central venous alimentation) and enteral (button gastrostomy) feedings are the mainstay of therapy for short bowel syndrome.*
- *The first priority is to adequately replace fluid, electrolyte and mineral losses and to provide sufficient amino acids and non-nitrogen energy sources, using standard parenteral nutrition solutions to support the growth and development of the infant.*
- *The second priority is to initiate enteral feedings as soon as possible in a continuous infusion of a protein hydrolysate, glucose polymer, and long-chain fat formula, to stimulate intestinal hyperplasia.*
- *Oral feedings should be attempted early in the refeeding process to minimize oral food aversions.*
- *Periodic screening for vitamin, mineral, trace mineral and protein deficiencies is mandatory.*

Inflammatory Bowel Disease

Inflammatory bowel disease represents two disorders of the gastrointestinal tract, Crohn's disease and ulcerative colitis, both of which are characterized by inflammation, ulceration and scar formation in the intestinal tract. Although these disorders affect various sites of the gut, extra-intestinal manifestations of each disease may precede or occur simultaneously with intestinal symptoms. Nevertheless, these entities are considered distinct because of the differences in their presentation, pathophysiology and management. The etiology of Crohn's disease and ulcerative colitis is unknown; however, a genetic predisposition has been postulated.[61-63] Other factors such as infectious agents, environmental toxins, abnormal immune regulation, dietary factors including cow milk proteins, neuroendocrine abnormalities and psychological factors also have been implicated in the pathogenesis of the disease.[64]

The pathologic features of Crohn's disease are characterized by aphthous ulcers or linear, serpiginous ulcerations, intestinal wall thickening and stenosis, fistula formation, mesenteric thickening with enlarged lymph nodes, and indurated fat that migrates over the serosal surface of the small intestine. In contrast, the pathologic features of ulcerative colitis are characterized by superficial or deep ulcers separated by mounds of inflamed, non-ulcerated tissue, or pseudopolyps. Approximately one-half of children with Crohn's disease have involvement of the terminal ileum and colon, one-third have small bowel involvement alone, and the remainder have disease limited to the colon. In contrast, ulcerative colitis is confined to the colon and rarely extends into the terminal ileum. As a result of the localization of the inflammatory process in various parts of the gastrointestinal tract, a number of different nutritional abnormalities such as fat and carbohydrate malabsorption, impaired electrolyte, mineral, vitamin, and water absorption, a protein-losing enteropathy, a bile salt-losing enteropathy, and gastrointestinal bleeding, may be diagnosed.

The most common presenting clinical features of Crohn's disease are abdominal pain, diarrhea and weight loss. Less common symptoms include rectal bleeding, perianal disease, malnutrition and growth failure; extraintestinal manifestations include joint and musculoskeletal symptoms, cutaneous manifestations, oral mucosal lesions, ocular complications, vascular symptoms, renal disease and hepatobiliary manifestations. The most common presenting clinical features of ulcerative colitis are diarrhea, rectal bleeding and abdominal pain. Less common symptoms include weight loss, anemia and extraintestinal manifestations similar to those of Crohn's disease.

The nutritional complications of inflammatory bowel disease include protein-energy malnutrition (wasting), linear growth failure (stunting) and individual vitamin and mineral deficiencies, particularly folate and vitamin B_{12} deficiency, iron deficiency anemia and osteopenia.[65] Approximately one-third of children are stunted and as many as 50% are wasted,[66] with the greatest deficit appearing in the fat-free (muscle) mass.[67] One-half to three-fourths of these children have individual nutrient deficiencies. The nutritional complications persist into adulthood in that one-third of adults are stunted, 60% have persistent weight loss, and three-fourths have nutritional anemias (iron, folate, vitamin B_{12}). Nutritional disorders are diagnosed at least twice as frequently in Crohn's disease as in ulcerative colitis.

There are many factors that cause the nutritional complications of inflammatory disease. Insufficient dietary nutrient intake relative to increased metabolic need occurs as a consequence of malabsorption; so do increased enteric losses, drug-nutrient interactions and the increased nutrient requirements associated with the inflammatory process itself and the metabolic cost of growth. Dietary intakes may be reduced because of anorexia, disease-related symptoms or iatrogenic dietary restriction. Malabsorption of dietary carbohydrate, particularly lactose or fat may occur because of small bowel bacterial overgrowth associated with intestinal stenosis or fistulas, reduced surface area from intestinal resection or a bile salt-losing enteropathy. Increased enteric losses of electrolytes, minerals and trace metals may occur with diarrhea or a protein-losing enteropathy. Drug-nutrient interactions such as those that occur with sulfasalazine or cholestyramine increase dietary folate and fat-soluble vitamin needs.

The inflammatory response associated with fever, villous damage and repair, abscess formation or sepsis increases nutrient needs. Although significant increases in resting metabolic rates have not been documented, total daily energy expenditure is approximately 200 kcal greater in patients with inflammatory bowel dis-

In regard to treatment of diarrheal diseases, Mike Farrell, M.D. Chief of Staff, Children's Hospital Medical Center in Cincinnati, Ohio, states, "Name one disease for which starvation is therapeutic." Another quip by Dr. Farrell: "Avoid stool vs. child disease."

abstracted by
Reginald C. Tsang M.D.

ease than in healthy individuals.[68] Rates of whole body protein synthesis are increased also with greater inflammatory activity,[69,70] as are fractional protein synthesis rates in the colon and liver.[71] Urinary nitrogen losses increase threefold above the normally augmented nitrogen losses that occur with disease-induced anorexia.[72] Increased urinary losses of vitamins (A and C) and minerals (potassium, magnesium, phosphorus, zinc, and sulfur) are associated with the inflammatory response.[73] Thus, no matter how limited or severe the inflammatory response, there will be some adverse effect on nutritional status with respect to nearly all nutrients.[74] Finally, children also have increased nutrient needs by virtue of their growth requirements. With peak weight velocities of 2 to 7 kg per six months, and an energy cost of tissue growth estimated to be 5 kcal per gram of tissue accreted,[75] this gain represents an additional energy requirement of 50 to 190 kcal/d.

Nutritional support is indicated to treat disease activity, the nutrient deficiencies associated with drug-nutrient interactions or detected by specific laboratory tests, and malnutrition and growth failure. With nutritional therapy alone or combined with corticosteroids, symptoms resolve, body weight increases, laboratory measures of disease activity normalize and corticosteroid requirements decrease.[76-78] In this setting, nutritional therapy may be useful in treating newly diagnosed disease or chronic disease unresponsive to medical management. Nutritional therapy can also help in the closure of fistulas, the resolution of partial bowel obstruction associated with inflammatory strictures, or the healing of inflamed tissue surrounding high output ostomies; it can be helpful in cases where surgical intervention results in the short bowel syndrome.

Enteral nutrition is as effective as parenteral nutrition in reducing disease activity, although this comparison has not been well-studied in children. The mechanisms by which elemental diets or parenteral nutrition reduce disease activity are unknown, although several possibilities are likely. Elemental or elimination diets are thought to reduce the intraluminal antigenic load, and thereby diminish the inflammatory response of the intestine.[79-81] Specific foods that are high in essential fatty acids, such as fish oils, are thought to modulate the immune response of the gut by synthesizing the selective inflammatory mediators.[82-84] Although the use of parenteral nutrition or a low-residue diet is thought to provide bowel rest to the diseased gut, the clinical outcome does not differ between these diets and the consumption of habitual foods.[85] Individual nutrients, such as glutamine, are thought to improve tissue regeneration and function because they serve as primary metabolic fuels for the intestinal tract.[86, 87]

The most common single nutrient deficiencies include serum iron and folate, although combined macronutrient (hypoalbuminemia, lactose intolerance, fat malabsorption) and micronutrient (calcium, magnesium, zinc, folate, and vitamins D and B_{12}) abnormalities are more likely to occur. Folate deficiency may develop readily, particularly in children who are treated with sulfasalazine, because this drug impairs folate absorption.[88] The interpretation of individual laboratory abnormalities must be reviewed carefully because blood plasma or serum values may not reflect the status of body nutrient stores.

Growth failure is one of the major complications of inflammatory bowel disease and may precede clinical evidence of bowel disease, often by years.[89] Height-for-age and weight-for-height measurements should be obtained to assess the degree of linear stunting and ponderal wasting, respectively.[90, 91] Skeletal bone age also may be reduced in children with height and weight deficits. Skeletal demineralization may occur, although few studies have examined the status of the bone mineral and matrix composition in this disease.[92, 93] Alterations of body composition occur during active disease such that visceral proteins and body fat are mobilized initially, followed by the fat-free mass, to meet the protein and energy demands imposed by the inflammatory process.[94] The use of corticosteroids is particularly bothersome because of their ability to induce a protein catabolic response, although children may be somewhat protected in this

respect.[66] Nevertheless, many children demonstrate improved growth rates when corticosteroid therapy is initiated because this treatment reduces the inflammatory activity of the disease.

The goals of nutritional therapy in inflammatory bowel disease are to increase dietary intakes sufficiently enough to replace nutrient losses, to correct body deficits, to sustain normal metabolic function, and to promote catch-up growth. The easiest way to increase dietary intakes is to use commonly available foods. No specific diet has been shown to alter the course of Crohn's disease or ulcerative colitis in remission. Children should be encouraged to eat an adequate, well-balanced diet and to avoid food fads. There is no evidence that eating or avoiding specific foods influences the severity of disease, the frequency of relapses or induces a remission. When disease is active, when specific foods exacerbate symptoms, or when laboratory tests suggest specific abnormalities such as lactose intolerance, the diet should be modified accordingly. Multivitamins with minerals should be administered routinely to replace potential deficits in the diet. Supplemental iron or folic acid therapy may be appropriate depending on laboratory findings. Zinc therapy has not been prescribed uniformly because anecdotal reports have failed to confirm a beneficial effect on growth from this treatment. Although significant decreases in total body calcium have been documented in adults with inflammatory bowel disease,[95] specific recommendations, including the use of calcium, vitamin D, estrogen, sodium fluoride, calcitonin or bisphosphonates, have not been forthcoming for the treatment of osteopenia in children with this disorder.[96]

When the child is unable to increase dietary intake with palatable snacks, commercially available liquid formulas should be prescribed. However, many children will not increase their total daily nutrient intake because they experience early satiety with these formulas. In this setting, intragastric feedings using a nasogastric tube or gastrostomy button should be recommended. The advantage of the nasogastric tube is that it can be placed in the evening for the overnight administration of a liquid formula and removed upon awakening, thereby avoiding interference with school attendance and the social development of the child. Nevertheless, compli-

Recommended Daily Energy Allowances for Infants and Children*	
Age (years)	Energy (kcal • kg⁻¹ • day⁻¹)
0.0-0.5	110
0.5-1	100
1-3	100
4-6	90
7-10	70
11-14 (male)	55
15-18 (male)	45
11-14 (female)	45
15-18 (female)	40

* Adapted from Subcommittee on the Tenth Edition of the RDAs, National Academy of Sciences - National Research Council. *Recommended Dietary Allowances.* 10th ed. Washington, DC: National Academy Press; 1989.

Table 1: Recommended dietary energy allowances for infants and children.

ance may be difficult. The advantage of the gastrostomy button is that it is cosmetically acceptable, is easily cared for, and the administration of large amounts of formula can be achieved readily. However, the disadvantage of this device is that its placement requires an invasive procedure. The amount of nutritional supplement administered enterally varies, depending on the nutritional needs and tolerance of the child. Overall, the volume of supplemental formula, in addition to usual meals and snacks, should provide energy intakes of 85 to 95 kcal·kg⁻¹·d⁻¹.

In children who are unable to achieve adequate enteral intakes because of increased disease activity, diarrhea or intestinal obstruction, parenteral alimentation may provide substantial benefit. However, parenteral nutrition has been less effective in children with frank rectal bleeding, abdominal masses or fistulas. Although peripheral parenteral nutrition is an option, central venous alimentation is a more suitable choice because of the likelihood that parenteral nutrition will be administered for a prolonged period of time. Central venous alimentation should be administered using a standard solution pro-

viding 20% glucose, 3% amino acids, vitamins and minerals, accompanied with a 20% lipid emulsion. Cyclical parenteral alimentation is available for children who require long-term nutritional support while maintaining their educational and social activities. Children may be monitored by their local hospital programs or by a commercial nutritional maintenance company.

Practical Points

- *Inflammatory bowel disease represents two disorders, Crohn disease and ulcerative colitis, both of which are characterized by inflammation, ulceration, and scar formation in the gastrointestinal tract.*
- *The nutritional complications of inflammatory bowel disease include protein-losing enteropathy, lactose intolerance, fat malabsorption, folate and vitamin B_{12} deficiency, iron deficiency anemia, osteopenia, malnutrition and growth failure.*
- *The cause of the nutritional complications of inflammatory bowel disease is multifactorial and includes inadequate dietary intakes, malabsorption, increased enteric nutrient losses and increased nutrient requirements associated with inflammatory and growth processes.*
- *Nutritional support is indicated for the treatment of disease activity, individual nutrient deficiencies, and malnutrition and growth failure.*
- *Nutritional therapy alone or in combination with corticosteroid therapy induces remission of disease activity.*
- *Enteral nutrition is as effective as parenteral nutrition in reducing disease activity.*
- *The most common single nutrient deficiencies include iron deficiency anemia and folate deficiency, although all vitamins and minerals potentially may be deficient.*
- *Linear growth failure, skeletal demineralization and alterations of body composition, particularly the fat-free mass, are common abnormalities of inflammatory bowel disease.*

- *No specific diet alters the course of Crohn's disease or ulcerative colitis in remission, nor does the consumption or avoidance of specific foods influence the induction of remission.*
- *A well-balanced, oral diet and a vitamin and mineral supplement should be provided routinely; supplemental iron, folic acid and zinc should be added to the diet when clinically indicated.*
- *Intragastric feedings, using a nasogastric tube or button gastrostomy, may be necessary to adequately augment dietary intakes to meet metabolic needs.*
- *Parenteral nutrition may be necessary in the presence of increased disease activity and chronically severe diarrhea or intestinal obstruction.*

Nutritional Therapy and Its Complications

The treatment of nutritional deficits in infants and children with gastrointestinal diseases is accomplished by enteral or parenteral nutritional therapy. The enteral route is the method of choice, unless intestinal obstruction, atony or total villous atrophy precludes the use of the intestinal tract. The presence of specific malabsorptive or secretory defects does not prohibit the use of the gastrointestinal tract for nutritional support. Nevertheless, oral refeeding alone may be unsatisfactory because some children refuse or are unable to comply with the nutritional repletion program.

As a general rule, dietary energy is the first limiting nutrient in the nutritional rehabilitation of children. The first priority, therefore, is to estimate the dietary energy needs of the child. This estimate is determined on the basis of the recommended dietary allowances for the child's age-specific ideal body weight (Table 1) as follows:

$$\text{Estimated energy needs for nutritional support } (\text{kcal·kg}^{-1}\text{·d}^{-1}) = \frac{\text{Ideal body weight (kg) for chronologic age} \times \text{Recommended dietary energy intake } (\text{kcal·kg}^{-1}\text{·d}^{-1})}{\text{Actual body weight (kg)}}$$

Adequate nutritional repletion in infants can be achieved with dietary energy intakes in the range of 160 to 180 kcal·kg^{-1}·d^{-1}. In the older child, satisfactory nutritional repletion can be accomplished with energy intakes in the range of 85 to 95 kcal·kg^{-1}·d^{-1}.

The easiest way to provide nutritional therapy for infants is to increase their dietary intakes using standard infant formulas which may be concentrated and supplemented with glucose polymers and corn oil or medium-chain triglycerides to increase their caloric density. Older children should be encouraged to eat a well-balanced diet that mimics the pattern of the food pyramid (Fig. 1). Although the consumption of specific foods may aggravate disease symptoms, caution must be exerted to avoid iatrogenic malnutrition resulting from prescribed diets too limited in nutrients. When specific foods exacerbate symptoms or when laboratory tests suggest specific abnormalities, the diet should be modified accordingly. Milk substitutes (yogurt), food modifiers (Lactaid®, McNeil Consumer Products Co., Fort Washington, PA), nutrient alternatives (glucose polymers, medium-chain triglycerides) or drug therapy (pancreatic enzyme replacement) should be instituted when clinically indicated.

Oral refeeding programs are successful if commercially-prepared formulas are used as medical management. The choice of formulas depends on the age of the child and the type of absorptive defect. In general, it is prudent to choose a semi-elemental formula that consists of hydrolyzed protein, glucose polymers, long-chain triglycerides with some medium-chain triglycerides and a complete multivitamin and mineral mixture. Some infants and children may not tolerate this type of formula preparation, and an elemental formula that consists of amino acids, glucose polymers, and limited amounts of various fat sources may be required. Although the oral route should be used for daytime feedings, because of the volume of supplementation sometimes required, a portion of the prescribed energy will need to be administered as overnight tube feedings. Continuous feedings are better tolerated than intermittent bolus feedings in that fewer episodes of vomiting, cramping or diarrhea occur using this method.

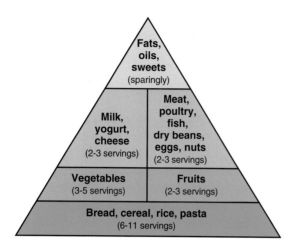

Age (years)	1-3	4-6	7-10
Milk, yogurt (cup)	1/2	3/4	1
Cheese (oz)	1/2	1	1-1/2
Meat, poultry, fish (oz)	1	1-1/2	3
Eggs	1	1	2
Peanut butter (tbsp)	1	2	3
Vegetables cooked or raw (cup)	3 T	1/3	1/2
Fruits			
Canned (cup)	3T	1/3	1/2
Fresh (small)	1/2	1	1 med
Juice (cup)	1/3	1/2	3/4
Bread (slice)	1/2	1	1
Dry cereal (cup)	1/2	3/4	1
Pasta, rice (cup)	1/3	1/2	3/4

Figure 1: Food pyramid and serving sizes.

Metabolic complications of refeeding programs are infrequent. However, in the early stages of refeeding, rapid shifts of fluid, electrolytes and minerals between intracellular and extracellular compartments of the body may lead to potentially fatal metabolic imbalances. Clinical and biochemical assessment should be performed whenever complications are suspected. Hypokalemia and hypophosphatemia are particularly ominous complications that warrant attention.

In the event that an infant or child is unable to tolerate sufficient amounts of enteral feeding, parenteral alimentation may provide substantial benefits. As a general rule, infants and children with hypoalbuminemia less than 30 g/L often benefit from a short (one- to two-week) course of combined enteral and intravenous alimentation. Parenteral alimentation with standard solutions that provide 10% (peripheral) or 20% (central) glucose and 2 to 3% amino acids, vitamins and minerals may be an acceptable primary or supplemental form of therapy. When parenteral alimentation is administered, it should be accompanied by an intravenous 20% lipid preparation to prevent the development of an essential fatty acid deficiency. Infants and children who receive parenteral alimentation should be monitored for potential metabolic, infectious, and mechanical complications associated with intravenous alimentation, including hyperglycemia; osmotic diuresis; postinfusion hypoglycemia; acidosis; hyperammonemia; amino acid toxicity; hypomagnesemia; hypercalcemia; hypophosphatemia; hypertriglyceridemia; trace element deficiencies; cholestasis, cardiac arrhythmias; venous perforation or thrombosis; air embolus; and bacterial or fungal septicemias.

Practical Points

- *Dietary energy is the first limiting nutrient in the nutritional rehabilitation of infants and children.*
- *Dietary energy needs can be estimated from the recommended dietary energy allowances for the child's age-specific ideal body weight.*
- *Standard infant formulas and well-balanced meals that are energy-dense are the best way to provide nutritional therapy for infants and children.*
- *Enteral (nasogastric tube, button gastrostomy) and parenteral (peripheral, central) techniques provide alternative methods for the nutritional rehabilitation of children with gastrointestinal disorders.*
- *The enteral route is the method of choice for refeeding unless intestinal obstruction, atony, or total villous atrophy is present.*
- *Regardless of the method of refeeding, careful monitoring for potential metabolic, infectious or mechanical complications is warranted.*

Case Histories

Case #1: A two-year-old female was referred for chronic diarrhea and failure to thrive. On physical exam, she appeared wasted and had a protuberant abdomen that was tympanitic to percussion. Her height was plotted on the growth curve at the 50th percentile, but her weight had fallen from the 50th to the 5th percentile. Laboratory tests were noteworthy for a hemoglobin content of 90 g/L and a serum albumin concentration of 27 g/L. Stool cultures and smears for bacterial pathogens and parasites were negative. A 72-h fecal fat study for malabsorption was positive (coefficient of absorption=85%). A hydrogen breath test for lactose intolerance was positive. A small bowel biopsy showed a flat villous lesion consistent with the diagnosis of celiac disease.

Question: What type of dietary treatment should be instituted in this child?

Answer: The child was placed on a gluten-free, low-lactose diet, with a multivitamin and mineral supplement. One month later, she showed marked clinical improvement.

Question: How should this child's nutritional progress be monitored?

Answer: Resolution of clinical symptoms and improvement in growth measurements and related laboratory tests constitute the mainstay of nutritional monitoring in this child. As a result of dietary intervention, this child's weight increased to the 25th percentile on the growth curve, her problems of diarrhea and abdominal bloating resolved, her hemoglobin and serum albumin levels normalized, and she tolerated milk and milk products. A repeat intestinal biopsy obtained after three months of dietary therapy showed normal villi. A gluten challenge and repeat intestinal biopsy were being planned after six months of dietary intervention.

Case #2: A 20-month-old male with short gut syndrome secondary to necrotizing enterocolitis was referred for evaluation of weight loss and recurrent fevers of 103° to 105°F, despite repeatedly negative blood cultures for aerobic, anaerobic and fungal organisms and replacement of the central venous catheter. On physical examination, the child appeared thin and somewhat dehydrated. His abdominal exam was remarkable for increased abdominal distention and hyperactive bowel sounds; his enterostomy output doubled and contained visible blood. Laboratory blood tests were noteworthy for electrolyte deficits (sodium, 132 mEq/L; potassium, 3.6 mEq/L), a

mild acidosis (bicarbonate, 15 mEq/L), and hypoalbuminemia (albumin, 30 g/L). Stool cultures and smears were negative for bacterial pathogens and parasites but positive for Clostridium difficile toxin.

Question: What should be the initial approach to the treatment of this child?

Answer: The child was treated initially with an intravenous glucose and electrolyte solution to correct his fluid and electrolyte deficits. Oral vancomycin therapy was instituted for the treatment of his intestinal problem. The fever defervesced and his enterostomy output returned to normal.

Question: What factors might explain this child's weight loss?

Answer: Inadequate nutrient intakes may account for this child's poor weight gain. A review of this child's enteral and parenteral feeding regimen revealed that 50% of his daily nutrient needs were derived from a protein hydrolysate formula supplemented with carbohydrate and fat to meet his energy and fluid requirements. However, inspection of his parenteral nutrition label revealed the contents of his bag to contain the following: glucose 20g/CTR, amino acids 3 g/CTR, NaCl 3.8 mEq/CTR, KHPO4 1.0 mmol/CTR, Ca gluconate 0.85 mmol/CTR, MgSO4 0.8 mEq/CTR, KCl 1.3 mEq/CTR, where CTR=480 ml, i.e., the remaining 50% of his fluid requirement, but not his nutrient requirement. After adjustments were made to standardize the formulation of his parenteral nutrition solution to 20% glucose, 3% amino acids and subsequent correction of electrolytes and minerals, the infant resumed appropriate weight gain.

Case #3: A 10-year-old male was referred with a two-year history of intermittent episodes of diarrhea, vomiting and abdominal pain. His parents noted that he had become the shortest child in his class at school, although previously he was much taller than most of his peers. On physical examination the child was pale and thin. His height had fallen from the 75th to the 50th percentile and his weight had fallen from the 25th to the 5th percentile on the growth curve. The abdominal findings included tenderness and a palpable mass in the right lower quadrant. Laboratory tests were noteworthy for anemia (hemoglobin 100 g/L), an elevated erythrocyte sedimentation rate (ESR 40 mm/hr), hypoalbuminemia (albumin 30 g/L) and normal folate and vitamin B$_{12}$ levels. Stool cultures and smears for bacterial pathogens and parasites were negative, but were positive for occult blood. A hydrogen breath test for small bowel bacterial overgrowth and lactose intolerance was positive. An upper gastrointestinal series with small bowel follow-through showed narrowing and "cobblestoning" of the terminal ileum. Colonoscopy showed aphthous ulcers of the ascending and transverse colon; biopsies showed inflammation and granuloma, the pathognomonic feature of Crohn's disease.

Question: What should be the initial approach to the medical and nutritional treatment of this child?

Answer: Corticosteroid and metronidazole therapy were instituted and a low-fat, low-lactose diet supplemented

with multivitamins and minerals was recommended. Symptoms resolved and the laboratory abnormalities normalized. Despite an improved appetite, however, weight gain was minimal.

Question: What additional nutritional intervention would be useful to improve this child's poor weight gain?

Answer: Nutritional supplementation using nighttime nasogastric tube feedings of a standard commercial formula was added to his habitual dietary regimen. Total daily dietary energy intakes averaged 140% of the recommended dietary allowance for age. After three months of nutritional support, height and weight velocities improved, and early catch-up growth was apparent.

Historical Perspective...

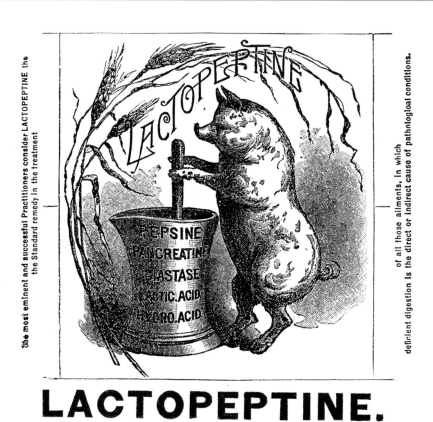

The most eminent and successful Practitioners consider LACTOPEPTINE the Standard remedy in the treatment

of all those ailments, in which deficient digestion is the direct or indirect cause of pathological conditions.

PEPSINE
PANCREATINE
DIASTASE
LACTIC ACID
HYDRO ACID

LACTOPEPTINE.

References

1. Ulshen MH, Lichtman SN. Basic aspects of digestion and absorption. In: Wyllie R, Hyams JS, eds. *Pediatric Gastrointestinal Diseases. Pathophysiology, Diagnosis, Management.* Philadelphia: WB Saunders Co; 1993:17-30.

2. Schmitz J. Digestive and absorptive function. In: Walker WA, Durie PR, Hamilton JR, Walker-Smith JA, Watkins JB, eds. *Pediatric Gastrointestinal Diseases.* Philadelphia: BC Decker Inc; 1991:266-280.

3. Auricchio S, Greco L, Troncone R. Gluten-sensitive enteropathy in childhood. *Pediatr Clin N Am.* 1988; 35:157-187.

4. Greco L, Auricchio S, Mayer M, Grimaldi M. Case control study on nutritional risk factors in celiac disease. *J Pediatr Gastroenterol Nutr.* 1988;7:395-399.

5. Auricchio S, Follo D, de Ritis G, Giunta A, Marzorati D, Prampolini L, Ansaldi N, Levi P, Dall'Olio D, Bossi A. Working hypothesis. Does breast-feeding protect against the development of clinical symptoms of celiac disease in children? *J Pediatr Gastroenterol Nutr.* 1983;2:428-433.

6. Ascher H, Holm K, Kristiansson B, Maki M. Different features of coeliac disease in two neighbouring countries. *Arch Dis Child.* 1993;69: 375-380.

7. Weile B, Cavell B, Nivenius K, Krasilnikoff PA. Striking differences in the incidence of childhood celiac disease between Denmark and Sweden: a plausible explanation. *J Pediatr Gstroenterol Nutr.* 1995;21:64-68.

8. Bosio L, Barera G, Mistura L, Sassi G, Bianchi C. Growth acceleration and final height after treatment for delayed diagnosis of celiac disease. *J Pediatr Gastroenterol Nutr.* 1990;11:324-329.

9. Maki M, Kallonen K, Lahdeaho ML, Visakorpi JK. Changing pattern of childhood celiac disease in Finland. *Acta Pediatr Scand.* 1988;77:408-412.

10. Stene-Larsen G, Mosvold J, Ly B. Selective vitamin B12 malabsorption in adult celiac disease. Report on three cases with associated autoimmune diseases. *Scand J Gastroenterol.* 1988;23:1105-1108.

11. Savilahti E, Simell O, Koskimes S, Rilva A, Akerblom HK. Celiac disease in insulin-dependent diabetes mellitus. *J Pediatr.* 1986;108:690-693.

12. Helin H, Mustonen J, Reunala T, Pasternack A. IgA nephropathy associated with celiac disease and dermatitis herpetiformis. *Arch Pathol Lab Med.* 1983;107:324-327.

13. Bai JC, Sambuelli A, Niveloni S, Sugai E, Mazure R, Kogan Z, Pedreira S, Boerr L. Alpha 1-antitrypsin clearance as an aid in the management of patients with celiac disease. *Am J Gastroenterol.* 1991;86:986-991.

14. Fine KD. The prevalence of occult gastrointestinal bleeding in celiac sprue. *N Engl J Med.* 1996;334: 1163-1191.

15. Bonamico M, Vania A, Monti S, Ballati G, Mariani P, Pitzalis G, Benedetti C, Falconieri P, Signoretti A. Iron deficiency in children with celiac disease. *J Pediatr Gastroenterol Nutr.* 1987;6: 702-706.

16. Frisancho AR. New norms of upper limb fat and muscle areas for assessment of nutritional status. *Am J Clin Nutr.* 1981;34:2540-2545.

17. Valletta EA, Mastella G. Adherence to gluten-free diet and serum antigliadin antibodies in celiac disease. *Digestion.* 1990;47:20-23.

18. Weile B, Krasilnikoff PA, Giwercman A, Skakkebaek NE. Insulin-like growth factor-I in celiac disease. *J Pediatr Gastroenterol Nutr.* 1994;19: 391-393.

19. Rakover Y, Hager H, Nussinson E, Luboshitzky R. Celiac disease as a cause of transient hypocalcemia and hypovitaminosis D in a 13 year-old girl. *J Pediatr Endocrinol.* 1994;7:53-55.

20. Mora S, Weber G, Barera G, Bellini A, Pasolini D, Prinster C, Bianchi C, Chiumello G. Effect of gluten-free diet on bone mineral content in growing patients with celiac disease. *Am J Clin Nutr.* 1993;57:224-228.

21. Molteni N, Caraceni MP, Bardella MT, Ortolani S, Gandolini GG, Bianchi P. Bone mineral density in adult celiac patients and the effect of gluten-free diet from childhood. *Am J Gastroenterol.* 1990; 85:51-53.

22. Damen GM, Boersma B, Wit JM, Heymans HS.

Catch-up growth in 60 children with celiac disease. *J Pediatr Gastroenterol Nutr.* 1994;19: 394-400.

23. Anson O, Weizman Z, Zeevi N. Celiac disease: parental knowledge and attitudes of dietary compliance. *Pediatrics.* 1990;85:98-103.

24. Vanderhoof JA. Short bowel syndrome in children. *Curr Opinion Pediatr.* 1995;7:560-568.

25. Thompson JS. Management of the short bowel syndrome. *Gastroenterol Clin N Am.* 1994;23: 403-420.

26. Kurkchubasche AG, Rowe MI, Smith SD. Adaptation in short-bowel syndrome: reassessing old limits. *J Pediatr Surg.* 1993;28:1069-1071.

27. Chaet MS, Farrell MK, Ziegler MM, Warner BW. Intensive nutritional support and remedial surgical intervention for extreme short bowel syndrome. *J Pediatr Gastroenterol Nutr.* 1994;19: 295-298.

28. Dorney SFA, Ament ME, Berquist WE, Vargas JH, Hassall E. Improved survival in very short small bowel of infancy with use of long-term parenteral nutrition. *J Pediatr.* 1985;107:521-525.

29. Grosfeld JL, Rescorla FJ, West JW. Short bowel syndrome in infancy and childhood. *Am J Surg.* 1986;151:41-46.

30. Caniano DA, Starr J, Ginn-Pease ME. Extensive short-bowel syndrome in neonates: outcome in the 1980's. *Surgery.* 1989;105:119-124.

31. Goulet OJ, Revillon Y, Jan D, De Potter S, Maurage C, Lortat-Jacob S, Martelli H, Nihoul-Fekete C, Ricour C. Neonatal short bowel syndrome. *J Pediatr.* 1991:18-23.

32. Grosfeld JL, Rescorla FJ, West KW. Gastrointestinal injuries in childhood: Analysis of 53 patients. *J Pediatr Surg.* 1989;24:580-583.

33. Feldman EJ, Dowling RH, McNaughton J, Peters TJ. Effects of oral versus intravenous nutrition on intestinal adaptation after small bowel resection in the dog. *Gastroenterology.* 1976;70:712-719.

34. Morin CL, Ling V, VanCaillie M. Role of oral intake on intestinal adaptation after small bowel resection in growing rats. *Pediatr Res.* 1978;12: 268-271.

35. Grey VL, Garofalo C, Greenberg GR, Morin CL. The adaptation of the small intestine after resection in response to free fatty acids. *Am J Clin Nutr.* 1984; 40:1235-1242.

36. Weser E, Babbitt J, Hoban M. Intestinal adaptation: Different growth responses to disaccharides compared with monosaccharides in rat small bowel. *Gastroenterology.* 1986;91:1521-1527.

37. Vanderhoof JA, Grandjean CJ, Burkley KT, Antonson DL. Effect of casein versus casein hydrolysate on mucosal adaptation following massive bowel resection in infant rats. *J Pediatr Gastroenterol Nutr.* 1984;3:262-267.

38. Spector MH, Levine GM, Deren JJ. Direct and indirect effects of dextrose and amino acids on gut mass. *Gastroenterology.* 1977;72:706-710.

39. Byrne TA, Persinger RL, Young LS, Ziegler TR, Wilmore DW. A new treatment for patients with short-bowel syndrome. Growth hormone, glutamine, and a modified diet. *Ann Surg.* 1995;222:243-254.

40. Hanhkard R, Goulet O, Ricour C, Rongier M, Colomb V, Darmaun D. Glutamine metabolism in children with short-bowel syndrome: a stable isotope study. *Pediatr Res.* 1994;36:202-206.

41. Uauy R, Stringel G, Thomas R, Quan R. Effect of dietary nucleotides on growth and maturation of the developing gut in the rat. *J Pediatr Gastroenterol Nutr.* 1990;10:497-503

42. Leleiko NS, Bronstein AD, Baliga S, Munro HN. *De novo* purine nucleotide synthesis in the rat small and large intestines. Effect of dietary protein and purines. *J Pediatr Gastroenterol Nutr.* 1983;2:313-319.

43. Gleeson MH, Bloom SR, Polak JM, Henry K. Endocrine tumor in kidney affecting small bowel structure, motility and absorptive function. *Gut.* 1971;12:773-782.

44. Hughes CA, Bates T, Dowling RH. Cholecystokinin and secretin prevent the intestinal mucosal hypoplasia of total parenteral nutrition in the dog. *Gastroenterology.* 1987;74:34-41.

45. Marti U, Burwen SJ, Jones AL. Biological effects of epidermal growth factor with emphasis on the gastrointestinal tract and liver. An update. *Hepatology.* 1989;9:126-138.

46. Weber TR. Enteral feeding increases sepsis in infants with short bowel syndrome. *J Pediatr Surg.* 1995;30:1086-1088.

47. Swaniker F, Fonkalsrud EW. Superior and inferior vena caval occlusion in infants receiving total parenteral nutrition. *Am Surg.* 1995;61:877-881.

48. Moukarzel AA, Haddad I, Ament ME, Buchman AL, Reyen L, Maggioni A, Baron HI, Vargas J. 230 patient years of experience with home long-term parenteral nutrition in childhood: natural history and life of central venous catheters. *J Pediatr Surg.* 1994;29:1323-1327.

49. Purdum PP, Kirky DF. Short-bowel syndrome: A review of the role of nutrition support. *J Parent Ent Nutr.* 1991;15:93-101.

50. Parker P, Stroop S, Greene H. A controlled comparison of continuous versus intermittent feeding in the treatment of infants with intestinal disease. *J Pediatr.* 1981;99:360-364.

51. Schwartz SM, Gewitz MH, Sec CC, Berezin S, Glassman MS, Medow CM, Fish BC, Newman LJ. Enteral nutrition in infants with congenital heart disease and growth failure. *Pediatr.* 1990;86:368-373.

52. Messing B, Pigot F, Rongier M, Morin MC, Ndeindoum U, Rambaud JC. Intestinal absorption of free oral hyperalimentation in the very short bowel syndrome. *Gastroenterol.* 1991;100:1502-1508.

53. Woolf GM, Miller C, Kurian R, Jeejeebhoy KN. Nutritional absorption in short bowel syndrome. Evaluation of fluid, calorie, and divalent cation requirements. *Dig Dis Sci.* 1987;32:8-15.

54. Arrigoni E, Marteau P, Briet F, Pochart P, Rambaud JC, Messing B. Tolerance and absorption of lactose from milk and yogurt during shortbowel syndrome in humans. *Am J Clin Nutr.* 1994;60: 926-929.

55. Zimmaro DM, Rolandelli RH, Koruda MJ, Settle RG, Stein TP, Rombeau JL. Isotonic tube feeding formula induces liquid stool in normal subjects: Reversal by pectin. *J Parent Ent Nutr.* 1989;13:117-123.

56. Bochenek W, Rodgers JB, Balint JA. Effects of changes in dietary lipids on intestinal fluid loss in the short-bowel syndrome. *Ann Intern Med.* 1970; 72:205-213.

57. Andersson H, Isaksson B, Sjogren B. Fat-reduced diet in the symptomatic treatment of small bowel disease. *Gut.* 1974;15:351-359.

58. Simko V, McCarroll AM, Goodman S, Weesner RE, Kelley RE. High-fat diet in the short-bowel syndrome. Intestinal absorption and gastroenteropancreatic hormone responses. *Dig Dis Sci.* 1980;25:333-339.

59. Oveson L, Chu R, Howard L. The influence of dietary fat on jejunostomy output in patients with severe short bowel syndrome. *Am J Clin Nutr.* 1983;38:270-277.

60. Galeano NF, Leroy C, Belli D, Levy E, Roy CC. Comparison of two special infant formulas designed for the treatment of protracted diarrhea. *J Pediatr Gastroenterol Nutr.* 1988;7:76-83.

61. Bennett RA, Rubin PH, Present DH. Frequency of inflammatory bowel disease in offspring of couples both presenting with inflammatory bowel disease. *Gastroenterology.* 1991;100:1638-1643.

62. Lashner BA, Evans AA, Kirsner JB, Hanauer SB. Prevalence and incidence of inflammatory bowel disease in family members. *Gastroenterology.* 1986; 91:1396-1400.

63. Orholm M, Munkholm P, Langholz E, Nielsen OH, Sorensen IA, Binder V. Familial occurrence of inflammatory bowel disease. *N Engl J Med.* 1991; 324:84-88.

64. Shanahan F. Current concepts of the pathogenesis of inflammatory bowel disease. *Irish J Med Sci.* 1994;163:544-549.

65. Motil KJ, Grand RJ. Inflammatory bowel disease. Nutritional aspects of specific disease states. In: Walker WA, Watkins JB, eds. *Pediatric Gastrointestinal Diseases. Pathophysiology, Diagnosis, Mangement.* 2nd ed. Hamilton, Ontario: BC Decker Inc; 1996:508-525.

66. Motil KJ, Grand RJ, Davis-Kraft L, Ferlic L, Smith EO. Growth failure in children with inflammatory bowel disease: a prospective study. *Gastroenterology.* 1993;105:681-691.

67. Motil KJ, Grand RJ, Matthews DE, Bier DM, Maletskos CJ, Young VR. Whole body leucine metabolism in adolescents with Crohn's

disease and growth failure during nutritional supplementation. *Gastroenterology.* 1982;82: 1359-1368.

68. Kushner RF, Schoeller DA. Resting and total energy expenditure in patients with inflammatory bowel disease. *Am J Clin Nutr.* 1991;53:161-165.

69. Powell-Tuck J, Garlick PJ, Lennard-Jones JE, Waterlow JC. Rates of whole body protein synthesis and breakdown increase with the severity of inflammatory bowel disease. *Gut.* 1984;25:460-464.

70. Thomas AG, Miller V, Taylor F, Maycock P, Scrimgeour CM, Rennie MJ. Whole body protein turnover in childhood Crohn's disease. *Gut.* 1992; 33:675-677.

71. Heys SD, Park KGM, McNurlan MA, Keenan RA, Miller JD, Eremin O, Garlick PJ. Protein synthesis rates in colon and liver: stimulation by gastrointestinal pathologies. *Gut.* 1992;33:976-981.

72. Beisel WR. Effect of infection on human protein metabolism. *Fed Proc.* 1966;25:1682-1687.

73. Scrimshaw NS, Taylor CE, Gordon JE. *Interactions of nutrition and infection.* Geneva: World Health Organization: 1968. WHO Monograph Series No. 57.

74. Scrimshaw NS. Effect of infection on nutrient requirements. *Am J Clin Nutr.* 1977;30:1536-1544.

75. Spady DW, Payne PR, Picou D, Waterlow JC. Energy balance during recovery from malnutrition. *Am J Clin Nutr.* 1976;29:1073-1088.

76. Morin CL, Roulet M, Roy CC, Weber A. Continuous elemental and enteral alimentation in the treatment of children and adolescents with Crohn's disease. *J Parent Ent Nutr.* 1982;6:194-199.

77. O'Moráin C, Segal Am, Levi AJ, Valman HB. Elemental diet in acute Crohn's disease. *Arch Dis Child.* 1983;53:44-47.

78. Navarro J, Vargas J, Cezard JP, Charritat JL, Polonovski C. Prolonged constant rate elemental enteral nutrition in Crohn's disease. *J Pediatr Gastroenterol Nutr.* 1982;1:541-546.

79. Giaffer MH, North G, Holdsworth CD. Controlled trial of polymeric versus elemental diet in treatment of active Crohn's disease. *Lancet.* 1990: 1:816-819.

80. Royall D, Jeejeebhoy KN, Baker JP, Allard JP, Habal FM, Cunnane SC, Greenberg GR. Comparison of amino acid v peptide based enteral diets in active Crohn's disease: clinical and nutritional outcome. *Gut.* 1994;35:783-787.

81. Jones VA, Dickinson RJ, Workman E, Wilson AJ, Freeman AH, Hunter JO. Crohn's disease: maintenance of remission by diet. *Lancet.* 1985;2: 177-180.

82. Lorenz R, Weber PC, Szimnau P, Heldwein W, Strasser T, Loeschke K. Supplementation with n-3 faty acids from fish oil in chronic inflammatory bowel disease—a randomized, placebo-controlled, double-blind cross-over trial. *J Intern Med.* 1989; 225S:225-232.

83. Aslan A, Triadafilopoulos G. Fish oil fatty acid supplementation in active ulcerative colitis: a double-blind, placebo-controlled, crossover study. *Am J Gastroenterol.* 1992;87:432-437.

84. Stenson WF, Cort D, Rogers J, Burakoff R, De Schryver-Kecskemeti K, Gramlich TL, Beeken W. Dietary supplementation with fish oil in ulcerative colitis. *Ann Intern Med.* 1992;116:609-614.

85. Greenberg GR, Fleming CR, Jeejeebhoy KN, Rosenberg IH, Sales D, Tremaine WJ. Controlled trial of bowel rest and nutritional support in the management of Crohn's disease. *Gut.* 1988;29: 1309-1315.

86. Souba WW, Smith RJ, Wilmore DW. Glutamine metabolism by the intestinal tract. *J Parent Ent Nutr.* 1985;9:608-617.

87. Tremel H, Kienle B, Weilemann LS, Stehle P, Furst P. Glutamine dipeptide-supplemented parenteral nutrition maintains intestinal function in the critically ill. *Gastroenterology.* 1994;107: 1595-1601.

88. Selhub J, Dhar GJ, Rosenberg IH. Inhibition of folate enzymes by sulfasalazine. *J Clin Invest.* 1978; 61:221-224.

89. Burbidge EJ, Huang S, Bayless TM. Clinical manifestations of Crohn's disease in children and adolescents. *Pediatrics.* 1975;55:866-871.

90. Waterlow JC. Classification and definition of protein calorie malnutrition. *BMJ.* 1972;3:566-569.

91. Waterlow JC. Note on the assessment and classification of protein-energy malnutrition in children. *Lancet.* 1973;2:87-89.

92. Issenman RM, Atkinson SA, Radoja C, Fraher L. Longitudinal assessment of growth, mineral metabolism, and bone mass in pediatric Crohn's disease. *J Pediatr Gastroenterol Nutr.* 1993;17: 401-406.

93. Genant HK, Mall JC, Wagonfeld JB, Horst JV, Lanzi LH. Skeletal demineralization and growth retardation in inflammatory bowel diseases. *Invest Radiol.* 1976;11:541-549.

94. Hill GL, Blackett RL, Pickford IR, Bradley JA. A survey of protein nutrition in patients with inflammatory bowel disease—a rational basis for nutritional therapy. *Br J Surg.* 1977;64:894-896.

95. Ryde SJS, Clements D, Evans WS, Motley R, Morgan WS, Evans C, Rhodes J, Compston JE. Total body calcium in patients with inflammatory bowel disease: a longitudinal study. *Clin Sci.* 1991; 80:319-324

96. Compston JE. Review article: osteoporosis, corticosteroids and inflammatory bowel disease. *Aliment Pharmacol Ther.* 1995;9:237-250.

Building Better Bones:
Calcium, Magnesium, Phosphorus and Vitamin D

Winston W. K. Koo M.B.B.S.[1], Reginald C. Tsang M.B.B.S.[2]

Department of Pediatrics and Obstetrics/Gynecology, Wayne State University School of Medicine, Detroit, Michigan,[1] Department of Pediatrics, Pediatric Bone Research Center, University of Cincinnati Medical Center, Cincinnati, Ohio[2]

Reviewed by Stephanie A. Atkinson Ph.D., Stanley Zlotkin M.D., Ph.D. and Steve Abrams M.D.

Introduction

The word calcium is derived from Latin calx, *limestone, and from Greek,* khalix, *pebble. Magnesium is derived from Latin* magnesia; *and from Greek* magnesia, *name of various minerals, and from Magnesia, a metalliferous region of Thessaly. Phosphorus is derived from Latin and Greek,* phosphoros, *"light bearing" (so named because white phosphorus is phosphorescent in air);* phos *indicates the presence of light;* phoros *indicates* pherein, *to bear.* (The American Heritage Dictionary of the English Language, 1975)

The physiology and metabolism of calcium (Ca), magnesium (Mg), phosphorus (P) and vitamin D are intimately related and of critical importance in maintaining good bone health and mineral homeostasis. Historical descriptions of clinical symptoms and signs of skeletal disorders, and research on this subject, indicate a keen appreciation of the importance of these nutrients in tissue function and structure. Even in 1879, Routh described:

Phosphate of lime in breast milk: deformity of every kind in the skeleton may depend on an insufficient quantity of this salt in the blood for it should be remarked first that not only is it useful because it is itself appropriated into the system, but, secondly, phosphate of lime, when present in a fluid which in the present case is milk and by subsequent assimilation becomes blood, has the property of enabling that fluid to take up more carbonic acid. Now, when carbonic acid in its turn is in excess, it dissolves carbonate of lime, hence the quantity of carbonate of lime held in solution in the blood is thereby made greater and is in this way from time to time more easily and largely deposited in bone. (Infant Feeding and Its Influence on Life, 3rd ed. CHF Routh, 1879)

Howland's and Marriott's paper, "The Calcium Content of the Blood in Rachitis and Tetany," showed that in the former disease, there was no more than a "very slight" reduction in calcium, but that in tetany (seven cases) the reduction was marked during the active stage, returning to normal with recovery. They had devised a method applicable to one to two cc of serum, a significant step in the direction of microchemistry. (Proceedings, 31st meeting of the American Pediatric Society, Atlantic City, NJ, June 1919).

Glisson in 1660 had established rickets as a clinical entity and believed it was the result of overeating.[1] The derivation of the word "rickets" is obscure. One possibility is that the Greek word for spine, "rhachis", was converted into the word rachitis and then rickets. Another view is that the word arose from the Dorset dialect, to rucket (breathe with difficulty). Rucket in turn is possibly a derivation of the Scandinavian word ruckle (make a rattling noise in the throat). It may also be an eponym from the name of one Rickets who, in 1620, was active by treating the disease in Dorset.[2] Another possibility is the early English wrick or wrikken (twist or sprain). By 1634, however, the word was generally used as if it was general knowledge, although the medical profession called it rachitis.[3]

Physiology
Body Content

The skeleton is the major reservoir of Ca, Mg and P. It contains about 99% of total body Ca, 60%-65% of total body Mg, and 80%-85% of total body P. Soft tissue also contains large amounts of Mg and P. For example, skeletal muscle contains approximately 27%

	Birth	6 Months	12 Months	24 Months
Body weight (g)	3270	7850	10150	12590
Length (cm)	50.50	67.80	76.10	87.60
Calcium (g)	31.18	37.47	47.36	54.45
Magnesium (g)	0.82	1.78	2.97	6.54
Phosphorus (g)	17.13	21.19	26.89	31.37

Adapted from references 5, 11 and based on fiftieth percentile of male reference population reference 16.
Conversion: Calcium 1 mmol=40mg, magnesium 1 mmol=24mg, phosphorus 1 mmol=31 mg.

Table 1: Estimated average body content of calcium, magnesium and phosphorus from birth to 2 years.

of total body Mg and 9% of total body P; viscera contain approximately 7% of Mg and 5% of P.[4-9] After birth, circulating concentrations of Ca, Mg and P constitute less than one % of their total body content.

In the fetus, Ca, Mg and P build up increases rapidly from 24 weeks to term gestation. The reported range of peak accretion for Ca is between 102 to 151 mg (conversion 1 mmol=40 mg); for Mg is between 2.5 to 3.7 mg (conversion 1 mmol=24 mg); and for P is between 65 to 85 mg (conversion 1 mmol=31 mg) /kg/day at 34 to 36 weeks' gestation. At term, the body content of Ca, Mg and P, as determined by chemical analyses,[4-6] neutron activation analysis,[8] or dual energy X ray absorptiometry,[9] are quite comparable and approximately 28 to 30 g, 0.6 to 0.8 g, and 17 to 19 g, respectively.

The rate of mineral accretion relative to body weight remains rapid in infants when compared with older children by chemical estimation[10,11] or by single photon absorptiometry.[12-15] The estimated content of Ca, Mg and P between birth and two years is shown in Table 1. These data are based on the bone Ca content with proportional changes in P and Mg; higher soft tissue P and Mg content compared with bone; and they are adjusted to the fiftieth percentile of National Center for Health Statistics growth chart[16] for male infants.

Direct quantitative measurement of vitamin D stores in human infants is lacking. Vitamin D status, as indicated by serum 25 hydroxyvitamin the level consistent with vitamin D (25 OHD) concentrations, the major circulating vitamin D metabolite, can be depleted to the level consistent with vitamin D deficiency within eight weeks after birth in breast-fed infants without vitamin D supplementation or adequate sunshine exposure.[17] However, serum 25 OHD concentrations can remain normal for many months in infants receiving parenteral nutrition[18] with minimal amounts of vitamin D (approximately 30 IU/kg/day). In ambulatory young children between four and 13 years who are receiving home total parenteral nutrition, serum 25 OHD concentration apparently can be maintained in the low normal range for up to one year following withdrawal of vitamin D from parenteral nutrition solutions.[19]

Circulating Concentrations

The normal ranges of circulating total and ionized Ca, Mg, P and vitamin D metabolite concentrations are shown in Table 2. Serum mineral concentrations are maintained within a narrow range; physiologic factors such as age, race, season and diet normally account for less than 5% variability in the mean serum Ca, Mg and P concentrations.[20-23] However, different dietary intake or dietary supplement may markedly affect serum P and 25 OHD concentration. Thus, the average serum P concentration of infants fed cow milk is at least 20% greater than the values for infants fed human milk;[24] the average serum 25 OHD concentration of infants receiving "routine" vitamin D supplement is at least 50% greater than that of infants without vitamin D supplement;[25] and the average serum 1,25 dihydroxyvitamin D ($1,25(OH)_2D$) concentration of infants fed cow milk-based infant formula is about 20% higher than human milk-fed infants.[21] Similarly, seasonal variations in sunlight exposure can directly affect the level of serum 25 OHD concentration with values during summer up to two to three times the values during winter.[26-29] The differences between plasma and serum values of these minerals and vitamin D metabolites are minimal and of no practical significance.

Acute transient fluctuations of serum concentrations of Ca, Mg and P may occur in response to compartmental shifts of these elements, without major clinical consequences. However, acute changes in serum concentrations of minerals beyond the normal ranges may be associated with disturbances in physiologic function.[24, 30-32] A change in serum concentration of one of the minerals also may reflect a change in the status of

	n	mean	Normal Range (± 2SD)
Ionized Calcium† (mg/dl)	150	5.2	4.7-5.8
Total Calcium† (mg/dl)	144	9.7	8.4-11.0
Magnesium† (mg/dl)	145	2.1	1.7-2.5
Phosphorus† (mg/dl)	145	6.6	4.6-8.6
25-Hydroxyvitamin D‡ (ng/ml)	149	52	16-88
1,25 dihydroxyvitamin D§ (pg/ml)	141	64	18-122

* No gender differences in any variable.
† Age, race, season and diet normally account for <5% of variablity of mean serum concentrations.
‡ Season, diet and vitamin D supplementation may result in 2 to 3 fold differences in serum concentrations.
§ Age, diet and physiologic mineral need may result in >20% difference in mean serum concentrations.
Conversion: Calcium 1 mmol/L=40 mg/dl, magnesium l mmol/L=2.4 mg/dl, phosphorus 1 mmol/L=3.1 mg/dl, 25 hydroxyvitamin D
   1 nmol/L=0.4 ng/ml, 1,25 dihydroxyvitamin D 1 pmol/L=0.4 pg/ml
Adapted from references 20 and 21.

Table 2: Normal serum ranges* of minerals and vitamin D metabolites between birth to 18 months.

another mineral. For example, low P intake as occurs in breast-fed infants may be associated with "physiologic hypercalcemia," with serum Ca in apparently healthy infants reaching as high as 11 mg/dl;[22, 33] whereas a higher P intake, as with the ingestion of cow milk-based infant formula[24, 30, 34] may have lower serum Ca, and higher serum P and PTH concentrations compared with human milk-fed infants. Chronic and severely lowered serum mineral concentrations may reflect the presence of a deficiency state.[35]

Quantitatively, serum 25 OHD concentration is generally regarded as the best indicator of vitamin D status. It is normally present in wide ranges and depends on endogenous production and dietary intake[21, 25] with values in the summer up to about twice that of the winter.[26-29] In the Ca-deficient state, increased metabolic clearance of 25 OHD may lead to low serum 25 OHD concentrations.[36, 37] There is also overlap in serum 25 OHD concentrations for infants and children who are clinically well[21, 25-29] and those suffering from rickets.[38-43] However, the lower limit of normal range is generally considered to be approximately 11 ng/ml (conversion 1 nmol/L=0.4 ng/ml).

Intestinal Absorption of Ca, Mg and P

Is it not possible for infants to thrive upon other foods than those containing fresh milk? Answer: They may do so for a short time but never permanently. The long continued use of other foods as a sole diet is attended with great risk. What are the dangers of such foods? Answer: Frequently scurvy is produced, often rickets ... The child does not thrive, is pale, and his muscles are soft and flabby. (Holt E. The Care and Feeding of Children: A Catechism for the Use of Mothers and Children's Nurses. New York, D. Appleton & Co., 1904: 45-46.)

The regulation of body Ca content is primarily by way of the gastrointestinal tract. Ca absorption occurs by a saturable, active, transcellular process, primarily in the duodenum and upper jejunum, and is vitamin D dependent, probably related to the effect of vitamin D on modulating the complex, sequentially-integrated process involving Ca entry into the cell, intracellular transport and extrusion from intestinal cells.[44, 45] The primary mechanism of vitamin D-dependent transport is direct interaction of $1,25(OH)_2D$ at the level of cellular genome via specific receptors for vitamin D metabolites,[46-48] although there is a more rapid onset (within two to four minutes) non-genomic effect of $1,25(OH)_2D$ on intestinal Ca transport.[47] There is also a non-saturable paracellular transport that occurs throughout the small bowel, dependent on a concentration and voltage differential.[49] The solubility of Ca salts is maintained in the lower small bowel, partly by binding to taurine-conjugated bile acid to allow for Ca to be

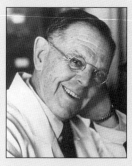

Edwards A. Park M.D. (1878-1969) was a graduate of Columbia's College of Physicians and Surgeons. He served as a resident under Howland at the New York Foundling Hospital and moved with Howland to St. Louis and Baltimore. At Hopkins, Park began a collaboration with McCollum which resulted in the identification of vitamin D deficiency rickets. Park accepted the first Chairmanship of Pediatrics at Yale in 1921. He was a vigorous proponent of women in medicine and he appointed Jews to his housestaff and faculty when other departments would not. Park returned to Hopkins as the second Chairman of Pediatrics where he established the first pediatric specialty clinics. He retired in 1947 but continued to publish about nutritional disturbances of bone until 1964. First Howland Award, Pediatrics, 1952;10:82-107 (Photo courtesy of J. Hopkins).

absorbed.[50] Normally the colon plays no significant role in Ca absorption; however, significantly increased Ca absorption may occur through the colon in patients with long segment small bowel resection.[51] Endogenous secretion, i.e., the flux of Ca across the intestinal cell into the lumen, also occurs. From stable isotope studies, the endogenous fecal Ca excretion in adults is estimated to be 70 to 80 mg/day at a Ca intake of <200 mg/day, and increases directly with increase in Ca intake;[52] in one study of five children aged 3-14 years, it was reported as 1.0-1.9 mg/kg/day.[53]

There are marked variations in endogenous losses of Ca and true Ca absorption in preterm infants. Based on stable isotope studies, the former averages 10% to 20% of intake,[54, 55] with the latter reported between 40% to 90%.[54-57] These values are consistent with data from standard "balance studies" (a net balance of intake minus all losses) at levels of nutrient intake approximating normal requirements.[58] Stable isotope studies on mineral metabolism in children born at term are limited.[59] In one report using dual-tracer stable isotope technique, calcium absorption averaged 61.3 ± 22.7 (SD)% in five to seven month infants fed human milk and solid foods.[60] Multiple balance studies reported average Ca absorption as between 30% and 58%, with the highest values reported for infants fed human milk,

and lowest for infants fed whole cow milk.[11]

The major determinant of mineral retention for enterally-fed infants, particularly for Ca and Mg, is the amount of mineral intake and mineral absorption. However, differences in the distribution and concentration of minerals (and vitamin D) between human milk and infant formulas theoretically may affect mineral absorption and retention. Approximately half of the Ca and Mg is found in the protein fraction of milk. The majority of Ca and Mg is present in the whey protein of human milk, in contrast to the casein fraction of bovine milk.[61, 62] Another one-third of Ca content and one-half of Mg content are bound to low molecular weight compounds. The final 20% of the Ca is found in the fat fraction of human milk.[61, 63] There are differences in the content of Ca, Mg and P in milk between mothers from different geographic regions delivering term and preterm infants.[64-66] Maternal diet,[67] calcium supplementation[68] or smoking[69] has no effect on milk Ca content. In a case report, maternal ingestion of pharmacologic doses of vitamin D (100,000 IU daily) did not affect breast milk content of Ca, Mg and P.[70] Variations in individuals and study design and assay methods account for some of the differences in the reported human milk contents of Ca, Mg and P.[71, 72] In longitudinal studies, human milk Ca, Mg and P contents varied by 10% to 20% during the first six months of lactation,[33, 66, 68, 73] with Ca being the only mineral achieving a statistically significant decrease by about 25% beyond the first three months of lactation. The reported range of mean content of minerals in human milk is 270 to 320 mg Ca, 30-40 mg Mg, and 130-150 mg P per liter, with Ca:P ratios ranging from 1.8:1 to 2.2:1 by weight.

Vitamin D,[44, 45] dietary lactose[74] and phosphate[75] can increase Ca absorption and retention. Contrary to a report that glucose and glucose polymer result in increased Ca absorption in adults,[76] complete substitution of glucose polymer for lactose in term infant formula results in slightly lower Ca retention when compared with lactose-containing infant formulas.[74, 77] Phytate[78] in soy formula theoretically may impair Ca absorption, although infants fed current (mineral fortified) preparations of soy formula have normal serum biochemistry and distal radial bone mineralization.[79-81] The absorption of fat does not appear to be a major determinant of Ca absorption under most conditions in normal infants. A threefold increase in Ca intake results in a decrease in fat absorption of about 5% from infant formulas with well-absorbed fat blends, but has no significant effect on absorption or retention of nitrogen, magnesium, copper and zinc.[82] Fourfold increase in Ca and P intake for up to 9 months did not adversely affect iron status of healthy term infants fed iron fortified formulas.[83]

The net effect of bidirectional Mg flux across the intestine supports the concept that Mg absorption occurs predominantly in the distal small bowel and colon, although Mg absorption can occur throughout the intestine. In the usual range of intake, intestinal absorption of Mg is a linear function of intake, which is consistent with a passive diffusion process. However, decreased fractional absorption with increasing intake up to 960 mg elemental Mg,[84, 85] is consistent with facilitated diffusion, possibly via "solvent drag". Normally, vitamin D metabolites have little or no effect on Mg absorption. Pharmacologic doses of vitamin D may increase Mg absorption. There is no consistent effect of dietary Ca and P on Mg absorption, although some studies of human adults have reported Mg absorption may be depressed when intakes of Ca and P are about double the normal dietary range.[85-87] In the rat, Mg absorption decreases in the presence of phytate[88] and at high intakes of Ca and P.[89]

Endogenous fecal excretion of Mg for adults appears small and is approximately 0.6 mg/kg/day.[90] It appears to be highly variable for infants and is reported to range from zero to 6.2 mg/kg/day.[91] However, the Mg content of gastrointestinal secretion may be as high as 16.8 mg/dl[92] and is a significant source of Mg loss in pathological situations.

In suckling rat pups, bioavailability of Mg from human milk, whole cow milk, and cow milk- or soy protein-based infant formulas are comparable in spite of the differences in the distribution and the form of Mg salt in these milks.[93] In suckling rat pups, the mean whole body tissue retention for Mg from various dietary sources is between 51% to 79%.[93] The average net Mg absorption in infants fed human milk or formulas is 40% to 52%; is 30% to 38% in infants fed whole cow milk; and the mean net Mg retention rate

varies between 11% and 40%, with a higher percent retention in younger infants fed human milk.[11, 75] In infants received 20 mg of [25]Mg orally, the mean fractional absorption of [25]Mg increases from 54.3% to 64% if the isotope is given in divided doses versus a single bolus. With the dose of [25]Mg increased from 20 mg to 60 mg, the fractional absorption was reduced, although the absolute isotope absorption was at least doubled.[91] However, the net Mg absorption and retention were uninfluenced by total Mg intake.[91] In breast-fed term infants, doubling the normal P intake with phosphate supplementation improves Mg retention.[75] In humans[94] and rats,[95] vitamin D action in promoting Mg absorption probably occurs only in the vitamin D-deficient state.

Phosphate absorption occurs throughout the small intestine, but most efficiently in the duodenum and jejunum. It is absorbed by paracellular diffusion and by an active transfer process dependent on sodium potassium ATPase. The latter is subjected to adaptive hormonal control including vitamin D metabolites, modulators of vitamin D action including thyroid and steroid hormones, and peptide hormones such as insulin.[96] In normal circumstances, most P is absorbed independent of Ca.[97] The vitamin D-dependent active transfer mechanism may not be important except in vitamin D-deficient states.[98]

Intestinal P absorption generally is more complete than Ca absorption, and the average P absorption or retention when expressed as percentage of intake is usually higher than that for Ca. The average intestinal net absorption of P is reported to vary between 56% and 85% in infants.[11, 75] P appears to be similarly well absorbed for infants fed human milk or whole cow milk, and is lowest for infants fed soy protein-based formula, presumably because of the presence of poorly absorbed phytate P. The average net P retention in infants fed different milk varies between 25% and 55%.[11] Infants fed human milk have the highest net percent P retention because of the milk's low P content.

An excess of either Ca or P may reduce the absorption of the other mineral because of precipitation of insoluble Ca phosphate. Binding of P within the gastrointestinal tract by aluminum and Mg has been responsible for antacid-induced phosphate deficiency.[32]

	Ca	Mg	P
Proximal convoluted tubule	80%	20%-30%	75%-80%
Loop of Henle	10%-20%	50%-60%	---
Distal nephron		10%	10%-15%
Mean daily excretion mg/d in infants*	15-36 (2.8-7.6)	13-28 (13.1-34.6)	29-409 (22.2-50.2)

* Data obtained from healthy infants fed various milk preparations during standard balance studies.[11] Infants fed human milk has lowest urine P and those fed whole cow milk has highest urine P.
Numbers in parenthesis = % of intake.
Conversion: Ca 1 mmol=40 mg, Mg 1mmol=24 mg, P 1 mmol=31 mg.

Table 3: Renal handling of Ca, Mg and P.

Urinary Excretion of Ca, Mg and P

The sites of renal reabsorption of Ca, Mg, and P are shown in Table 3. The kidney filters large amounts of Ca, Mg, and P daily; for example, in an infant with a glomerular filtration rate of 20 ml/min (28.8 L/day) and 60% of serum Ca (100 mg/L) being ultra-filtrable, the daily amount of filtered Ca would be 1728 mg. Similarly, the daily amount of filtered Mg and P would be 442 mg and 1445 mg, respectively. However, only 1% to 2% of filtered Ca, 3% to 4% of Mg, and 10% to 15% of P are excreted. Thus, a small percent increase in renal loss of any of these minerals may significantly affect mineral balance, particularly at low ranges of intake.

The amount of Ca, Mg and P excreted in urine varies with dietary intake. Some common factors of clinical importance that may increase urinary excretion of Ca, Mg and P include increased loading of the respective minerals; increased sodium intake with resulting positive sodium balance and extracellular fluid expansion; and intravenous and oral glucose loading.[99, 100] Similar mechanisms are at work in increased urinary excretion of Ca and possibly Mg during total parenteral nutrition (PN). In addition, excessive amino acid (particularly sulfur amino acids), glucose and vitamin D intake contributes to increased urine Ca loss during PN.[101]

The effect of vitamin D and its metabolites on ion transport is much less marked in the kidney than in the intestine. 1,25 Dihydroxyvitamin D [1,25(OH)$_2$D] receptors and vitamin D-dependent Ca binding protein are found in distal renal tubule, and 1,25(OH)$_2$D stimulation of sodium-dependent P transport in brush border membrane of proximal renal tubule is also present, thus supporting the possible role of vitamin D metabolite in renal Ca conservation. Non-genomic, receptor-mediated action of 1,25(OH)$_2$D is reported for intestinal transport of Ca, but its effect on renal tubule is unclear. Large doses of 1,25(OH)$_2$D produce hypercalcemia, hyperphosphatemia and phosphaturia[102] presumably, in part, secondary to its effect on mobilization of bone minerals and increased intestinal absorption of Ca and P. Hypercalcemia inhibits Mg reabsorption, while Mg infusion inhibits Ca reabsorption in the loop of Henle. P intake, either orally or intravenously, decreases urinary Ca and Mg excretion, particularly in the phosphate-deficient state. The kidney in the human infant adapts well to retaining P, particularly under conditions of low P intake such as with human milk feeding and during increased need, such as for bone growth and mineralization[35, 99, 100] when urine P excretion is negligible.

Vitamin D Metabolism

Vitamin D is either derived exogenously from diet or is produced endogenously in the epidermis. Two chemical forms of vitamin D exist: vitamin D$_2$ (ergocalciferol), which is of plant origin, and vitamin D$_3$ (cholecalciferol), which is of animal origin (Figure 1). In the mammal, vitamins D$_2$ and D$_3$ appear to be metabolized along the same pathway, and there is little functional difference between their metabolites. The term vitamin D is frequently used generically to describe vitamins D$_2$ and D$_3$ and their corresponding metabolites.

Hess and Weinstock in 1925 irradiated excised human skin with a mercury-vapor lamp, fed it to rats, and were

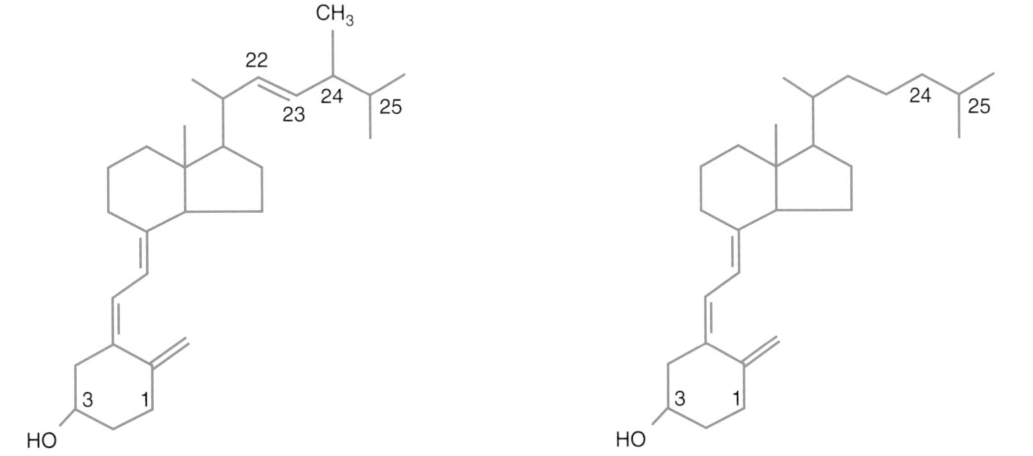

Figure 1: Two chemical forms of vitamin D exist: vitamin D$_2$ (ergocalciferol), which is of plant origin, and vitamin D$_3$ (cholecalciferol), which is of animal origin.

able to prevent rickets. They concluded therefore that the anti-rachitic factor was formed from the human skin.

Vitamin D is produced endogenously in the skin from provitamin D$_3$ (7 dehydrocholesterol), an intermediate in cholesterol biosynthesis. It undergoes chemical photolysis under ultraviolet B irradiation at 280 to 300 nm wavelength to produce previtamin D$_3$. Under thermal ionization, previtamin D$_3$ is isomerized to vitamin D$_3$,[103] which is then released into the circulation bound to vitamin D binding protein (DBP).[104] Excessive amounts of previtamin D$_3$ in the skin can undergo further photoconversion to lumisterol or tachysterol, which are stored in the skin and are in equilibrium with previtamin D$_3$[103] (Figure 2). In addition, these metabolites have a low affinity for DBP and tend to remain in the skin. Thus skin may provide a storage site for vitamin D and possibly a protective mechanism against vitamin D toxicity from ultraviolet exposure.

The diet is generally a poor source of vitamin D except in countries where fortification of foodstuffs with vitamin D is practiced or where oily fish is routinely consumed. In general, the rate of absorption of vitamin D is linearly related to the dose, suggesting that absorption takes place by passive diffusion.[105] Intestinal absorption of vitamin D and its major metabolite, 25 OHD, is facilitated by the presence of bile salts.[106, 107]

In normal adults an absorption of vitamin D between 62% and 91% (mean 78%) has been reported,[108] but in adults with T tube biliary drainage after elective cholecystectomy, the absorption rate of vitamin D is only 3.9%.[106] In three to 21-days-old term infants with inoperable brain deformities, Kodicek[109] reported that between 77% and 87% of an oral dose of labeled vitamin D$_2$ was absorbed within three days. Recent data in normal infants show that non-esterified vitamin D$_2$ is better absorbed than vitamin D$_3$ palmitate. Both compounds are better absorbed by two-to-threefolds in 10-days-old versus one day-old infants.[110]

The somewhat more polar 25 OHD appears to be better absorbed by subjects with liver disease; i.e., those with low bile salt production[111, 112] compared with its parent compound, vitamin D. After absorption through the intestine, vitamin D is carried in chylomicrons through the lymphatics into the blood. Most of the vitamin D is then bound to DBP in the blood before uptake by the liver.[113] Enterohepatic circulation of vitamin D and its metabolites exists, but is probably of little importance quantitatively with respect to vitamin D nutritional status.[106]

Vitamin D is more properly considered a steroid hormone than a vitamin in the classic sense; D$_3$ itself may be regarded as a prohormone or precursor.

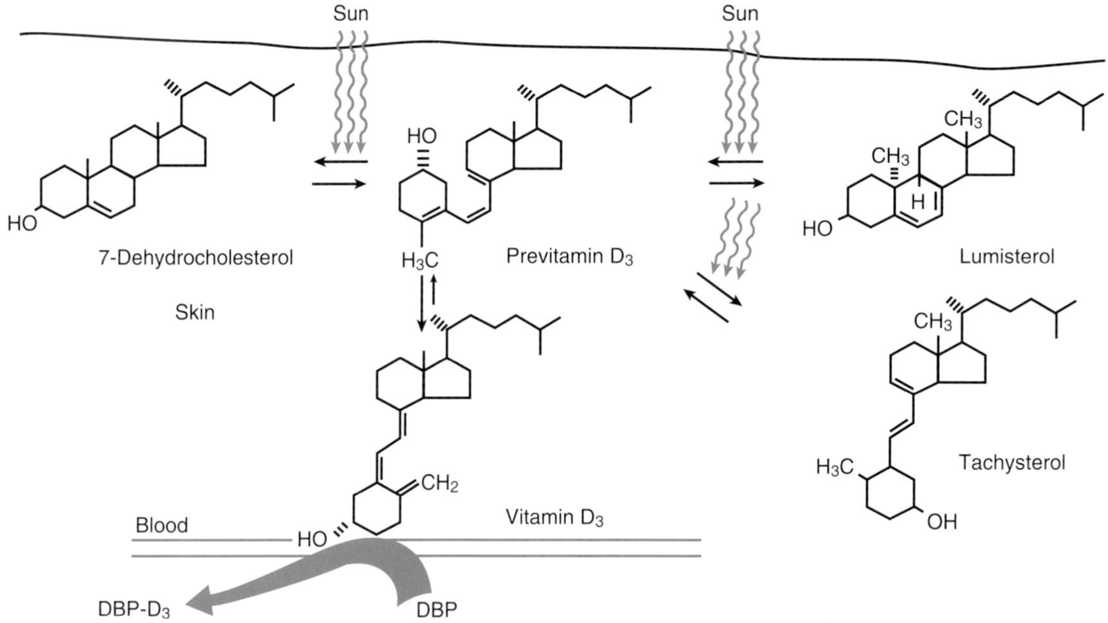

Figure 2: Formation of vitamin D₃ in skin. 7-Dehydrocholesterol is converted to pre-vitamin D₃ following ultraviolet radiation. Pre-vitamin D₃ undergoes thermal isomerization to vitamin D₃ which is carried in the blood bound to vitamin D binding protein. During continual exposure to the sun, pre-vitamin D₃ also photoisomerizes to lumisterol and tachysterol, which are biologically inert photoproducts; that is, they do not stimulate intestinal calcium absorption. As soon as pre-vitamin D₃ stores are depleted (because of thermal isomerization to vitamin D₃), exposure of lumisterol and tachysterol to ultraviolet radiation will promote the photoisomerizaiton of these isomers to pre-vitamin D₃. (From Reference 103, with permission)

Vitamin D is catalyzed to 25 OHD in the liver and is further metabolized to $1,25(OH)_2D$. Quantitatively, 25 OHD is the major metabolite of vitamin D, and its serum concentration is generally regarded as an indicator of vitamin D status whereas $1,25(OH)_2D$, the hormonal form of vitamin D, is biologically the most active metabolite of vitamin D and plays a major role in mineral, especially Ca, metabolism. Its production and circulating concentrations are raised by parathyroid hormone (PTH) and by deficiencies in Ca and P; and are lowered by Ca and P sufficiency and $1,25(OH)_2D$ itself. The primary role of $1,25(OH)_2D$ is to stimulate intestinal absorption of Ca and P,[44, 45, 114] and it also appears to promote renal reabsorption of Ca and P.[102] Its action on the bone involves both bone resorption and bone formation, and is important in bone remodeling.[114-117] For growing children with sufficient Ca and P, its net effect on bone is to increase

formation and mineralization. PTH is an important trophic stimulator of the renal synthesis of $1,25(OH)_2D$. Conversely, $1,25(OH)_2D$ inhibits the synthesis of PTH directly through an interaction with the preproparathyroid hormone gene[118, 119] or secondarily, through an increase in circulating ionized Ca.[120]

The molecular effects of $1,25(OH)_2D$ are mediated by vitamin D receptors [VDR].[46, 47, 118, 119] The VDRs are ligand-inducible intracellular transcription factors. Its gene is localized to the long arm of chromosome 12[122] and the VDR cDNA has been cloned.[123] Free receptors occur in the cytoplasm with occupied receptors located in the nuclei. The $1,25(OH)_2D$-VDR complex regulates the expression of vitamin D-sensitive genes by interaction with specific DNA fragments (vitamin D responsive elements, VDRE)[124] to initiate the $1,25(OH)_2D$ action on transcription and translation of specific genes. Specific $1,25(OH)_2D$ receptors

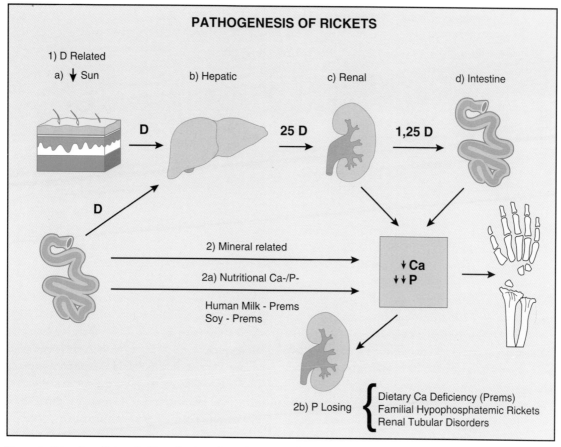

PATHOGENESIS OF RICKETS

1) D Related

a) ↓ Sun   b) Hepatic   c) Renal   d) Intestine

D   25 D   1,25 D

D

2) Mineral related

2a) Nutritional Ca-/P-

Human Milk - Prems
Soy - Prems

↓Ca
↓↓P

2b) P Losing { Dietary Ca Deficiency (Prems)
Familial Hypophosphatemic Rickets
Renal Tubular Disorders

Figure 3: Disorders of vitamin D and mineral metabolism in the pathogenesis of rickets. Endogenously produced vitamin D_3 from the skin and dietary intake of vitamins D_2 and D_3, are converted by 25-hydroxylation in the liver to 25 hydroxyvitamin D (25 OHD). 25 OHD is the major vitamin D metabolite and is often used as an indicator of vitamin D status. It is further converted to either 24,25-dihydroxyvitamin D or 1,25-dihydroxyvitamin D ($1,25(OH)_2D$). The renal conversion of 25 OHD to $1,25 (OH)_2 D$ is stimulated by calcium lack, phosphate lack and parathyroid hormone (PTH). $1,25 (OH)_2 D$ results in stimulation of intestinal calcium and phosphate absorption and mobilization of calcium from bone. Calcium and phosphorus intake, absorption and loss also are critical to bone health.

are present in intestinal mucosa and many other tissues and organs.[118, 119] Specific binding for $1,25 (OH)_2D$ is present in the small intestine of human fetus as early as 13 weeks gestation and in the large intestine by 19 weeks gestation,[125] and the list of potential target organs and functional effects of $1,25(OH)_2D$ are many and varied. However, there are two basic clinical functions that define the major classic action of vitamin D. The first is that vitamin D is required to prevent rickets in children and osteomalacia in adults. The second is the prevention of hypocalcemic tetany (Figure 3).

Rickets is indeed a price paid by man for his abandonment of a life out of doors and a natural diet for a life in houses and a diet of denatured food stuffs; it is a sign of the operation of the immutable law of nature that nothing out of accord with her shall flourish. Edwards A. Park, 1923

Bone mineralization of the skeleton is thought to be the result of $1,25(OH)_2D$ in increasing the intestinal absorption of Ca, and independently, of P absorption;[44, 45, 114-117] these two actions thereby elevate circulating Ca and P concentrations and facilitate bone mineralization. In addition, $1,25(OH)_2D$ appears to

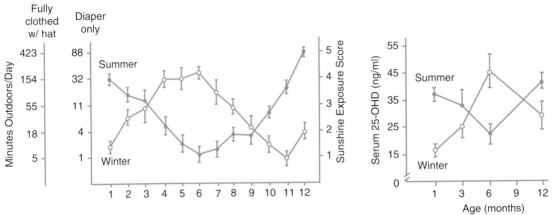

Figure 4: Significant changes in sunshine exposure occur throughout the year and correlate with changes in serum 25-hydroxyvitamin D concentrations. These changes are significantly different for infants born during winter months (o) when compared with infants born during summer months (l). (From reference 29, with permission.)

have direct effects on osteoblasts with resulting synthesis of bone matrix and increased bone mineralization; $1,25(OH)_2D$ also activates osteoclasts with resultant bone resorption and release of bone minerals.[114-117] Its actions are modulated by PTH and other hormones: glucocorticoid, thyroid hormone, insulin,[118, 119, 126-128] and nutrients such as vitamin A.[129] Thus, it appears that $1,25 (OH)_2D$ can have both anabolic and antianabolic effects, with the former predominating in well nourished growing children.

Sources of Vitamin D for Infants

In infants, vitamin D may be derived from three sources: transplacental, endogenous synthesis and exogenous intake.

Normally there is very little vitamin D that crosses the placenta to the fetus, and the small amounts of vitamin D in the cord sera cannot be measured reliably.[130] An anecdotal report of a pregnant woman with post-surgical hypoparathyroidism given large amounts of vitamin D_2 (100,000 IU/day) resulted in a cord blood vitamin D_2 at about 8%, and 25 OHD_2 at about 50% of maternal values of 551 ng/ml and 545 ng/ml, respectively.[70]

The major vitamin D metabolite to cross the placenta from mother to fetus appears to be 25 OHD. A direct relationship between maternal and cord blood 25 OHD has been demonstrated[17, 130-134] and most reports show cord blood values about 20% to 30% below the maternal value. Cord blood concentrations of 25 OHD also

may be affected by race (higher in whites compared with blacks)[130] and season (higher in summer)[131, 132] and increased by maternal vitamin D supplementation.[132-134]

It is unknown to what extent the fetus is able to store vitamin D or its metabolites for use after birth. Vitamin D is stored in fat in the rat[135] and may be in muscle and other tissues in the adult human.[136] In any case, vitamin D stores of most infants born to mothers with normal vitamin D status are depleted by about eight weeks after birth.[17]

Infants are capable of vitamin D synthesis upon exposure to ultraviolet (UV) light. This is reflected in the marked seasonal variation in serum 25 OHD concentrations observed in infants[27, 29] and in children.[26, 28] There is a direct relationship between sunlight exposure as quantitated by UV dosimeter, or a sunshine diary (coupled with a clothing diary to estimate surface area exposed to sunlight), and measured serum 25 OHD concentrations in exclusively breast-fed infants.[137] High serum 25 OHD concentrations found in summer-born infants decreases to about half this value in winter; with the opposite pattern in winter- born infants, reflecting the pattern of sunshine exposure[29] (Figure 4). It has been estimated that half an hour to two hours of sunshine exposure per week in fully clothed (head and hands exposed) breast-fed white infants in Cincinnati (latitude 39° North) will maintain a serum 25 OHD concentration >11 ng/ml.[29, 137] This estimate has been confirmed in a study in Beijing, China (latitude 40° North), where infants were randomly assigned to experimental sunshine (taken outside two hours per day) compared with conventional sunshine exposure.[138] Thus, a brief period of sunshine exposure in temperate climate appears sufficient to maintain adequate vitamin D status for a large proportion of the population. However, sunshine exposure varies with geographic location, season and cultural habits, and exclusively breast-fed infants, particularly those older than six months, with inadequate sunshine exposure are at risk for vitamin D deficiency.[27, 139, 140]

Other sources of vitamin D for infants are from exogenous dietary intake, or from direct supplementation. Human milk and naturally occurring whole cow milk have low vitamin D content.[141] The average total vitamin D activity in human milk is about 50 IU/L[141-146] and may be < 20 IU/L during winter months[144, 146] particularly in the milk from dark-skinned, lactating mothers.[144] Most of the vitamin D activity in human milk is accounted for by the vitamin D parent compound and 25 OHD.[141, 143, 145] The concentration of $1,25(OH)_2D$ in human milk is negligible.[141, 142] Total vitamin D activity in human milk is affected by race (higher in whites)[144] and season (higher in summer)[146] but not by the duration of lactation[146] or preterm delivery.[147] Milk vitamin D but not 25 OHD content, is correlated with maternal dietary vitamin D intake up to 706 IU/day.[144]

It is not known exactly how vitamin D and 25 OHD gain access to human milk. Vitamin D binding protein (DBP) may play a role, as it is found in human milk at 1% to 3% of concentrations in plasma.[141, 145] Vitamin D and its metabolites bind to DBP with varying affinities, 25 OHD being more tightly bound than vitamin D.[148] One could speculate that the weaker interaction between vitamin D and the plasma carrier as compared to 25 OHD allows vitamin D to be more easily diffusible into human milk. This is supported by the demonstration that 1.5 minimal erythemal doses (MED) of total body UV-B exposure (about 90 seconds of irradiation) of lactating mothers results in a tenfold increase in milk vitamin D_3 concentration with little change in milk 25 OHD concentration.[149]

In addition to UV-B exposure, oral vitamin D supplementation at 1000 to 2000 IU daily for lactating mothers can raise the total vitamin D activity of breast milk[146] although the extent of elevation in milk vitamin D activity varies widely. Anecdotal report of a mother taking 100,000 IU of vitamin D_2 per day, show a vitamin D_2 concentration in her milk samples at 25% to 30% of her serum values and milk 25 OHD_2 concentrations were <2% of her serum concentrations. The total vitamin D concentration of her milk was 7,000 IU/L, which contained almost exclusively vitamin D_2 and 25 OHD_2.[70]

Direct supplementation of vitamin D (as vitamin D_2 or D_3), either alone or as part of multivitamin preparation, is freely available for infant use.[150] All commercial standard infant formulas in the U.S. are fortified with 400 IU of vitamin D_3/L.

Calcium, Magnesium and Phosphorus Requirements
Enteral Requirement

The requirements for Ca, Mg and P in an infant vary with growth rate, and primarily concern the need to meet the demands for bone mineralization and maintain serum concentrations of these minerals within a defined range. During early infancy, the daily intake for infants born at term may be based on those fed primarily on human milk. The recommended daily requirement for Ca is about 45-60 mg/kg, with a total daily intake of about 400 mg by six months, 600 mg by one year of age, and 800 mg between one to two years; for Mg is 6-8 mg/kg, with a total daily intake of about 40 mg by six months, 60 mg by one year and 80 mg between one to two years; and for P is 25-40 mg/kg with a total daily intake of about 300 mg by six months, 500 mg by 1 year, and 800 mg between one to two years.[151-153]

These amounts of minerals are likely to be met by consumption of about 150-250 ml of human milk/kg/day during early infancy. Currently available infant formulas contain a greater quantity of minerals to compensate for the lower mineral absorption compared to human milk. Cow-milk based infant formula with intact or partially hydrolyzed protein have an average Ca content of 420 to 490 mg/L (63-73 mg/100 kcal), Mg content of 41 to 53 mg/L (6-7.8 mg/100 kcal), and P content of 190-380 mg/L (28-56 mg/100 kcal). Cow-milk based infant

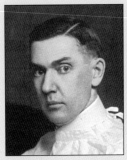

Elmer V. McCollum PhD
(1879-1967) obtained his graduate degree under Johnson, a pupil of Liebig, at Yale in 1906. He was a postdoctoral fellow under Mendel. His first position was at the University of Wisconsin where he demonstrated that rats did not thrive on purified diets and discovered that " fat-soluble A" and "water-soluble B" factors were required to restore growth. In 1917 he moved to Hopkins where he collaborated with one of Howland's faculty, Edwards Park, in the discovery of vitamin D. McCollum objected to the use of the word vitamin because the suffix was chemically inaccurate. J. Nutr. 100,1-10, 1970 (Photo courtesy of CNRC)

formula with extensively hydrolyzed protein, and soy protein-based infant formulas generally contain greater amounts of mineral with Ca content of 600 to 710 mg/L (90-105 mg/100 kcal), Mg content of 51 to 134 mg/L (7.5-20 mg/100 kcal), and P content of 370 to 510 mg/L (55-75 mg/100 kcal) to compensate for the potential of further lowering of calcium absorption for example, secondary to the phytate content of soy formulas. (See Appendix)

There is no clear evidence that the mineral needs of six to 12 month old infants cannot be met entirely by breast-feeding, although vitamin D deficiency may become an issue under certain circumstances (see vitamin D deficiency section). There are no balance or other studies to specifically evaluate the amount or the need for additional Ca, Mg, or P containing solids in this age group. However, it seems prudent to introduce a variety of supplemental foods as additional sources of minerals when the volume of milk intake begins to decrease beyond six to nine months of age.

For infants beyond one year, dairy products including vitamin D-fortified whole cow milk remain excellent sources of minerals and vitamins. Availability of cow milk- or soy-based "toddler" milk formula provide theoretically advantages related to iron and multiple vitamin fortification, altered fatty acid composition and lower renal solute load compared to whole cow milk.[154] However, the benefits of a "toddler" milk formula remains to be proven. Until more data become available, the most

prudent approach is to encourage a balanced diet in the second year of age that includes human milk or natural dairy products as major source of minerals.

Numerous balance studies indicate that, in spite of reported differences in the percent absorption of Ca between human milk and milk formulas, the absolute amount of Ca, Mg and P retained by the body from milk-based or soy-based formula are similar to or greater than those reported for human milk-fed infants.[11, 58, 74, 75, 77, 82]

Bone mineral content (BMC) from single photon absorptiometry measurement of infants receiving cow milk formulas and the newer formulation of soy formula appears to be comparable to[79-81, 155] or greater than[25] that of human milk-fed infants.

Serum mineral concentrations are generally comparable among groups with various types of milk feedings,[79, 81] although urine excretion of Ca and P tends to reflect the higher intake of these minerals in infant formulas compared to human milk. Hormonal indicators of mineral homeostasis, specifically serum $1,25(OH)_2D$ concentrations, appear to be higher in formula-fed infants[79, 81] and particularly those fed soy formula,[81] when compared with human milk-fed infants. This pattern appears to be a compensatory change to increase the absorption of Ca and possibly other minerals, presumably secondary to differences in bioavailability of minerals in infant formulas as compared to human milk. Serum PTH concentrations may be higher in cow milk formula-fed infants, associated with lower serum ionized Ca and higher serum P concentrations in the first few weeks after birth.[34] Occasionally, cow milk-fed infants may still suffer from hypocalcemic tetany.[30]

There are extremely limited data to determine the mineral requirement of infants over one year of age. One study of clinically healthy infants and young children, at the mean ages of 21 to 33 months with daily Ca and P intake in the range of 600 to 1200 mg, reports distal radius BMC;[156] this is comparable to other reports of distal radius BMC from healthy subjects of the same age range but with no dietary intake information.[14, 15] The estimated average increase in BMC at distal radius between birth and one year is about 80%, and between one and two years is about 27%.[12, 13, 15] The serum biochemical and vitamin D metabolite concentrations in the former study are also comparable to the values obtained in other healthy infants.[21]

There are wide ranges in intake of minerals in infants and young children. The Third US National Health Nutrition Examination Survey (NHANES), performed between 1988 and 1991, showed the median daily intake at ages two to 11 months for Ca was 665 mg; for Mg was 106 mg; and for P was 541 mg. The median intakes for these respective minerals between one and two years were 800 mg, 174 mg and 900 mg, respectively, with a very wide range of intakes noted at all ages.[157] Based on this population survey, it appears that the majority of the infants up to two years in the U.S. would achieve an intake of Ca, Mg and P near or above the current recommended dietary allowance.[151-153] However, the minimum mineral intake necessary for normal growth and bone mineralization is not known.

Parenteral Requirement

Extensive clinical and research data have demonstrated that parenteral mineral needs for term infants can be easily met by currently available commercial preparations.[58, 101] Clinically stable, large preterm and term infants requiring parenteral nutrition (PN) can maintain normal biochemistry and hormonal indices of mineral homeostasis, as indicated by normal serum Ca, Mg and P, and normal and stable tubular reabsorption of P and serum $1,25(OH)_2D$ concentrations, while receiving PN solution with 600 mg Ca and 470 mg P/L.[158] As the rate of growth and bone mineralization is slower in older infants and young children[12, 13, 15, 16] compared with early infancy, a lower Ca content may be more suited for infants between one and two years. P and Mg contents in PN solutions probably need not be adjusted down at this age because of the increased need for soft tissue growth at this stage. The parenteral requirement for Mg in infancy has been estimated to be 10-25 mg/day.[159] In one report,[160] PN solutions containing 24 mg of Mg/L resulted in hypomagnesemia in 11 of 42 infants. Serum Mg concentrations were normal in infants studied after the Mg content of the solution was increased to 48 to 72 mg/L; the Mg delivered was 7.2 to 10.8 mg/kg/day. In another report,[158] PN solutions with 96 mg of Mg/L delivering an average of 12 mg of Mg/kg/day resulted in transient episodes of hypermagnesemia in five of 18 infants studied. In neither of the reports was Mg lost from gastrointestinal fluid losses replaced separately. The exact requirement for Mg given intravenously is difficult to define, since it is not usual practice for the clinician to replace Mg losses from the gastrointestinal fluid, which may contain varying amounts of Mg from five to 170 mg/L; in addition, urinary Mg losses may be influenced by other nutrients delivered in PN (see section on urinary excretion). However, it would appear that a PN solution with a Mg content of 48 to 60 mg/L delivering approximately 4.8 to 7.8 mg/kg/day would be sufficient for most infants.

Other factors may affect the parenteral requirement for minerals. For example, any factor that predisposes to increased urine mineral loss (see above) can decrease mineral retention. Furthermore, infants requiring PN frequently have abnormal gastrointestinal fluid losses secondary to intestinal motility disorders or fistulas which could be a significant source of loss for many electrolytes, minerals and trace metals. Substantial disturbances of Mg and zinc status have been reported if fistula losses are not specifically replaced[91, 160, 161] and it is possible that acid base and electrolyte disturbances also can occur under these circumstance.[162] It is therefore imperative that specific nutrient replacement be undertaken whenever a large amount of gastrointestinal fluid loss is present, ideally based on direct measurement of the nutrient content of gastrointestinal fluid losses.

Calcium:Phosphorus Ratio

The Ca:P ratio varies widely in foods, from a high of 2.8:1 (gm:gm) in green vegetables to a low of 0.06:1 in meat. The approximate ratio by weight for human milk is 2:1, for cow milk is 1.2:1, for commercial infant formula is 1.3-1.5:1, and for commercial preterm infant formula is 2:1.[152, 163] The high P content of cow milk ("evaporated") formula with its lower Ca:P ratio is one factor in the pathogenesis of "late" neonatal tetany, a situation not encountered in the human milk-fed infant.[24, 164]

It is likely there are higher numbers of asymptomatic hypocalcemic infants related to cow milk formula feeding. Even though cow milk formula has

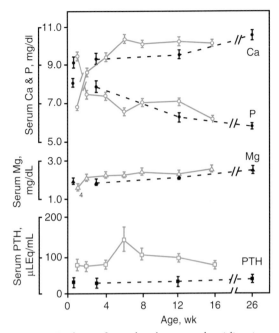

Figure 5: Evidence of secondary hyperparathyroidism in infants after hypocalcemic tetany. Sequential changes in serum Ca, P, Mg and parathyroid hormone (PTH) concentrations in tetanic infants (open symbols) versus 18 control infants (closed symbols) fed human milk. All five infants were studied for the duration of the study but samples were not available from all time points. Serum Ca and Mg concentrations were initially corrected in tetanic infants but subsequently became higher relative to control infants. Serum phosphate concentration was initially high in tetanic infants vs. control infants but subsequently declined, with no significant difference between the two groups. Serum PTH concentrations were consistently high in tetanic infants vs control infants. Values depicted as mean ±SEM. (From reference 30, with permission)

been "humanized", the P load of such milks (Ca:P ratio 1.3:1 by weight), though lower than that of cow milk (Ca:P ratio 1.2:1), is still higher than that of human milk. Hypocalcemic tetany and convulsions in infants fed these cow milk formulas is associated with hyperphosphatemia, and presumably compensatory elevation of serum parathyroid hormone concentrations.[30, 34] (Figure 5)

The Archives of Pediatrics was the first American journal entirely devoted to pediatrics. In the first issue published in 1884, practical hints were given on convulsions

in children. The young physician was urged to evoke order from chaos when he made a house call to see a convulsing child. The secret was to keep everyone busy in preparing a warm bath, moving the patient to a larger bedroom, removing his clothing, wrapping him in a flannel blanket, and looking for mustard to put in the hot bathwater. By the time all these had been done the convulsion would probably have abated. (Cone TE Jr. History of American Pediatrics, Little, Brown & Co., Boston, 1979;127). One assumes that if the convulsions were due to cow milk ingestion, the convulsions would have been generally self-resolving and the management "appropriate".*

In general, infants are remarkably tolerant of a wide range of Ca:P ratios in their diet. A number of factors may influence the development of symptoms in infants receiving varying dietary intakes of Ca and P. First, the absolute quantity of Ca and P delivered in the diet: even if a grossly "imbalanced" Ca:P ratio occurs in a single food item (e.g., green leafy vegetable or meat), as long as it is ingested in limited quantities, there will be little impact on Ca and P homeostasis. Second, intestinal absorption and maturity of the renal excretory system: the more mature infant theoretically will have greater capacity to excrete excess minerals and thus minimize the disturbance to the body's homeostasis. Human milk with its low P content and a Ca:P ratio of approximately 2:1 by weight appears most appropriate for Ca and P homeostasis, especially for the term infant.

In theory, the Ca:P ratio and the absolute quantity of each mineral in the diet should allow for normal bone mineralization and soft tissue growth. *In utero* bone Ca and P accretion occur in the ratio of 2:1 by weight (1.7:1 molar ratio). The greater soft tissue accretion of Mg and P results in a whole body Ca:P ratio of about 1.7:1 by weight (1.3:1 molar ratio). The optimum dietary Ca:P ratio thus depends on the absolute amount of Ca and P in the nutrient. It relies as well on the possibility for interaction of Ca and P to form insoluble and therefore non-absorbable compounds, for example, in a cross over study design of infants fed formulas with a fat blend of soy (60%) and coconut (40%) oils to a fat blend of soy (47%) and palm olein (57%), there was an increase in fecal fat excretion particularly in palmitic acid, and the average absorption of fat and Ca was about 4.6% and 9.4% lower, respectively, when the infants were fed the latter formula.[165] The optimal Ca:P ratio also depends on other factors affecting intestinal absorption and the renal regulation of minerals, as described above. For younger infants, dietary intake from various milk sources probably should have a Ca:P ratio resembling human milk at about 2:1. For older infants who might receive whole cow milk and a mixed diet with ubiquitous phosphate content, the dietary Ca:P ratio presently in the U.S. is close to 1:1 by weight, as reported by the NHANES III survey of nutrient intake for children in this age range.[157]

For infants requiring parenteral nutrition, widely varying Ca:P ratios of the infusate from 4:1–1:8 have been reported.[166, 167] However, in addition to the factors described above, Ca and P needs and ratios will be affected by factors that influence urinary Ca and P excretion, and by intercompartmental shifts of P that may occur with injudicious use of intravenous nutrients. For example, excess glucose infusion, particularly after a period of "starvation," can result in severe hypophosphatemia because of a rapid shift (from fat) to glucose as the predominant fuel and the high demand for phosphate ion in the production of phosphorylated intermediates of glycolysis, and the intracellular "trapping" of phosphate.[35, 168, 169]

> *Bone mineral capital is at least a consequence of the greater calcium and phosphate dietary cashflow."*
>
> Manuel Moya, MD
> Alicante, Spain

Thus, P requirement of infants receiving PN is likely to be somewhat higher than enterally-fed in-fants. PN solutions with a Ca:P ratio of 1.3:1 by weight (1:1 molar ratio) appear to maintain biochemical and hormonal measurements indicative of normal mineral homeostasis in both term[158] and preterm[170] infants. It is theoretically possible that, in infants undergoing rapid "catch up" growth, in particular small preterm infants, the Ca:P ratio probably could be lowered further. However, there is probably no indication for a Ca:P ratio of <1:1 by weight, because of the potential risk for hyperphosphatemia and hypocalcemia.[58, 101, 158]

Vitamin D Requirement
Enteral Requirement

The requirement for vitamin D is based on preventing vitamin D deficiency rickets, and maintaining mineral homeostasis, specifically the prevention of hypocal-cemia. Adequacy of vitamin D status is generally considered to be associated with a serum 25 OHD concentration >10 ng/ml.

Exclusively human milk-fed infants without vitamin D supplementation are at risk for vitamin D deficiency, if there is insufficient sunshine exposure, regardless of geographic region or race.[137-140, 171-174] Maternal supplementation of 1,000 IU vitamin D per day during lactation is unable to prevent a decrease in serum 25 OHD concentrations to very low levels in breast-fed offspring.[139, 140] However, direct daily supplementation of 400 IU vitamin D[25, 139, 140] as well as 1,000 IU vitamin D per day[140] to the breast-fed infant appears to maintain adequate serum 25 OHD concentrations.

In a double-blind randomized study conducted in Madison, Wisconsin (latitude 43° North) of infants mostly born in winter, at the end of six months of human milk feeding, the total serum 25 OHD concentrations were significantly higher in the vitamin D supplemented (400 IU vitamin D2/day) versus unsupplemented infants (mean values 37 vs 24 ng/ml), but serum 25 OHD$_3$ concentrations were significantly higher in the unsupplemented group (mean values 23 vs 12 ng/ml).[25] It appears that endogenous synthesis of vitamin D$_3$ is able to maintain relatively normal vitamin D status even in human milk-fed infants unsupplemented with vitamin D. In the same study, a separate group of infants fed cow milk-based formula fortified with vitamin D$_3$ had serum 25 OHD$_3$ levels similar to or higher than the levels produced endogenously by the human milk-fed infants (Figure 6). It appears that the vitamin D supplement as D$_2$ or D$_3$, is absorbed and metabolized to 25 OHD, and a daily supplementation of 400 IU of vitamin D can prevent the occurrence of vitamin D deficiency in human milk-fed infants. Body weight, body length, serum Ca, P, PTH and 1,25(OH)$_2$D and distal radial BMC were not significantly different between human milk-fed infants with and without vitamin D supplementation.

In another report,[155] BMC of distal radius also was not significantly different between vitamin D (400 IU/day) supplemented and non supplemented human

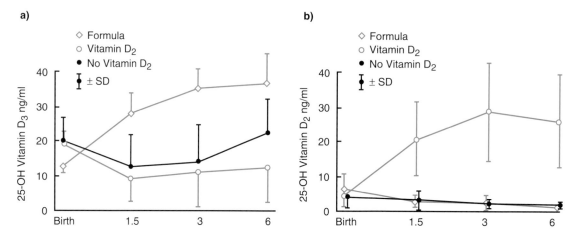

Figure 6: Serum concentrations of 25-hydroxyvitamin D_3 and 25-hydroxyvitamin D_2 from birth to six months in infants fed cow milk-based formula, human milk with and without supplementation of 400 IU of vitamin D_2 per day. Endogenous synthesis of vitamin D_3 is able to maintain relatively normal vitamin D status even in human milk-fed infants without vitamin D supplementation (a). However, direct supplementation of vitamin D to breast-fed infants (b) or vitamin D fortification of infant formulas (a) assures the maintenance of normal vitamin D status in infants. (From reference 25, with permission)

milk fed infants, in spite of a significantly lower (but within the normal range) of serum 25 OHD values in the latter group.

In infants fed human milk or other milks unfortified with vitamin D, who were randomized to receive 100, 200 or 400 IU vitamin D supplementation, serum 25 OHD concentrations were directly related to the amount of vitamin D supplementation.[174] This study was performed in infants living at latitude 40°-47° North, and 95% of the infants who received vitamin D supplementation of 400 IU/day had serum 25 OHD concentrations within the normal range. None of the infants in the three vitamin D-supplemented ranges had clinical or radiographic changes of rickets in spite of the low serum 25 OHD concentrations in some infants, and all had normal serum Ca, P and alkaline phosphatase values.

There is no documented report of vitamin D deficiency in infants fed regular vitamin D fortified commercial infant formula in the U.S., even though the volume of formula consumed usually results in a daily vitamin D intake of <400 IU. There is no indication for additional vitamin D supplementation for infants receiving vitamin D-fortified standard commercial

infant formulas, and there is no data to indicate that any modification to this approach is needed for infants from different races or geographic regions.

BMC of distal radius in infants fed standard formula is reported to be comparable[79-81] or higher than human milk-fed infants.[25] However, transient hyperphosphatemia and hypocalcemia may be associated with the use of standard infant formula.[30, 34] This is presumably related to the relatively greater P load from infant formula, lower renal excretory capacity for P, and relatively immature parathyroid gland response, rather than being secondary to vitamin D deficiency.

Adequate and consistent sunshine exposure is required for normal vitamin D production,[175] and rickets is an end-stage disease occurring after months of sustained vitamin D deficiency. It seems reasonable to maintain the current recommendation of daily vitamin D intake of 300 IU for infants <six months and 400 IU at >six months of age.[176] For human milk-fed infants, daily supplementation of 200-300 IU vitamin D is recommended[176] to provide a margin of safety in view of the low vitamin D content of human milk and the vagaries of sunshine exposure. The current practice of fortification of standard infant formulas with 400 IU vitamin D/L generally meets these recommendations and there is no evidence that additional vitamin D supplementation is needed. A daily intake of about 400 IU of vitamin D probably should be continued throughout childhood since vitamin D deficient rickets in infants and young children has been reported even in southern U.S. with a subtropical climate.[172, 173]

Parenteral Requirement

The predominant action of vitamin D metabolites is to increase Ca and P absorption from the gut. Thus, when Ca and P are supplied intravenously in PN (i.e., bypassing the intestine), the intravenous requirement for vitamin D might be minimal. Furthermore, it has been suggested that occasionally vitamin D in the nutrient infusate may cause hypercalcemia, hypercalciuria and metabolic bone disease in adults on long-term PN.[177] In these instances, the discontinuation of vitamin D in PN[177] or the discontinuation of PN[178] apparently resulted in resolution of hypercalcemia, decreased urinary Ca loss, and symptomatic improvement in the patients.

Systematic study of vitamin D and mineral homeostasis in infants receiving PN has demonstrated an intravenous vitamin D intake as low as 30 IU/kg to be adequate to maintain normal vitamin D status.[18] A higher dose of 160 IU of vitamin D/kg/day with a maximum of 400 IU/day has not been associated with complications, and maintains serum 25 OHD concentrations within the reference range for term infants fed orally;[179] this intake is currently recommended for infants requiring PN.[180] In young children ages four to 13 years requiring long-term PN, serum 25 OHD concentrations are halved within 12 months after discontinuation of vitamin D in the nutrient infusate. After 12 months of vitamin D free nutrient infusate, four of the six subjects in this study had serum 25 OHD concentrations < 11 ng/ml, i.e., in the vitamin D deficient range. Six of the seven subjects had persistent radiographic bone demineralization and three had delayed bone age, although the discontinuation of vitamin D intake apparently had no significant impact on these changes.[19]

Based on current evidence, the vitamin D requirement is minimal for patients requiring total PN and does not appear to be greater than the recommended dose for children receiving a normal diet, i.e., 400 IU/day.[180] However it is also possible that vitamin D deficiency as indicated by a very low or undetectable serum 25 OHD can occur in children[19] and adults[177] receiving vitamin D free PN solutions. It is well known that chronic vitamin D deficiency can result in bone disease and it would seem prudent to maintain normal vitamin D status in patients receiving PN. In addition, the maintenance of normal vitamin D status may be advantageous even for patients receiving PN, since maintenance of normal vitamin D status will theoretically maximize the absorption and retention of any enteral Ca and P intakes tolerated by these patients or minerals secreted into the intestinal tract. Thus, until further supportive evidence becomes available, it is premature to recommend complete discontinuation of vitamin D supplementation for patients requiring PN. The parenteral dose of vitamin D in the commonly used preparations for PN is available only as part of standard multivitamin preparations, and any adjustment in this dose would also affect the concomitant delivery of other vitamins.

Deficiency
Calcium, Magnesium and Phosphorus

In 1803 Johnson stated, "Bonhomme found that chickens fed lime phosphate had harder bones. This had also been fed profitably to children with rickets and was claimed as a means of improving dentition and the healing of fractures. In mothers at the time of delivery of infants, the softness of bones was recognized and the failure of fractures to heal was appreciated." (Verzar F (ed). Clive M. McCay. Notes on the History of Nutrition Research. Berne, Hans Huber Publishers, 1973; page 173.)

Specific nutritional "deficiency" of Ca alone is rarely diagnosed. It may in part contribute to the cause of early neonatal hypocalcemia and to bone demineralization and rickets of small preterm infants.[35, 181] Ca deficiency is a potential hazard for older infants and young children who are weaned from the breast and are receiving a vegetarian or fad diet with little or no intake of dairy products. The dietary goal for Ca intake is difficult to achieve without the inclusion of dairy foods, fortified foods or supplements.[182] Both Ca and vitamin D deficiency are independent factors contributing to the development of rickets in infants receiving macrobiotic diets.[183] Although children receiving a predominantly vegetarian diet are generally in good health, they may be at risk for a number of other nutritional deficiencies including energy, protein, iron, vitamin B12, riboflavin and possibly also long chain n3 fatty acid because the abundant plant derived linoleic acid (18:2n-6) may inhibit the syn-thesis of docosahexanoic acid (DHA) from linolenic acid (18:3n-3).[184, 185]

Unreplaced Mg losses from chronic gastrointestinal or biliary fistula and injudicious use of fluid and electrolyte therapy probably are the major situations in which infants are predisposed to nutritional Mg deficiency. Congenital selective intestinal Mg malabsorption and congenital Mg-losing nephropathies are rare conditions that predispose the infant to Mg deficiency.[181]

Extreme hypophosphatemia (serum P <2 mg/dl) may occur in infants receiving intravenous fluid or parenteral nutrition, usually associated with inadequate or no P administration, and is aggravated by injudicious use of fluid and electrolyte therapy which increases urinary P loss and intercompartmental shifts of P. Rapid increase in nutrient delivery after a prolonged period of inadequate nutrition is responsible for a relative deficiency in P, and resultant hypophosphatemia, as a part of the "refeeding" syndrome.[168, 169] Phosphorus deficiency is often only one facet of the typical "hypophosphatemic syndrome",[32] since the condition usually occurs in the sick infant with complex disorders and multiple nutrient deficiencies. Rickets in association with chronic P deficiency, as occurs with inherited hypophosphatemic rickets, is thought to contribute to decreased stature.[186]

Vitamin D

The original description of rickets, as well as the first hint that it was a disease of urban dwellers, is due to Soranus of Ephesus (about A.D. 100), who ascribed the crooked legs of Roman toddlers both to maternal neglect and to the hardness of the street pavement which bent their soft bones.[186] It was Claudius Galenus (A.D. 132-210), in his De morborumcausis, who noticed thoracic deformities as well as genu varus or valgus in overfed children.

The first description of rickets in the modern age is the medical thesis, written in 1645, by Daniel Whistler.[188] The classical treatise De Rachitide of Francis Glisson appeared in 1650.[189] Glisson coined the word "rachitis" for rickets.

Rickets was common in industrialized cities in the nineteenth century and its incidence reported to be as high as 90% in British infants and children up to four to five years of age.[190] The Civil War in the U.S. also brought its rachitic toll. Already in 1870, as a consequence of the flight of blacks to cities of the North, in Philadelphia 25% of all black children of less than five years of age had rickets.[191] As early as 1884, it was noted that there was a cyclical pattern to the incidence of rickets and tetany with increases during the winter months and decreases during summer and autumn.[192] In 1885, Pommer established the pathology of rickets through histological studies.[193]

Theobald A. Palm, an English medical missionary in Japan, studied the geographic distribution of rickets in 1890 and reported that "rickets came about as a result of lack of sunlight" and that its incidence was inversely related to the amount of sunshine at a given latitude. He even stated that "the important factor in the sunshine was the chemical activity of the sun's rays rather than its heat" and proposed a systematic use of sun baths as a preventive and therapeutic measure in rickets. Palm was astute enough also to point out that rickets was related to air pollution.[3]

In the early 1900s several hypotheses regarding the etiology of rickets were developed. Siegert had a theory of inheritance[194, 195] which was supported by Sambon, who noted that pigmented skin increased the susceptibility to rickets and that a predisposition in that sense may be inherited.[196] In the late 1800s and early 1900s, rickets also was thought to be a result of infectious disease. Koch felt he was able to produce rickets by means of inoculation with bacteria[197] and Edlefsen thought that the enlarged spleen in rickets was significant and regarded fever as an early manifestation of this infectious disease.[198] The occurrence of rickets in certain houses further suggested that it was related to an infectious agent.[197]

In 1909, Schmorl demonstrated seasonal variations in rickets in pathological studies and found the highest inci-

dence of early manifestations of the disease to be between November and May.[199] In 1914, Funk published the following: "It is very probable that rickets occurs only when certain substances in the diet essential for normal metabolism are lacking or supplied in insufficient amount. Substances occur in good breast milk, also in good cod liver oil, but are lacking in sterilized milk and in cereals."[200]

Despite Funk's observation that rickets was a result of a substance missing in the diet, the credit for establishing the relationship between the development of rickets and a deficiency of vitamin D belongs to Mellanby, who in 1918 announced the production of rickets by means of a diet lacking in "an accessory factor."[201] In 1919 the British Medical Research Committee publicly stated that rickets was a deficiency disease due to a lack in the diet of an "antirachitic factor".[202]

Clinical signs of advanced rickets include craniotabes, frontal skull bossing, rachitic rosary (enlarged costochondral junctions), widened ribs, bowed legs, and muscle weakness. Laboratory findings vary during the course of vitamin D deficiency rickets[38-43] (Figure 7). In infants and young children there is overlap of serum 25 OHD concentration between clinically normal subjects and those with vitamin D deficient rickets.[38, 39, 41] However, serum 25-OHD concentrations less than 15 ng/ml are usually observed in cases with severe rickets.[38-43] In the early stage of rickets, serum Ca concentration is low with normal serum P concentration. Increases in PTH, stimulated by the low serum Ca, result in an increase in serum 1,25(OH)$_2$D, a normalization of serum Ca, phosphaturia and a decrease in serum P. It is at this stage that there are typical radiographic rachitic bone features: generalized osteopenia, and widening, cupping and fraying of metaphyses (Figure 8) are present; serum 25-OHD concentrations are decreased but serum 1,25(OH)$_2$D concentrations are usually elevated.[40, 41, 43] Although concentrations of 1,25(OH)$_2$D may be elevated above the normal ranges, they still may be too low to maintain adequate mineral homeostasis if dietary intake of minerals is also inadequate. The muscle hypotonia is probably in part the result of a decrease in intracellular phosphorus pool of skeletal muscle.[203]

It is likely that the 1 α-hydroxylase enzyme in the kidney is highly active in rickets, presumably stimu-

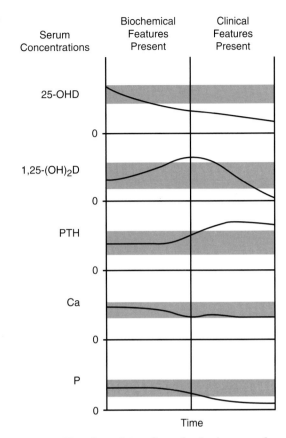

Figure 7: Hypothetical time frame for development of vitamin D deficiency rickets.

lated by increased PTH concentration and Ca and P deficiency. This suggestion is supported by consistent findings of increases in serum 1,25(OH)$_2$D to supranormal concentrations following the initiation of vitamin D therapy, even when vitamin D therapy is only 400 IU/day.[40] Presumably, supply of the substrate 25-OHD to a highly active 1 α-hydroxylase, produces marked elevation of serum 1,25(OH)$_2$D concentrations and there is a continued need for increase in intestinal absorption of Ca and P for continued bone mineralization.

Management of Vitamin D Deficiency

The first report of ultraviolet irradiation in the cure of rickets was made by Kurt Huldschinsky in 1919, a Berlin pediatrician who used a mercury-vapor quartz lamp, which emits ultraviolet irradiation, on four cases of

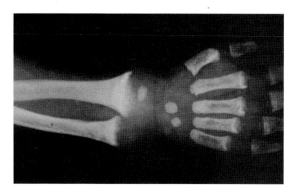

Figure 8: Radiograph of the wrist of a child showing classical signs of vitamin D deficiency rickets. "Fraying" and cupping of the metaphyses of the long bones are present.

advanced rickets, resulting in cures within two months. He even anticipated the current emphasis on vitamin D as a hormone by irradiating one arm of a rachitic child with ultraviolet light. X-rays showed that the Ca salts were deposited not only in the irradiated arm but in the other arm as well.[3]

Vitamin D deficiency rickets is rapidly responsive to various doses (400 to 10,000 IU) of vitamin D per day.[39-41, 43] Serum 25 OHD concentrations return rapidly to normal ranges as early as one week after commencement of treatment[40, 41] and have returned to normal ranges in all subjects by two months after starting treatment[39] after which normal vitamin D supplements should be continued. A single day vitamin D (100,000 IU q 4 hrs) therapy with a total dose of 600,000 IU given orally has been used for the treatment of vitamin D deficient rickets if there was uncertainty of the family's adherence to daily administration of vitamin D to the subject.[42] Hypocalcemia and hypophosphatemia may occur if there is insufficient mineral intake with the high dose vitamin D therapy,[42] and vitamin D toxicity is possible particularly if there is concomitant high Ca intake (see Toxicity section). In view of the possibility of side effects, it is much more preferable to treat rickets with lower doses of vitamin D.

In young children with vitamin D deficiency rickets, it is equally important to be cognizant of the possibility of coexistent deficiency of other nutrients, in particular Ca, iron, and vitamins B_{12} and E, since some of these children are subjected to the faddist diets of their

parents (strict vegan diet or dietary practices excluding dairy products). Sibling involvement also may be found and needs to be treated. Extensive nutritional and social counseling for these families is also needed.

Toxicity
Calcium, Magnesium, Phosphorus

Under normal circumstances, toxicity associated with Ca, Mg and P is usually iatrogenic. Fortunately most of the potential toxicity associated with disturbed serum concentrations and tissue content of these elements is preventable by meticulous attention to details of fluid and electrolyte management, mechanical ventilatory efforts (to minimize acid-base disturbances), and diuretic therapy.

Excessive administration of Ca, Mg or P results in abnormally elevated circulating concentrations of these minerals and their clinical sequelae.[181, 204] The intestinal tract and the physicochemical dietary interactions described earlier are to some extent effective barriers to excessive absorption of orally administrated Ca.

The major source of potential toxicity occurs with parenteral administration of these minerals. Alternate infusion of Ca and P as a means of avoiding Ca-P precipitation in intravenous fluid is an inefficient means of mineral delivery; hyperphosphatemia, and hypocalcemia and phosphaturia during P infusion, and hypercalcemia and hypercalciuria during Ca infusion have been reported with its use.[205] It is therefore essential that serum concentrations of these minerals be measured regularly. Hypermagnesemia is a well-known complication of parenteral nutrition (see earlier comments).

Frequently, Ca, Mg and P toxicity result from therapeutic maneuvers, unrelated directly to the administration of these minerals. For example, enteric fluid restriction in association with high Ca and P supplement apparently can cause intestinal milk curds and intestinal obstruction.[206] Chronic furosemide administration may result in Ca-containing nephrolithiasis,[207] cholelithiasis[208] and bone demineralization in infants.[209] Chronic furosemide administration has a growth-inhibitory effect associated with low bone mineral content in nursing young rat pups.[210] Thiazide diuretics are effective in reducing the calciuric effect of furosemide in adults[211] and some[207] but not all[212]

	Calcium*		Magnesium*		Phosphorus*		Vitamin D‡
	mg	mg/kg	mg	mg/kg	mg	mg/kg	IU
0-6 months	400	45-60†	40	6-8†	300	25-40†	300
7-12 months	600		60		500		400
13-24 months	800		80		800		400

* Infant formulas usually contain about 50-100% higher Ca content to compensate for lower absorption, and higher Mg (about 50 to 100%) and P (about 100 to 350%) content compared to human milk.
† Estimated from human milk fed infants.
‡ Total daily intake as part of diet or as daily supplement.
Conversion: Ca 1 mmol=40 mg, Mg 1mmol=24 mg, P 1 mmol=31 mg.

Table 4: Suggested daily enteral intake for Ca, Mg, P.

infants. Chronic thiazide diuretic use also may be associated with hypokalemia, hypercalcemia and other metabolic disturbances,[213] and its efficacy and safety in the neonate require further study. Toxins, for example, aluminum[214] also may be given to infants incidental to the delivery of Ca, Mg and P.

Vitamin D

Most reports of vitamin D toxicity are iatrogenic in origin or associated with accidental overfortification of food products. Overuse of vitamin D supplementation for infants in Europe, with intakes between 3000 to 4000 IU daily, is believed to be related to high frequencies of "idiopathic" hypercalcemia of infancy during and after World War II. The disease became extremely rare after the dietary intake of vitamin D was reduced to 400 IU daily.[215]

Asymptomatic[216] and symptomatic[217, 218] complications of hypervitaminosis D have been reported from high dose vitamin D (600,000 IU single dose) therapy or accidental overfortification of vitamin D in drinking milk. Hypercalcemia occurred on at least one occasion in 34% of infants who received high dose (600,000 IU) vitamin D prophylaxis;[216] hypercalcemia with failure to thrive, anorexia, vomiting and constipation[212] and possible nephrocalcinosis[218] have been associated with vitamin D intoxication.

In an anecdotal report, a healthy infant at term was delivered to a mother with hereditary resistance to $1,25(OH)_2D$. The mother was treated with pharmacologic doses (17 to 36 µg/day) of $1,25(OH)_2D$ and maintained extraordinarily high serum $1,25(OH)_2D$ concentrations (170 to 500+ pg/ml) throughout pregnancy. The cord serum $1,25(OH)_2D$ (410 pg/ml) was similar to the maternal level (430 pg/ml) at delivery and the postnatal course of the infant over seven months of follow up was normal, except for a transient episode of mild hypercalcemia (serum Ca 11.6 mg/dl) on the first day after birth.[219] High dose (100,000 IU daily) vitamin D treatment for maternal hypoparathyroidism has been reported to result in normal offspring.[70, 220] The only complication appears to be transient (asymptomatic) hypercalcemia in a breast-fed infant consuming maternal milk containing high vitamin D (7,000 IU/L) activity.[70]

Recommendations

Enteral requirements are listed in Table 4. Parenteral requirements can be met by the use of PN solution with 500-600 mg of Ca, 48-60 mg of Mg, and 400-470 mg of P per liter. The lower Ca content may be sufficient for infants between one and two years because of the slower rate of bone mineralization in these infants. There may not be a need at this age to change Mg and P content because of increased soft tissue growth. Ca:P ratio of PN solutions also may be lowered from 1.3:1 to 1:1 by weight because of increased soft tissue growth, and depending on the results of standard biochemical laboratory measurements.[221] Parenteral vitamin D requirement may be met by 160 IU/kg/day up to a maximum total intake of 400 IU daily.

Specific clinical conditions may adversely affect infant bone mineralization. For example, in subjects with cystic fibrosis, there is a need to improve fat malabsorption to optimize mineral and vitamin D absorption and bone mineralization. Preterm infants with bronchopulmonary dysplasia (BPD) frequently receive pharmacotherapy such as chronic diuretic therapy and corticosteroids, which are both well known to adversely affect mineral metabolism. A frequent clinical review of the necessity for the use of pharmacotherapy, coupled with optimization of general nutritional status appears to be most appropriate for the maintenance of adequate growth and bone mineralization in these infants. Additional mineral and vitamin D intake, if needed, should be prescribed on an individual basis and monitored closely for its intended benefits and side effects.

There are limited information on the outcome of bone mineralization in infants fed milk formulas containing highly processed protein and modified fat composition. Thus the nutritional adequacy of these formulas should be monitored[222] particularly if they are used on a long-term basis. Specific management of infants with chronic illnesses is discussed in the Chapter by Wilson and Pencharz.

Case Histories

Case #1: A male infant was born at term weighing 3.6 kg, without birth asphyxia or maternal diabetes. Apgar scores were 9 and 10 at one and five minutes respectively. A family history of parathyroid adenoma was present in the maternal aunt. After a relatively benign immediate postnatal course, complicated only by hyperbilirubinemia and managed with phototherapy, the child was sent home on the sixth of day of life, while receiving a standard cow milk formula.

On the seventh day, the mother noted "twitching" of the left arm and leg. Bilateral jerking movements ensued intermittently and five of these episodes were noted. On the eighth day, the pediatrician saw the infant and referred him to a pediatric neurologist. While an electroencephalogram was being done, the infant had a seizure and convulsion activities recorded on electroencephalogram. The infant was then admitted to the Neonatal Intensive Care Unit.

On admission the infant's weight was 3.61 kg, head circumference was 36 cm, and length was 51 cm. Physical examination was essentially normal, except for some "jitteriness" while the infant was quiet without seizures.

Serum sodium was 136 mmol/L, glucose 63 mg/dl, blood urea nitrogen 5 mg/dl, calcium 7.3 mg/dl, magnesium 1.6 mg/dl, and phosphorus 9.2 mg/dl. Twelve hours after admission the serum calcium concentration was 6.2 mg/dl. The next day it was 6.1 mg/dl.

Questions and Answers

Question: What are the considerations for diagnosis?

Answer: Maternal hyperparathyroidism can be associated with neonatal hypoparathyroidism and tetany. Other forms of primary hypoparathyroidism can occur at this age; for example, DiGeorge's syndrome also should be considered and cardiac and thymic abnormalities should be sought. Magnesium deficiency can also lead to secondary hypoparathyroidism. Cow milk formulas have high phosphate contents relative to human milk, and neonatal tetany occurring at one week of age is a classic time for presentation.

Question: Is a serum calcium 7.3 mg/dl low enough to be considered as hypocalcemia?

Answer: Yes, in a term infant. Normal term infants rarely have total serum Ca concentration of < 8 mg/dl. Ideally, a serum ionized Ca concentration also should be measured since it is the physiologically active fraction of circulating Ca concentration. The normal range of serum ionized Ca in term infants is 4.4 to 5.6 mg/dl.[223]

Question: How would you treat this infant?

Answer: Parathyroid related disorders should be considered through serum PTH measurements in the mother and infant, especially at the time of hypocalcemia and prior to therapy. Acute correction with calcium salts intravenously may be needed to control seizures. If parathyroid disorders are ruled out, changing to a low-phosphate infant formula with phosphate content similar to human milk theoretically might be of help, or to human milk if it is still available. Supplementation with calcium may be required for a short period. In general these infants appear to adapt to the phosphate load and the disorder is transitory.

Case #2: A one-year-old black male was noted to be "falling off" the growth curve from six to seven months of age. Height, weight and head circumference measures at birth were between the 40th and 50th percentile. His development was normal except that he was not walking on his own. He had frequent upper respiratory tract infections. The child had been exclusively breast-fed since birth.

At presentation he was just below the 5th percentile in head circumference, height, and weight. Complete blood count and serum electrolytes, albumin, and total protein were determined and were normal. X-rays showed a three-month bone age, "fraying" and cupping of the metaphyses of the long bones and peribronchial thickening. He had a serum calcium concentration of 7.9 mg/dl (infant normal values 8.4-11.0 mg/dl), and alkaline phosphatase 792 IU/l (infant normal <360 IU).

His 25-hydroxyvitamin D (25 OH$_2$D) concentrations were undetectable (normal 16-68 ng/ml). Serum 1,25-dihydroxyvitamin D (1,25-(OH)$_2$D) concentration was 97 pg/ml (infant normal 18-122 pg/ml) and intact PTH concentration was high (121 pg/ml; normal 10-65 pg/ml). Mother's serum 25-OHD concentration was 8 ng/ml and subsequent analysis of her milk revealed undetectable amounts of vitamin D and 25-OHD.

The infant was considered to have vitamin D deficiency rickets and was started on 400 IU of vitamin D/day in the form of a commercial infant multivitamin preparation. Two weeks following the beginning of treatment, his serum 25-OHD rose to 16 ng/ml, 1,25(OH)$_2$D was further elevated at 198 pg/ml, and intact PTH remained high at 113 pg/ml. Five weeks following treatment, his serum 25-OHD had risen to 26 ng/ml, 1,25(OH)$_2$D concentration had fallen to 76 pg/ml, PTH was 60 pg/ml, and alkaline phosphatase had fallen to 180 IU/l. Dietary counselling was also provided for the family.

Questions and Answers

Question: Could the infant have vitamin D resistant rickets?

Answer: The largest number of subjects with so-called vitamin D "resistant" rickets have X-linked hypophosphatemic vitamin D resistant rickets (HPDR) involving a renal defect of phosphate wasting with altered 1,25(OH)$_2$D synthesis, and a bone defect that decreases mineral deposition in the matrix. Serum 25 OHD concentrations are normal. These patients have phosphaturia, hypophosphatemia, and usually "normal" serum

1,25(OH)$_2$D concentrations although it may be relatively low for the extent of hypophosphatemia. These patients are best treated with a combination phosphate therapy and modest doses of 1,25(OH)$_2$D.[224]

Rickets secondary to the autosomal recessive renal 1 alpha hydroxylase deficiency which blocks the conversion of 25 OHD to 1,25(OH)$_2$D, is associated with extremely low serum 1,25(OH)$_2$D concentrations. Hypocalcemia, hyperparathyroidism and normal serum 25 OHD concentrations are also present. These patients usually respond efficiently to lifelong replacement with physiologic doses of 1,25(OH)$_2$D.[224]

True vitamin D "resistant" rickets or end organ resistance to 1,25(OH)$_2$D is rare. At the molecular level, this condition potentially can involve each step from binding of 1,25(OH)$_2$D to VDR and to the various steps that may affect the genomic expression of 1,25(OH)$_2$D effect. End organ resistance to 1,25(OH)$_2$D is autosomal recessive in inheritance and some patients may have alopecia in addition to rickets. Biochemically, these patients frequently have hyperparathyroidism and elevated serum 1,25(OH)$_2$D secondary to hypocalcemia. Serum 25 OHD concentrations are normal. These patients may be responsive to extremely high doses of 1,25(OH)$_2$D and Ca therapy.[225]

Rickets associated with nutritional vitamin D deficiency is the only rachitic condition that is responsive to the vitamin D parent compound at or close to the physiologic daily requirement.

Question: Why was only 400 IU/day given to treat rickets and not more?

Answer: Many traditional textbooks recommend large doses of vitamin D as treatment, often as a single intramuscular injection. However, there is always a potential of toxicity with the use of pharmacologic doses of vitamin D (see Toxicity section) and low-dose vitamin D therapy combined with nutritional counseling for a normal diet (as described above) is the safest management of nutritional vitamin D deficient rickets.

We elected to treat with a dose of vitamin D that is thought to be close to the "physiologic" dose, on the assumption that it would be logical that a physiologic dose would be appropriate and sufficient for a condition of presumed vitamin D deficiency. We speculated that a highly active renal 1 α-hydroxylase activity, stimulated by hypocalcemia, hypophosphatemia, and high serum PTH concentrations would allow for maximal production of $1,25(OH)_2D$, provided sufficient 25 OHD substrate was available.

In this situation, supra physiologic serum concentrations of $1,25(OH)_2D$ are produced with the administration of a physiologic dose of 400 IU vitamin D/day. The normalized serum 25 OHD and the elevated $1,25(OH)_2D$ concentrations would maximize intestinal calcium and phosphorous absorption, and rickets should be resolved. This dose of vitamin D also serves as a test to rule out rickets due to deficiency of renal 1 α-hydroxylase and target organ unresponsiveness to $1,25(OH)_2D$; in both these instances, there would be no response to 400 IU of vitamin D.

Question: Was the infant's race contributory to the etiology of rickets?

Answer: In the United States at the present time most of the cases of vitamin D deficient rickets in breast-fed infants occur in black infants (although all races are susceptible to vitamin D deficiency if there is insufficient sunshine exposure) or in groups with unusual dietary practices. Compared to the white population, African-American mothers and infants have lower serum 25 OHD concentrations and there are lower vitamin D concentrations in breast milk, but there is no clear evidence that black breast-fed infants are substantially at higher risk for development of rickets, provided infants are taken outdoors or receive vitamin D supplements. It is theoretically possible also that the use of sunscreens blocking out UV-B exposure can increase the risk for vitamin D deficiency.

Historical Perspective...

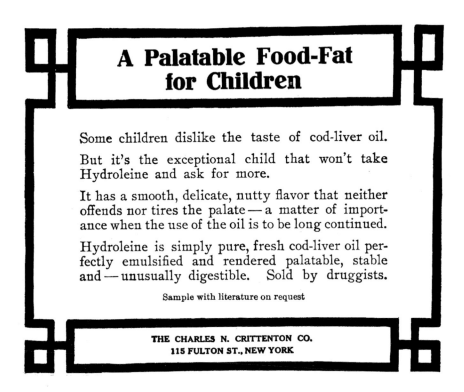

References

1. Glisson F. De rachitide, sive morbo puerili qui vulgo "The rickets" dicitur, tractatus. 2nd ed. London: 1660.

2. Ell B. Rickets and rachitis. *Lancet.* 1977;1:113-114.

3. Cone TE. *200 years of feeding infants in America.* Columbus, OH: Ross Laboratories; 1976.

4. Widdowson EM, McCance RA. The metabolism of calcium, phosphorus, magnesium and strontium. *Pediatr Clin North Am.* 1965;12:595-614.

5. Ziegler EE, O'Donnell AM, Nelson SE, Fomon SF. Body composition of the reference fetus. *Growth.* 1976; 40:320-341.

6. Sparks JW. Human intrauterine growth and nutrient accretion. *Semin Perinatol.* 1984;8:74-93.

7. Greer FR, Tsang RC. Calcium, phosphorus, magnesium, and vitamin D requirements for the preterm infant. In: Tsang RC, ed. *Vitamin and Mineral Requirements in Preterm Infants.* New York: Marcel Dekker Inc; 1985:99-136.

8. Ellis KJ, Shypailo RJ, Schanler RJ. Body composition of infants: Human cadaver studies. In: Ellis KJ, Eastman JD, eds. *Human Body Composition. In Vivo Methods, Models, and Assessment.* New York: Plenum Press; 1993: 147-160.

9. Koo WWK, Steichen JJ. Osteopenia and rickets of prematurity. In: Polin R, Fox W, eds. *Fetal and Neonatal Physiology.* 2nd ed. Phildelphia: WB Saunders Company; In press.

10. Fomon SJ, Haschke F, Ziegler EE, Nelson SE. Body composition of reference children from birth to age 10 years. *Am J Clin Nutr.* 1982;35:1169-1175.

11. Fomon SJ, Nelson SE. Calcium, phosphorus, magnesium, and sulfur. In: Fomon SJ, ed. *Nutrition of Normal Infants.* St. Louis: Mosby; 1993:192-218.

12. Minton SD, Steichen JJ, Tsang RC. Bone mineral content in term and preterm appropriate-for-gestational-age infants. *J Pediatr.* 1979;95:1037-1042.

13. Greer FR, Lane J, Weiner S, Mazess RB. An accurate and reproducible absorptiometric technique for determining bone mineral content in newborn infants. *Pediatr Res.* 1983;17:259-262.

14. Specker BL, Brazerol W, Tsang RC, Levin R, Searcy J, Steichen J. Bone mineral content in children 1 to 6 years of age. Detectable sex differences after 4 years of age. *Am J Dis Child.* 1987;141:343-344.

15. Li J-Y, Specker BL, Ho ML, Tsang RC. Bone mineral content in black and white children 1 to 6 years of age. Early appearance of race and sex difference. *Am J Dis Child.* 1989;143:1346-1349.

16. Hamill PVV, Drizd TA, Johnson CL, Reed RB, Roche AF, Moore WM. Physical growth: National Center for Health Statistics percentiles. *Am J Clin Nutr.* 1979;32: 607-629.

17. Hoogenboezem T, Degenhart HJ, De Muinch Keizer-Schrama SMPF, et al. Vitamin D metabolism in breast-fed infants and their mothers. *Pediatr Res.* 1989;25:623-628.

18. Koo WWK, Tsang RC, Steichen JJ, et al. Vitamin D requirement in infants receiving parenteral nutrition. *J Parenter Enteral Nutr.* 1987;11:172-176.

19. Larchet M, Grabedian M, Bourdeau A, Gorski A-M, Goulet O, Ricour C. Calcium metabolism in children during long-term total parenteral nutrition: The influence of calcium, phosphorus, and vitamin D intakes. *J Pediatr Gastroenterol Nutr.* 1991;13:367-375.

20. Specker BL, Lichtenstein P, Mimouni F, et al. Calcium regulating hormones and minerals from birth to 18 months: A cross sectional study. II. Effects of sex, race, age, season and diet on serum minerals, parathyroid hormone, and calcitonin. *Pediatrics.* 1986;77:891-896.

21. Lichtenstein P, Specker BL, Tsang RC, et al. Calcium-regulating hormones and minerals from birth to 18 months of age: A cross-sectional study I. Effects of sex, race, age, season, and diet on vitamin D status. *Pediatrics.* 1986;77:883-890.

22. Fomon SJ, Ziegler EE, Filer LJ Jr, Anderson TA, Edwards BB, Nelson SE. Growth and serum chemical values of normal breast-fed infants. *Acta Paediatr Scand.* 1978;suppl273:1-29.

23. Meites S, ed. *Pediatric Clinical Chemistry. Reference (Normal) Values.* Washington, DC: Amer Assoc Clin Chem Inc; 1989.

24. Cockburn F, Brown JK, Belton NR, Forfar JO. Neonatal convulsions associated with primary disturbance of calcium, phosphorus, and magnesium metabolism. *Arch Dis Child.* 1973;48:99-108.

25. Greer FR, Marshall S. Bone mineral content, serum vitamin D metabolite concentrations, and ultraviolet B light exposure in infants fed human milk with and without vitamin D2 supplements. *J Pediatr.* 1989;114:204-212.

26. Chesney RW, Rosen JF, Hamstra AJ, et al. Absence of seasonal variation in serum concentrations of 1,25-dihydroxyvitamin D despite a rise in 25-hydroxyvitamin D in summer. *J Clin Endocrinol Metab.* 1981;53:139-142.

27. Markestad T. Plasma concentrations of vitamin D metabolites in unsupplemented breast-fed infants. *Eur J Pediatr.* 1983;141:77-80.

28. Taylor AF, Norman ME. Vitamin D metabolite levels in normal children. *Pediatr Res.* 1984;18:886-890.

29. Specker BL, Tsang RC. Cyclical serum 25-hydroxyvitamin D paralleling sunshine exposure in exclusively breast-fed infants: mirror image in summer vs winter born. *J Pediatr.* 1987;110:744-747.

30. Venkataraman PS, Tsang RC, Greer FR, Noguchi A, Laskarzewski P, Steichen JJ. Late infantile tetany and secondary hyperparathyroidism in infants fed humanized cow milk formula. Longitudinal follow-up. *Am J Dis Child.* 1985;139:664-668.

31. Reinhart RA. Magnesium metabolism: A review with special reference to the relationship between intracellular content and serum levels. *Arch Intern Med.* 1988;148:2415-2420.

32. Berner YN, Shike M. Consequences of phosphate imbalance. *Annu Rev Nutr.* 1988;8:121-148.

33. Greer FR, Tsang RC, Levin RS, Searcy JE, Wu R, Steichen JJ. Increasing serum calcium and magnesium concentrations in breast-fed infants: longitudinal studies of minerals in human milk and in sera of nursing mothers and their infants. *J Pediatr.* 1982;100:59-64.

34. Specker BL, Tsang RC, Ho ML, et al. Low serum calcium and high parathyroid hormone levels in neonates fed "humanized" cow's milk-based formula. *Am J Dis Child.* 1991;145:941-945.

35. Koo WWK, Tsang RC. Bone mineralization in infants. *Prog Food Nutr Sci.* 1984;8:229-302.

36. Clements MR, Johnson L, Fraser DR. A new mechanism for induced vitamin D deficiency in calcium deprivation. *Nature.* 1987;325:62-65.

37. Bell NH, Shaw S, Turner RT. Evidence that calcium modulates circulating 25-hydroxyvitamin D in man. *J Bone Miner Res.* 1987;2:211-214.

38. Arnaud SB, Stickler GB, Haworth JC. Serum 25-hydroxyvitamin D in infantile rickets. *Pediatrics.* 1976;57:221.

39. Garabedian M, Vainsel M, Mallet E, et al. Circulating vitamin D metabolite concentrations in children with nutritional rickets. *J Pediatr.* 1983;103:381-386.

40. Venkataraman PS, Tsang RC, Buckley DD, Ho M, Steichen JJ. Elevation of serum 1,25-dihydroxyvitamin D in response to physiologic doses of vitamin D in vitamin D-deficient infants. *J Pediatr.* 1983;103:416-419.

41. Markestad T, Halvorsen S, Seeger Halvorsen K, Aksnes L, Aarskog D. Plasma Concentrations of vitamin D metabolites before and during treatment of vitamin D deficiency rickets in children. *Acta Paediatr Scand.* 1984;73:225-231.

42. Shah BR, Finberg L. Single-day therapy for nutritional vitamin D-deficiency rickets: a preferred method. *J Pediatr.* 1994;125:487-490.

43. Kruse K. Pathophysiology of calcium metabolism in children with vitamin D-deficiency rickets. *J Pediatr.* 1995;126:736-741.

44. Norman AW. Intestinal calcium absorption: a vitamin D-hormone-mediated adaptive response. *Am J Clin Nutr.* 1990;51:290-300.

45. Bronner F. Current concepts of calcium absorption: an overview. *J Nutr.* 1992;122:641-643.

46. Ozono K, Sone T, Pike JW. Perspectives: the genomic mechanism of action of 1,25-dihydroxyvitamin D3. *J Bone Mineral Res.* 1991;6:1021-1027.

47. Norman AW, Nemere I, Zhou L-X, et al. 1,25(OH)2-Vitamin D3, a steroid hormone that produces biologic effects via both genomic and nongenomic pathways. *J Steroid Biochem Mol Biol.* 1992;41:231-240.

48. Delvin EE. Vitamin D: metabolism, and effects on growth and development. *Acta Paediatr Scand.* 1994;405(suppl):105-110.

49. Karbach U. Paracellular calcium transport across the small intestine. *J Nutr.* 1992;122:672-677.

50. Hofmann AF, Roda A. Physicochemical properties of the bile acids and their relationship to biological properties, an overview of the problem. *J Lipid Res.* 1984;25:1477-1489.

51. Hylander E, Ladefoged K, Jarnum S. The importance of the colon in calcium absorption following small-intestine resection. *Scand J Gastroenterol.* 1980;15:55-60.

52. Abrams SA, Yergey AL, Heaney RP. Relationship between balance and dual tracer isotopic measurements

of calcium absorption and excretion. *J Clin Endocrinol Metab.* 1994;79:965-969.

53. Abrams SA, Sidbury JB, Muenzer J, Esteban NV, Vieira NE, Yergey AL. Stable isotope measurement of endogenous fecal calcium excretion in children. *J Pediatr Gastroenterol Nutr.* 1991;12:469-473.

54. Moore LJ, Machlan LA, Lim MO, Yergey AL, Hansen JW. Dynamics of calcium metabolism in infancy and childhood. I. methodology and quantification in the infant. *Pediatr Res.* 1985;19:329-334.

55. Hillman LS, Johnson LS, Lee DZ, Vieira NE, Yergey AL. Measurement of true absorption, endogenous fecal excretion, urinary excretion, and retention of calcium in preterm infants by using a dual tracer, stable isotope method. *J Pediatr.* 1993;123:444-456.

56. Ehrenkranz RA, Ackerman BA, Nelli CM, Janghorbani M. Absorption of calcium in premature infants as measured with a stable isotope [46]Ca extrinsic tag. *Pediatr Res.* 1985; 19:178-184.

57. Liu Y-M, Neal P, Ernst J, et al. Absorption of calcium and magnesium from fortified human milk by very low birth weight infants. *Pediatr Res.* 1989;25:496-502.

58. Koo WWK, Tsang RC. Calcium, magnesium, phosphorus, and vitamin D. In: Tsang RC, Lucas A, Uauy R, Zlotkin S, eds. *Nutritional Needs of the Preterm Infant: Scientific Practice and Practical Guidelines.* New York: Williams and Wilkins; 1993:135-155.

59. Abrams SA. Clinical studies of mineral metabolism in children using stable isotopes. *J Pediatr Gastroenterol Nutr.* 1994;19:151-163.

60. Abrams SA, Wen J, Stuff JE. Absorption of calcium, zinc and iron from breast milk by five to seven month old infants. *Pediatr Res.* 1997;41: 384-390.

61. Fransson GB, Lonnerdal B. Distribution of trace elements and minerals in human and cow's milk. *Pediatr Res.* 1983;17:412-415.

62. Abrams SA, Vieira NE, Yergey AL. Unequal distribution of a stable isotopic calcium tracer between casein and whey fractions of infants formulas, human milk and cow's milk. *J Nutr.* 1990;120:1672-1676.

63. Fransson GB, Lonnerdal B. Zinc, copper, calcium, magnesium in human milk. *J Pediatr.* 1982;101:504-508.

64. Sann L, Bienvenu J, Bienvenu F, Lahet C, Bethenod M. Comparison of the composition of breast milk from mothers of term and preterm infants. *Acta Paediatr Scand.* 1981;70:115-160.

65. Lemons JA, Moye L, Hall D, Simmons M. Differences in the composition of preterm and term human milk during early lactation. *Pediatr Res.* 1982;16:113-117.

66. Laskey MA, Prentice A, Shaw J, et al. Breast milk calcium concentrations during prolonged lactation in British and rural Gambian mothers. *Acta Paediatr Scand.* 1990;79:507-512.

67. Specker BL. Nutritional concerns of lactating women consuming vegetarian diets. *Am J Clin Nutr.* 1994; 59(suppl):S1182-S1186.

68. Prentice A, Jarjou LMA, Cole TJ, Stirling DM, Dibba B, Fairweather-Tait S. Calcium requirements of lactating Gambian mothers: effects of a calcium supplement on breast milk calcium concentration, maternal bone mineral content, and urinary calcium excretion. *Am J Clin Nutr.* 1995;62:58-67.

69. Hopkinson JM, Schanler RJ, Fraley JK, Garza C. Milk production by mothers of premature infants: influence of cigarette smoking. *Pediatrics.* 1992;90:934-938.

70. Greer FR, Hollis BW, Napoli JL. High concentrations of vitamin D2 in human milk associated with pharmacologic doses of vitamin D2. *J Pediatr.* 1984;105: 61-64.

71. Picciano MF. What constitutes a representative human milk sample? *J Pediatr Gastroenterol Nutr.* 1984;3:280-283.

72. Lonnerdal B, Smith C, Keen CL. Analysis of breast milk: current methodologies and future needs. *J Pediatr Gastroenterol Nutr.* 1984;3:290-295.

73. Allen JC, Keller RP, Archer P, Neville MC. Studies in human lactation: milk composition and daily secretion rates of macronutrients in the first year of lactation. *Am J Clin Nutr.* 1991;54:69-80.

74. Ziegler EE, Fomon SJ. Lactose enhances mineral absorption in infancy. *J Pediatr Gastroenterol Nutr.* 1983; 2:288-294.

75. Widdowson EM, McCance RA, Harrison GE, Sutton A. Effect of giving phosphate supplements to breast-fed babies on absorption and excretion of calcium, strontium, magnesium and phosphorus. *Lancet.* 1963;2:1250-1251.

76. Wood RJ, Gerhardt A, Rosenberg IH. Effects of glucose and glucose polymers on calcium absorption in healthy subjects. *Am J Clin Nutr.* 1987;46:699-701.

77. Moya M, Cortes E, Ballester MI, Vento M, Juste M. Short-term polycose substitution for lactose reduces calcium absorption in healthy term babies. *J Pediatr Gastroentero Nutr.* 1992;14:57-61.

78. Allen LA. Calcium bioavailability and absorption: a review. *Am J Clin Nutr.* 1982;35:783-808.

79. Hillman LS, Chow W, Salmons SS, Weaver E, Erickson M, Hansen J. Vitamin D metabolism, mineral homeostasis, and bone mineralization in term infants fed human milk, cow milk-based formula, or soy-based formula. *J Pediatr.* 1988;112:864-874.

80. Hillman LS. Bone mineral content in term infants fed human milk, cow milk-based formula, or soy-based formula. *J Pediatr.* 1988;113:208-212.

81. Mimouni F, Campaigne B, Neylan M, Tsang RC. Bone mineralization in the first year of life in infants fed human milk, cow-milk formula, or soy-based formula. *J Pediatr.* 1993;122:348-354.

82. DeVizia B, Fomon SJ, Nelson SE, Edwards BE, Ziegler EE. Effect of dietary calcium on metabolic balance of normal infants. *Pediatr Res.* 1985;19:800-806.

83. Dalton MA, Sargent JD, O'Connor GT, Olmstead EM, Klein RZ. Calcium and phosphorus supplementation of iron-fortified infant formulas: no effect on iron status of healthy full-term infants. *Am J Clin Nutr.* 1997;65: 921-926.

84. Fine KD, Santa Ana CA, Porter JL, Fordtran JS. Intestinal absorption of magnesium from food and supplements. *J Clin Invest.* 1991;88:396-402.

85. Hardwick LL, Jones MR, Brautbar N, Lee DBN. Magnesium absorption: mechanisms and the influence of vitamin D, calcium and phosphate. *J Nutr.* 1991;121: 13-23.

86. Norman DA, Fordtran JS, Brinkley LJ, et al. Jejunal and ileal adaptation to alterations in dietary calcium: changes in calcium and magnesium absorption and pathogenic role of parathyroid hormone and 1,25-dihydroxyvitamin D. *J Clin Invest.* 1981;67:1599-1603.

87. Karbach U, Feldmeier H. New clinical and experimental aspects of intestinal magnesium transport. *Magnesium Research.* 1991;4:9-22.

88. Brink EJ, Dekker PR, Van Beresteijn ECH, et al. Inhibitory effect of dietary soybean protein vs casein on magnesium absorption in rats. *J Nutr.* 1991;121:1374-1381.

89. Brink EJ, Beynen AC, Dekker PR, et al. Interaction of calcium and phosphate decreases ileal magnesium solubility and apparent magnesium absorption in rats. *J Nutr.* 1992;122:580-586.

90. Shils ME. Experimental human magnesium depletion. *Medicine.* 1969;48:61-85.

91. Schuette SA, Ziegler EE, Nelson SE, Janghorbani M. Feasibility of using the stable isotope ^{25}Mg to study magnesium metabolism in infants. *Pediatr Res.* 1990;27: 36-40.

92. Thoren L. Magnesium deficiency in gastrointestinal fluid loss. *Acta Chir Scand.* 1963;306(Suppl):1-65.

93. Lönnerdal, Yuen M, Glazier C, Litov RE. Magnesium bioavailability from human milk, cow milk, and infant formula in suckling rat pups. *Am J Clin Nutr.* 1993;58: 392-397.

94. Wilz DR, Gray RW, Dominguez JH, Lemann J Jr. Plasma 1,25(OH)2 vitamin D concentrations and net intestinal calcium, phosphate, and magnesium absorption in humans. *Am J Clin Nutr.* 1979;32:2052-2060.

95. Levine BS, Brautbar N, Walling MW, et al. Effects of vitamin D and diet magnesium on magnesium metabolism. *Am J Physiol.* 1980;239:E515-E523.

96. Cross HS, Debiec H, Peterlik M. Mechanism and regulation of intestinal phosphate absorption. *Miner Electrolyte Metab.* 1990;16:115-124.

97. Wasserman RH. Intestinal absorption of calcium and phosphorus. *Fed Proc.* 1981;40:68-72.

98. Senterre J, Putet G, Salle B, Rigo J. Effects of vitamin D and phosphorus supplementation on calcium retention in preterm infants fed banked human milk. *J Pediatr.* 1983;103:305-307.

99. Koo WWK, Tsang RC. Calcium and magnesium metabolism. In: Werner M, ed. *CRC handbook of clinical chemistry.* Boca Raton, FL: CRC Press; 1989;2:51-91.

100. Senterre J, Salle B. Renal aspects of calcium and phosphorus metabolism in preterm infants. *Biol Neonate.* 1988;53:220-229.

101. Koo WWK. Parenteral nutrition-related bone disease. *J Parenteral Enteral Nutr.* 1992;16:386-394.

102. Kawashima H, Kurokawa K. Metabolism and sites of action of vitamin D in the kidney. *Kidney Internat.* 1986; 29:98-107.

103. Holick MF, MacLaughlin JA, Doppelt SH. Regulation

of cutaneous previtamin D3 photosynthesis in man: skin pigment is not an essential regulator. *Science.* 1981; 211:590-593.

104. Franceschi RT, Simpson RU, DeLuca HF. Binding proteins for vitamin D metabolites: serum carriers and intracellular receptors. *Arch Biochem Biophys.* 1981;210: 1-13.

105. Hollander D. Intestinal absorption of vitamin A, E, D, and K. *J Lab Clin Invest.* 1981;97:449-462.

106. Clements MR, Chalers TM, Fraser DR. Enterohepatic circulation of vitamin D: a reappraisal of the hypothesis. *Lancet.* 1984;1:1376-1379.

107. Lo CW, Paris PW, Clemens TL, et al. Vitamin D absorption in healthy subjects and in patients with intestinal malabsorption syndromes. *Am J Clin Nutr.* 1985;42:644-649.

108. Thompson GR, Lewis B, Booth CC. Absorption of vitamin D3-3H in control subjects and patients with intestinal malabsorption. *J Clin Invest.* 1960;45:94-102.

109. Kodicek E. The fate of 14C-labeled vitamin D2 in rats and infants. In: Garattini S, Paoletti G, eds. *Drugs Affecting Lipid Metabolism.* Amsterdam: Elsevier; 1961: 515-519.

110. Hollis BW, Lowery JW, Pittard WBIII, Guy DG, Hansen JW. Effect of age on the intestinal absorption of vitamin D3-palmitate and nonesterified vitamin D2 in the term infant. *J Clin Endocrinol Metab.* 1996;81: 1385-1388.

111. Sitrin MD, Bengoa JM. Intestinal absorption of cholecalciferol and 25-hydroxycholecalciferol in chronic cholestatic liver disease. *Am J Clin Nutr.* 1987;46: 1011-1015.

112. Heubi JE, Hollis BW, Specker B, Tsang RC. Bone disease in chronic childhood cholestasis. I. Vitamin D absorption and metabolism. *Hepatology.* 1989;9:258-264.

113. Dueland S, Helgerud P, Pederson JI, et al. Plasma clearance, transfer, and tissue distribution of vitamin D3 from rat intestinal lymph. *Am J Physiol.* 1983;245: E326-E331.

114. Suda T, Shinki T, Takahashi N. The role of vitamin D in bone and intestinal cell differentiation. *Annu Rev Nutr.* 1990;10:195-211.

115. Maierhofer WJ, Gray RW, Cheung HS, Lemann J Jr. Bone resorption stimulated by elevated serum 1,25(OH)2

vitamin D concentrations in healthy men. *Kidney Int.* 1983;24:555-560.

116. Stern PH. Vitamin D and bone. *Kidney Internat.* 1990; 38:S17-S21.

117. DeLuca HF. Osteoporosis and the metabolites of vitamin D. *Metabolism.* 1990;39:3-9.

118. Haussler MR. Vitamin D receptors: nature and function. *Ann Rev Nutr.* 1986;6:527-562.

119. Pike JW. Vitamin D3 receptors: structure and function in transcription. *Annu Rev Nutr.* 1991;11:189-216.

120. Lundgren S, Hjalm G, Hellman P, et al. A protein involved in calcium sensing of the human parathyroid and placental cytotrophoblast cells belongs to the LDL-receptor protein superfamily. *Experimental Cell Res.* 1994;212:344-350.

121. Tsang RC, Greer F, Steichen JJ. Perinatal Metabolism of Vitamin D. Transition from fetal to neonatal life. *Clin Perinatol.* 1981;8:287-306.

122. Labuda M, Fujiwara TM, Ross MV, et al. Two hereditary defects related to vitamin D metabolism map to the same region of human chromosome 12q13-14. *J Bone Mineral Res.* 1992;7:1447-1453.

123. Baker AR, McDonnell DP, Hughes M, et al. Cloning and expression of full-length cDNA encoding human vitamin D receptor (1,25-dihydroxyvitamin D3). *Proc Natl Acad Sci.* 1988;85:3294-3298.

124. Carson-Jurica MA, Schrader WT, O'Malley BW. Steroid receptor family: structure and functions. *Endoc Rev.* 1990;11:201-220.

125. Delvin EE, Richard P, Pothier P, et al. Presence and binding characteristics of calcitriol receptors in human fetal gut. *FEBS Lett.* 1990;262:55-57.

126. Reichel H, Koeffler HP, Norman AW. The role of the vitamin D endocrine system in health and disease. *N Eng J Med.* 1989;320:980-990.

127. DeLuca HF, Krisinger J, Darwish H. The vitamin D system: 1990. *Kidney Int.* 1990;38:S2-S8.

128. Lee S, Clark SA, Gill RK, Christakos S. 1,25-Dihydroxyvitamin D3 and pancreatic-cell function: vitamin D receptors, gene expression, and insulin secretion. *Endocrinol.* 1994;134:1602-1610.

129. Carlberg C, Bendik I, Wyss A, et al. Two nuclear signaling pathways for vitamin D. *Nature.* 1993;361:657-660.

130. Hollis BW, Pittard WB III. Evaluation of the total

fetomaternal vitamin D relationships at term: evidence for racial differences. *J Clin Endocrinol Metab.* 1984;59: 652-657.

131. Bouillon R, Van Assche FA, Van Baelen H, et al. Influence of the vitamin D-binding protein on the serum concentration of 1,25-dihydroxyvitamin D3. Significance of the free 1,25-dihydroxyvitamin D3 concentration. *J Clin Invest.* 1981;67:589-596.

132. Verity CM, Burman D, Beadle PC, Holton JB, Morris A. Seasonal changes in perinatal vitamin D metabolism maternal and cord blood biochemistry in normal pregnancies. *Arch Dis Child.* 1981;56:943-948.

133. Markestad T, Aksnes L, Magnar U, Aarskog D. 25-Hydroxyvitamin D and 1,25-dihydroxyvitamin D of D2 and D3 origin in maternal and umbilical cord serum after vitamin D2 supplementation in human pregnancy. *Am J Clin Nutr.* 1984;40:1057-1063.

134. Delvin EE, Salle BL, Glorieux FH, Adeleine P, David LS. Vitamin D supplementation during pregnancy: effect on neonatal calcium homeostasis. *J Pediatr.* 1986;109: 328-334.

135. Rosenstreich SJ, Rich C, Volwiler W. Deposition in and release of vitamin D3 from body fat. Evidence for a storage site in the rat. *J Clin Invest.* 1971;50:679-687.

136. Mawer EB, Schaefer K. The distribution of vitamin D3 metabolites in human serum and tissue. *Biochem J.* 1969; 114:P74-P75.

137. Specker BL, Valanis B, Hertzberg V, et al. Sunshine exposure and serum 25-hydroxyvitamin D concentrations in exclusively breast-fed infants. *J Pediatr.* 1985;107: 372-376.

138. Ho ML, Yen HC, Tsang RC, et al. Randomized study of sunshine exposure and serum 25-OHD in breast-fed infants in Beijing, China. *J Pediatr.* 1985;107:928-931.

139. Rothberg AD, Pettifor JM, Cohen DF, et al. Maternal-infant vitamin D relationships during breast-feeding. *J Pediatr.* 1982;101:500-503.

140. Ala-Houhala M. 25-Hydroxyvitamin D levels during breast-feeding with or without maternal or infantile supplementation of vitamin D. *J Pediatr Gastroenterol Nutr.* 1985;4:220-226.

141. Hollis BW, Roos BA, Draper HH, Lambert PW. Vitamin D and its metabolites in human and bovine milk. *J Nutr.* 1981;111:1240-1248.

142. Greer FR, Ho M, Dodson D, Tsang R. Lack of 25-hydroxyvitamin D and 1,25-hydroxyvitamin D in human milk. *J Pediatr.* 1981;99:233-235.

143. Reeve LE, Chesney RW, DeLuca HF. Vitamin D of human milk: identification of biologically active forms. *Am J Clin Nutr.* 1982;36:122-126.

144. Specker BL, Tsang RC, Hollis BW. Effect of race and diet on human milk vitamin D and 25-hydroxyvitamin D. *Am J Dis Child.* 1985;139:1134-1137.

145. Hollis BW, Pittard WB III, Reinhardt TA. Relationships among vitamin D, 25-hydroxyvitamin D, and vitamin D-binding protein concentrations in the plasma and milk of human subjects. *J Clin Endocrinol Metab.* 1986; 62:41-44.

146. Ala-Houhala M, Koskinen T, Parviainen MT, Visakorpi JK. 25-hydroxyvitamin D and vitamin D in human milk: effects of supplementation and season. *Am J Clin Nutr.* 1988;48:1057-1060.

147. Atkinson SA, Reinhardt TA, Hollis BW. Vitamin D activity in maternal plasma and milk in relation to gestational stage at delivery. *Nutr Res.* 1987;7:1005-1011.

148. Hollis BW, Lambert PW, Horst RL. Factors affecting the antirachitic sterol content of native milk. In: Holick MF, Gray JK, Anast CS, eds. *Perinatal Calcium and Phosphorus Metabolism.* New York: Elsevier; 1983:157-182.

149. Greer FR, Hollis BW, Cripps DJ, Tsang RC. Effects of maternal ultraviolet B irradiation on vitamin D content of human milk. *J Pediatr.* 1984;105:431-433.

150. Vitamin D. In: Golshahr VE, Neubauer DJ, Reinert AE, eds. *Drug facts and comparisons.* St. Louis: Wolters Kluwer Company; 1996:8-13.

151. *Minerals. In Recommended Dietary Allowances.* Washington, DC. Subcommittee on the Tenth Edition of the RDAs, Food and Nutrition Board, Commission on Life Sciences, National Research Council: 1989 National Academy Press; 174-194.

152. Committee on Nutrition. American Academy of Pediatrics. Calcium, phosphorus and magnesium. In: Barness LA, ed. *Pediatric Nutrition Handbook.* 3rd ed. Elk Grove Village, IL: American Academy of Pediatrics; 1993:115-124.

153. National Institutes of Health Consensus Development Panel on Optimal Calcium Intake. Optimal calcium intake. *JAMA.* 1994;272:1942-1948.

154. Committee on Nutrition. American Academy of Pediatrics. The use of whole cow's milk in infants. *Pediatrics.* 1992;89:1105-1109.

155. Roberts CC, Chan GM, Folland D, Rayburn C, Jackson R. Adequate bone mineralization in breast-fed infants. *J Pediatr.* 1981;99:192-196.

156. Koo WWK, Succop PA, Bornschein RL, et al. Serum vitamin D metabolites and bone mineralization in young children with chronic low to moderate lead exposure. *Pediatrics.* 1991;87:680-687.

157. Alaimo K, McDowell MA, Briefel RR, et al. Dietary intake of vitamins, minerals, and fiber of persons ages 2 months and over in the United States. *Third National Health and Nutrition Examination Survey, Phase 1, 1988-91.* National Center for Health Statistics: 1994. 258:1-28.

158. Koo WWK, Tsang RC, Steichan JJ, et al. Parenteral nutrition for infants: effects of high versus low calcium and phosphorus content. *J Pediatr Gastroenterol Nutr.* 1987;6:96-104.

159. Committee on Nutrition. American Academy of Pediatrics. Commentary on parenteral nutrition. *Pediatrics.* 1983; 71:547-552.

160. Koo WWK, Fong T, Gupta JM. Parenteral nutrition in infants. *Aust Paediatr J.* 1980;16:169-174.

161. Wolman SL, Anderson GH, Marliss EB, Jeejeebhoy KN. Zinc in total parenteral nutrition: requirement and metabolic effects. *Gastroenterology.* 1980;76:458-467.

162. Randall HT. Water and electrolyte balance in surgery. *Surg Clin North Am.* 1952;32:445-469.

163. Leveille GA, Zabick ME, Morgan KJ. *Nutrients in Foods.* Massachusetts: The Nutrition Guild; 1983:2-283.

164. Gittleman IJ, Pincus JB. Influence of diet on the occurrence of hyperphosphatemia and hypocalcemia in the newborn infant. *Pediatrics.* 1951;8:778-787.

165. Nelson SE, Rogers RR, Frantz JA, Ziegler EE. Palm olein in infant formula: absorption of fat and minerals by normal infants. *Am J Clin Nutr.* 1996;64:291-296.

166. Adamkin DH. Nutrition in very low birth weight infants. *Clin Perinatol.* 1986;13:419-443.

167. Heird WC, Winters RW. Total parenteral nutrition. *J Pediatr.* 1975;86:2-16.

168. Derr R, Zieve L. Intracellular distribution of phosphate in the underfed rat developing weakness and coma following total parenteral nutrition. *J Nutr.* 1976;106: 1398-1403.

169. Weinsler RL, Krumdieck CL. Death from overzealous total parenteral nutrition: the refeeding syndrome revisited. *Am J Clin Nutr.* 1980;34:393-399.

170. Koo WWK, Tsang RC, Succop P, Krug-Wispe SK, Babcock D, Oestreich AE. Minimal vitamin D and high calcium and phosphorus needs of preterm infants receiving parenteral nutrition. *J Pediatr Gastroenterol Nutr.* 1989;8:225-233.

171. Markestad T, Kolmannskog S, Arntzen E, Toftegaard L, Haneberg B, Aksnes L. Serum concentrations of vitamin D metabolites in exclusively breast-fed infants at 70° North. *Acta Paediatr Scand.* 1984;73:29-32.

172. Hayward I, Stein MT, Gibson MI. Nutritional rickets in San Diego. *Am J Dis Child.* 1987;141:1060-1066.

173. Bhowmick SK, Johnson KR, Rettig KR. Rickets caused by vitamin D deficiency in breast-fed infants in the southern United States. *Am J Dis Child.* 1991;145:127-130.

174. Specker BL, Ho ML, Oestreich A, et al. Prospective study of vitamin D supplementation and rickets in China. *J Pediatr.* 1992;120:733-739.

175. Webb AR, Kline L, Holick MF. Influence of season and latitude on the cutaneous synthesis of vitamin D3: exposure to winter sunlight in Boston and Edmonton will not promote vitamin D3 synthesis in human skin. *J Clin Endocrinol Metab.* 1988;67:373-378.

176. *Vitamin D. In Recommended Dietary Allowances.* Washington, DC. Subcommitte on the Tenth Edition of the RDAs, Food and Nutrition Board, Commission on Life Sciences, National Research Council: 1989. National Academy Press; 92-98.

177. Shike M, Sturtridge WC, Tam CS, et al. A possible role of vitamin D in the genesis of parenteral nutrition-induced metabolic bone disease. *Ann Intern Med.* 1981; 95:560-568.

178. Klein GL, Targoff CM, Ament ME, et al. Bone disease associated with total parenteral nutrition. *Lancet.* 1980; 11:1041-1044.

179. Baeckert PA, Greene HL, Fritz I, et al. Vitamin concentrations in very low birth weight infants given vitamins intravenously in a lipid emulsion: measurement of vitamins A, D, and E and riboflavin. *J Pediatr.* 1988; 113:1057-1065.

180. Greene HL, Hambidge KM, Schanler R, Tsang RC.

Guidelines for the use of vitamins, trace elements, calcium, magnesium, and phosphorus in infants and children receiving total parenteral nutrition: Report of the Subcommittee on Pediatric Parenteral Nutrient Requirements from the Committee on Clinical Practice Issues of the American Society for Clinical Nutrition. *Am J Clin Nutr.* 1988;48:1324-1342. (Revised reprint, December, 1990).

181. Mimouni F, Koo WWK. Neonatal Mineral Metabolism. In: Tsang RC, ed. *Calcium and Magnesium Metabolism in Early Life.* Boca Raton, FL: CRC Press Inc: 1995;71-89.

182. Weaver CM, Plawecki KL. Dietary calcium: adequacy of a vegetarian diet. *Am J Clin Nutr.* 1994;59(suppl): S1238-S1241.

183. Dagnelie PC, Vergote FJVRA, van Staveren WA, van den Berg H, Dingjan PG, Hautvast JGAJ. High prevalence of rickets in infants on macrobiotic diets. *Am J Clin Nutr.* 1990;51:202-208.

184. Sanders TAB, Reddy S. Vegetarian diets and children. *Am J Clin Nutr.* 1994;59(suppl):S1176-S1181.

185. Dagnelie PC, van Staveren WA. Macrobiotic nutrition and child health: results of a population-based, mixed-longitudinal cohort study in The Netherlands. *Am J Clin Nutr.* 1994;59(suppl):S1187-S1196.

186. Herweijer TJ, Steendijk R. The relation between attained adult height and the metaphyseal lesions in hypophosphatemic vitamin D resistant rickets. *Acta Pediatr Scand.* 1985;74:196-200.

187. Peiper A. Quellen zur geschichte der kinderheilkunde. Bern: Verlaf Hans Huber; 1966:104.

188. Whistler D. Morbo puerili anglorum, quem patrio idiomate indigenae vocant the rickets. *Lugduni Batavorum.* 1645.

189. Glisson F. De rachitide sive morbo puerili qui vulgo the rickets dicitur. *Londinium.* 1650.

190. Parks EA. The etiology of rickets. *Physiol Rev.* 1923;3: 106-163.

191. Weick MT. A history of rickets in the United States. *Am J Clin Nutr.* 1967;20:1234-1241.

192. Kassowitz M. Tetanie and autointoxication im kindersalter. *Wien Med Presse.* 1887;38:97:139. Also in: Kassowitz M. *Gesammelte abhandlungen.* Berling: 1914: 192.

193. Pommer G. Untersuchungen ueber osteomalacie and rachitis, etc. Leipzig: 1885.

194. Siegert F. Beitrag zur lehr von de rachitis. *Jahrb Kinderh.* 1903;58:929.

195. Siegert F. Die aetiologie der rachitis auf grund neuerer untersuchungen. *Munchen Med Wochenschr.* 1905;52:622.

196. Sambon LW. Tropical clothing. *J Trop Med.* 1907;10:67.

197. Koch J. Untersuchungen ueber die lokalisation der bakterien, das verhalten des knochenmarkes und die veranderungen der knochen, insbesondere der epiphysen, bei infektionskrankheiten. Mit bemerkungen zur theorie der rachitis. *Zeitschr Hyg Infetionskrankh.* 1911;69:436.

198. Edlefsen G. Ueber die entstehungsursachen der rachitis und ihre verwandschaft mit gewissen infektionskrankheiten. *Deutsch Aerzte Zeitg.* 1902;169: 200.

199. Schmorl G. Die pathologische anatomie der rachitischen knochenerkrankung mit besonderer berucksichtigung ihrer histologie und pathogenese. *Ergebn Med Kinderh.* 1909;4:403.

200. Funk C. Die vitamine, ihre bedeutung fur die physiologie und pathologic, etc. Wiesbaden: 1914.

201. Mellanby E. The part played by an "accessory factor" in the production of experimental rickets. (*Proc Physiol Soc.* Jan 26, 1918). *J Physiol.* 1918;52:xi.

202. Report on the present state of knowledge concerning accessory food factors (vitamins). Compiled by a committee appointed jointly by the Lister Institute and the Medical Research Committee. London: 1919. H.M. Stat Off Med Research Comm. Spec Rep No. 38.

203. Mize CE, Corbett JT, Uauy R, Nunnally RL, Williamson SB. Hypotonia of rickets: A sequential study by P-31 magnetic resonance spectroscopy. *Pediatr Res.* 1988;24:713-716.

204. Bainbridge RR, Koo WWK, Tsang RC. Neonatal calcium and phosphorus disorders. In: Lifshitz F, ed. *Pediatric Endocrinology: A Clinical Guide.* 3rd Edition. New York: Marcel Dekker Inc; 1996:473-496.

205. Kimura S, Nose O, Seino Y, et al. Effects of alternate and simultaneous administration of calcium and phosphorus on calcium metabolism in children receiving total parenteral nutrition. *J Parenter Enteral Nutr.* 1986; 10:513-516.

206. Cleghorn GJ, Tudehope DI. Neonatal intestinal obstruction associated with oral calcium supplementation. *Aust Paediatr J.* 1981;17:298-299.

207. Hufnagle KG, Khan SN, Penn D, et al. Renal calcifications: a complication of long term furosemide therapy in preterm infants. *Pediatrics.* 1982;70:360-363.

208. Barth RA, Brasch RC, Filly RA. Abdominal pseudotumor in childhood: distended gallbladder with parenteral hyperalimentation. *Am J Roentgenol.* 1981;136:341-343.

209. Venkataraman PS, Han BK, Tsang RC, Daugherty CC. Secondary hyperparathyroidism and bone disease in infants receiving long term furosemide therapy. *Am J Dis Child.* 1983;137:1157-1161.

210. Koo WWK, Guan ZP, Tsang RC, et al. Growth failure and decreased bone mineral of newborn rats with chronic furosemide therapy. *Pediatr Res.* 1986;20:74-78.

211. Wasnich RD, Benfante RJ, Yano K, et al. Thiazide effect on the mineral content of bone. *N Engl J Med.* 1983;309:344-347.

212. Atkinson SA, Shah JK, McGee C, Steele BT. Mineral excretion in premature infants receiving various diuretic therapies. *J Pediatr.* 1988;113:540-545.

213. Diuretics. In: McEvoy GK, Litvak K, Welsh OH Jr, eds. *Drug Information. American Hospital Formulary Service.* Bethesda, MD: Amer Soc Health System Pharmacists; 1995:1776-1821.

214. Koo WWK, Kaplan LA. Aluminum and bone disorders: with specific reference to aluminum contamination of infant nutrients. *J Am Coll Nutr.* 1988;7:199-214.

215. Committee on Nutritional Misinformation. Hazards of overuse of vitamin D. *Am J Clin Nutr.* 1975;28:512-513.

216. Markestad T, Hesse V, Siebenhuner M, et al. Intermittent high-dose vitamin D prophylaxis during infancy: effect on vitamin D metabolites, calcium, and phosphorus. *Am J Clin Nutr.* 1987;46:652-658.

217. Jacobus CH, Holick MF, Shao Q, et al. Hypervitaminosis D associated with drinking milk. *N Engl J Med.* 1992; 326:1173-1177.

218. Misselwitz J, Hesse V, Markestad T. Nephrocalcinosis, hypercalciuria and elevated serum levels of 1,25-dihydroxyvitamin D in children. *Acta Paediatr Scand.* 1990; 79:637-643.

219. Marx SJ, Swart EG, Hamstra AJ, Deluca HF. Normal intrauterine development of the fetus of a woman receiving extraordinarily high doses of 1,25-dihydroxyvitamin D3. *J Clin Endocrinol Metab.* 1980;51: 1138-1142.

220. Goodenday LS, Gordon GS. No risk from vitamin D in pregnancy. *Ann Intern Med.* 1971;75:807-808.

221. Koo WWK. Laboratory assessment of nutritional metabolic bone disease in infants. *Clin Biochem.* 1996; 29:429-438

222. Rigo J, Senterre J. Metabolic balance studies and plasma amino acid concentrations in preterm infants fed experimental protein hydrolysate preterm formulas. *Acta Paediatr Scand.* 1994;405(suppl):98-104.

223. Loughead JL, Mimouni F, Tsang RC. Serum ionized calcium concentrations in normal neonates. *Am J Dis Child.* 1988;142:516-518.

224. Glorieux FH. Calcitriol treatment in vitamin D-dependent and vitamin D-resistant rickets. *Metabolism.* 1990;39:10-12.

225. Kruse K, Feldmann E. Healing of rickets during vitamin D therapy despite defective vitamin D receptors in two siblings with vitamin D-dependent rickets type II. *J Pediatr.* 1995;126:145-148.

Recognizing Deficiencies and Excesses
of Zinc, Copper and Other Trace Elements

Stephanie A. Atkinson Ph.D.[1], Stanley Zlotkin M.D., Ph.D.[2]

Department of Paediatrics, McMaster University, Hamilton, Ontario,[1]
Department of Paediatrics, University of Toronto, Division of Gastroenterology and Nutrition,[2]
The Hospital for Sick Children, Research Institute, Toronto, Ontario

Reviewed by Winston W. Koo M.B.B.S., Reginald C. Tsang M.B.B.S. and Michael Hambidge M.D., Sc.D.

Introduction

Quantitatively, trace elements make up a small fraction of the total mineral content of the human body, but they play key functional roles in numerous metabolic pathways. The current recommendations from Canadian[1] and U.S. agencies[2] for dietary intake of microelements for infants to two years of age are shown in Table 1. Recommendations vary between the countries and are not available for all microelements owing to lack of appropriate data upon which to base an estimate of physiologic need.

For infants in the first year of life, the micromineral content of human milk is the accepted "gold standard" upon which recommended intakes are based. However, when setting the standards for the micromineral content of formulas or other foods to be consumed by infants, consideration has to be given to the availability or coefficient of absorption of individual elements relative to human milk. Most microelements are more highly available for absorption from human milk than from cow's milk-based formula or other foods. Thus, the value based on breast milk composition is often adjusted upwards to account for a lower availability of mineral elements when the source of nutrition is cow's milk or soy-based formulas rather than breast milk.

Because of the ubiquitous nature of microelements, dietary deficiencies in normal free-living populations of infants in developed countries are uncommon. From a global perspective, however, deficiencies of iodine, zinc and perhaps selenium affect segments of the infant population that are concentrated in developing or emerging countries.

Clinical deficiencies have been described for zinc, copper, selenium, chromium, fluoride, iodine and manganese but not for molybdenum or cobalt. When deficien-cies occur, they are usually associated with specific clinical conditions that lead to malabsorptive losses due to a mal-functioning biliary tract or intestine; or to increased losses through urine or skin exudates. Excessive intakes of microelements are most often related to presence of the ele-ment due to contamination of the food source or environ-mental exposure. This chapter will discuss only those microelements that are of clinical relevance to the nutri-tional care of infants: zinc, copper, fluoride, selenium, iodine, chromium and manganese. We will also discuss aluminum and lead, which are of relevance to infant diets because of their potentially toxic effect .

Key Points

- *Globally, micronutrient deficiencies of iodine, zinc and perhaps selenium are responsible for a significant amount of morbidity among infants. In North America, such microelement deficiencies can occur in infants but diagnosis requires careful clinical detective work.*

- *Zinc deficiency should be considered a cause of growth restriction in premature infants, as well as in cases of severe chronic malabsorption, and in populations whose diets contain excessive iron or fiber. Copper deficiency, although rare, may be confused with iron deficiency and must be carefully investigated in populations at risk.*

- *Striking a balance of fluoride from dietary intake and dentifrices in growing children is important; both too little and too much can have significant clinical effects.*

- *Selenium, manganese and aluminum are potentially toxic microelements. Although clinical toxicity in infants is relatively uncommon,*

Element	Canadian			American		
Age mo.:	0-4	5-12	12-24	0-6	6-12	12-36
Zinc, mg/d	2	3	4	5	5	10
Fluoride, mg/d	0.25[4]	0.25	0.25	0.1-1[3]	0.1-1	0.5-1.5
Iodine, µg/d	30	40	55	40	50	70
Copper, mg/d	0.31-0.25[1]	–	–	0.4-0.6[3]	0.6-0.7	0.7-1.0
Selenium, µg/d	14[1]	–	–	10-40[3]	15	20
Chromium, µg/d	15[1]	–	–	0-40[3]	20-60	20-80
Manganese, mg/d	0.9-0.5[1]	–	–	0.3-0.6[1]	0.6-0.1	1.0-1.5
Molybdenum, mg/d	–[2]	–	–	15-30[3]	20-40	25-50

[1] Based on intakes from human milk
[2] No data to base a recommendation
[3] Range of intake reflects average reported intakes which are judged to be adequate and safe. In some
   cases, the values for infants are extrapolated from data in adults by adjusting for body weight.
[4] Fluoride is only recommended if the household water supply contains <0.3 mg/L of fluoride.

*Table 1: Current recommended dietary intakes for microelements for infants of two years of age based on Canadian[1]
and American[2] standards.*

Causes of Zinc Deficiency in Infants
Acrodermatitis enteropathica (genetic)
Reduced dietary intake from parenteral or synthetic diets
Prolonged malabsorption: • celiac disease • Crohn's disease
Low birthweight infants due to: • poor zinc sores • increased requirement for growth • prolonged intravenous nutrition containing inadequate zinc • abnormally low zinc content of mother's milk • supplements of Fe or Cu which compete with Zn for absorption

Table 2: Causes of zinc deficiency in infants.

*the situations in which infants might be subject to
excessive exposure are easily identifiable.*

• *Lead toxicity continues to be a clinical problem
in a large percentage of young children
(under age six years). Avoiding excessive lead
exposure from environmental contamination
(especially paint chips) should be stressed.*

Zinc

Zinc is an essential nutrient for growth and development; it plays major roles in bone structure, the structure and function of transcription factors and steroid receptors, and as a metalloenzyme. Zinc is contained in DNA-binding proteins in a formation called a zinc finger, where its function is to maintain the structure of the DNA-binding domain of the protein. Thus, zinc is essential for regulation of gene expression.[3] Regulatory proteins that contain these zinc fingers include estrogen and glucocorticoid receptors. Over two hundred zinc-metalloenzymes have been identified associated with carbohydrate and energy metabolism, protein catabolism and synthesis, nucleic acid synthesis, heme biosynthesis and other biological processes.[4]

Zinc is essential for embryogenesis and fetal growth, with most zinc being accrued in the fetus during the third trimester of pregnancy.[5] Fetal storage of zinc occurs principally in the liver bound to metallothionein – the major zinc-binding protein in both liver and intestinal mucosa.[6] Hepatic metallothionein appears to be mobilized in early life, since concentrations are lower in older compared to newborn infants.[6] Thus, this storage source of zinc may protect infants

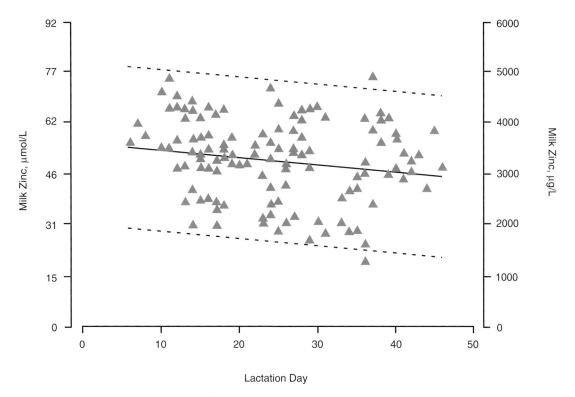

Figure 1: The concentration of zinc in milk of mother's giving birth prematurely with the mean + 2SD values indicated by the hatched lines. The decline in milk zinc (n=122 samples from 22 mothers) over time of lactation is described by the equation y=3592 (μg/L) - 14.0x, r=-0.18, p=0.05) (SA Atkinson, unpublished data).

from zinc deficiency during the first weeks of life when dietary intake of zinc is limited. Under normal circumstances, zinc homeostasis appears to be maintained primarily by changes in the fecal excretion of endogenous zinc through bile and pancreatic secretions; zinc secretion from intestinal cells; mucosal sloughing of desquamated cells; and dietary factors that influence the fractional absorption of zinc. The primary route of excretion of endogenous zinc is in the feces, with smaller quantities being excreted in the urine. The only exception is in the parenterally-fed infant, where the primary route of excretion is via the kidneys.[7]

The adequacy of dietary zinc depends on both the quantity and the relative availability of zinc for absorption. The concentration of zinc in human milk declines precipitously (60 to 22 μmol/L) over the first three months of lactation. Maternal intake of zinc does not appear to influence milk zinc content at least when maternal zinc intakes are adequate.[8] The availability of

dietary zinc for absorption is negatively influenced by the presence of phytate and fiber,[9] and the presence of other mineral elements[10] or exogenous glucocorticoid,[11] which might compete for uptake mechanisms across the brush border membrane. Zinc absorption from the intestine is enhanced by the presence of amino acids like histidine or cysteine.[12] At alkaline pH, phytate, zinc and calcium form an insoluble complex that retards zinc absorption. Thus, soy formulas containing phytate will inhibit dietary zinc absorption.[9] Zinc is better absorbed from human milk than from formula or cow milk.[13, 14] The difference in availability is likely due to the tight binding of zinc to casein, which is the predominant protein in cow milk.[15]

The now classic identification of zinc deficiency was in young boys in Iran and Egypt who demonstrated severe growth retardation, skin lesions and impaired sexual development.[16] In a recent review, Sanstead[17] concluded that on a global basis there is evidence to

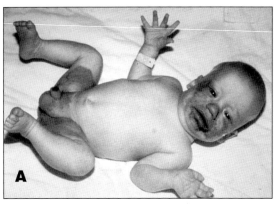 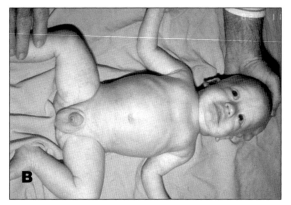

Figure 2: Infant of 2.5 months of age adjusted to term date who had been prematurely born at 33 weeks of gestation and fed primarily mother's milk from birth. Milk zinc content was 4.5 μmol/(293 μg)/L (normal value for stage of lactation (135 days post-partum) is 22±10 μmol (1430±650 μg)/L.[8] A. The extensive dermatitis over the cheeks, chin, nasolabial folds and pinnae and well demarcated and symmetrical erythema in the perineal region are classic signs of skin deficiency. An unhealed circumcision wound is also present. B. The same infant as in A. two weeks after receiving oral zinc supplements (Zinc sulfate providing 1 mg elemental zinc/kg/d) for one week.

support the hypothesis that zinc deficiency is sufficiently prevalent to be a public health problem, but more research is needed. The problems in identifying zinc deficiency relate to the difficulties in assessing zinc intake and bioavailability, the influence of host and environmental factors on zinc status, and the insensitivity of available laboratory methods to measure zinc status. The mechanisms by which zinc deficiency involves growth retardation are unknown. Zinc plays a possible role in cell proliferation, protein synthesis or somatogenic binding of growth hormone to liver cells.[3]

The most common causes of zinc deficiency observed in clinical pediatrics are listed in Table 2. In hospital populations, zinc deficiency should be contemplated in infants who have chronic diarrhea caused by malabsorptive states due to gastric or intestinal surgery. It should also be considered in infants who have excessive loss of endogenous zinc through intestinal secretions due to exocrine pancreatic insufficiency, biliary obstruction, ileostomy or hepatic disease. In diarrheal states, the deficiency occurs because gut proteases are metalloproteins that bind zinc, and these are lost with rapid intestinal transit. Excessive non-intestinal zinc losses may occur with high output renal failure and diuretic therapy or severe exfoliative dermatoses. In these cases zinc intakes may have to be doubled or even tripled, depending on the volume and concentration of the losses.[18]

Inadequate dietary intake of zinc is not a common cause of zinc deficiency in North America. There are case reports of both preterm[19] and term infants,[20-22] who developed frank zinc deficiency while being breast-fed. In most cases the zinc content of the mother's milk was found to be about 30% of the normal value expected for mature human milk.[19] Figure 1 depicts the mean and 95% confidence interval for milk zinc over the first six weeks of lactation in mothers of prematurely born infants (Atkinson SA, unpublished). Infants weaned to pure vegan (non-animal product) diets[23] or those who have been fed for extensive periods by zinc-free intravenous nutrition or refined enteral diets may also be at risk for zinc deficiency. In the latter instance, most commercial products now contain zinc in amounts to meet normal infant needs. If there are increased demands for zinc because of rapid growth or excessive losses as described above, then supplemental zinc may be required.

The clinical effects of zinc deficiency include growth failure, diminished food intake, skin lesions, poor wound healing, hair loss, decreased protein synthesis and depressed immune function. Disturbances of smell and taste are attributed to zinc deficiency. Figure 2 shows an infant who has zinc deficiency symptoms before and after oral zinc supplementation.[19] This picture typifies the classic presentation of zinc deficiency

Clinical Evaluation		
	Mild	Extreme
Skin Manifestations	None	Typical rash
Dietary Intake	Decreased	Very low
Losses (urine or stool)	Increased	Excessive
Laboratory Evaluation		
	Mild	Extreme
Serum zinc	Normal or borderline low	Low (< 10.7 µmol/L)
Alkaline phosphatase	Normal	Low (< 175 U/L)
Urine excretion	Normal	Low

Table 3: Clinical and laboratory evaluation of zinc deficiency.

associated with the genetic disorder acrodermatitis enteropathica of a periorifical and extensor dermatitis, which is vesiculobullour, pustular and hyperkeratotic in nature.[14] Delayed healing of a circumcision in this case suggests impaired immune function.

Cases of severe zinc deficiency are relatively easy to diagnose because of the severity of the clinical and biochemical presentation (Table 3). In addition to the symptoms described above, plasma zinc concentrations and alkaline phosphatase activity are usually below normal. A low serum zinc may also reflect zinc sequestration in tissue due to infections or other stressors such as endotoxins, starvation or glucocorticoids. This redistribution of body zinc is likely mediated by interleukin-1, which stimulates the synthesis of metallothionein; metallothionein in turn sequesters zinc in tissues such as liver and bone.[24] Unfortunately, biochemical confirmation of subclinical zinc deficiency is not easy. The only definitive method of diagnosing zinc deficiency is to carefully consider the plasma zinc concentration in relation to other metabolic and clinical indicators and to monitor the clinical and biochemical response to zinc supplementation.

The treatment of zinc deficiency is oral zinc sulfate at 0.05 mmol (3 mg)/kg bodyweight/day until serum zinc returns to the normal range and clinical symptoms resolve.

Toxicity of zinc is rare but has been described in one 18-month-old girl who ingested tinning paint which caused almost total necrosis of her stomach wall with some perforations.[25] The tinning paint contained 19% zinc chloride that can be corrosive to the gastrointestinal tract when ingested in large quantities. Gastric lavage with water or milk to remove the ingested zinc salts and maintaining fluid and electrolyte balance are the most important therapies.[26] In adults, zinc toxicity has occurred after food poisoning due to presumed leaching of zinc from galvanized pots used to prepare foods or liquid refreshments[27] or due to ingestion of large doses of zinc salts.[28] The acute symptoms include nausea, vomiting, fever, irritability and drowsiness.[29] Caution is advised in not over-treating zinc deficiency in infants with careful monitoring to keep serum zinc within normal limits. If toxicity does occur it should be treated with chelation therapy such as desferroxamine.

Copper

Fetal accretion of copper is approximately 50 µg/kg/day.[5] The fetal liver concentration is reported to be 16 times greater than that found in the adult,[5] providing a reserve of copper that is available to the term infant in early post-natal life. Other than in the fetus, concentrations of copper in the liver are constant throughout life, except in disease states or deficiency. Copper homeostasis is regulated via absorption and excretion through the pancreas and gastric mucosa. Although the exact mechanisms for copper absorption have not been delineated, it appears to share

Etiologies of Copper Deficiency
Menkes' disease - genetic defect in copper absorption by the intestine and the liver
Low birth weight: • low body stores at birth and failure to accrue copper at intrauterine rates
Extended parenteral nutrition if copper added in insufficient amounts
Early feeding with cow milk
Severe antecedent malnutirition due to malabsorption and diarrhea, giardiasis, short bowel syndrome or celiac disease
Excess dietary zinc or iron causing reduced absorption of copper (metal-metal interaction)

Table 4: Etiologies of copper deficiency.[41]

Clinical Manifestations	Laboratory Evaluation
Skin hypopigmentation	Osteoporosis of bones on X-ray
Bone fractures	Retarded bone age
Hepatosplenomegaly	Neutropenia
	Hypochromic microcytosis
	Low plasma copper (< 6.3 µmol/L)
	Low ceruloplasmin (< 130 mg/L)

Table 5: Clinical and laboratory evaluation of copper deficiency.

some of the transport and mucosal cell storage (on metallothionein) steps with zinc, a cation with similar coordination chemistry.[30] The liver also plays a key role in copper homeostasis. Excess albumin-bound copper from the intestine enters the liver where it induces metallothionein, a metal-binding protein with high affinity for copper. When copper is needed by tissues, the liver releases it bound to ceruloplasmin for transport.

Copper, like zinc, is an essential constituent of many enzymes. Of special importance are the copper-dependent oxidative enzymes, including cytochrome oxidase, the terminal oxidase in the electron transport chain. The most abundant copper-containing enzymes are the superoxide dismutase enzymes which protect cell membranes against oxidative damage. Ceruloplasmin, which has ferroxidase activity, accounts for about 60% of the copper in plasma and interstitial fluids. Its main function is copper transport; but it also has important antioxidant and enzymatic functions. Copper deficiency can lead to anemia since ceruloplasmin appears to play a role in iron transport from hepatic storage sites to transferrin; it functions as a ferroxidase for the conversion of ferric to ferrous iron prior to the attachment of iron to transferrin.[31, 32] While the ferroxidase role of copper-containing ceruloplasmin has not been accepted universally, new clinical evidence for mutations of the ceruloplasmin gene has demonstrated an aceruloplasminemia that is associated with low serum iron and high tissue iron stores.[33] This rare genetic defect in ceruloplasmin biosynthesis offers the opportunity for further investigations of the interrelationships between iron and copper.[34]

In the United States and presumably all developed countries, copper deficiency is not a major public health problem, and occurs only in overt dietary deficiency such as parenteral nutrition or general malnutrition.[35] High dietary zinc can also induce excessive loss of copper through the intestine; this has been described in one infant.[36] Other etiologies of copper deficiency in infants less than two years of age are summarized in Table 4. Early feeding of cow's milk[37] or use of copper-free parenteral formulations[38, 39] have been the cause of copper depletion in infants. Most reported cases of copper deficiency are in premature infants.[40, 41]

Antagonistic interactions between iron, zinc and copper have the potential to reduce copper absorption. Iron-fortified formulas (at 7-14 mg iron/L) fed to infants in the first six months of life have been associated with significantly reduced copper absorption[42] and lower plasma copper[43]; in preterm infants, these formulas have resulted in a significant reduction in erythrocyte copper zinc superoxide dismutase.[44] Although prolonged high iron intakes might precipitate clinical manifestations of copper deficiency, this has never been described.

Menkes' disease is probably the most recognized cause of copper deficiency. Although rare, this x-linked defect in absorption, utilization and transport of dietary copper leads to cerebral and cerebellar degeneration, deficiency of melanin in skin and abnormalities in connective tissue associated with arterial aneurism and steely, spiky hair.[45] At present, there is no treatment for Menkes' disease and children die in their early years.[45]

As noted above, hereditary ceruloplasmin deficiency as a rare autosomal recessive condition has recently been described.[33] Clinical presentation includes diabetes, retinal degeneration, galactorrhea, mental confusion, cerebrallar ataxia and dementia. Curiously, low serum iron and excessive storage of iron in liver, brain, pancreas and other tissues were not associated with abnormal hemoglobin.[33]

Neutropenia and anemia are the two most prominent symptoms of copper deficiency, although other manifestations can occur (Table 5). Copper deficiency-induced neutropenia, (usually $<1.0 \times 10^9/L$) first described in 1966,[37] may result from altered cellular differentiation or turnover, but more research is required to clarify copper's role in this immune process.[35] Anemia results when ceruloplasmin is unavailable as a transporter of the ferrous form of iron from stores to the bone marrow. The hypochromic anemia of copper deficiency is unresponsive to iron therapy . Early radiological features are osteoporosis of the metaphysis and retarded bone age. The bone changes are a consequence of impaired collagen and elastin synthesis, because the enzyme involved, lysyl oxidase, is copper-dependent, it limits collagen synthesis. Hypopigmentation is likely a result of impaired melanin synthesis due to low tyrosinase activity – a copper-dependent enzyme.

Nutritional copper deficiency can be reversed with oral intakes of about 4-5 µmol/kg/d (290 µg/kg/d).[41] Intravenous copper treatment has been given at 0.79 µmol/kg/d (50 µg/kg/d).[41] A response in erythropoiesis has been observed within one to two weeks after initiating copper supplementation and a rise in neutrophil count within five days.[41] Healing of osteoporosis or fractures has been seen after only one month of therapy. In deficiency, the plasma copper concentration is usually < 6.3 µmol/L (<40 µg/dl) and ceruloplasmin is < 130 mg/L.

Age, year	Fluoride Concentration of Principal Drinking Water Source (ppm)		
	< 0.3	0.3-0.6	> 0.6
6 mo - 3	0.25	0	0
>3-6	0.5	0.25	0
>6-16	1.0	0.5	0

Table 6: Dosage schedule for dietary fluoride supplements (mg/day).[54]

Accidental copper toxicity has not been described in infants. Since copper's main route of excretion is bile, hepatic cholestasis is an indication to eliminate copper from parenteral or enteral feeding.[46]

Wilson's disease, an autosomal recessive disorder of copper accumulation in liver, brain, kidney and the eye, represents a copper toxicity state. The excessive copper in tissue occurs because of a defect in the hepatic excretion of copper through the bile. To attenuate the neurological manifestations of Wilson's disease, D-penicillamine was used since the late 1950s[47] as a copper-chelating agent which enhances copper excretion from the urine; unfortunately there are many toxic side effects with penicillamine.[48] Brewer, working in the lab of Ananda Prasad,[48] discovered that large doses of zinc reduced 24-urinary copper excretion, non-ceruloplasmin copper and liver copper.[49] Zinc acts as a copper detoxicant by inducing intestinal cell metallothionein; this complexes copper with high affinity, preventing it from being absorbed into the blood and ensuring that it is lost in the feces through mucosal sloughing.[50]

Fluoride

Fluoride in drinking water, toothpaste, mouthwash and processed food is credited with major reductions in cavities.[51] Fluoride concentration in breast milk is relatively constant (< 5 µg/L) and not influenced by the fluoride intake of lactating women.[52] It has been well demonstrated that infants who ingest fluoride from any source from an early age have fewer dental caries (including caries of deciduous teeth) than those who do not ingest fluoride at all or who start fluoride at a later age.[53] There is controversy about the degree of protection offered

---

Fluoride Supplementation Guidelines[55]

1) The Nutritional Committee continues to support the principle of universal community water fluoridation.

2) Supplementation is recommended (at the dosage schedule outlined in Table 6) for infants from age six months living in homes which do not have access to fluoridated community water supplies.

3) All parents should be warned of the dangers of excessive fluoride ingestion.

4) Manufacturers of fluoride containing dentifrices targeted to infants and children should be encouraged to:
   - lower the concentration of fluoride in the product manufacture tubes which make it more difficult to place excessive amounts of dentifrice on a toothbrush
   - label fluoride products with the specific fluoride concentration
   - include a warning that children under six years of age should use only a pea-sized portion,
   - should spit out after brushing, should avoid swallowing the paste, and should rinse thoroughly afterward.

Table 7: Fluoride supplementation guidelines.[55]

when fluoride is started at different ages; however, if fluoride is not given in the first three years of life, there will likely be a small increase in the prevalence of dental caries in school-aged children living in households with unfluoridated water supplies.[54]

The supplemental fluoride dosage schedule is shown in Table 6.[54-56] Compared with earlier schedules,[57] the age of introducing fluoride supplements is later (six months versus first few months), the initial dose is lower (0.25 mg/day) and continues for a longer period of time (three versus two years); an intermediate dose (0.5 mg/day) is recommended for children three to six years of age; the dose for older children is unchanged, but continues until an older age (16 versus 12 years). The later introduction of fluoride supplements at lower dosages reflects a recognition that mild dental fluorosis (Figure 3) is increasing in North America.[53, 58, 59] Similar to the previous recommendations, the general principles for avoiding toxicity yet providing an appropriate

amount of dietary fluoride were reaffirmed in the 1994 and 1995 reports. These principles are outlined in Table 7.

The new dosage schedule recognizes the potential impact of increased fluoride intake on dental fluorosis during this vulnerable age, yet acknowledges the need to provide fluoride for caries prevention in populations without fluoridated water supplies. Monitoring trends in dental fluorosis is important. If the rate of moderate/severe fluorosis increases, a further modification of the dosage schedule may be necessary.

Selenium

Selenium is an element which is essential for its antioxidant activity in biological systems, as part of the selenium-dependent enzyme glutathione peroxidase. This enzyme is one of the body's principal cellular defense mechanisms against cytotoxic active oxygen species (H_2O_2, $\cdot O_2^-$, $HO_2\cdot$) which are produced as part of normal metabolism. Selenium, through this enzyme, is involved in cell membrane protection from peroxidase damage by detoxification of these peroxides and free radicals.[60] Thyroid function is dependent on another selenoprotein, the deiodenase enzyme, that converts thyroid hormone (T4) to triiodothyroxine (T3 – the active form of the hormone).[61]

It was only in the early 1960s that selenium was first recognized as an essential nutrient. This microelement has gained prominence in the clinical nutrition field in recent years because of the recognition that there are areas where the earth is selenium-deficient; thus, transfer of this element through foods and up the food chain into major food products such as milk can be affected by the selenium available in agricultural areas. Selenium is now recognized to be a protective factor against oxidative stress, particularly in relation to heart disease and drug metabolism.[62] Selenium may also be a dietary factor that plays a preventive role in cancer.[63]

Selenium from human and cow milk and infant formula is well-absorbed by infants. Plasma selenium appears to decrease from birth to four months and then rise to a plateau at about 20 years,[64] although infants who are born premature appear to have a greater nadir in plasma selenium and glutathione peroxidase activity compared to infants born at term.[65, 66] In some areas of the world the selenium content of infant formula may be lower than that of human milk because the milk protein source comes from cows grazing in areas of low selenium soil content; in such situations there may be differences in selenium status among infants fed breast milk, commercial formula or cow's milk.[67, 68] Selenium intakes from North American infant formulas may be lower (0.09 µmol/d) than from breast milk (0.12 µmol/d), and the breast-fed infant generally has higher plasma selenium and glutathionine peroxidase activities.[69] However, the lower intakes have not been associated with clinical signs of selenium deficiency.[70, 71] Some formula manufacturers add selenium salts during processing, but the need for this in areas where there is adequate selenium in the soil remains questionable. The exception to this is for therapeutic formulas of low protein content (see discussion of selenium deficiency that follows.) The amount of selenium in human milk should be used as a guide for the concentration of selenium in commercial formulas.

Selenium deficiency is associated with Keshan's disease, which presents as a cardiomyopathy of endemic proportions in selenium-deficient zones of China. The first severe outbreak of this disease was in 1935 in Keshan County, Heilongjiang Province.[72] Keshan's disease presents as acute or chronic bouts of heart disorder with cardiogenic shock and/or congestive heart failure.

Aside from the Keshan form found in populations living in areas of low selenium soil content, selenium deficiency has been described in several clinical case reports[73-80] associated with the clinical situations outlined in Table 8. Because of the purity of the crystalline amino acid solutions and of the components of current hyperalimentation solutions, selenium does not occur even in small amounts as a contaminant. Current recommendations for trace elements required for parenteral nutrition for infants do not include selenium as a standard addition.[46] However, based on recent case reports,[79, 81] there is reason to add selenium to parenteral nutrition solutions of infants who require long-term intravenous support (see problem set on selenium deficiency at the end of the chapter).

In infants and young children maintained on low protein diets to treat phenylketonuria or maple syrup urine disease, or in those with general malnutrition,

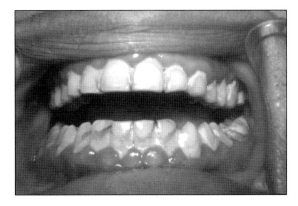

Figure 3: Dental flourosis. Note opaque appearance of the enamel, as well as the extensively discolored, pitted areas.

plasma selenium is lower than that of healthy infants and children.[82, 83] Therapeutic formulas to treat such disorders should have selenium added in the same amount as present in the human milk of selenium-sufficient mothers. Selenium deficiency was also observed in association with generalized protein-energy malnutrition in hospitalized patients[84] and children with kwashiorkor and marasmus.[85, 86]

Selenium deficiency presents clinically with loss of skin and hair pigmentation (pseuodoalbinism) and sometimes motor function difficulties indicative of skeletal myopathy (Table 8). Macrocytosis,[77] and abnormalities in the biochemistry and functioning of red cells and granulocytes,[76, 87] are the biochemical indices of selenium deficiency (Table 8). The molecular basis of the pseudoalbinism and macrocytosis is currently unknown. Whether the selenoprotein glutathione peroxidase which is an antioxidant protector of cells has a role in bone marrow or the melanocyte is open to speculation.

Plasma selenium is the most practical and widely used measure to assess selenium status (Tables 8 and 9). Activity of selenium glutathione peroxidase in whole blood (which contains about 12 to 15% of the total plasma selenium in humans[88]) is also a sensitive indicator of selenium status,[43] although it can be derived in part from the peroxidase activity of hemoglobin.

Achieving the appropriate balance of selenium in the diet is important since it can also be a toxic element. In fact, selenium was regarded as a toxic element[89] long before it was accepted as nutritionally essential. Most

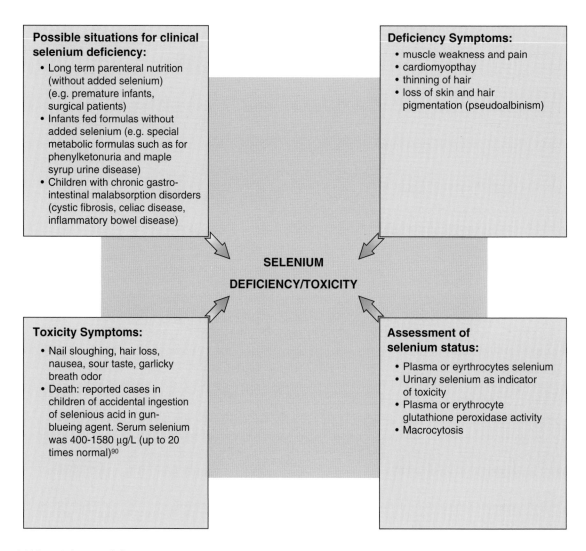

Possible situations for clinical selenium deficiency:

- Long term parenteral nutrition (without added selenium) (e.g. premature infants, surgical patients)
- Infants fed formulas without added selenium (e.g. special metabolic formulas such as for phenylketonuria and maple syrup urine disease)
- Children with chronic gastro-intestinal malabsorption disorders (cystic fibrosis, celiac disease, inflammatory bowel disease)

Deficiency Symptoms:

- muscle weakness and pain
- cardiomyopthay
- thinning of hair
- loss of skin and hair pigmentation (pseudoalbinism)

SELENIUM DEFICIENCY/TOXICITY

Toxicity Symptoms:

- Nail sloughing, hair loss, nausea, sour taste, garlicky breath odor
- Death: reported cases in children of accidental ingestion of selenious acid in gun-blueing agent. Serum selenium was 400-1580 µg/L (up to 20 times normal)[90]

Assessment of selenium status:

- Plasma or eyrthrocytes selenium
- Urinary selenium as indicator of toxicity
- Plasma or erythrocyte glutathione peroxidase activity
- Macrocytosis

Table 8: Selenium deficiency/toxicity.

selenium toxicity relates to occupational exposure to selenium aerosols in copper smelters or selenium-rectifier plants,[62] but accidental ingestion of gun blueing solutions containing 2% selenious acid did result in non-fatal acute poisoning in a two-year-old child.[90] The clinical signs of selenium toxicity include: garlic odour of the breath, skin eruptions, pathologic nails, hair loss, dyspepsia, diarrhea and anorexia.[64] To protect infants and children against selenium toxicity, one must guard against inappropriate use of selenium supplements or accidental consumption of concentrated selenium products such as gun blueing solutions or selenium sulfide-containing antidandruff shampoos.[64]

Chromium

Chromium is involved in preventing glucose intolerance as it is part of, or necessary for, a "glucose tolerance factor." This chromium-containing glucose tolerance factor (GTF) is described as being a water-soluble component of liver, blood and plasma as well as other biologic cells, where it appears to take up glucose and potentiate insulin action. The role of chromium in glucose homeostasis is the only biological role currently known.

There have been no studies on chromium absorption by infants and only a few in adults. Adults are said to absorb less than 2% of a chromium load.

Chromium is excreted primarily via the urine, with excretion rates reflecting dietary intake.[92]

The concentration of chromium in cow milk and formula based on cow milk (15 μg (288 nmol) /L) is considerably higher than human milk which is 0.3-0.5 μg (5-10 nmol) /L.[92, 93] Since infants fed formula with significantly higher amounts of chromium have not developed overt toxicity, there is likely a wide "safe range of intake."

The recommended parenteral intake of chromium is 0.2 μg (3.8 nmol) /kg/day for the preterm infant.[46] This recommendation was based on the dose known to prevent chromium deficiency in adults on long-term parenteral nutrition (0.3 μg (5.7 nmol) /kg/day), and the realization that infants fed human milk only receive about 0.05 μg (1 nmol) /kg/day. No adverse effects have been reported in infants receiving this amount of chromium. Since chromium is primarily excreted via the kidneys, the dosage should be lowered in the presence of decreased renal output.

Although chromium deficiency has been described in three adult patients on long-term chromium-free parenteral nutrition,[94, 95] no documentation of chromium deficiency has been described in the pediatric population. There are no satisfactory laboratory methods to assess chromium status because contamination of samples readily occurs.

Trivalent chromium has a very low order of toxicity.[96] However, elevated urinary losses and/or serum chromium occurred in young children receiving long-term supplemental chromium, and values did not return to normal even one year after discontinuation of the high chromium intake.[97] The physiological significance of prolonged excessive accumulation of chromium in the body is not known. Thus, chromium in intravenous solutions should be monitored.

Manganese

Manganese is an essential element because of its role in several metabolic functions: 1) activation of the gluconeogenic enzymes pyruvate carboxylase and isocitrate dehydrogenase; 2) part of superoxide dismutase, which functions to protect mitochondrial membranes; and 3) activation of glycosyl transferase, which is involved in mucopolysaccharide synthesis.

Although it is difficult to accurately measure manganese absorption (stable isotope tracers are not available), estimates derived from classical balance studies are about 43% for mean relative retention of dietary manganese.[98] This may underestimate true absorption, since manganese is primarily excreted through the biliary tract with urine excretion only a minor route.

Manganese deficiency has not been identified in children except for the case of a female infant with short-bowel syndrome.[99] There is no readily available laboratory test that measures manganese status.

Intake of manganese from infant formula is more than ten times that from breast milk.[98] The few studies of manganese balance in infants have determined that retention of manganese from formula is positive[98, 100] but from human milk is negative.[101] However, there is no evidence that the higher manganese retention from formula is in any way deleterious to human infants.

The only clinical indication to limit manganese intake (usually from parenteral nutrition solutions) is in neonates with immature liver function or hepatic cholestasis.[46] Since bile is the major excretory route for manganese, cholestasis could lead to excessive accumulation. There is concern that excessive body burden with manganese may lead to an accumulation in the brain, possibly causing a Parkinson-like syndrome.[102]

Iodine

The only known role of iodine is in thyroid function where it is part of the tri- and tetraidothyronines (T3 and T4) which are 60% iodine by weight. In the intestinal tract, dietary iodine is converted to I⁻ prior to absorption. Iodine is stored in the thyroid gland and, following peroxidation, becomes attached to the tyrosine residues of thyroglobulin. Iodine deficiency

> *The ornithologists have long recognized that they cannot learn much by studying birds in cages. But doctors and nurses are still doing that.*
>
> Primary Health Care Pioneer
> The Selected works of
> Dr. Cicely D. Williams
> Naomi Baumslag, Editor
> World Federation of
> Public Health Associations
> and UNICEF

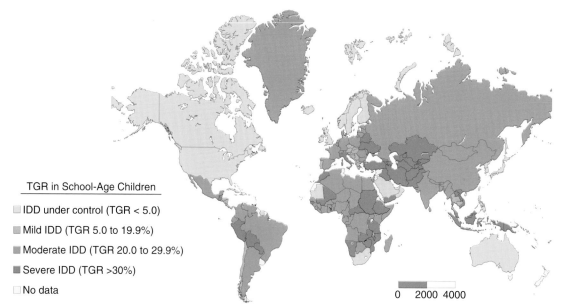

Figure 4: Global distribution of the prevalence of iodine deficiency disorders (IDD). Note that iodine deficiency disorders are under control only in the highly developed countries comprising North America, Scandinavia, United Kingdom, Australia, New Zealand, Japan and the Middle East. (reprinted with permission from Global Prevalence of Iodine Deficiency Disorders, MDIS Working Paper #1, WHO, Geneva, Switzerland). TGR = Total Goiter Rate.

depresses the production of thyroid hormones, especially T4. The physiological response to iodine deficiency in humans is increased thyroid-stimulating hormone (TSH) secretion, thyroid hyperplasia and hypertrophy, increased thyroid iodine uptake, and increased secretion ratio of triiodothyronine (T3) relative to T4.

The content of iodine in human milk is variable depending on the dietary intake of the mother. The average iodine content of mature human milk in European mothers is 70-90 µg (0.5-0.7 µmol)/L, while in the United States the iodine content is higher at 140-180 µg (1.1-1.4 µmol)/L. An American infant ingesting 150 mL/kg/day of breast milk will receive iodine at about 24 µg (0.2 µmol)/kg/day. Formulas based on cow milk are said to contain about (335 µg (2.6 µmol)/L) or 50 µg(0.4 µmol)/100 kcal as recently recommended.[103] The average iodine content of cow milk (415 µg (3.3 µmol)/L) is about three times higher than that found in human milk, but may vary from <100 to >1,300 µg (0.8-10 µmol)/L.[104] Much of the iodine present in milk comes from ethylenediamine dihydroiodide (EDDI), added to feed to pre-

vent footrot in cattle[105] and from improper use of iodophor sanitizers.[106]

Endemic goiter occurs in specific areas (Figure 4) throughout the world when dietary iodine intake is less than 15 µg(0.12 µmol)/day. Maternal iodide deficiency during pregnancy leads to cretinism in infancy. Overt cretinism is said to occur in about 5 to 15% of cases of endemic neonatal goiter. Milder degrees of iodine deficiency both *in utero* and after birth may occur and have detrimental effects on growth and intellectual performance, even in the absence of more severe manifestations.[107] Endemic goiter is not a problem in North America due to the mandatory addition of iodine to table salt.

Excess iodine intake can cause hypothyroidism, and newborn infants may be particularly sensitive to the effects of iodine excess. Even in the infant who receives no iodine by mouth (or parenterally), excessive iodine may be absorbed through the skin from topical disinfectants, detergents and other sources.[108, 109] Cutaneous application of povidone-iodine at the time of delivery resulted in excess transfer of iodine to the infant via breast milk with resulting compensated hypothyroidism.[108] Despite this theoretical risk of toxicity,

Element	Laboratory Test	Acceptable Range
Aluminum	Serum aluminum	<13.5 µg/L (0.5 µmol)
Chromium	None readily available	
Flouride	None readily available	
Iodine	T3, T4, TSH for thyroid function	T3, 1.4-4.1 nmol/L T4, 65-200 nmol/L TSH <5 mU/L
Lead	Plasma lead	<10 µg/dl (0.48 µmol/L)
Manganese	None readily available	
Selenium	Plasma/serum selenium Red blood cell glutathione peroxidase	40-100 ng/ml (0.5-0.75 µmol/L) 6-9 U/g HB

Table 9: Biochemical assessment of trace elements.

iodine intakes of up to 1,000 µg(7.8 µmol)/day in children have not resulted in deleterious outcomes. In view of the potential detrimental effects of high intakes of iodine on thyroid function, intakes in excess of 1,000 µg(7.8 µmol)/day should be avoided.

Biochemical assessment of iodine status includes measures of the hormones T3, T4 and TSH (Table 9).

Aluminum

Aluminum is well known to be toxic when excessive amounts accumulate within the body. The low rate of intestinal absorption of aluminum (about 2% of intake in adults) acts as a protective barrier when aluminum is orally ingested. Aluminum excreted in the urine, the major excretory site, usually represents about 1% of oral intake.[110] In theory, the more permeable immature intestines of infants may facilitate greater absorption of aluminum, but this has never been proven in studies. The kidneys are the main route for aluminum excretion. The combination of "low output" renal failure and high aluminum intake (as is aluminum-containing phosphate binders) may lead to a toxic accumulation of aluminum in the body. The issues with respect to aluminum in pediatric populations were sufficient to warrant a statement from the American Academy of Pediatrics in 1986.[111]

The major source of dietary aluminum in infant diets is from parenteral nutrition solutions. Crystalline amino acid solutions are relatively free of aluminum (in contrast to higher concentrations found in casein hydrolysate solutions used in the past).[112, 113] The major sources of parenteral aluminum currently are calcium and phosphorus salts, since they contain relatively high amounts of aluminum derived as a contaminant from the native sources for the salts (Table 10). An alternate calcium/phosphorus salt, calcium glycerophosphate, has been found to have one-fifth the concentration of aluminum found in commercially available salts,[101] but this product is not marketed by any pharmaceutical company. In a study by Atkinson et al,[101] aluminum intake and excretion were significantly lower in prematurely born infants receiving calcium glycerophosphate than with intravenous calcium gluconate and potassium mono and dibasic phosphate salts.

While the amount of aluminum absorbed by infants from orally ingested foods is unknown, it should be noted that some infant formulas are significantly higher in their aluminum content. The data summarized in Table 10 demonstrate that human milk and cow milk have similar aluminum concentrations and that standard cow milk-based infant formula is only slightly higher in aluminum. However, specialty formulas (e.g., soy) and premature infant formulas, which have calcium and phosphorus added to them, have considerably higher amounts of aluminum.[114] Indirect evidence is available that despite much higher intakes from premature infant formulas, the amount of aluminum absorbed is minimally different, since renal excretion of

Parenteral Solutions	µg/L (µmol/L)	Reference
Potassium phosphate (3 mmol/L)	16,598 (615)	112
Sodium phosphate (3mmol/L)	5,977 (222)	112
Calcium gluconate (10%)	5,056 (187)	112
Calcium glucoheptonate	3.645 (135)	113
Magnesium sulphate	944	115
Multivitamin infusate	890 (33)	113
Heparin (1000 U/mL)	684 (25)	112
Calcium gluconate + potassium phosphate (in parenteral nutrition solution)	304 (11)	101
Calcium glycerophosphate (in parenteral nutrition solution)	50 (1.8)	101
Enteral Feedings		
Human milk	9.9±6.8 (0.36±0.25)	114
Cow milk	<50 µg/L (1.8)	114
Soy formula	1,478±103 (55±3.8)	114
Premature formula (Ross LBW)	699±321 (26±12)	114
Standard cow milk-based formula	266±92 (10±3)	114

Table 10: Aluminum content of nutrient sources used for the parenteral and enteral feeding of infants (mean±SD).

aluminum did not respond as it did with higher intravenous infusions of this element (Atkinson SA, unpublished). The American Academy of Pediatrics[111] recommends an intake of elemental aluminum <30 mg/kg/day, pending further evaluation of safe doses.

From a clinical perspective, only infants who have been maintained on long-term parenteral nutrition may be at risk of a high body burden of aluminum. This is easily detected by measuring serum aluminum concentrations. Values for serum aluminum greater than 0.5 µmol/L (13.5 µg/L) should be considered abnormal.[115] The major organ involved in aluminum toxicity is the brain, leading to encephalopathy (degenerative disease of the brain), although this condition has only been found in association with renal disease and not parenteral feeding. In the bone where aluminum interferes with normal mineralization, aluminum has been shown to accumulate at the mineralization front in infants.[116, 117] Aluminum-induced osteomalacia was observed in infants and children maintained on long-term parenteral nutrition.[112, 117] The only known treatment to decrease body aluminum is the use of deferoxamine.[118, 119] The efficacy of this treatment can be assessed by measuring for an increase in urinary aluminum and/or fall in serum aluminum (Table 9). However, deferoxamine must be used with caution because chelation of other essential trace elements may also occur, and hypocalcemia has been reported.[120]

Lead

In children as young as two years, lead absorption was measured at 32% of intake.[121] The toxic effects of lead are manifest in abnormalities in haeme synthesis, the kidney and the nervous system.[122] The latter include damage to the peripheral nervous system as well as cognitive deficits and encephalopathy.[123-126] As illustrated in Table 11, the severity of the neurologocal effects are directly related to blood lead levels. Higher levels are associated with more severe neurological, renal and gastrointestinal pathology. Lead (Pb^{2+}) has the ability to displace Ca^{2+} from cell membranes, causing loss of structured and functional integrity. Lead may interact with sulfhydryl groups on enzymes[127] and is readily transported into cells.[128] Lead may also act directly on neurons, blood vessels, blood brain barrier and synaptic functions.[129]

There are no known specific physiologic needs for lead. Thus, toxicity rather than deficiency is of greatest clinical concern.

> *Zinc has finally gained intrauterine and extrauterine respectability.*
> Robert M. Suskind M.D.
> Louisiana State University
> School of Medicine
> New Orleans, Louisiana

Lowest observed effect level (PbB)[a] (ug/dL)	Heme synthesis and hematological effects	Neurological and related effects	Renal system effects	Gastrointestinal effects
80-100		Encephalopathic signs and symptoms	Chronic nephropathy (aminoaciduria, etc.)	Colic and other overt gastrointestinal symtpoms ↓
70	Frank anemia			
60		Peripheral neuropathies		
50		↓ ?		
40	Reduced hemoglobin synthesis	Peripheral nerve dysfunction (slowed NCVs) CNS cognitive effects (IQ deficits, etc.)		
30			Vit. D metabolism interference	
15	Erythrocyte protoporphyrin elevation	Altered CNS electro-physiological responses		
10	ALA-D inhibition ↓ Py-5-N[b] activity ↓ ?	Mental Development Index deficits, reduced gestational age and birth weight (prenatal exposure) ↓		

[a] PbB = Blood lead concentration
[b] Py-5-N = Pyrimidine-5-nucleotidase
Source: US Department of Health and Human Services Agency for Toxic Substances and Disease Registry, 1990; ATSDR publ TP-88/17 (Reproduced from Reference 126) (Reproduced with permission)

Table 11: Summary of lowest observed effect levels of key lead-induced health effects in children.

Low-level lead exposure is the most common environmental threat during childhood. Lead is ubiquitous in our environment: air, water, dust, and soil contain varying amounts. Ingestion from lead-containing folk remedies and cooking utensils has also been associated with elevated body lead levels.[130] Prospective studies in children have identified deleterious clinical outcomes resulting from low lead exposure (reviewed in AAP).[131]

National estimates from the USA suggest that 17% of all children under the age of six have blood lead concentrations >7.2 μmol/L (150 μg/L).[132] There is controversy regarding the blood levels at which lead adversely alters neurobehavioural development. The current blood lead concentration identified with low dose lead exposure in children by the Centers for Disease Control is >0.48 μmol/L (10 μg/dl) (Table 9). Previously, blood lead >2 μmol/L (40 μg/dl) was the cut-off for association with harmful side effects. Excessive lead exposure in children is primarily related to environmental contamination from pica, especially where paint chips are being consumed.[133]

Approaches to Assessment of Trace Element Status

Although eight trace minerals are known to be nutritionally essential to man, trace mineral deficiencies are not commonly detected in clinical practice. To determine whether a child is at risk of a trace mineral defi-

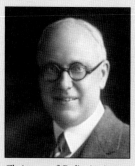

Williams McK. Marriott Ph.D., M.D.

(1885-1936) received his degrees from Cornell Medical School. Marriott joined the Department of Biochemistry at the Medical School of Washington University in 1910. Howland came to Washington U. as Chairman of Pediatrics in 1911 but left for Hopkins after six months. Marriott joined Howland at the Harriet Lane Home in 1914. The collaboration with Howland resulted in discovery of the acidosis of diarrhea and hypocalcemia of tetany. Marriott returned to Washington U. in 1917 as Chairman of Pediatrics. His book *Infant Nutrition* was published in 1930 and the fourth edition, with Jeans, appeared in 1947. The "Marriott Method" of infant feeding was to dilute evaporated cow milk with Karo syrup. Marriott taught, "Infant feeding, there is nothing to it." After the introduction of evaporated milk formulas, artificial infant feeding was no longer the chief problem of pediatrics. Pediatric Profiles editor B. S. Veeder, Mosby, St. Louis, 1957, 218-228 (Photo courtesy of St. Louis CH)Bethesda, MD 1963

ciency, history is most important. There are four situations where one may suspect a trace mineral deficiency in infants and young children:

1. Children with low trace mineral stores due to premature birth and rapid growth in the first months of life.

2. Children on a restricted or incomplete diet (e.g., strict vegans, PKU with a nutritionally incomplete formula). Children eating a sampling of foods from the food pyramid should not be at risk of deficiencies.

3. Children with increased mineral losses, usually through the gastrointestinal tract, although occasionally via urinary losses. Examples would include children with malabsorption syndromes such as cystic fibrosis; those with increased stool output such as with inflammatory bowel disease; or those on chronic diuretic therapy who would be at risk of excessive urinary zinc losses.

4. Children on total parenteral nutrition (TPN) where the TPN does not contain the recommended amounts of trace minerals.

Global Issues of Microelements

Deficiencies of the microelements iron and iodine (as well as vitamin A) are a major impediment to the health and nutritional status of a significant proportion of the world's population, many of whom are infants. The World Summit for Children in 1990 and the International Conference on Nutrition[134] endorsed goals from which evolved the International Micronutrient Initiative. The Initiative's aim is to eliminate iodine deficiency disorders and reduce iron deficiency anemia in women to 30% by the year 2000. The global elimination of micronutrient deficiencies will be attained through interventions that include promotion of breast-feeding, improvements in food security, food fortification, and supplementation and improved nutrition education.

Sixteen to eighteen percent of the world's population or about 1.5 billion people live in iodine-deficient areas and are at risk of iodine deficiency. Iodine deficiency disorder (IDD) affects about 650 million people. Twenty million suffer varying degrees of mental deficiency caused by lack of iodine, while about six million have overt cretinism.[135] All age groups are susceptible to IDD, but the most vulnerable groups are women in their reproductive years and their babies. Developing fetus and infants up to the age of two years are most susceptible to the effects of IDD, and although IDDs are preventable, most of the effects are irreversible after the second year of life,[136] emphasizing the need for addressing iodine deficiency in reproductive age women.[137] (Figure 4). The use of iodized salt in developed countries prevents the occurrence of such devastating developments during fetal development and early infancy. Concurrent selenium deficiency may exacerbate goiter and the hypothyroidism that is associated with iodine deficiency.[138] The true prevalence of selenium deficiency in all parts of the world is not well delineated.

Zinc deficiency, while not included as one of the main micronutrient deficiencies in the current initiative, is known to be widespread in developing countries.[17] Growth faltering, especially in linear growth, is the major clinical observation in nutritional zinc deficiency. Fortifying food with zinc is the prime intervention approach to eliminating this dietary deficiency, since for many populations food choices with high natural zinc content are not possible.

Problem Sets
Nutritional Zinc Deficiency

A male infant was referred to a tertiary care hospital at the age of four and a half months by the family physician because of a dermatitis. He had been born after a 33-week gestation at a birthweight of 1760 g. With the exception of the occasional feeding of formula in the hospital when breast milk was unavailable, this infant was fed exclusively his mother's milk, either expressed or suckled. No mineral supplements had been prescribed at any time.

A rash was first noted as small red spots on the thighs, buttocks and face at three months of age. As the rash worsened, it was treated by the family physician with several antibacterial agents, both topical (clotrimazole, bactracin) and oral (cloxacillin sodium, cefaclor), but without response. The rash began to peel with bleeding and then appeared on the eyelids, feet, and fingers. Hexachlorophene cream and 1% hydrocortisone were administered without effect. At three and a half months of age, the infant was circumcised, and healing was incomplete a month later. He displayed occasional irritability but otherwise nursed reasonably well until two weeks before admission, when his mother noted a decrease in appetite and weight loss. On admission, his weight was 4.1 kg (5th to 10th percentile for a corrected age of two and a half months), length was 37 cm (25th to 50th percentile), and head circumference was 40 cm (75th percentile).

By the time of his admission to the hospital (at four and a half months of age), the inflammation was distributed over the cheeks, chin, nasolabial folds and pinnae, the dorsa of the fingers and both big toes. In the perineal area, there were punctate erosions and a diffuse erythema that was symmetrical and well demarcated with an erythematous border. There were a few satellite lesions but no scales. The center blanched to pressure. The pattern of the rash was similar to that classically associated with familial acrodermatitis

enteropathica (Figure 2A). Pertinent biochemical investigations on admission and our laboratory normal values for infants were as follows:

Biochemical Investigations:		
On Admission		Normal Values
Serum zinc	9.6 µmol/L	11.5 to 18.5 µmol/L
Hemoglobin	96 g/L	113 to 177 g/L
Alkaline		
phosphatase	241 U/L	30 to 120 U/L
Phosphorus	0.98 mmol/L	1.8 to 2.1 mmol/L

His mother had normal serum zinc (14.0 µmol/L) but low milk zinc concentrations. Oral supplements of zinc sulfate providing 1 mg of elemental zinc per kilogram of body weight per day were prescribed. After one week of therapy, the dermatitis had cleared on his face and fingers, and only minor remnants of the marginating rash in his buttock area remained (Figure 2B). Because of a low blood hemoglobin content, an iron supplement was prescribed providing two mg of elemental iron per kilogram per day. A bone density measurement of the one-third distal radius done at this time measured 77 mg/cm. The normal range for infants of this corrected postnatal age is 75 to 100 mg/cm.

At a follow-up visit, six weeks after the initiation of zinc therapy his skin was clear. He had been breast-fed, with only zinc and iron supplements and a small amount of rice cereal with 2% cow milk daily. Most blood biochemistry values had returned to the normal range: zinc, 18 µmol/L; phosphorus, 1.69 mmol/L; and hemoglobin, 100 g/L. The alkaline phosphatase level, was elevated at 807 U/L following zinc supplementation. Bone mineral density had also increased to 92 mg/cm, which is within the cited normal range. Review the pictures in Figure 2 and consider the following questions:

1. What are the most obvious clinical signs of zinc deficiency?
2. Why would prematurely born infants be "at risk" of zinc deficiency?

The acrodermatitis observed in the facial area is identical to that seen in the classic presentation of

Acrodermatitis Enteropathica in which there is a genetic defect in mucosal absorption of zinc.

Selenium Deficiency

A 12-month-old boy had been maintained on total parenteral nutrition since having major resection of the upper small intestine due to necrotizing enterocolitis with perforation in the early neonatal period. Following discharge from hospital at two months of age (adjusted to term date), the boy had received parenteral nutrition support from a commercial company that followed the nutrient prescription provided by the hospital pediatric gastroenterologist. Protein was provided as free amino acids (Aminosyn, Abbott Laboratories), glucose (Travenol Laboratories) and lipid as Intralipid (Pharmacia Ltd.). A standard vitamin mix (MVI Pediatric) and the trace elements zinc, copper, iodine, chromium and manganese were added.

The parents inquired at a routine follow-up visit to their pediatrician as to whether they should be concerned that their infant was not yet crawling or walking. Attempts to make him bear weight caused him to cry. On examining the infant the physician noted that his leg and foot muscles were tender, but power, tone, reflexes, coordination and cranial nerves appeared normal. The parents also thought it unusual for the infant's hair to be very blond, sparse and coarse. Their two previous children had masses of dark hair by this age.

Biochemical Investigations:

On Admission		Normal Values
Hemoglobin	120 g/L	95 to 118 g/L
Plasma toal		
protein	55 g/L	45-75 g/L
Plasma albumin	35 g/L	30 -48 g/L
Serum zinc	13 µmol/L	11.5-18.5 µmol/L
Serum copper	18 µmol/L	10-25 µmol/L
Plasma		
tocopherol	15 µmol/L	11.5-35 µmol/L
Plasma selenium	non-detectable	0.8-1.6 µmol/L
RBC glutathione		
peroxidase	non-detectable	13-25 U/g hemoglobin
Plasma glutathione		
peroxidase	6 U/L	90-350 U/L

Because of the biochemistry suggesting selenium deficiency, a cardiology consult was made.

Cardiology Findings:[79]

- electromylogram showed a myopathic process with increased polyphase and reduced amplitude of potentials
- electrocardiogram was normal
- echocardiogram was normal
- chest x-ray film was normal

Follow-up

Sodium selenite was added to the intravenous solution at 20 nmol/kg/d. Within six weeks the infant was crawling of his own accord and enjoying the challenges of standing unaided in his playpen.

At two months after the intravenous selenium was started, the infant's plasma selenium was 0.73 µmol/L and RBC glutathione peroxidase was 17 U/g Hb. An EMG repeated after four months of selenium infusions was normal.

Questions:

1. What is the link between selenium deficiency and cardiomyopathy?
2. How do you classify the clinical state noted by the condition of the hair?
3. Is selenium deficiency likely to be diagnosed in an infant who had always been orally fed.

Historical Vignettes
Zinc

In 1961, Prasad and others first identified zinc deficiency as the cause of dwarfism and hypogonadism among zinc- and iron- deficient adolescent Iranian village boys. In 1995, Sandstead[17] declared that zinc deficiency is an unrecognized public health problem that may be prevalent in western cultures as well as in developing countries.

Copper

Neutropenia – a persistent and early clinical sign of copper deficiency – was first described in 1964. The genetic disorders of Wilson's (defective copper excretion) and Menkes (defective copper absorption, transport and utilization) diseases have been recognized since the middle of this century, but treatment has not been satisfactory. For Wilson's disease the efficacy of chelation therapy with zinc (rather than with penacillamine) was only accepted in the late 1980s,[48, 49] although it was first proposed in 1961.[139]

Selenium

The biological significance of selenium was first recognized in 1934 when it was identified as the cause of lameness and death of livestock in parts of the Dakotas and Wyoming. These areas were subsequently shown to have high levels of selenium in soils and forage plants. Signs of what is now known as selenium toxicity were described in livestock in Tibet and western China by Marco Polo in 1295 and in Colombia in 1560 by early Spanish explorers. In 1957, Schwartz and Foltz gave a completely new direction to research on sele-

nium in nutrition when they showed it to be an essential nutrient for animals. An apparent interaction with vitamin E in several species suggested that selenium had an antioxidant function. The biochemical function of selenium was not elucidated until 1973, when it was discovered separately by Rotruck et al[140] in Wisconsin and Flohe's group[47] in West Germany that glutathione peroxidase was a seleno-enzyme.

Keshan's disease is often defined as an endemic cardiomyopathy observed in women of child-bearing age and infants living in areas with selenium-deficient soils. A severe outbreak of Keshan's disease was first reported in 1935 in Keshan county, Heilongjiang Province, China. While selenium deficiency due to inadequate dietary intakes is widely accepted as a major etiological factor in Keshan disease, other substances such as mycotoxins, inorganic elements and organic substances have been proposed but not fully investigated.[72]

Historical Perspective...

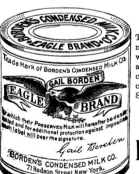

References

1. Health and Welfare Canada. *Nutrition Recommendations. The Report of the Scientific Review Committee.* Ottawa: National Department of Health and Welfare: 1990.

2. National Research Council. *Recommended dietary allowances.* 10th ed. Washington, DC: National Academy Press; 1990.

3. Prasad AS. Zinc: An Overview. *Nutrition.* 1995;11:93-99.

4. Vallee BL, Galdes A. The metallobiochemistry of zinc enzymes. *Adv in Enzymol.* 1984;56:283-430.

5. Widdowson EM, Dauncey J, Shaw JCL. Trace elements in fetal and early postnatal development. *Proc Nutr Soc.* 1974;33:275.

6. Zlotkin SH, Cherian G. Hepatic metallothionein as a source of zinc and cysteine during the first year of life. *Pediatr Res.* 1988;24:326-329.

7. Zlotkin SH, Casselman C. Urinary zinc excretion in normal subjects. *J Trace Elem Exp Med.* 1990;3:13-21.

8. Krebs NF, Reidinger CJ, Hartley S, Robertson AD, Hambidge KM. Zinc supplementation during lactation: effects on maternal status and milk zinc concentrations. *Am J Clin Nutr.* 1995;61:1030-1036.

9. Lonnerdal B, Sandberg AS, Sandstrom B, Kunz C. Inhibitory effects of phytic acid and other inositol phosphates on zinc and calcium absorption. *J Nutr.* 1989; 119:211-214.

10. Atkinson SA, Shah JK, Webber CE, Gibson IL, Gibson RS. A multi-element assessment of mineral bioavailability and utilization from formula with increased content of calcium, phosphorus, zinc, copper and iron in a piglet model. *J Nutr.* 1993;123:1586-1593.

11. Wang Z, Atkinson SA, Bertolo R, Polberger S, Lonnerdal B. Alterations in intestinal uptake and compartmentalization of zinc in response to short-term dexamethasone therapy or excess dietary zinc in piglets. *Pediatr Res.* 1993;33:118-124.

12. Zlotkin SH. Nutrient interactions with TPN: The effect of histidine and cysteine intake on urinary zinc excretion. *J Pediatr.* 1989;114:859-864.

13. Sandstrom B, Davidson L, Lederblad A, Lonnerdal B. Zinc absorption from human milk, cow's milk and infant formulas. *Am J Dis Child.* 1983;137:726-729.

14. Hambidge KM, Walravens PA, Casey CE, Brown RM, Bender C. Plasma zinc concentration of breast-fed infants. *J Pediatr.* 1979;94:607-608.

15. Lonnerdal B, Keen CL, Bell JG, Hurley LA. Zinc uptake and retention from chelates and milk fractions. In: Mills CF, Bremner I, Chesters JK, eds. *Trace Elements in Man and Animals.* Farnham Royal, UK: Commonwealth Agricultural Bureau; 1985:5;427-430.

16. Prasad AS, Meale A, Farid Z, et al. Zinc metabolism in patients with the syndrome of iron deficiency anemia, hypogonadism, and dwarfism. *J Lab Clin Med.* 1963; 61:537.

17. Sandstead HH. Is zinc deficiency a public health problem? *Nutrition.* 1995;11:87-92.

18. Stec J, Podracka L, Pavkovcekova O, Kollar J. Zinc and copper metabolism in nephrotic syndrome. *Nephron.* 1990;56:186-187.

19. Atkinson SA, Whelan D, Whyte RK, et al. Abnormal zinc content in human milk: Risk for development of nutritional zinc deficiency in infants. *Am J Dis Child.* 1989;43:608-611.

20. Khoshoo V, Kjarsgaard J, Krafchick B, Zlotkin SH. Zinc deficiency in a full-term breast-fed infant: unusual presentation. *Pediatrics.* 1992;89:1094-1095

21. Bye AME. Transient zinc deficiency in a full-term breast-fed infant of normal birth weight. *Pediatr Dermatol.* 1985;2:308-311.

22. Kuramoto Y, Igarashi Y, Kato S, Tagami H. Acquired zinc deficiency in two breast-fed mature infants. *Acta Derm Venereol.* 1986;66:359-361.

23. Shinwell ED, Gorodischer R. Totally vegetarian diets and infant nutrition. *Pediatrics.* 1982;70:582-586.

24. Cousins RJ, Leinart AS. Tissue-specific regulation of zinc metabolism and metallothionein genes by interleukin 1. *FASEB J.* 1988;2:2884-2890.

25. Finney DCW, Schnaufer L, Stafford ES. Total gastrectomy in an infant made necessary by ingestion of tinning paint. *Ann Surg.* 1960;151:891.

26. Dreisbach RH. *Handbook of Poisoning: Diagnosis and Treatment.* 2nd ed. Los Altos, CA: Lange; 1959:304-305.

27. Brown MA, Thom JV, Orth GL, Cova P, Juarez J. Food poisoning involving zinc contamination. *Arch Environmental Health.* 1964;8:657-660.

28. Murphy JV. Intoxication following ingestion of elemental zinc. *JAMA.* 1970;212:2119-2120.

29. National Research Council, Subcommittee on Zinc. Toxicity of zinc. In: *Zinc.* Baltimore: University Park Press; 1979:10;249-253.

30. Mills CF. Dietary interactions involving the trace elements. *Ann Rev Nutr.* 1985;5:173-193.

31. Osaki S, Johnson DA, Frieden E. The mobilization of iron from the perfused mammalian liver by a serum copper enzyme, ferroxidase I. *J Biol Chem.* 1971;246: 3018-3023.

32. Evans JL, Abraham PA. Anemia, iron storage and ceruloplasmin in copper nutrition in the growing rat. *J Nutr.* 1973;103:196-201.

33. Logan JI, Harveyson KB, Wisdom GB, Hughes AE, Archbold GPR. Hereditary caeruloplasmin deficiency, dementia and diabetes mellitus. *Q J Med.* 1994;87: 6630-6670.

34. Harris ED. The iron-copper connection: The link to ceruloplasmin grows stronger. *Nutr Rev.* 1995;53(6):170-173.

35. Percival SS. Neutropenia caused by copper deficiency: Possible mechanisms of action. *Nutr Rev.* 1995;53:59-66.

36. Botash AS, Nasca J, Dubowy R, Weinberger HL, Oliphant M. Zinc-induced copper deficiency in an infant. *Am J Dis Child.* 1992;146:709-711.

37. Graham GG, Cordano A. Copper depletion and deficiency in the malnourished infant. *John Hopkins Med J.* 1966;124:139.

38. Karpel JT, Peden VH. Copper deficiency in long-term parenteral nutrition. *J Pediatr.* 1972;80:83.

39. Tokuda Y, Yokoyama S, Tsuji M, Sugita T, Tajima T, Mitomi T. Copper deficiency in an infant on prolonged total parenteral nutrition. *J Parent & Enteral Nutr.* 1986;19:242-244.

40. Seely J, Humphrey G, Matler B. Copper deficiency in a premature infant fed on iron fortified formula. *N Eng J Med.* 1972;286:109.

41. Shaw JCL. Copper deficiency in term and preterm infants. In: Fomon SJ, Zlotkin S, eds. *Nutritional Anemias.* Nestle Nutrition Workshop Series, Vol. 30. New York: Raven Press Ltd; 1992:105-119.

42. Haschke F, Zeigler EE, Edwards BB. Effect of iron fortification of infant formula on trace mineral absorption. *J Pediatr Gastroenterol Nutr.* 1986;5:768-773.

43. Lonnerdal B, Hernell O. Iron, zinc, copper and selenium status of breast-fed infants and infants fed trace element fortified milk-based infant formula. *Acta Paediatr.* 1994; 83:67-73.

44. Barclay SM, Aggett PJ, Lloyd DJ, Duffty P. Reduced erythrocyte superoxide dismutase activity in low birth weight infants given iron supplements. *Pediatric Res.* 1991;29:297-301.

45. Petrukhin K, Gilliam TC. Genetic disorders of copper metabolism. *Curr Opin Pediatr.* 1994;6:698-701.

46. Greene H, Hambidge K, Schanler R, Tsang R. Guidelines for the use of vitamins, trace elements, calcium, magnesium, and phosphorus in infants and children receiving total parenteral nutrition: report of the Subcommittee on Pediatric Parenteral Nutrient Requirements from the Committee on Clinical Practice Issues of the American Society for Clinical Nutrition. *Am J Clin Nutr.* 1988;48:1324-1342.

47. Danks DM. Hereditary disorders of copper metabolism in Wilson's disease and Menkes' disease. In: Stanbury JB, Wyngaarden JB, Frederickson DS, eds. *The Metabolic Basis of Inherited Disease.* 5th ed. New York: McGraw-Hill; 1983:1251-1268.

48. Brewer GJ, Hill GM, Prasad AS, Cossack ZT, Rabbani P. Oral zinc therapy for Wilson's disease. *Ann Intern Med.* 1983;99:314-320.

49. Brewer GJ, Yuzbasiyan-Gurkan V, Lee Doh-Yeel. Use of zinc-copper metabolic interactions in the treatment of Wilson's disease. *J Am College Nutr.* 1990;9:487-491.

50. Fischer PWF, Giroux A, L'Abbe MR. Effects of zinc on mucosal copper binding and on the kinetics of copper absorption. *J Nutr.* 1983;113:462-469.

51. Hennon DK, Stookey GK, Muskler JC. The clinical anticariogenic effectiveness of supplementary fluoride-vitamin preparations. Results at the end of three years. *J Dent Child.* 1966;33:3-12.

52. Esala S, Vuori E, Helle A. Effect of maternal fluorine intake on breast milk fluoride content. *Br J Nutr.* 1982; 48:210-214.

53. Newbrun E. Current regulations and recommendations concerning water fluoridation, fluoride supplements, and topical fluoride agents. *J Dent Res.* 1992;71(5):1255-1265.

54. American Dental Association Council on Dental Therapeutics. New Fluoride schedule adopted. *Amer Dent Assoc News.* 1994;12-14.

55. Nutrition Committee, Canadian Pediatric Society. Statement on the use of fluoride in infants and children. *Pediatr Child Health* 1996;1:141-145.

56. American Dietetic Association Reports. Position of the American Dietetic Association: The impact of fluoride on dental health. *J Am Diet Assoc.* 1994;94(12):1428-1431.

57. Nutrition Committee, Canadian Pediatric Society. Fluoride supplementation. *Contemp Pediatr.* 1987:50-56.

58. Levy SM. Review of fluoride exposures and ingestion. *Community Dent Oral Epidemiol.* 1994;22(3):173-180.

59. Clark DC. Appropriate uses of fluorides for children: guidelines from the Canadian Workshop on the Evaluation of Current Recommendations Concerning Fluorides. *Can Med Assoc J.* 1993;149(12):1787-1793.

60. Flohe L, Gunzler WA, Schock HH. Glutathoine peroxidase: a selenoenzyme. *FEBS Lett.* 1973;32:132-134.

61. Arthur JR, Beckett GJ. *7th International symposium on trace elements in Man and Animals (TEMA-7).* Dubrovnik: 1990.

62. Combs GF Jr, Combs SB. *The Role of Selenium in Nutrition.* New York, NY: Academic Press; 1986.

63. Combs GF Jr. Selenium. In: Moon TE, Micozzi MS, eds. *Nutrition and Cancer Prevention.* New York, NY: Marcel Dekker; 1989:389-420.

64. Litov RE, Combs GF. Selenium in Pediatric Nutrition. *Pediatrics.* 1991;87:339-351.

65. Friel JK, Andrews WL, Long DR, L'Abbe MR. Selenium status of very low birth weight infants. *Pediatr Res.* 1993; 34:293-296.

66. Smith AM, Chan GM, Boyer-Mileu LJ, Johnson CE, Gardner BR. Selenium status of preterm infants fed human milk, preterm formula or selenium-supplemented preterm formula. *J Pediatr.* 1991;119:429-433.

67. Kumpulainen J, Salmenpera L, Siimes MA, Koivistoinen P, Lehto J, Perheentupa J. Formula feeding results in lower selenium status than breast-feeding or selenium supplemented formula feeding: a longitudinal study. *Am J Clin Nutr.* 1987;45:49-53.

68. Gropper SAS, Anderson K, Landing WM, Acosta PB. Dietary selenium intakes and plasma selenium concentrations of formula-fed and cow's milk-fed infants. *J Am Diet Assoc.* 1990;90:1547-1550.

69. Smith AM, Picciano MF, Milner JA, Hatch TF. Influence of feeding regimens on selenium concentrations and glutathione peroxidase activities in plasma and erythrocytes of infants. *J Trace Elem Exp Med.* 1988;1:209-216.

70. Lombeck I, Ebert KH, Kasperek K, Feinendegen LE, Bremer H. Selenium intake of infants and young children, healthy children and dietetically treated patients with phenylketonuria. *Eur J Pediatr.* 1984;143:99-102.

71. Kumpulainen J, Vuori E, Kuitunen P, Makinen S, Kara R.

Longitudinal study on the dietary selenium intake of exclusively breast-fed infants and their mothers in Finland. *Int J Vitam Nutr Res.* 1983;53:420-426.

72. Ge K, Yang G. The epidemiology of selenium deficiency in the etiological study of endemic diseases in China. *Am J Clin Nutr Suppl.* 1993;57:S259-S263.

73. Van Rij AM, Thomson CD, McKenzie JM, et al. Selenium deficiency in total parenteral nutrition. *Am J Clin Nutr.* 1979;32:2076-2085.

74. Collipp PJ, Chen SY. Cardiomyopathy and selenium deficiency in a two-year old girl. *N Eng J Med.* 1981;304: 1304-1305.

75. Fleming CR, Lie JT, McCall JT, et al. Selenium deficiency and fatal cardiomyopathy in a patient on home parenteral nutrition. *Gastroenterology.* 1982;83: 689-693.

76. Baker SS, Lerman RH, Krey SH, et al. Selenium deficiency with total parenteral nutrition: Reversal of biochemical and functional abnormalities by selenium supplementation: A case report. *Am J Clin Nutr.* 1983; 38:769-774.

77. Vinton NE, Dahlstrom KA. Macrocytosis and pseudoalbinism: manifestations of selenium deficiency. *J Pediatr.* 1987;111:711-717.

78. Kien L, Ganther HE. Manifestations of chronic selenium deficiency in a child receiving total parenteral nutrition. *Am J Clin Nutr.* 1983;37:319-328.

79. Kelly DA, Coe AW, Sheakin A, Lake BD, Walker-Smith JA. Symptomatic selenium deficiency in a child on home parenteral nutrition. *J Pediatr Gastroenterol Nutr.* 1988;7:783-786.

80. Van Caillie-Bertrand M, Degenhart HJ, Fernandes J. Selenium status of infants on nuritional support. *Acta Pediatr Scand.* 1984;76:816-819.

81. Johnson RA, Baker SS, Fallon JT, et al. An accidental case of cardiomyopathy and selenium deficiency. *N Eng J Med.* 1981;30:1210-1212.

82. Lombeck I, Kasperek K, Feinendegen LE, et al. Serum-selenium concentrations in patients with maple-syrup-urine-disease and phenylketonuria under dietotherapy. *Clin Chim Acta.* 1975;64:57-61.

83. Lombeck I, Kasperek K, Harbisch HD, et al. The selenium state of children, II: selenium content of serum, whole blood, hair and the activity of erythrocyte glutathione peroxidase in dietetically treated patients with phenylketonuria and maple-syrup-urine-disease. *Eur J Pediatr.* 1978;128:213-223.

84. Smith DK, Teague RJ, McAdam PA, et al. Selenium status of malnourished hospitalized patients. *J Am Coll Nutr.* 1986;5:243-252.

85. Burk RF, Pearson WN, Wood RP, et al. Blood-selenium levels and in vitro red blood cell uptake of ^{75}Se in kwashiorkor. *Am J Clin Nutr.* 1967;20:723-733.

86. Levine RJ, Olson RE. Blood selenium in Thai children with protein-calorie malnutrition. *Proc Soc Exp Biol Med.* 1970;134:1030-1034.

87. Lombeck I, Kasperek K, Harbisch HD, Feinendegen LE, Dremer HJ. The selenium state of healthy children. *Eur J Pediatr.* 1977;125:87-88.

88. Avissar N, Whitin JC, Allen PZ, et al. Antihuman plasma glutathione peroxidase antibodies; immunologic investigations to determine plasma glutathione peroxidase protein and selenium content in plasma. *Blood.* 1989;73: 318-323.

89. Yang G, Wang S, Zhou R, Sun S. Endemic selenium intoxication of humans in China. *Am J Clin Nutr.* 1983; 37:872-881.

90. Lombeck I, Menzel H, Frosch D. Acute selenium poisoning of a 2 year old child. *Eur J Pediatr.* 1987;146: 308-312.

91. Bayliss PA, Buchanan BE, Hancock RGV, Zlotkin SH. Tissue selenium accretion in premature and full-term human infants and children. *Biol Trace Element Res.* 1985;7:755-761.

92. Casey CE, Hambidge KM. Trace Minerals. In: Tsang RC, ed. *Vitamin and mineral requirements in preterm infants.* New York: Marcel Dekker Inc; 1985:152-184.

93. Kumpulainen JT, Vuori E. Longitudinal study of chromium in human milk. *Am J Clin Nutr.* 1980;33: 2299-2302.

94. Freund H, Atamian S, Fischer JE. Chromium deficiency during total parenteral nutrition. *JAMA.* 1979;241:496-499.

95. Kien CL, Veillon C, Patterson KY, et al. Mild peripheral neuropathy but biochemical chromium sufficiency during 16 months of chromium free total parenteral nutrition. *JPEN.* 1987;10:662-664.

96. Casey CE, Hambidge KM, Neville MC. Studies in human lactation: zinc, copper, manganese and chromium in human milk in the first month of lactation. *Am J Clin Nutr.* 1985;41:1193-1200.

97. Moukarzel AA, Song MK, Buckman AL, et al. Excessive chromium intake in children receiving total parenteral nutrition. *Lancet.* 1992;339:385.

98. Dorner K, St. Dziadzka Oldigs H-D, Schulz-Lell G, Schaub J. Manganese balances in term infants. In: *Composition and Physiological Properties of Human Milk.* Schaub J, ed. Elsevier Science Publishers; 1985:117-130.

99. Norose N, Araki K. Clinical studies on manganese deficiency during long-term parenteral nutrition in a child. *Jap J Parent Ent Nutr.* 1987;9:978.

100. Atkinson SA, Shah JK. Calcium and phosphorus fortification of preterm formulas: Drug-mineral and mineral-mineral interactions. In: Hillman L, ed. *Mineral Requirements for the Premature Infant.* Wyeth-Ayerst Nutritional Seminar Series. New York: Elsevier Press; 1990:58-75.

101. Widdowson, EM. Trace elements in human development. In: Barltrope D, Burlund WL, ed. *Mineral Metabolism in Pediatrics.* Oxford: Blackwell Scientific Publications; 1976:88-95.

102. Ejima A, Imamura T, Nakamura S, et al. Manganese intoxication during total parenteral nutrition. *Lancet.* 1992;339:426.

103. Fisher DA. Upper limit of iodine in infant formulas. *J Nutr.* 1989;119:1865-1868.

104. Fisher DA, Giroux A. Iodine content of Canadian retail milk samples. *Can Inst Sci Technol J.* 1987;20:166-169.

105. Beng JN, Padgitt D. Iodine concentrations of milk of dairy cattle fed various levels of iodine as ethylenediamine dihydroiodide (EDDI). *J Dairy Sci.* 1985;68 (Suppl 1): 139.

106. Dunsmore DG, Wheeler SM. Iodophors and iodine in dairy products. VIII. The total industry situation. *Aust J Dairy Technol.* 1977;32:166.

107. Delange FM. Endemic cretinism. In: SH, Braverman LE, eds. *Werner's the thyroid: a fundamental and clinical text.* 5th edition. Philadelphia: Ingbar Lippincott; 1986: 722-734.

108. Chabrolle JP, Rossier A. Goiter and hypothyroidism in the new born after cutaneous absorption of iodine. *Arch Dis Child.* 1978;53:495-498.

109. Castaing H, Fournet JP, Lager FA, et al. Thyroide au nouveau - ne et surcharge en iode apres la naissance. *Arch Fr Pediatr.* 1979;36:356-368.

110. Greger JL, Baier MJ. Excretion and retention of low or moderate levels of aluminum by human subjects. *Food Chem Toxic.* 1983;21:473-477.

111. Committee on Nutrition. Aluminum toxicity in infants and children. *Pediatrics.* 1986;78:1150-1154.

112. Sedman AB, LKlein GL, Merritt RJ, et al. Evidence of aluminum loading in infants receiving intravenous therapy. *N Eng J Med.* 1972;286:109.

113. Koo WWK, Kaplan LA, Bendon R, Succop P, Tsang RC, Horn J, Steichen JJ. Response to aluminum in parenteral nutrition during infancy. *J Pediatr.* 1986;109:877-883.

114. Weintraub R, Hams G, Meerkin M, Rosenberg AR. High aluminum content of infant formulas. *Arch Dis Child.* 1986;61:914-916.

115. Moreno A, Bornin C, Ballabriga A. Aluminum in the neonate related to parenteral nutrition. *Acta Paediatr.* 1994;83:25-29.

116. Koo WWK, Kaplan LA. Aluminum and bone disorders: With specific reference to aluminum contamination of infant nutrients. *J Am College Nutr.* 1988;7:199-214.

117. Koo WWK, Krug-Wispe SK, Succop P, Bendon R, Kaplan LA. Sequential serum aluminum and urine aluminum: Creatinine ratio and tissue aluminum loading in infants with fractures/rickets. *Pediatrics.* 1992;89: 877-881.

118. Klein GL. Aluminum in parenteral solutions revisited - again. *Am J Clin Nutr.* 1994;61:449-465.

119. Swartz RD. Deferoxamine and aluminum removal. *Am J Kidney Dis.* 1985;6:358-364.

120. Klein GL, Snodgrass WR, Griffin P, Miller NL, Alfrey AC. Hypocalcemia complicating deferoxamine therapy in an infant with parenteral nutrition-associated aluminum overload: Evidence for a role of aluminum in the bone disease of infants. *J Pediatr Gastro Nutr.* 1989;9:400-403.

121. Ziegler EE, Edwards BB, Jensen RL, Mahaffey KR, Fomon SF. Absorption and retention of lead by infants. *Pediatr Res.* 1978;12:29-34.

122. Cullen MR, Robins JM, Eskenazi B. Adult inorganic lead intoxication: Presentation of 31 new cases and a review of recent advances in the literature. *Medicine.* 1983;62:221.

123. Baghurst RA, McMichael AJ, Wigg NR, Vimpani GV, Robertson EF, Roberts RJ, Tong S. Environmental exposure to lead and children's intelligence at the age of seven years. *New Engl J Med.* 1992;327:1279-1284.

124. Needleman HL, Schell A, Billinger D, Leviton A, Allved E. The long-term effects of exposure to low doses of lead in childhood: an 11-year follow-up report. *New Eng J Med.* 1990;322:83-88.

125. McMichael AJ, Baghurst PA, Wigg NR, Vempani GV, Robertson ER, Roberts RJ. Port Pieie Cohort Study: environmental exposure to lead and children's abilities at the age of four years. *New Engl J Med.* 1988:319: 468-475.

126. Bellinger D, Leviton A, Waternaux C, Needleman H, Robinowitz M. Longitudinal analyses of prenatal and postnatal lead exposure and early cognitive development. *N Eng J Med.* 1987;316:1037-1043.

127. Nieboer E, Sanford WE. Essential, toxic and therapeutic functions of metals (including determinants of reactivity). In: Hodgson E, Bend JR, Philpot RM, eds. *Reviews in Biochemical Toxicology.* Elsevier Science Publishing Co Inc; 1985:7;205-245.

128. Ong CN, Lee RW. Interaction of calcium and lead in human erythrocytes. *Br J Ind Med.* 1980;37:70.

129. Spencer PS, Schaumburg HH, eds. *Experimental and Clinical Neurotoxicology.* Baltimore: Williams and Wilkins; 1980:490.

130. Gellert GA, Wagner GA, Maxwell RM, Moore D, Foster L. Lead poisoning among low-income children in Orange County. *JAMA.* 1993;270:69-71.

131. American Academy of Pediatrics. Lead Poisoning: From screening to primary prevention. *Pediatrics.* 1993;92: 176-182.

132. Bar-Or ME, Boyle RM. Are pediatricians ready for the new guidelines on lead poisoning? *Pediatrics.* 1994;93(2): 178-182.

133. Shannon MW, Graef JW. Lead intoxication in infancy. *Pediatrics.* 1992;89:87-90.

134. WHO and FAO. *Nutrition and Development - A Global Assessment. International Conference on Nutrition.* 1992.

135. Hetzel BS. The prevention and control of iodine deficiency disorders. ACC/SCN State-of-the-art series. March 1988. (Reprinted June 1993). Nutrition policy discussion paper No. 3.

136. Hetzel BS, Mayberly GF. Iodine. In: Mertz C, ed. *Trace Elements in Human and Animal Nutrition.* New York: Academic Press; 1986;139-208.

137. Levine MH, Pollitt E, Galloway R, McGuire J. Micronutrient deficiency disorders. In: Jameson DT, Mosley WH, Meashan AR, Bohadilla, eds. *Disease Control Priorities in Developing Countries.* Oxford University Press; 1993.

138. Beckett GJ, Nicol F, Rae PWH, Beech S, Guo Y, Arthur JR. Effects of combined iodine and selenium deficiency on thyroid hormone metabolism in rats. *Am J Clin Nutr.* (suppl). 1993;57:240-2435.

Color Atlas

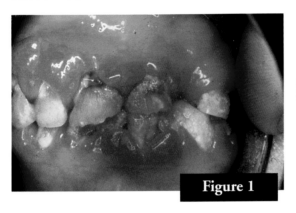

Figure 1

Figure 1: In scurvy hemorrhage is common. Impaired collagen formation fails to support the matrix of the capillary bed. The gingiva at the base of the teeth become hemorrhagic and finally necrotic. The interdental papillae become swollen, blood supply is compromised and eventually teeth fall out. Slide courtesy of Hospital for Sick Children, Toronto, library.

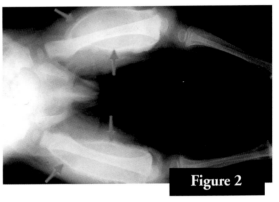

Figure 2

Figure 2: Clinical presentation of scurvy reflects the role of the vitamin in the metabolism of mesenchymal cells which form connective tissue, osteoid and dentin. This x-ray shows massive subperiosteal hemorrhage with calcification of the raised periosteum (arrow) after the start of vitamin C therapy. Slide courtesy of ICNND.

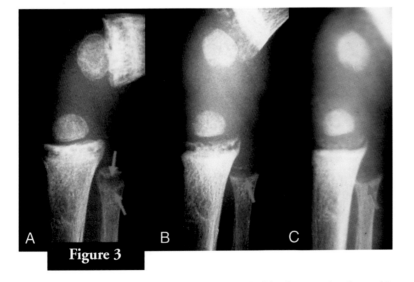

Figure 3

Figure 3: (a). The diagnosis of rickets is established by the typical radiographic changes in the growing ends of long bones which demonstrate a widened radiolucent zone in the epiphyseal plate (due to uncalcified preosseous cartilage) and also by the general rarefaction and coarse trabecular pattern of cancellous bones. (b) Healing is occurring after appropriate treatment. (c) Note increasing ossification of the metaphyseal regions and increasing density of bones. Slide courtesy of ICNND.

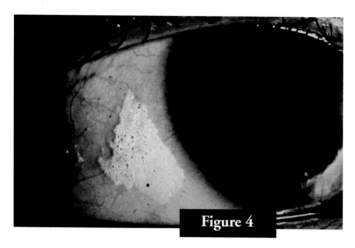

Figure 4

Figure 4: Bitot's Spot. Silver-gray shiny, foamy triangular spots consisting of dried epithelium. Results from xerosis (drying) of the conjunctiva secondary to vitamin A deficiency. Slide courtesy of ICNND.

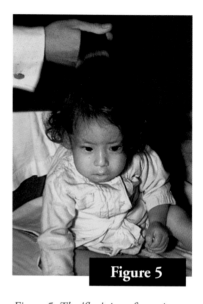

Figure 5

Figure 5: The 'flag' sign of protein malnutrition. The light hair coloring reflects the period of severe protein deficiency. Hair pigment changes are reversed with refeeding, thus the dark-light-dark hair coloring. Slide courtesy of ICNND.

Figures 6-9: Manifestations of pellagra (niacin deficiency). With chronic pellagra, the skin over exposed surfaces and pressure points may be thickened, hyperkeratotic and hyperpigmented without evidence of inflammation. In Figures 7 and 8 note skin changes on neck (Casal's necklace) and over extensor surfaces of the knees. Note the scalloped, atrophied tongue with swollen papillae. Slides courtesy of ICNND and Dr. T. Spies.

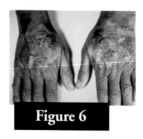

Figure 6

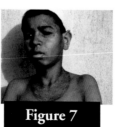

Figure 7

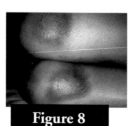

Figure 8

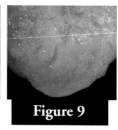

Figure 9

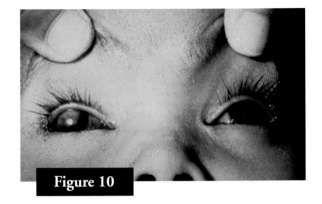

Figure 10

Figure 10: Keratomalacia (softening of the cornea). With more severe and prolonged vitamin A deficiency, xerosis of the cornea appears, followed by corneal distortion, and ultimately prolapse of the iris. The corneal structure literally becomes a soft gelatinous mass. Slide courtesy of ICNND.

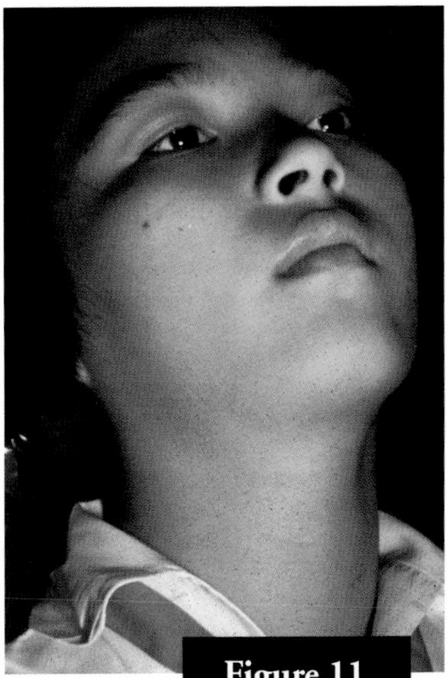

Figure 11

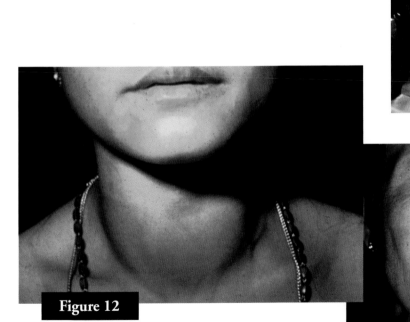

Figure 12

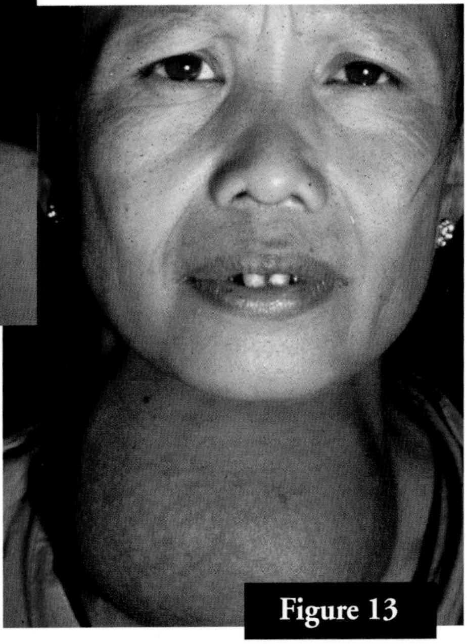

Figure 13

Figures 11-13: Goitrous manifestations of iodine deficiency, from mild (figure 11) to severe (figure 13). Slide courtesy of ICNND.

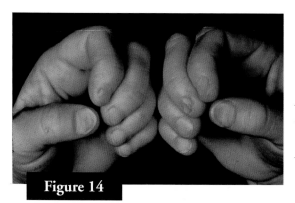

Figure 14

Figure 14: Nails in iron anemia. The fingernails may become dull colored, flattened and then spoon-shaped (kooilonychia) as is shown in the figure. Slide courtesy of ICNND.

Figure 15: Xerosis and skin keratinization with vitamin A deficiency. Normal columnar epithelial cells in the skin are replaced by thick layers of horny, stratified epithelium. Slide courtesy of ICNND.

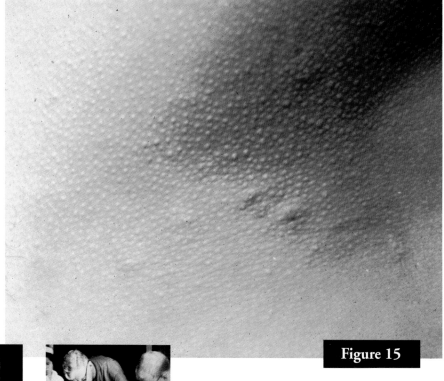

Figure 15

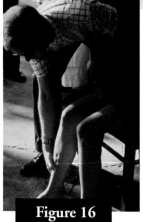

Figure 16

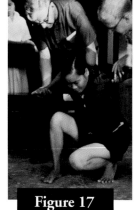

Figure 17

Figures 16 and 17: Manifestations of beriberi (thiamin deficiency). Note the pitting edema in figure 16. Muscle weakness and atrophy are typical signs of beriberi (Figure 17). Slide courtesy of ICNND.

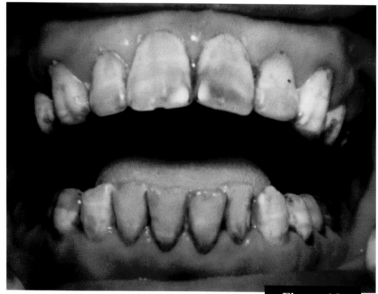

Figure 18

Figure 18: Staining and pitting of teeth with severe dental fluorosis. Note bands across lower teeth. Slide courtesy of ICNND.

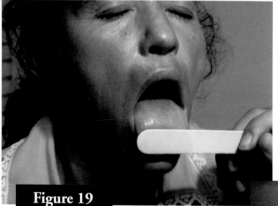

Figure 19

Figure 19: Advanced chronic glossitis with marked papillary atrophy typical of vitamin B complex deficiencies. Slide courtesy of Dr. B. Nichols.

Figure 20. Note follicular hyperkeratosis over nose with vitamin A deficiency. Slide courtesy of Dr. B. Nichols.

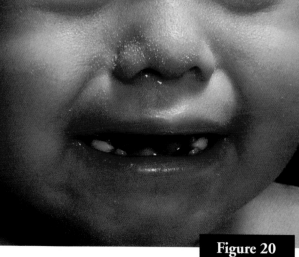

Figure 20

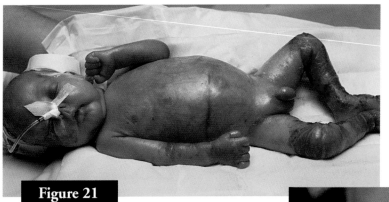

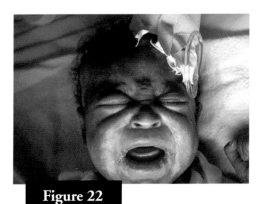

Figure 21: Severe protein deficiency in a post-operative child. Note the collodion type of hyperpigmentation. Slide courtesy of Dr. B. Nichols.

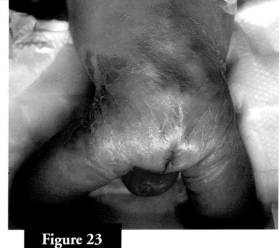

Figure 22: Severe protein deficiency with hypoalbuminemia. Note periorbital edema, angular cheilitis and hyperkeratosis of facial skin. Slide courtesy of Dr. B. Nichols.

Figure 23: Protein-energy malnutrition with possible B-vitamin deficiency. Note gluteal atrophy, collodion-type friable skin, patulous anus and scrotal edema. Slide courtesy of Dr. B. Nichols.

Figure 24: Rickets. Note flaring of distal ends of radius and ulna and frayed appearance of epiphysis. Slide courtesy of Dr. B. Nichols.

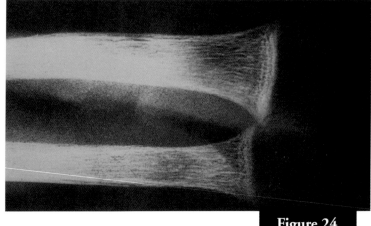

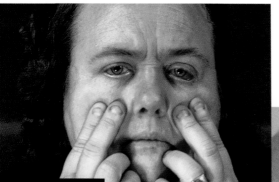

Figure 25

Figure 25: Capillary injection of sclera of eyes associated with riboflavin deficiency. Slide courtesy of Dr. T. Spies.

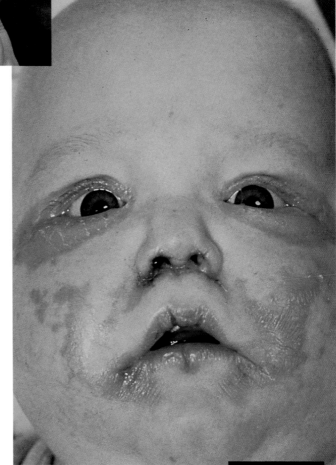

Figure 26: Biotin deficiency. Note unusual mask-like distribution around eyes, angular cheilosis and severely cracked lips. There is also significant involvement of all mucous membranes (including nose and anus), face and diaper area. Courtesy of Dr. S. Zlotkin and Dr. D. Mock.

Figure 26

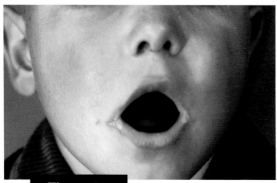

Figure 27

Figure 27: Angular cheilitis typical of many vitamin B complex deficiencies. Slide courtesy of Dr. T. Spies.

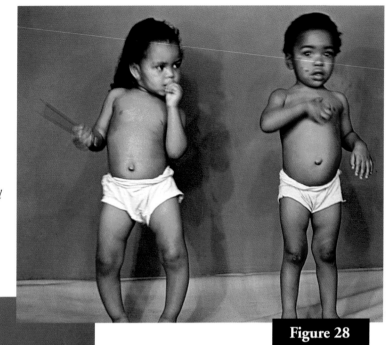

Figure 28: Rickets. Child on left has typical 'bowed' legs of rickets. Slide courtesy of Dr. T. Spies.

Figure 28

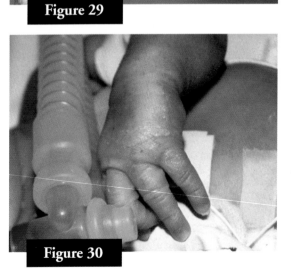

Figure 29

Figure 29: Note hemorrhage and petechiae on legs and ankles associated with scurvy. Slide courtesy of Dr. T. Spies.

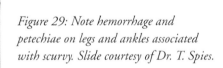

Figure 30: Scaly, dry dermatitis in an 8 day old newborn infant with confirmed essential fatty acid deficiency. The infant suffered from tracheoesophageal fistula treated surgically on day 2 of life, and from aspiration pneumonia, and received fat free parenteral nutrition. See uncropped photo (p.145).

Figure 30

Anemia: A Persistent Problem
Ferdinand Haschke M.D.

Department of Pediatrics,
University of Vienna,
Vienna, Austria

Reviewed by Stanley Zlotkin M.D., Ph.D., Reginald C. Tsang M.B.B.S.
and Peter R. Dallman M.D.

Introduction

It is evident that iron deficiency is the most common micronutrient deficiency in the world: approximately 2.5 billion people suffer from it (Table 1).[1] Severe iron deficiency produces ferropenic anemia, and is associated with poor health and serious functional impairments that diminish infant and child development. However, the substantial literature on iron deficiency and other nutritional anemias (Figure 1) in infants and children is difficult to interpret because of uncertainties about definitions, variable reports of prevalence in different age and socio-economic groups, and disagreement about dietary micronutrient requirements and interactions.

Over the past two decades, iron requirements for infants have become more precisely defined. Studies of food iron absorption have emphasized the importance of dietary composition in determining the amount of absorbable iron, and have led to strategies for improving food iron availability. Prevalence studies in industrialized and third world countries are available, and programs for iron supplementation and iron fortification of infant and toddler food have been instituted. However, there are additional discussions on macrocytic nutritional anemia, copper deficiency, vitamin A deficiency, vitamin E deficiency, infection and anemia of prematurity.

Physiology - Fe Deficiency

Not until physicians begin to think of anemia as a physiologic or biochemical derangement rather than a mere reduction in red cell mass, will they be able to answer the seemingly simple question, "Is the patient anemic?"[2]

Indeed, it was argued until the early 70s that a moderately decreased concentration of hemoglobin is of little consequence unless it causes decreased capacity for physical work by imposing an increased load on cardio-respiratory mechanisms.[3] Clinical data on systemic manifestations of iron deficiency anemia are available now. In infants, alterations in cognitive performance have been described. Such findings, even though limited, cannot be ignored and must be the basis for preventive measures.

Iron ranks among the most abundant elements in our environment. The concentrations of iron in the milk of those animals whose young are relatively mature at birth are generally low. The young of these animals generally have ready access to iron in the environment (dirt etc). The human infant is mature enough during the early months of life to be expected to have access to dirt. However, during the last decades, strong efforts to exclude sources of contamination from the diet and to raise infants in a clean environment have been made in the industrialized countries. Therefore, for most infants from industrialized countries, food is the only iron source.[4]

Function

As a part of hemoglobin, heme (and therefore iron) is necessary for the transport of oxygen from the lungs to the tissues, and as a component of myoglobin, heme is required for the storage of oxygen for use during muscle contraction.[5,6] Examples for iron-containing enzymes and their functions in the body are summarized in Table 2.

Absorption

Iron absorption takes place in the duodenum and the proximal jejunum from two distinct pools, (a) the heme iron pool (hemoglobin, myoglobin), and (b) the non-heme iron pool, which includes all other forms of iron.

Region	0-4 years Percentage	0-4 years Number[b]
Africa	56	48.0
Latin America	26	13.7
East Asia[c]	20	3.2
South Asia	56	118.2
World[c]	43	193.5
Developed regions[d]	12	10.3
Developing regions	51	183.2

a From United Nations, 1987[1]
b Numbers=millions
c Excluding China
d According to United Nations: regions including North America, Japan, Europe, Australia, New Zealand, and the Union of Soviet Socialist Republics.

Table 1: Estimated prevalence of anemia in children by geographic region (1980)[a].

Absorption of Heme Iron

Heme iron is absorbed as an iron-porphyrin complex directly into the mucosal cells.[7] Twenty to 25% of the heme- iron in a meal is absorbed. Only calcium has been identified as an inhibitor of heme iron so far (Figure 2).[8] A well-known enhancer of absorption of heme iron is meat.[9] Heme iron is generally better absorbed than non-heme iron. Although heme iron provides only 5 to 10% of the iron in the Western adults diet, it accounts for more than one third of the iron absorbed.[10] In infants between 6 and 12 months of age who were fed formulas non-fortified or fortified with iron, heme iron (from meat) accounted for 8 to 9% and 3 to 5% of total iron intake.[11]

Absorption of Non-heme Iron

Most dietary iron for children and adults is in the form of non-heme iron. Absorption depends on the iron nutritional status of the infant, the quantity consumed, and the presence or absence of inhibitors or enhancers of iron absorption.[12] Iron is better absorbed by iron-deficient than by iron sufficient infants: mean geometric absorp-

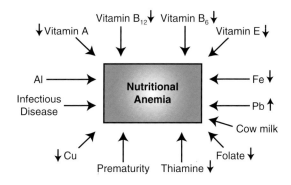

Figure 1: Factors contributing to nutritional anemia.

tion of 5 mg of ferrous iron given with food to 5 to 18 month old infants with or without iron deficiency was 8.5% and 3.8%.[13] When iron of a specified bioavailability is present in a meal, the percentage of iron absorbed is inversely related to the iron content of that meal.[14]

The major inhibitors of non-heme iron absorption are indicated in Figure 2.[15] Infants and young children fed commercially available formulas or cow milk consume greater amounts of protein and calcium than do breast-fed infants. Substantial amounts of phytates are consumed by infants fed soy protein-based formulas. Phenolic compounds are present in tea and certain vegetables. Insoluble tannins which prevent the absorption of iron are formed when tea is consumed with or immediately after a meal. Because inhibitors of iron absorption are found in many food items, absorption of iron is lower when iron is given with meals.

Ascorbic acid is a potent enhancer of iron absorption (Figure 2). It allows the delivery of non-heme iron to the intestinal mucosa in an ionic form. The absorption of iron from infant formulas and cereals can be increased threefold by raising the ascorbic acid-to-iron ratio (wt:wt) from 1:1 to 5:1.[16] Citrate and animal tissue protein (meat, fish and poultry) also enhance iron solubility and absorption.

Metabolism

The major protein responsible for transporting iron within the body is transferrin (Figure 3). Transferrin releases its iron to transferrin receptors located on the cell surface, which bring iron into the cells. Much of the iron delivered to the erythropoietic cells of the bone marrow is incorporated into heme. Iron from break-

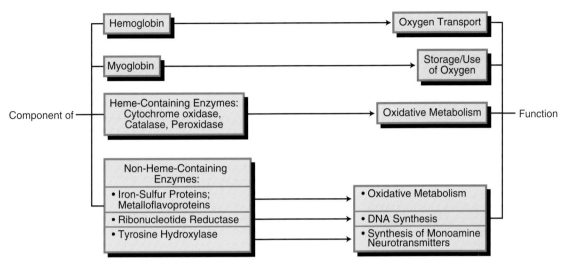

Table 2: Iron - Functions in the body.

down of senescent erythrocytes and iron absorbed by the intestinal tract is bound to circulating transferrin.

Iron is stored within tissues in two forms: (a) ferritin, a soluble mobile form and (b) hemosiderin, an aggregated insoluble form. Most of the body ferritin is found in the reticulo-endothelial-system (RES), but all body cells require the presence of ferritin. Hemosiderin is a mixture of protein, lipid and iron, consisting of degraded ferritin within a lysosomal membrane.[17]

Ferritin and the transferrin receptor, the major proteins involved in the regulation of iron homeostasis, are proteins which seem to be regulated by intracellular iron (Figure 3) at the level of translation and mRNA stability.[18] Transferrin receptor brings iron into the cell, where it is transferred to the iron-storage protein ferritin or to other cellular proteins requiring iron. Iron regulatory factors (IRF) are involved in posttranscriptional regulation of ferritin and transferrin-receptor, which is needed because of the toxicity of free iron in the cell. This toxicity is due to the ability to form reactive hydroxyls which can cause peroxidation of lipid membranes and other cellular elements. High free iron concentration in the cell mobilizes ferritin mRNAs onto polysomes for translation, but decreases transferrin receptor synthesis, which is controlled at the level of mRNA stability. The result of ferritin upregulation and transferrin receptor downregulation is a decrease in the free iron levels in the cell, thereby preventing iron toxicity. Iron starvation induces the expression of transferrin receptor, thereby increasing iron uptake, and represses the synthesis of protein involved in iron storage and utilization.

Iron Requirements and Intake

Relation between iron status of mother and newborn. It was long believed that iron nutritional status of the mothers had little influence on intrauterine iron acquisition by the fetus.[19] However, recent data indicate that iron deficiency during pregnancy can be associated with prematurity and low birth weight.[20]

Term Infants

To remain in satisfactory iron nutritional status, infants must absorb sufficient iron for growth and as replacement of losses that occur via the gastrointestinal tract, skin, and urine. By emptying iron stores, redistributing iron and lowering hemoglobin concentration, the healthy, term infant is able to double its birth weight without requiring an exogenous iron source.[21] However, beginning at 3 to 4 months of age, the term infant becomes dependent on an exogenous supply of iron to maintain adequate iron nutritional status. Estimated requirements for absorbed iron are approximately 0.55-0.75 mg/day during the first year of life and 0.8 mg/day during the second year of life.[4]

As already indicated, iron concentration in human milk is low (0.3-0.5 mg/l). The most detailed description of iron concentration in "term breast milk" between 14 and 183 days of age[22] indicates a logarithmic decline in

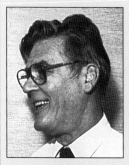

Calvin W. Woodruff M.D. (1920-1989) was a 1944 graduate of Yale Medical School. From 1947 until 1960, he was in the Department of Pediatrics at Vanderbilt, a period when this institution was the center of U.S. nutritional biochemistry and public health. Woodruff subsequently served at the American University of Beirut, University of Michigan and University of Missouri. He discovered the relationship between feeding of whole cow milk and iron depletion of infants. Woodruff, C.W. Anemias in History of Pediatrics 1850-1950, ed. by B.L.Nichols, A Ballabriga and N. Kretchmer Raven Press, NY. 1991, 181-187 (Photo courtesy of CNRC)

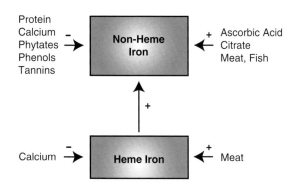

Figure 2: Enhancers (+) and inhibitors (-) of heme- and non-heme iron absorption.

iron during the lactational period. Concentrations of iron in breast milk of mothers delivering preterm infants are between 62 and 115% higher than those of mothers delivering at term during the first seven weeks of lactation,[23] but no data for comparison are available beyond that stage of lactation. It is generally believed[24, 25] that approximately 50% of the iron in breast milk is absorbed. If an infant consumes 0.5 liter of breast milk per day during the early weeks of life (when iron concentration is 0.5 mg/liter) and 0.75 l/d later (when iron concentration is 0.3 mg/l), the amount ingested will be only approximately 0.26 mg. If 50% is absorbed, the amount absorbed will be approximately 0.13 mg, an amount far less than the estimated requirement for absorbed iron of 0.55 to 0.75 mg/d.[4] Breast-fed infants who do not receive iron supplements or iron from beikost items are at risk of becoming iron-deficient between 6 and 12 months of age.[26]

Fortification of infant formulas with iron is an effective and convenient means of providing iron to infants (Table 3). The iron-fortification level in infant formulas ranges from 6 to 15 mg/l, and concentrations of ascorbic acid similar to those used in infant formulas (40-60 mg/l) enhance absorption of iron from milk.[16] Geometric mean absorption of iron from formulas providing 12 mg of iron and 50 mg of ascorbic acid per liter is 4 to 5% of intake. If 750 ml of formula are consumed per day, the amount of iron absorbed will be approximately 0.36 mg, an amount which corresponds to 48 to 65% of the estimated requirement for absorbed iron.[4]

Daily consumption of fortification iron from Beikost in infants between 6 and 12 months of age ranges from 0.25 to 0.45 mg/kg (Figure 4).[11] Clinical studies indicated that daily consumption of iron-fortified rice-cereal can contribute substantially to preventing iron deficiency anemia in breast-fed infants or infants fed non-iron fortified formulas between 8 and 15 months of age.[27]

Bioavailability of fortification iron in commercially prepared, iron-fortified beikost items such as cereals and vegetables is low. Studies in fasting nine-month-old infants indicated a geometric mean iron bioavailability of 3.0% from a proprietary dehydrated vegetable product, 3.0% from whole-heat breakfast cereal, 3.1% from wholemeal bread, and 4.3% from baked beans. When cereal, bread, or baked beans were taken with a drink containing ascorbic acid, there was a two-fold increase in iron bioavailability.[28] The iron in these foods is assumed to be of high bioavailability, because meat and ascorbic acid enhance the bioavailability of non-heme (i.e., fortification) iron.[15]

Preliminary data from the NHANES III[29] indicate iron intakes (mean, SD) of 11.50 (0.50) and 9.53 (0.24) mg/day for US infants between 2 to 11 months and one to two years, respectively. During the second year of life, less iron is required for growth and more highly bioavailable iron is offered with a mixed diet, which is less dominated by milk (Table 4).[30]

Iron Deficiency
Clinical Findings

In the case of severe iron deficiency anemia, pallor, fatigue, irritability and delayed motor development

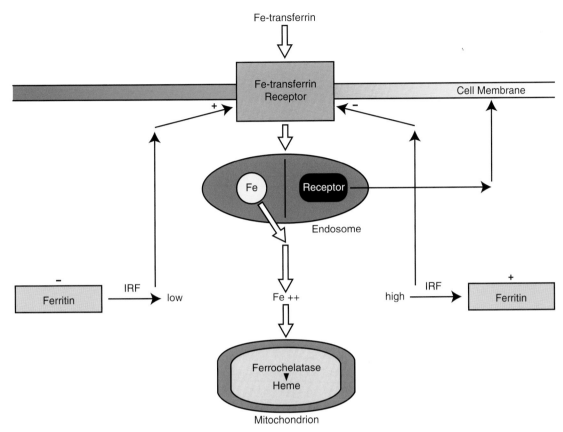

Figure 3: Intracellular regulation of ferritin and transferrin-receptor. Modified from Leibold and Guo.[18]

have been observed. The child is often fat and flabby, with poor muscle tone.

Systemic manifestations of iron deficiency anemia include behavioral and cognitive abnormalities, which were expressed as lower scores on tests of psychomotor development. The problem that arises in the interpretation of results is the common association of anemia with adverse health, environment, socio-economic background and nutrition. The studies suggest that iron deficiency causing anemia, but not iron deficiency without anemia, is associated with impaired performance of mental and psychomotor development. Follow-up studies demonstrate that the subjects who had been anemic as infants, even though they were in adequate iron nutritional status at 5 to 6 years of age, performed less well on tests of cognitive function than did their peers.[31, 32] Thus, it cannot be excluded that the effects of early iron deficiency anemia on brain development may be irreversible. The neuropharmacological and neurobiochem-

ical basis for the well-documented behavioral alterations seen during iron deficiency in experimental animals can be explained, at least in part, by an adverse effect of iron deficiency on the activity of the monoamine neurotransmitters dopamine, serotonine and norepinephrine.[33] These neurotransmitters are involved in learning, cognition and in neuropsychiatric disorders.

Although laboratory evidence indicates that iron deficiency adversely affects immune function and cellular resistance to infection,[5, 34] data from clinical studies so far are controversial. Andelman and Sered[35] reported fewer respiratory infections in infants fed iron-fortified formulas than in those fed non-iron-fortified formulas. However, Burman[36] found no difference between infants with or without iron treatment either in incidence of infections or in days of illness. Prospective studies with adequate experimental design are needed to answer the question whether the incidence and severity of infections in iron-deficient infants is higher.

IMPROVE IRON NUTRITION

PROPOSE	AVOID
• Breast-feeding (> 6 mo.) • Fe-fortified formulas • Meat • Ascorbic acid-rich foods • Fe-fortified Beikost	• Non-fortified formulas • Fresh cow milk (before 12 mo.)

Table 3: Strategies to improve iron nutritional status.

The urinary excretion of betain, a red pigment from beetroot, is referred to as beeturia, which has been mistaken for hematuria. Tunnessen et al[37] reported that 63% of infants and children with iron deficiency anemia developed marked beeturia after consumption of six tablespoons of homogenized beets.

Laboratory Indices (Table 5)

Hemoglobin Concentration and Hematocrit

Hemoglobin and/or hematocrit determinations are the most convenient screening methods, and are most useful when the prevalence of iron deficiency is high, as in infancy. The major limitation of hemoglobin measurement is low specificity. Normal values vary considerably with age, decreasing from high values after birth until 2 to 3 months of age, and then increasing.

Response to Iron Treatment

Screening for anemia at about 1 year of age has been proposed for high risk populations.[38, 39] Multiple tests do provide a greater degree of certainty with respect to iron-deficient infants, but are expensive. The hemoglobin determination alone may be a basis for a therapeutic trial of iron. However, only 35% of the infants with hemoglobin values below the selected cutoff value (11.5 g/dl) had a rise in hemoglobin concentration >1 g/dl during a three-month therapeutical trial.[39]

> *The feeding of Children properly is of much greater importance to them than their clothing. We ought to take great care to be right in this material article, and that nothing to be given them but what is wholesome and good for them, and in such quantity as the body calls for towards support and growth; not a grain more. Let us consider what Nature directs in this case: if we follow Nature, instead of driving it, we cannot err.*
>
> *Pediatrics of the Past*
> An anthology compiled and edited by John Ruhrah M.D.,
> 1925
> Paul B. Hoeber, Inc., Publishers,
> New York, NY

Mean Corpuscular Volume

A decrease in hemoglobin in erythrocytes is accompanied by a decrease in erythrocyte size. Low MCV strongly suggests iron deficiency, if thalassemia trait and infections can be excluded.

Erythrocyte Protoporphyrin

When insufficient iron is available to combine with protoporphyrin to form heme, the erythrocyte protoporphyrin increases. Raised erythrocyte protoporphyrin levels also occur in lead poisoning.

Transferrin Saturation

Nearly all of the serum iron is present in transferrin. Low transferrin saturation suggests that the delivery of iron to the hematopoietic tissues is insufficient to promote normal erythropoiesis.

Serum Ferritin

Although nearly all of the ferritin is present within cells, a small amount circulates in the serum. A decreased serum concentration of ferritin indicates depletion of body iron stores. The serum ferritin is of lesser value during or after an infection.

Transferrin Receptor

The protein plays a key role in receptor-mediated endocytosis, the process by which transferrin iron is delivered to the cytosol. When a cell perceives a need for additional iron, there is an upregulation of transferrin receptor synthesis, which allows the cell to compete more effectively for circulating transferrin iron. Small amounts of transferrin receptor can be detected in the serum. Elevated serum transferrin receptor concentration indicates increased tissue iron need. A great advantage of the serum transferrin receptor as an index of iron nutritional status is that it is unaffected by inflammation or infection.[40]

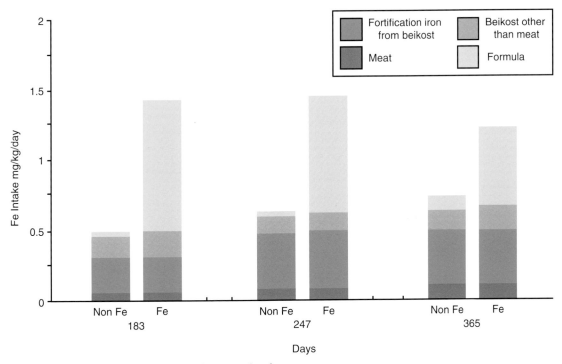

Figure 4: Feeding patterns between 6 and 12 months of age.[11]

Treatment

Treatment of confirmed iron deficiency anemia involves changes in the diet as well as the administration of iron, usually as ferrous sulfate. A dose of 3-5 mg/kg/day is recommended for term infants, but premature infants may need a higher dose. Parents should be informed about the danger of toxicity due to accidental ingestion and the dark color of the stool during treatment. Transient staining of teeth may occur. Infants respond rapidly to treatment, with half correction of the anemia, on the average, after two weeks. Hemoglobin determinations two or four weeks after initiation of treatment can confirm the therapeutic response. In order to build up sufficient iron stores in the body, treatment should be continued during three to four months.

Prevalence of Iron Deficiency

Data on U.S. children from 12 to 36 months collected in the Second National Health and Nutrition Examination Survey (NHANES II) are available. Iron deficiency was defined as an abnormality of two or more of the following indices: (i) MCV, (ii) transferrin satura-

tion and (iii) erythrocyte protoporphyrin. Prevalence of impaired iron status was 9.4%.[41] Among children from 12 to 36 months of age, 20.6% from low-income families and 6.7% from higher income families were iron deficient.[42]

Recent data from four Canadian cities indicate that 1.1% and 6.9% of the infants between 8 and 15 months of age had hemoglobin values <10 g/dl and between 10-11 g/dl, respectively. 33.9% had ferritin values <10 ng/ml. The proportion of iron deficient anemic infants (Hb<11 g/dl; ferritin<10 ng/ml; FEP>100 ug/l) was 4.3%.[43]

Detailed epidemiological data from different European regions (Table 6) collected in 1993/1994 indicate that iron deficiency is still a public health problem. Hemoglobin, MCV, transferrin saturation, serum ferritin and serum transferrin receptor values of 520 healthy term infants (age 12 months) from eleven European cities were measured as part of the Euro-Growth project.[44] Depletion of iron stores (serum ferritin <10 ng/ml) was present in one out of four European infants. The prevalence of anemia at 12 months of age was 9.8%, which corresponds to the data from the U.S.[41]

	Age (days)		
	365	548	730
total (mg/d)	9.1	7.0	7.9
meat, fish, poultry	0.6	1.2	1.6
fruits, vegetables	1.7	0.9	1.0
bread, cereals, potatoes	0.6	1.6	1.7
milk, yogurt	0.2	1.5	1.8
fortification iron	5.6	1.1	1.0
other sources	0.4	0.7	0.8

* Heil et al, 1986[30]

Table 4: Iron intake between 365 and 730 days of age (x;n=58). *

Prevention of Iron Deficiency (Table 3)

Canadian and U.S. proposals for prevention strategies[38, 45, 46] indicate that after six months of age, breast-fed infants should receive extra iron in the form of iron-fortified cereals and infant food. They should be offered iron-fortified infant formula after they have been weaned from breast milk (Figure 4). Term infants who are not breast-fed should be given an iron-fortified formula from birth. Cow milk should not be introduced before 12 months of age.[47] For children over one year of age, iron-containing foods such as meats, some vegetables, legumes, fruits and iron-fortified cereals provide iron in sufficient amounts.

Yip et al[48] reported a decline in prevalence of anemia in infants enrolled into the Special Supplemental Food Program for Women, Infants, and Children (WIC; low income groups) between 1973 and 1984. The decreasing prevalence of anemia was also observed in infants (9 to 23 months) visiting a pediatric practice in a middle class area of Minneapolis between 1969 and 1984. The only likely explanation for improved iron nutritional status is increased iron intake. Breast-feeding and the use of iron-fortified formulas at six months of age has become more popular between 1975 and 1995. Other feeding practices, such as the use of whole cow milk or non-iron-fortified formula, are less popular now than in the 70s. Iron intake with cow milk is low, iron absorption is inhibited by the high protein and calcium concentrations in cow milk,

and a substantial proportion of infants fed cow milk between 6 and 12 months of age suffers from gastrointestinal blood loss.[49] In Canada and Europe, early introduction of cow milk into the infants diet is a strong factor which negatively influences iron nutritional status between 8 and 15 months of age.[43, 44]

Iron Toxicity

Iron ions are powerful promoters of free radical damage, which accelerate lipid peroxidation and cause $OH°$ formation. The human body has a complex system of iron transport and storage proteins to ensure that iron is rarely allowed to be in the "free" state. For example, iron bound to transferrin will not catalyze damaging free radical reactions. The same is true of iron in breast milk which is bound to lactoferrin.[50]

However, in a high percentage of preterm infants, and a lower percentage of healthy term infants, circulating transferrin is iron-saturated and plasma contains iron that can catalyze damaging free radical reactions, such as $OH°$ formation.[51-53]

Iron is essential for the multiplication of most bacteria because the iron-containing enzyme ribonuclease reductase is needed for DNA synthesis.[54] Iron binding proteins (e.g. transferrin) bind the iron so tightly that it is not available to invading organisms.[34] The administration of iron to premature and term infants with high transferrin

Indices	Cutoff Value	Interpretation
Hemoglobin	<11 g/dl	Depletion of iron stores Erythropoiesis impaired (late)
Hematocrit	<32%	Depletion of iron stores Erythropoiesis impaired (late)
Erythrocytes: hypochromia, poikilocytosis, anisocytosis		Depletion of iron stores Erythropoiesis impaired (late)
Mean corpuscular volume	<70 fl	Depletion of iron stores Erythropoiesis impaired (late)
Erythrocyte protoporphyrin	>3µg/gHb (>100 µg/l)	Depletion of iron stores Erythropoiesis impaired (early)
Transferrin saturation	<10 %	Depletion of iron stores Erythropoiesis impaired (early)
Serum ferritin	<10 ng/ml	Depletion of iron stores Erythropoiesis normal
Transferrin receptor	↑**	Increased cellular iron need
Test normal		Normal iron nutritional Status

* age range six months to two years
** cutoff values not well established for age group six months to two years

Table 5: Indices of iron nutritional status.*

saturation has been advocated to be undesirable because of the possibility that transferrin would become saturated, thus promoting the growth of micro-organisms. However, with the possible exception of premature, malnourished infants or those with malaria, tuberculosis or brucellosis, there is no evidence that oral iron therapy increases the risk of infection or its severity.[55]

Of clinical importance is the presence of diseases that can lead to iron overload such as hemochromatosis.[56] The regulation of iron absorption from the diet is disturbed, so that the body becomes iron overloaded beyond childhood, and iron catalytic for free radical reactions is present in large amounts *in vivo*.

An adverse effect of iron intake on absorption of zinc and copper is unlikely under usual feeding circumstances.[57] It has been felt that infants fed iron-fortified formulas or receiving medicinal iron are prone to fussiness, regurgitation, loose stools, constipation, colic and flatus. Controlled studies failed to confirm those observations.[58-60]

Macrocytic Nutritional Anemia

Macrocytic anemia can be caused by folate or cobalamin (vitamin B12) deficiency. In the presence of folate deficiency, DNA synthesis is slowed because single-carbon transfers needed from nucleic acids are inadequate.[61] Because of this slow cell reproduction, erythrocytes are large, and maturation of cells in the mouth, tongue, and esophagus is likely to be abnormal. Major non-hematological manifestations of folate deficiency in infants and small children are failure to thrive, anorexia, weakness, pallor, glossitis and delayed brain development.[62] VLBW-infants, preterm infants receiving erythropoietin treatment, and term infants who receive most of their energy intake from goats milk are at risk to become deficient.[62-64] Folate deficiency occasionally is found in diseases affecting the upper portion of the small intestine (e.g. gluten-sensitive enteropathy), and in infants with heart disease.

	Cut off-value	% below/above
Hemoglobin	<11 g/dl	9.8
MCV	<70 fl	9
S-Ferritin	<10 ng/ml	24
Transferrin receptor	>4.2 ug/ml	10
Transferrin saturation	<10%	21

Male C. et al.[44]

Table 6: Iron nutritional status of European children at 12 months of age.

Because higher plants and animals are unable to synthesize vitamin B_{12}, they are dependent on the synthesis of this vitamin by bacteria, fungi and algae. Vitamin B_{12} deficiency has been described in breast-fed infants from industrialized and third-world countries whose mothers have become vitamin B_{12}-deficient through a strict vegetarian diet.[65, 66] In addition to megaloblastic anemia, the infants showed developmental delay, hypotonia and hyperpigmentation of the extremities. Concentrations of vitamin B_{12} in serum and in milk of the mothers were low.

Copper Deficiency

The anemia of copper deficiency is sideroblastic, microcytic, and hypochromic. It is explained in part by the decrease in ferroxidase activity of ceruloplasmin with consequent inability to release iron from tissue stores.[67] Ferrochelatase activity may be reduced in copper deficiency, with a negative effect on the final stage of heme synthesis, which involves the insertion of iron into protoporphyrin. Fifty-one cases of copper deficiency have been described in premature and term infants.[68] The clinical manifestations include psychomotor retardation, hypotonia, hypopigmentation, pallor, hepatosplenomegaly and increased risk for bone fractures due to osteoporosis. The sideroblastic anemia is resistant to iron therapy.

Vitamin E Deficiency

Erythrocytes of premature infants are susceptible to hemolysis in the presence of hydrogen peroxide, and vitamin E reduces this hemolytic tendency.[69] Tocopherols are the major source of natural protection against lipid peroxydation of the polyunsaturated fatty acids in biological membranes. The infants at greatest risk of vitamin E deficiency are those with primary fat malabsorption or cholestasis and those who receive intravenous lipid emulsions without adequate supplements of vitamin E. Premature infants are born with low vitamin E stores. If they were fed diets low in vitamin E and high in polyunsaturated fatty acids, hemolytic anemia was reported.[70] Medicinal doses of iron may increase hemolysis in vitamin E-deficient infants.[71] However, vitamin E deficiency is rare during enteral feeding with breast milk or modern vitamin E-fortified infant formulas. Small intravenous doses of vitamin E delivered in multivitamin preparations are generally sufficient to protect infants who receive parenteral nutrition.

Anemia Related to Infection

Chronic disease and severe infections are well-recognized causes of anemia,[72] but even mild infections may result in anemia.[48] During inflammatory diseases, it has been shown that pro-inflammatory and other cytokines are important mediators of intracellular iron metabolism, because they control expression of transferrin-receptor and ferritin as well as intracellular iron handling.[73, 74] Interleukin-1, a protein released from mononuclear phagocytes in response to microbial invasion, enhances synthesis of a number of acute phase proteins, among them ferritin. The result of increased ferritin synthesis is a block in iron release, resulting in reduced serum iron levels.[75]

In Europe, only 70% of the children with anemia at 12 months of age had laboratory parameters (low ferritin, elevated transferrin-receptor, and low MCV) which indicated iron deficiency.[44] Two out of three infants with anemia and no signs of iron deficiency had infections during the four weeks before blood sampling. Yip et al[48] compared the prevalence of anemia between healthy middle-class U.S. children and children with mild infections (age 9 to 83 months). Prevalence of anemia of the sick children measured at four times between 1969 and 1986 was significantly higher.

Anemia of Prematurity

The anemia of prematurity is commonly associated with low reticulocyte counts and deficient erythropoietin production.[76, 77] Diagnostic tests can also cause substantial blood loss,[78, 79] and premature infants receive frequent transfusions according to the amount of blood drawn.[79, 80] Iron deficiency plays a minor role at least during the first four to six weeks.

Recombinant human erythropoietin stimulates erythroid progenitors from preterm infants in a normal dose-response relation.[81, 82] A multicenter, controlled, blinded trial in 241 infants with birth weights below 1500g indicated that treatment with recombinant human erythropoietin (250 IU/kg body weight three times weekly from day 3 to day 42) resulted in lower need for transfusion. Absence of need for transfusions and a hematocrit that never fell below 32 percent was found in 27.5% of the infants treated with recombinant human erythropoietin, but only in 4.1% of the infants without treatment. Serum ferritin as the indicator of iron stores decreased rapidly during treatment with recombinant human erythropoietin.[63] Oral iron supplementation (2-6 mg/day) is needed for optimal erythropoiesis,[80, 83] because the high dose of recombinant human erythropoietin might increase the iron mobilization excessively relative to the stores available in very-low-birth-weight infants.[84] Folate and vitamin E supplements should also be considered during treatment with erythropoietin.

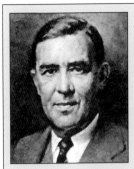

Kenneth D. Blackfan M. D. (1883-1941) was Howland's resident for ten years. He served as Chairman of Pediatrics at Harvard from 1921 until 1941. His research interests were in nutrition and hematology with an emphasis on anemia. He was a coauthor with Shohl in the 1939 description of first intravenous administration of hydrolyzed casein. Pediatric Profiles editor B. S. Veeder, Mosby St. Louis, 1957, 211-217 (Photo courtesy of BCH)

Historical Perspective...

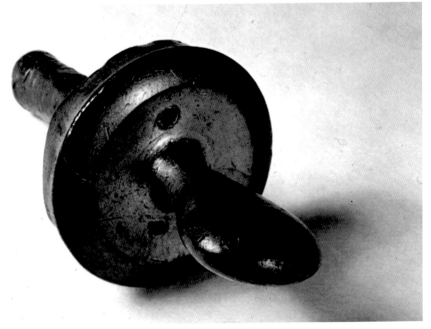

Pewter nipple, New England, early nineteenth century.

References

1. *United Nations: First Report on the World Nutrition Situation.* Rome; United Nations Administrative Committee on Coordination - Subcommittee on Nutrition: November 1987.

2. Oski FA. Designation of anemia on a functional basis. *J Pediatr.* 1973;883:353.

3. Elwood PC. Evaluation of the clinical importance of anemia. *Am J Clin Nutr.* 1973;26:958.

4. Fomon SJ, ed. *Nutrition of Normal Infants.* St. Louis: Mosby; 1993.

5. Dallman PR. Biochemical basis for manifestations of iron deficiency. *Ann Rev Nutr.* 1986;6:13-40.

6. Dallman PR. Iron. In: Brown ML, ed. *Present knowledge in nutrition.* 6th ed. Washington, DC: International Life Sciences Institute, Nutrition Foundation; 1990: 241-250.

7. Hallberg L, Sölvell L. Absorption of hemoglobin iron in man. *Acta Med Scand.* 1967;181:335-354.

8. Hallberg L, Brune M, Erlandsson M, et al. Calcium: effect of different amounts on non-heme- and heme-iron absorption in humans. *Am J Clin Nutr.* 1991;53: 112-119.

9. Hallberg L, Björn-Rasmussen E, Howard L, et al. Dietary heme iron absorption. A discussion of possible mechanisms for the absorption-promoting effect of meat and for the regulation of iron absorption. *Scand J Gastroenterol.* 1979;14:769-779.

10. Cook JD. Determinants of non-heme iron absorption in man. *Food Tech.* 1983;37:124-126.

11. Haschke F, Pietschnig B, Vanura H, Heil M, Steffan I, Hobiger G, Schuster E, Camaya Z. Iron intake and iron nutritional status of infants fed iron-fortified beikost with meat. *Am J Clin Nutr.* 1988;47:108-112.

12. Cook JD. Adaptation in iron metabolism. *Am J Clin Nutr.* 1990;51:301-308.

13. Heinrich HC, Gabbe EE, Whang DH, et al. Ferrous and hemoglobin-^{59}Fe absorption from supplemented cow milk in infants with normal and depleted iron stores. *Z Kinderheilk.* 1975;120:251-258.

14. Bezwoda WR, Bothwell TH, Charlton RW, et al. The relative dietary importance of haem and non-haem iron. *S Afr Med J.* 1983;64:552-556.

15. Hallberg L, Rossander-Hulten L, Brune M. Prevention of iron deficiency by diet. In: Fomon SJ, Zlotkin S, eds. *Nutritional Anemia.* Nestlé Nutrition Workshop Series. Vol. 30. New York: Raven Press; 1992:169-178.

16. Derman DP, Bothwell TH, MacPhail, et al. Importance of ascorbic acid in the absorption of iron from infant foods. *Scand J Haematol.* 1980;25:193-201.

17. Hoffmann KE, Yanelli K, Bridges KR. Ascorbic acid and iron metabolism: alterations in lysosomal function. *Am J Clin Nutr.* 1991;54:1188-1192.

18. Leibold EA, Guo B. Iron-dependent regulation of ferritin and transferrin receptor expression by the iron-responsive element binding protein. *Annu Rev Nutr.* 1992;12:345-368.

19. Dallman PR, Siimes MA, Stekel A. Iron deficiency in infancy and childhood. *Am J Clin Nutr.* 1980;33:86-118.

20. Scholl TO, Hediger ML, Fischer RL, et al. Anemia vs iron deficiency: increased risk of preterm delivery in a prospective study. *Am J Clin Nutr.* 1992;55:985-988.

21. Owen GM. Iron nutrition: growth in infancy. In: Filer LJ Jr, ed. *Dietary Iron: Birth to Two Years.* New York: Raven Press; 1989:103-117.

22. Siimes MA, Vuori E, Kuitunen P. Breast milk iron - a declining concentration during the course of lactation. *Acta Paediatr Scand.* 1979;68:29-31.

23. Harzer G, Haschke F. Micronutrients in human milk. In: Renner E, ed. *Micronutrients in Milk and Milk-Based Food Products.* London: Elsevier; 1989:125-237.

24. Cook JD, Bothwell TH. Availability of iron from infant foods. In: Stekel A, ed. *Iron nutrition in infancy and childhood.* New York: Raven Press; 1984:119-143.

25. Lönnerdal B, Glazier C. An approach to assessing trace element bioavailability from milk in vitro. Extrinsic labeling and proteolytic degradation. *Biol Trace Elem Res.* 1989;19:57-69.

26. Haschke F, Vanura H, Male C, Owen G, Pietschnig B, Schuster E, Krobath E, Huemer C. Iron nutrition and growth of breast- and formula-fed infants during the first 9 months of life. *J Pediatr Gastro Nutr.* 1993;16: 151-156.

27. Walter T, Dallman PR, Pizarro F, Velozo L, Perna G, Bartholmey SJ, Hertrampf E, Olivares M, Letelier A, Arredondo M. Effectiveness of iron-fortified infant cereal in prevention of iron deficiency anemia. *Pediatrics.* 1993;91:976-982.

28. Fairweather-Tait S, Fox T, Wharf SG, Eagles J. The bioavailability of iron in different weaning foods and the enhancing effect of a fruit drink containing ascorbic acid. *Pediatr Res.* 1995;37:389-394.

29. Alaimo K, McDowell MA, Briefel RR, et al. Dietary intake of vitamins, minerals, and fiber of persons aged 2 months and over in the United States. *Third National*

Health and Nutrition Examination Survey. Phase 1, 1988-1991. Advance data from vital and health statistics. Hyatsville, Maryland; National Center for Health Statistics: 1994. (no. 258).

30. Heil M, Haschke F, Steffan I, Vanura H, Hobiger G, Pietschnig B. Iron-, zinc-, and copper intake during infancy. *Infusionstherapie.* 1986;13:10-11.

31. Lozoff B, Jimenez E, Wolf AW. Long-term developmental outcome of infants with iron deficiency. *N Engl J Med.* 1991;325:687-694.

32. Walter T. Early and long-term effect of iron deficiency anemia on child development. In: Fomon SJ, Zlotkin S, eds. *Nutritional anemias.* Nestlé Nutrition Workshop Series. Vol. 30. New York: Raven Press; 1992:81-90.

33. Youdim MBH, Ben-Shachar D, Yehuda S. Putative biological mechanismus of the effect of iron deficiency on brain biochemistry and behavior. *Am J Clin Nutr.* 1989;50:607-617.

34. Dallman PR. Iron deficiency and the immune response. *Am J Clin Nutr.* 1987;46:329-334.

35. Andelman MB, Sered BR. Utilization of dietary iron by term infants. *Am J Dis Child.* 1966;111:45-55.

36. Burman D. Haemoglobin levels in normal infants aged 3 to 24 months, and the effect of iron. *Arch Dis Child.* 1972;47:261-271.

37. Tunnessen WW, Smith C, Oski FA. Beeturia. A sign of iron deficiency. *Am J Dis Child.* 1969;117:424-426.

38. Committee on Nutrition, American Academy of Pediatrics: Iron supplementation for infants. *Pediatrics.* 1976;58:765-768.

39. Dallman PR, Reeves JD, Driggers DA, Lo EY. Diagnosis of iron deficiency: the limitations of laboratory tests in predicting response to iron treatment in 1-year-old infants. *J Pediatr.* 1981;99:376-381.

40. Ferguson BJ, Skikne BS, Simpson KM, et al. Serum transferrin receptor distinguishes the anemia of chronic disease from iron deficiency anemia. *J Lab Clin Med.* 1992;19:389-390.

41. Dallman PR, Yip R, Johnson C. Prevalence and causes of anemia in the United States, 1976 to 1980. *Am J Clin Nutr.* 1984;39:437-445.

42. Pilch SM, Senti FR. Assessment of the iron nutritional status of the US population based on data collected in the Second Nutritional Health and Nutrition Examination Survey, 1976-1980. Bethesda, Md: Life Sciences Research Office, Federation of American Societies for Experimental Biology: 1984.

43. Zlotkin SH, Marie MS, Kopelman H, Jones A. The prevalence of iron depletion and iron-deficiency anemia in a randomly selected group of infants from four Canadian cities. Personal communication.

44. Male C, Barko E, Freeman V, Golser A, Guerra A, Haschke F, van't Hof M, Manrique M, Persson L, Radke M, Salerno C, Sanchez E, Tojo R, Zachou T. Iron status of European infants at 12 months of age. 7th European Nutrition Conference. 1995; (in press).

45. Committee on Nutrition, American Academy of Pediatrics. Iron-fortified infant formulas. *Pediatrics.* 1989; 84:1114-1115.

46. Canadian Pediatric Society, Nutrition Committee. Meeting the iron needs of infants and young children: an update. *CMAJ.* 1991;144:1451-1454.

47. Committee on Nutrition, American Academy of Pediatrics. The use of whole cow's milk in infancy. *Pediatrics.* 1992;89:1105-1109.

48. Yip R, Walsh KM, Goldfarb MG, et al. Declining prevalence of anemia in childhood in a middle-class setting: a pediatric success story? *Pediatrics.* 1987;80: 330-334.

49. Ziegler EE, Fomon SJ, Nelson SE, et al. Cow milk feeding in infancy: further observations on blood loss from the gastrointestinal tract. *J Pediatr.* 1990;116:11-18.

50. Aruoma OI, Halliwell B. Superoxide-dependent and ascorbate-dependent formation of hydroxyl radicals from hydrogen peroxide in the presence of iron. Are lactoferrin and transferrin promoters of hydroxyl-radical generation? *Biochem J.* 1987;241:273-278.

51. Moison RMW, Palinckx JJS, Roest M, Houdkamp E, Berger HM. Induction of lipid peroxidation of pulmonary surfactant by plasma of preterm babies. *Lancet.* 1993;341:79-82.

52. Evans PJ, Evans RW, Kovar IZ, Horton AF, Halliwell B. Bleomycin-detectable iron in the plasma of premature and full-term neonates. *FEBS Lett.* 1992;303:210-212.

53. Kaur H, Halliwell B. Aromatic hydroxylation of phenylalanine as an assay for hydroxyl radicals. Measurement of hydroxyl radical formation from ozone and in blood from premature babies using improved HPLC methodology. *Anal Biochem.* 1994;220:11-15.

54. Dallman PR. Upper limits of iron in infant formulas. *J Nutr.* 1989;119:1852-1855.

55. Hershko C. Iron and infection. In: Fomon SJ, Zlotkin S, eds. *Nutritional anemias.* Nestlé Nutrition Workshop Series. Vol. 30. New York: Raven Press; 1992: 53-61.

56. Edwards CQ, Griffen LM, Goldgar D, Drummond C, Skolnick MH, Hushner JP. Prevalence of hemochromatosis among 11, 6605 presumably healthy blood donors. *N Engl J Med.* 1988;318:1355-1362.

57. Haschke F, Ziegler EE, Edwards BB, et al. Effect of iron fortification of infant formula on trace mineral absorption. *J Pediatr Gastroenterol Nutr.* 1986;5:768-773.

58. Oski FA. Iron-fortified formulas and gastrointestinal symptoms in infants: a controlled study. *Pediatrics.* 1980;66:168-170.

59. Reeves JD, Yip R. Lack of adverse side effects of oral ferrous sulfate therapy in 1-year-old infants. *Pediatrics.* 1985;75:352-355.

60. Nelson SE, Ziegler EE, Copeland AM, et al. Lack of adverse reactions to iron-fortified formula. *Pediatrics.* 1988;81:360-364.

61. Herbert V. Biology of disease. Megaloblastic anemias. *Lab Invest.* 1985;52:3-19.

62. Anderson SA, Talbot JM. A review of folate intake, methodology, and status. Bethesda, Md. Life Science Research Office, Federation of American Societies for Experimental Biology: 1981.

63. Maier RF, Obladen M, Scigalla P, et al. The effect of epoetin beta (recombinant human erythropoietin) on the need for transfusion in very-low-birth-weight infants. *N Engl J Med.* 1994;330:1173-1178.

64. Hanna MD, Vogelsang SA, Carroll NL, et al. Dietary megaloblastic anemia in an infant. *SD J Med.* 1986;39: 7-9.

65. Baker SJ, Jacob E, Rajan KT, et al. Vitamin-B12 deficiency in pregnancy and the puerperium. *BMJ.* 1962;1:1658-1661.

66. Srikantia SG, Reddy V. Megaloblastic anemia in infancy and vitamin B12. *Br J Haematol.* 1967;13:949-953.

67. Danks DM. Copper deficiency in humans. *Annu Rev Nutr.* 1988;8:235-257.

68. Shaw JCL. Copper deficiency in term and preterm infants. In: Fomon SJ, Zlotkin S, eds. *Nutritional Anemias.* Nestlé Nutrition Workshop Series. Vol. 30. New York: Raven Press; 1992:105-117.

69. Gordon HH, de Metry JP. Hemolysis in hydrogen peroxide of erythrocytes of premature infants. *Proc Soc Exp Biol Med.* 1952;79:446-450.

70. Oski FA, Barness LA. Vitamin E deficiency: a previously unrecognized cause of hemolytic anemia in the premature infant. *J Pediatr.* 1967;700:211-220.

71. Melhorn DK, Gross S. Vitamin E-dependent anemia in the premature infant. 1. Effects of large doses of medicinal iron. *J Pediatr.* 1971;79:569-580.

72. Yip R, Dallman PR. The roles of inflammation and iron deficiency as causes of anemia. *Am J Clin Nutr.* 1988;48: 1295-1300.

73. Ward RJ, Kuhn LC, Kaldy P, Florence A, Peters TJ, Crichton RR. Control of cellular iron homeostasis by iron-responsive elements *in vivo. Eur J Biochem.* 1994; 220:927-931.

74. Seiser C, Teixeira S, Kuhn LC. Interleukin-2-dependent transcriptional and posttranscriptional regulation of transferrin receptor mRNA. *J Biol Chem.* 1993;268: 13074-13080.

75. Cook JD, Skikne BS, Baynes RD. Screening strategies for nutritional iron deficiency. In: Fomon SJ, Zlotkin S, eds. *Nutritional anemias.* Nestlé Nutrition Workshop Series. Vol. 30. New York: Raven Press; 1992: 159-165.

76. Brown MS, Garcia JF, Phibbs RH, Dallman PR. Decreased response of plasma immunoreactive erythropoietin to "available oxygen" in anemia of prematurity. *J Pediatr.* 1984;105:793-798.

77. Stockman JA III, Graeber JE, Clark DA, McClellan K, Garcia JF, Kavey REW. Anemia of prematurity: determinants of the erythropoietin response. *J Pediatr.* 1984;105:786-792.

78. Shannon KM. Anemia of prematurity: progress and prospects. *Am J Pediatr Hematol Oncol.* 1990;12:14-20.

79. Obladen M, Sachsenweger M, Stahnke M. Blood sampling in very low birth weight infants receiving different levels of intensive care. *Eur J Pediatr.* 1988;147: 399-404.

80. Shannon KM, Mentzer WC, Abels RI, et al. Recombinant human erythropoietin in the anemia of prematurity: results of a placebo-controlled pilot study. *J Pediatr.* 1991;118:949-955.

81. Shannon KM, Naylor GS, Torkildson JC, et al. Circulating erythroid progenitors in the anemia of prematurity. *N Engl J Med.* 1987;317:728-733.

82. Rhondeau SM, Christensen RD, Ross MP, Rothstein G, Simmons MA. Responsiveness to recombinant human erythropoietin of marrow erythroid progenitors from infants with the "anemia of prematurity." *J Pediatr.* 1988; 112:935-940.

83. Shannon KM, Mentzer WC, Abels RI, et al. Enhancement of erythropoiesis by recombinant human erythropoietin in low birth weight infants: a pilot study. *J Pediatr.* 1992; 120:586-592.

84. Halperin DS, Wacker P, Lacourt G, et al. Effect of recombinant human erythropoietin in infants with the anemia of prematurity: a pilot study. *J Pediatr.* 1990;116:

Who Needs Water-Soluble Vitamins?
Richard J. Schanler M.D.

Section of Neonatology and USDA/ARS Children's Nutrition Research Center,
Department of Pediatrics,
Baylor College of Medicine, Houston, TX

Reviewed by Frank R. Greer M.D., Helen K. Berry and Harry Greene M.D.

Introduction

Water-soluble vitamins function as cofactors for enzyme reactions of intermediary metabolism; they are therefore dependent upon the energy and protein content of an individual's diet, as well as on his rates of growth and energy use. First elucidated as etiologic agents of diseases now known to be deficiency syndromes, water-soluble vitamin needs were emphasized during the early development of commercial formula and parenteral nutrition mixtures.

At birth, the concentration of water-soluble vitamins is greater in the neonate than in the mother. Active transport of water-soluble vitamins during pregnancy results in concentration gradients (1:1.5 to 1:6) favoring the fetus.[1] Significant correlations between maternal and neonatal plasma water-soluble vitamin indices are reported.[2] Hypovitaminosis for many water-soluble vitamins can occur when a woman does not take vitamin supplements during pregnancy.[3]

Under usual circumstances in the United States, sufficient water-soluble vitamins tend to be maintained throughout the infancy of breast-fed, full-term infants. The mother's diet does affect milk concentration of water-soluble vitamins to some degree. Currently available commercial formulas in the United States satisfy the vitamin needs of infancy.

The gastrointestinal tract and liver modify orally-ingested water-soluble vitamins. Parenteral administration of these vitamins, bypassing this barrier, may present the kidney with a large quantity of vitamin for excretion. The kidney's ability to adapt to continuous parenteral administration of vitamins has not been determined.

This chapter addresses how infants and toddlers maintain sufficient intakes and avoid deficiencies of thiamin, riboflavin, niacin, vitamin B_6, pantothenic acid, biotin, folate, vitamin B_{12} and vitamin C.

Thiamin

In 1887, Dr. Takaki, a surgeon in the Japanese Navy, recognized that beriberi could be eliminated by modifying the diet.[4] The disease, which causes a paralysis of the hands and feet, had been known for centuries. The deficiency occurs most frequently in areas of the world where the diet consists of unenriched white rice or flour. Deficiency also may occur as a result of the consumption of large quantities of raw fish colonized with thiaminase-containing microorganisms.[5]

Physiology

Thiamin comprises a thiazole moiety joined by a methylene bridge to a pyrimidine ring (Figure 1). It is absorbed in the proximal small intestine by both active and passive mechanisms, and phosphorylated in the mucosal cells to yield the coenzyme thiamin pyrophosphate (TPP) and adenylic acid.[6, 7] The coenzyme TPP, with magnesium as a cofactor, functions in biochemical reactions related to carbohydrate metabolism, specifically, active aldehyde transfer of two general types.[7, 8, 9] The first type is catalyzed by dehydrogenase complexes for the oxidative decarboxylation of α-keto acids (pyruvate, α-ketoglutarate and the keto analogues of branched-chain amino acids). The dehydrogenase complexes are found in the mitochondria and are necessary for initiating the citric acid cycle. The second type of general reaction requiring TPP is the formation of α-ketols catalyzed by transketolase. This enzyme is located in the cytosol, especially in liver and

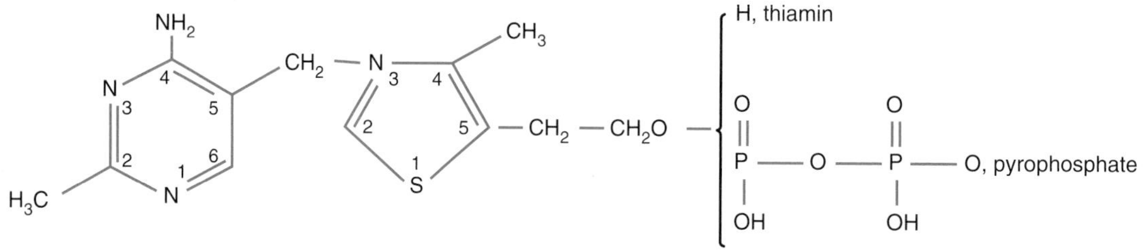

Figure 1: Thiamin and its pyrophosphate coenzyme.

red blood cells. Transketolase supplies NADPH needed for biosynthetic reactions in the pentose phosphate pathway. Because of its association with intermediary metabolism, thiamin deficiency usually manifests by abnormalities of carbohydrate metabolism, e.g., elevation of plasma and tissue pyruvate.[5] Marginal thiamin deficiency may be unmasked, therefore, by administering large carbohydrate loads.

In addition to its coenzyme functions, thiamin is thought to play a specific role in neurophysiology. Decreased concentrations of TPP and TTP (thiamin triphosphate) are observed with nerve stimulation. Thiamin and TPP are located in peripheral nerve membranes and may function as part of the sodium channel.[10]

Although a 30% incidence of thiamin deficiency has been reported during pregnancy and explained on the basis of increasing metabolism, decreasing appetite and persistent vomiting, thiamin deficiency is not observed in the infants.[11, 12] The fetomaternal gradient for thiamin favors the fetus and may protect it against maternal deficiency.[3, 12, 13]

Needs of Full-Term Infants

The thiamin concentration of human milk increases from approximately 20 µg/L in colostrum to an average of 220 µg/L (31 µg/100 kcal, range 21 to 36 µg/100 kcal) in mature milk.[14-21] The thiamin contents of human and bovine milk, commercial formulas, juices, and vitamin preparations for infants and toddlers are shown in Tables 1-4.[14, 22]

The classic studies of Holt[23] in infants of five to seven kg body weight reported marked decreases in urinary excretion of thiamin when intakes of the vitamin were below 140 to 200 µg/d; he proposed that range as the minimum intake of the vitamin.

The need for thiamin is directly related to the amount of metabolizable carbohydrate consumed. Practically, requirements are expressed in terms of energy content (µg/100 kcal).[24, 25] The Committee on Nutrition (CON) of the American Academy of Pediatrics, recommends 40 µg thiamin/100 kcal, which provides a safety margin for the advisable intake of the vitamin (Table 5). The thiamin intake of full-term, breast-fed infants, however, appears satisfactory. Thiamin deficiency in breast-fed infants of well-nourished mothers has not been reported. The CON recommendation is similar to the Recommended Dietary Allowance (RDA) for full-term infants.[5, 25]

The thiamin needs of infants receiving total parenteral nutrition (TPN) have not been described fully. Thiamin sufficiency was reported after parenteral daily doses of 1200 µg thiamin hydrochloride (130 µg/100 kcal) in full-term infants and children.[26, 27] Elevated whole blood thiamin concentrations after 50 and 115 days of TPN are reported in children receiving 1.5 to 4.5 mg/d.[28] The current recommendation for full-term infants, 1,200 µg/d, based on guidelines of the American Medical Association Nutritional Advisory Group, probably is appropriate (Table 6).[27] Thiamin status also is appropriate in adults receiving water-soluble vitamins as complete admixtures (glucose, amino acid, lipid and mineral solutions).[29]

Deficiency

A deficiency of thiamin results in beriberi. The signs of this disease relate to the chronic nature of the depletion, its severity, and associated stresses.[30] The illness has been described as "wet" or "dry," depending on the presence of edema or muscle wasting. Severe deficiency will produce cardiovascular changes progressing to fulminant cardiac failure ("cardiac beriberi").[31, 32] A high

	Human Milk*	Bovine Milk**	Enfamil	Similac	SMA
Thiamin (μg)	220 (150-250)	375	520	676	670
Riboflavin (μg)	400 (300-600)	1650	1000	1014	1000
Niacin (mg)	2.0 (1.8-2.3)	0.8	7.7	7.1	5.0
Vitamin B_6 (μg)	140 (90-200)	415	417	406	420
Pantothenic acid (mg)	4.0 (2.5-6.7)	3.2	3.1	3.0	2.1
Biotin (μg)	5.0 (4-8)	50#	15	30	15
Folate (μg)	50 (40-85)	50	105	100	50
Vitamin B_{12} (μg)	0.7 (0.5-1.2)	3.6	1.6	1.7	1.3
Vitamin C (mg)	50 (30-90)	12	54	60	55

*　See text for reference.
**　(22)
\#　(111)
　　Enfamil (Mead Johnson Nutritionals, Evansville, IN); Similac (Ross Laboratories, Columbus, OH);
　　SMA (Wyeth Laboratories, Philadelphia, PA)

Table 1: Milk concentrations of water-soluble vitamins (units/L).

intake of carbohydrate calories only, coupled with decreased intake of nutritionally adequate foods is thought to lead to the array of neurologic manifestations in thiamin deficiency.

Although thiamin deficiency in infants may be either acute or chronic, the acute cardiac symptoms and signs generally predominate.[31, 33] Anorexia, apathy, vomiting, restlessness and pallor progress to cardiomegaly and congestive heart failure, causing death in 24 to 48 hours. The infant with beriberi may have a striking characteristic cry: the infant is aphonic, he appears to be crying but no sound is uttered. A pseudomeningitic phase characterized by bulging fontanelle, seizures and coma also has been reported.[34-36]

"Infantile" beriberi may occur between one and four months of age in breast-fed infants whose mothers have deficient intakes of thiamin.[32] The nursing mother, however, may not have obvious signs of the deficiency.[33] Maternal alcoholism may be associated with infantile thiamin deficiency. King[37] reported that an infant born to a marginally thiamin-deficient mother demonstrated acute cardiac failure four days after birth and recovered following treatment with thiamin, five to ten mg/d. There are additional scattered case reports of infants presenting with encephalopathic signs of unknown etiology who had consumed formulas which presumably were improperly prepared or supplemented with thiamin.[35, 38]

A possible case of cardiac beriberi, determined by the transketolase assay, has been reported during total parenteral nutrition in a 12-year-old girl who received an inadequate dose of thiamin in relation to the glucose intake (16 μg/100 kcal glucose).[39] Asymptomatic thiamin deficiency has been demonstrated in 12% of hospitalized children in a Pediatric Intensive Care Unit and in four out of six children receiving chemotherapy in an Oncology Unit.[40] Shock, lactic acidosis and cardiac compromise have been prominent in the case reports of in-hospital thiamin deficiency.[41]

Large doses of thiamin have been effective in treating certain metabolic disorders, including a variant of maple syrup urine disease, Leigh's encephalopathy, thiamin-responsive megaloblastic anemia and an abnormality in pyruvate decarboxylase characterized clinically by severe lactic acidosis.[7]

The most common test for thiamin deficiency is the erythrocyte transketolase assay. In this assay, transketolase activity is measured before and after adding thiamin

	Human Milk*	Enfamil	Similac	SMA
Thiamin (μg)	31 (21-36)	78	100	100
Riboflavin (μg)	56 (42-85)	150	150	150
Niacin (mg)	0.29 (0.27-0.34)	1.1	1.1	0.75
Vitamin B$_6$ (μg)	20 (15-30)	62	60	63
Pantothenic acid (mg)	0.6 (0.3-1.0)	0.5	0.4	0.3
Biotin (μg)	0.7 (0.6-1.1)	2.2	4.5	2.2
Folate (μg)	7 (6-12)	15.6	15	7.5
Vitamin B$_{12}$ (μg)	0.10 (0.07-0.16)	0.23	0.25	0.20
Vitamin C (mg)	8 (5-13)	8	9	9

* See text for reference.
  Enfamil (Mead Johnson Nutritionals, Evansville, IN); Similac (Ross Laboratories, Columbus, OH);
  SMA (Wyeth Laboratories, Philadelphia, PA)

Table 2: Milk concentrations of water-soluble vitamins (units/100 kcal).

	Apple Juice	Orange Juice	White Grape Juice	Red Grape Juice	Mixed Fruit Juice	Grape Juice (Regular)
Thiamin (μg)	150	400-600	0	75	225-310	290
Riboflavin (μg)	150	230	0-240	150	150-225	375
Niacin (mg)	0.75	2.3	0.75-3.2	0.75	0.9-3.1	2.9
Vitamin B$_6$ (μg)	300	540	540	600	385-770	665
Vitamin C (mg)	325	325	325	300	325	0

From reference 22.

Table 3: Vitamin concentrations in juices for children (units/L).

pyrophosphate. The "TPP effect" refers to enhancement of transketolase activity. Severe thiamin deficiency exists when this ratio increases by more than 25%, mild or marginal deficiency occurs when the ratio is 15 to 25%, and adequate status is suggested by a ratio of <15%.[8] Whole blood and CSF thiamin concentrations, however, may be better quantitative measures of thiamin status.[42]

Urinary excretion of thiamin parallels dietary intake, except at low intake levels.[11] Thiamin not needed for tissue stores is excreted in the urine.[8] Conditions result-ing in large diureses, such as with diuretic therapy, may increase the urinary excretion of thiamin.[8, 31] Thiamin is destroyed or inactivated by heat, alkaline solutions and ionizing radiation. Loss of vitamin occurs during milk pasteurization and sterilization.[8, 13, 31]

Toxicity

No toxic effects of large oral doses of thiamin have been reported. Large intravenous doses, however, may produce respiratory depression and anaphylaxis.[31, 43]

	Poly-Vi-Sol Drops (units/ml)	Poly-Vi-Sol Chewable (units/tab)	Vi-Daylin Drops (units/ml)	Vi-Daylin Chewable (units/tab)
Thiamin (μg)	500	1050	500	1050
Riboflavin (μg)	600	1200	600	1200
Niacin (mg)	8.0	13.5	8.0	13.5
Vitamin B$_6$ (μg)	400	1050	400	1050
Pantothenic acid (mg)	0	0	0	0
Biotin (μg)	0	0	0	0
Folate (μg)	0	300	0	300
Vitamin B$_{12}$ (μg)	0	4.5	0	4.5
Vitamin C (mg)	35	60	35	60

Poly-Vi-Sol (Mead Johnson Nutritionals, Evansville, IN)
Vi-Daylin (Ross Laboratories, Columbus, OH)

Table 4: Water-soluble vitamin composition of commercial preparations for infants and children.

	AAP, CON* (units/100 kcal)	RDA† (units/d)			RDA (units·kg^{-1}·d^{-1})	
		0-6 mo	6-12 mo	1-3 y	0-6 mo	6-12 mo
Thiamin (μg)	40	300	400	700	50	44
Riboflavin (μg)	60	400	500	800	67	56
Niacin (mg)	.25(0.8**)	5**	6	9	0.8**	.7
Vitamin B$_6$ (μg)**	35	300	600	1000	50	67
Pantothenic acid (mg)	0.3	2	3	3	0.3	0.3
Biotin (μg)	1.5	10	15	20	1.7	1.7
Folate (μg)	4	25	35	50	4.2	3.9
Vitamin B$_{12}$ (μg)	0.15	0.3	0.5	0.7	0.05	0.06
Vitamin C (mg)	8	30	35	40	5	3.9

*   Committee on Nutrition of the American Academy of Pediatrics (25).
†   Recommended Dietary Allowances. Assume energy intake of 108 and 98 kcal·kg^{-1}·d^{-1}
    for 0-6 mo and 6-12 mo, respectively. Assumes body weight of 6 kg for 0-6 mo and 9 kg for 6-12 mo (5).
** As niacin equivalents.
*** Assumes vitamin B$_6$/protein ratio of at least 15 μg/g.

Table 5: Advisable intakes of water-soluble vitamins for full-term infants.

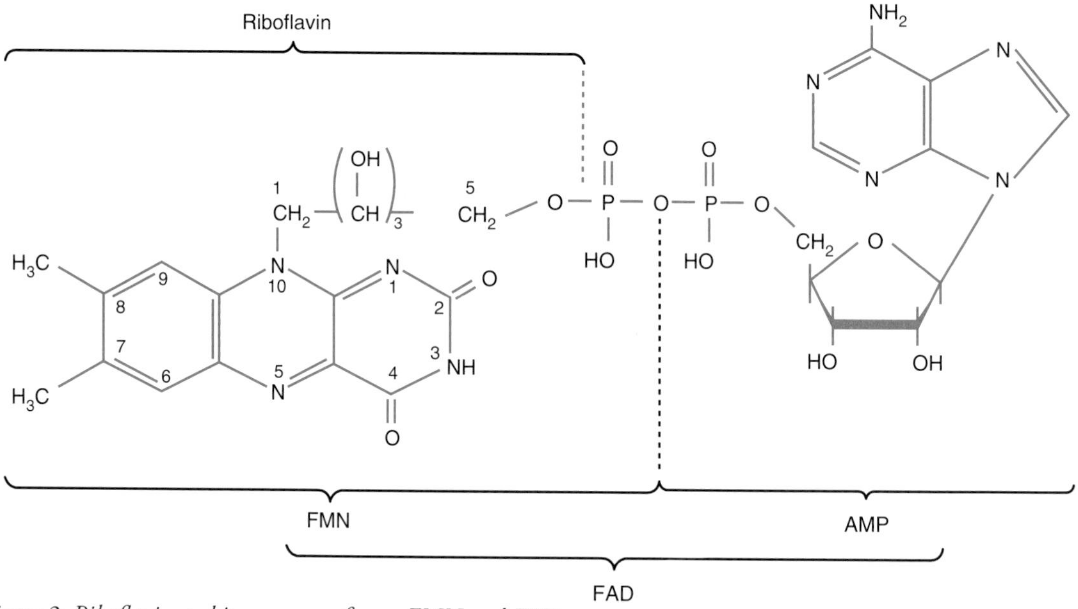

Figure 2: Riboflavin and its coenzyme forms, FMN and FAD.

Riboflavin

Not long after thiamin was isolated from yeast, the same water-soluble fraction was shown to contain a second, more heat-stable factor, identified as vitamin B$_2$.[44] This factor was shown to have both anti-pellagra and anti-dermatitis activity.

It contained a yellow compound found to be the same as a growth factor already identified in England called riboflavin. Once the compound was isolated by Warburg and Christian in 1932, its vitamin characteristics became clear.[45] Not long after riboflavin was isolated, its coenzyme derivatives were discovered.

Physiology

Riboflavin and its coenzymes, flavin mononucleotide (FMN) and flavin adenine dinucleotide (FAD), are shown in Figure 2. The vitamin is a tricyclic molecule that has a yellow color when synthesized. *In vivo*, it is phosphorylated (to FMN) and adenylated (to FAD). The coenzymes then function as electron donors and acceptors in biological oxidation-reduction systems. They are able to participate in both single and double electron transfers and can react directly with molecular oxygen. They are intimately involved with a number of enzymatic reactions, affecting glucose, fatty acid and amino acid metabolism.

After phosphorylation in the intestinal mucosa, riboflavin is readily absorbed from the small intestine. Absorption is reduced in biliary obstruction and in conditions that decrease intestinal transit time.[13] Urinary excretion of riboflavin depends upon dietary intake and saturation of tissue stores.[46] There is very little storage of the vitamin.

The placenta is permeable to riboflavin but not to its coenzymes. FAD is converted by the placenta to free riboflavin which is secreted into the fetal blood.[12] At 20 weeks of gestation, the fetal liver is able to convert riboflavin to FAD.[47] Cord blood concentrations of riboflavin are four times greater than maternal values at delivery.[3, 12, 47] At birth, therefore, riboflavin is the predominant form of the vitamin.[3]

Riboflavin and its phosphate are decomposed by exposure to light and in strong alkaline solutions.[48, 49, 50] The concentration of riboflavin-5-phosphate is reduced 50% after eight hours of indirect sunlight.[50] Phototherapy treatment for hyperbilirubinemia is reported to produce biochemical riboflavin deficiency in breast-fed newborn infants, as measured by activation of erythrocyte glutathione reductase.[46, 51-54] Riboflavin, however, is resistant to heat, acid and oxidation. The processes of pasteurization, evaporation and condensation of milk do not destroy the vitamin.[55]

Needs of Full-Term Infants

The riboflavin concentration in human milk, 400 µg/L (55 µg/100 kcal, range 40 to 85 µg/100 kcal), remains uniform throughout lactation.[14-16, 18, 20, 21, 56, 57] Vitamin supplementation is reflected in a greater milk riboflavin concentration only in situations where maternal riboflavin intake is below the RDA (1.7 mg/d) or when mothers receive almost three times the RDA.[5, 20, 57, 58] The riboflavin contents of human and bovine milk, commercial formulas, juices and vitamin preparations for infants and toddlers are shown in Tables 1-4.[14-16, 18, 20-22, 56, 57]

Breast-fed full-term infants have satisfactory riboflavin status.[25, 51] Serum riboflavin concentrations, however, are reported to be lower in breast-fed than in formula-fed infants, but neither group exhibits riboflavin deficiency.[59] Riboflavin deficiency was observed in unsupplemented children in The Gambia and intakes of 0.4 mg/d were needed to achieve riboflavin sufficiency.[60]

Riboflavin sufficiency is reported for full-term infants and children who receive 1,400 µg/d (150 µg/100 kcal) of the vitamin in TPN solutions.[26, 27] Because of the limitations of the assay, however, toxic levels could not be determined. Adequate whole blood riboflavin concentrations after 50 and 115 days of TPN are reported in children receiving 1.8 to 5.4 mg/d.[28] The TPN recommendation for riboflavin of 1,400 µg/d in full-term infants probably is appropriate (Table 6). Riboflavin status in adults receiving water-soluble vitamins in parenteral admixtures also appears appropriate.[29]

Deficiency

Generally, a deficiency of riboflavin occurs in conjunction with malnutrition and deficiencies of other vitamins. Ariboflavinosis is characterized by angular stomatitis, glossitis, cheilosis, seborrheic dermatitis around the nose and mouth, and eye changes which include reduced tearing, photophobia, corneal vascularization and cataracts. Riboflavin deficiency results in a reduction of the essential fatty acids, linoleic and linolenic acids, in liver and plasma.[55] Because the coenzymes are involved in the metabolism of vitamin B_6, the conversion of tryptophan to niacin also is impaired in riboflavin deficiency. Overt signs of deficiency are rare in

	Full-term Infants (units/d)
Thiamin (µg)	1200
Riboflavin (µg)	1400
Niacin (mg)	17
Vitamin B$_6$ (µg)	1000
Pantothenic acid (mg)	5
Biotin (µg)	20
Folate (µg)	140
Vitamin B$_{12}$ (µg)	0.75
Vitamin C (mg)	80

Greene et al (27).

Table 6: Parenteral intakes of water-soluble vitamins in full-term infants and children.

inhabitants of developed countries. Biochemical evidence of subclinical riboflavin deficiency, however, has been observed in women taking oral contraceptive agents, adults with diabetes, children from families of low socioeconomic status, children with chronic cardiac disease, the elderly and in infants during phototherapy for hyperbilirubinemia.[51, 52, 55, 61] Children hospitalized in Pediatric Intensive Care and Oncology Units also manifest biochemical evidence of riboflavin deficiency.[40]

The urinary excretion of riboflavin decreases in the early stages of deficiency, but the best correlation with a deficiency state is the activity of the enzyme erythrocyte glutathione reductase (EGR) before and after FAD administration. An activation coefficient of 1.2 or greater strongly suggests a deficient state.[24] Methods to quantitate serum riboflavin concentrations (FMN and FAD) have been reported recently.[62]

Toxicity

There are no reports of riboflavin toxicity. Riboflavin ingestion does produce a yellow discoloration of the urine.[43]

Niacin

The investigations of the disease "pellagra," initially considered to be due to a toxin, led to the discovery of the vit-

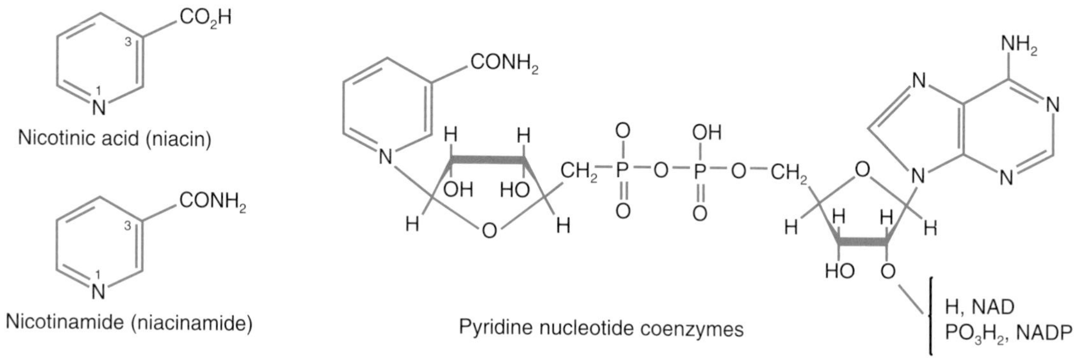

Figure 3: Niacin, niacinamide and the pyridine nucleotide coenzymes.

amin niacin. *The disease had appeared in the 1700s following the introduction of corn to Western Europe.*

The compound, nicotinic acid, had been isolated in 1867, but it was 1937 before Elvehjem demonstrated that nicotinic acid could cure pellagra in dogs.[63] Other investigators[64] also reported that tryptophan was curative, and in 1946 the transformation of tryptophan to "niacin equivalents" was demonstrated.

Physiology

The term niacin refers to the compound nicotinic acid and its amide form, nicotinamide (niacinamide), shown in Figure 3. The vitamin is biologically active as a component of the coenzymes nicotinamide adenine dinucleotide (NAD) and nicotinamide adenine dinucleotide phosphate (NADP). The coenzymes are important in two-electron transfers and are involved in multiple metabolic processes, including fat synthesis, intracellular respiratory metabolism and glycolysis.[65, 66] The physiologic need for niacin is related to energy expenditure, because of the involvement of NAD and NADP in the respiratory chain.

Because excess dietary tryptophan is converted to niacin, the tryptophan content of the diet must be considered when ascertaining niacin requirements. Tryptophan pyrrolase converts tryptophan eventually to kynurenine and after multiple additional conversions to niacin. The conversion is catalyzed by riboflavin and vitamin B_6. In adults, approximately 3% of administered tryptophan is converted to niacin and one niacin equivalent (NE) equals 60 mg tryptophan or one mg niacin.[5, 67] There are no data available to determine the appropriate conversion factor for infants. Tryptophan accounts for 1.5% of the amino acids in proteins of animal origin.[67] Niacin is stable in foods and can withstand heating and prolonged storage.[66]

Needs of Full-Term Infants

The concentration of niacin in human milk 2.0 mg/L (0.29 mg/100 kcal, range 0.27 to 0.34 mg/100 kcal) remains stable throughout lactation.[14, 68] If the mother is malnourished, niacin supplementation will increase the concentration in the milk.[58] Approximately 70% of the total niacin equivalents (NE) in human milk are derived from tryptophan. The tryptophan content of human milk, 22 mg/dL, provides 3.8 NE/L. The sum of preformed niacin and niacin equivalents derived from tryptophan in human milk is approximately 5.7 NE/L.[5] In bovine milk, 90% of the niacin equivalents are derived from tryptophan.[22, 64, 66, 67] The niacin contents of human and bovine milk, commercial formulas, juices, and vitamin preparations for infants and toddlers are shown in Tables 1-4.

Niacin status, as assessed by the urinary excretion of niacin metabolites, was normal in infants fed six NE but not in those receiving four NE per day.[69] The recommended allowance for full-term infants is based on the niacin equivalents in human milk. The distribution of preformed niacin vs tryptophan-derived niacin in milks has not been studied in relation to the estimated needs of this vitamin. The best estimate for niacin needs is given in Table 5.

Parenteral nicotinamide administration has been investigated in full-term infants and children who received 17 mg/d.[26, 27] No evidence for deficient or excessive intake of the vitamin was observed. Adequate whole blood niacin concentrations at 15 to 90 days of TPN are reported in children who receive 20 to 60 mg/d.[28] The latter studies also observed that whole blood niacin concentrations increased with the duration of TPN (from 0 to 90 days) and with increases in dosage of the vitamin (20 to 60 mg/d)[28]. Although exogenous niacin needs may decrease if dietary tryptophan is excessive, the small amount of tryptophan available in pediatric parenteral nutrition formulations probably would not alter recommendations. The recommendation for parenteral niacin intake in full-term infants and children, 17 mg/d, is appropriate (Table 6).[27]

Deficiency

A deficiency of niacin results in the clinical syndrome pellagra, a disease endemic to areas where corn is the primary staple.[66, 67, 70, 71] Pellagra is observed in people on a corn diet because corn is deficient in the amino acid tryptophan. The disease is characterized by weakness, lassitude, dermatitis, inflammation of mucous membranes, diarrhea, vomiting, dysphagia, and in severe cases, dementia. Initially, cutaneous inflammation looks like a sunburn because only areas exposed to light are affected (Figure 4). A familial disorder of tryptophan-niacin metabolism, Hartnup's disease, is caused by impaired absorption of monoamino/monocarboxylic acids, including tryptophan.[13, 31, 66, 71, 72]

In the liver, niacin is converted to multiple metabolites prior to its excretion in the urine. Measuring the urinary excretion of niacin metabolites, N^1-methylniacinamide and N^1-methyl-6-pyridone-3-carboxamide ("pyridone"), is considered a good method for diagnosing niacin deficiency.[31, 66, 70] Although the excretion of the pyridone decreases earlier in niacin deficiency, it is the most difficult metabolite to assay. The ratio of N^1-methylniacinamide to creatinine in random urine samples is easy to use; values below 0.5 mg/g creatinine suggest deficiency in adults.[31] Serum N^1-metabolites and nicotinamide can be assayed fluorimetrically.[66]

Toxicity

Because nicotinic acid is often used as a cholesterol-lowering agent, data are available describing the effects of its excessive intake. Excessive doses of nicotinic acid

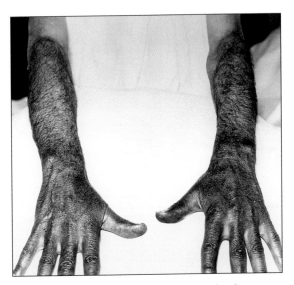

Figure 4: Manifestation of pellagra. Note the glove distribution of the keratotic skin changes on sun exposed surfaces.

in adults can cause cutaneous vasodilation, cardiac arrhythmias, pruritis, liver disease, skin disease, gout, gastrointestinal ulcers, and impaired glucose tolerance.[31, 73] Excessive doses of nicotinamide (niacinamide), however, do not produce the same side effects.[31, 43] The latter form is used in pediatric diets and is not effective as a cholesterol-lowering agent.

Vitamin B$_6$

The existence of vitamin B$_6$ was established in the 1920s when a disease was described in rats called acrodynia, a dermatitis ("rat pellagra") caused by a diet deficient in B-complex vitamins but not cured by supplementation with thiamin, riboflavin, or niacin. The term vitamin B$_6$ was assigned to this factor, which was isolated in 1938.[49]

Physiology

Vitamin B$_6$, shown in Figure 5, refers collectively to three naturally occurring pyridines--pyridoxine (PN, pyridoxol), pyridoxal (PL), and pyridoxamine (PM)--and their phosphorylated derivatives.[74] The vitamins are absorbed passively by intestinal mucosa cells, primarily in the proximal jejunum. There is rapid transfer to the liver, where phosphorylation occurs via a cytoplasmic pyridoxal kinase.[49] The liver also converts pyridoxine to pyridoxal and 4-pyridoxic acid (4-PA), the

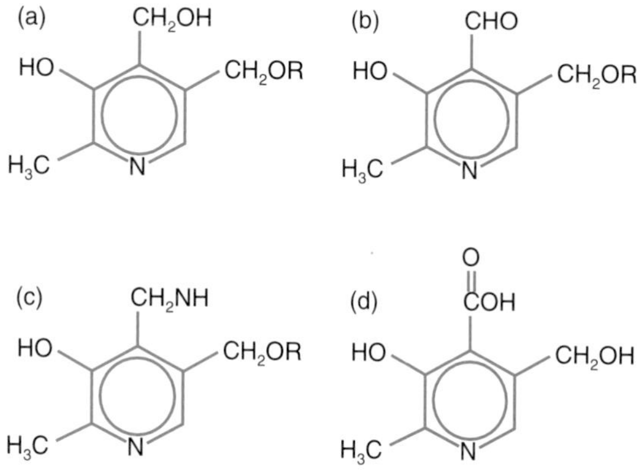

Figure 5: Forms of vitamin B₆: a) R=H, pyridoxine;
R=PO₃H₂, pyridoxine 5'-phosphate,
b) R=H, pyridoxal; R=PO₃H₂, pyridoxal 5'-phosphate,
c) R=H, pyridoxamine; R=PO₃H₂, pyridoxamine 5'-
phosphate, d) 4-pyridoxic acid.

major excretory product. In the blood, the dominant forms of the vitamin are PL, PN, PLP (pyridoxal-5-phosphate) and 4-PA.[75]

In the phosphorylated form (primarily PLP), vitamin B_6 plays a key role in metabolism by acting as a coenzyme in interconversion reactions of amino acids, the conversion of tryptophan to niacin and serotonin, neurotransmitter synthesis, carbohydrate metabolism, immune system development and in the biosynthesis of heme and prostaglandins. Because of the relationship between vitamin B_6 and protein metabolism, it is customary to consider the ratio of vitamin B_6 to protein when assessing needs. Ratios of vitamin B_6/protein of 15 µg/g are appropriate and the two standard deviation lower limit is 11 µg/g.[76] In adults with vitamin B_6 deficient diets, abnormalities of tryptophan and methionine metabolism develop faster and vitamin B_6 concentrations decline more rapidly when protein intakes are high (80-160 vs 30-50 g/d).[76] During repletion studies, tryptophan and methionine metabolism and plasma vitamin concentrations normalize faster at low protein intakes. Studies in infants with seizures due to vitamin B_6 deficiency observed some symptomatic improvement with high carbohydrate diets, but exacerbations of symptoms with high protein diets.[76]

Vitamin B_6 needs are increased with high dietary protein intakes and exposure to intense light. Heat

destruction may occur with the PL and PM forms, and partial destruction was responsible for vitamin B_6 deficiency and seizures in infants fed improperly processed formulas.[77, 78] For this reason, the heat-stable vitamer, pyridoxine hydrochloride, is used to fortify commercial infant formulas. The concentration of vitamin B_6 in human milk also may decline during enteral tube feeding.[78]

Transport of vitamin B_6 becomes more active during the last trimester of pregnancy, as assessed by the increased ratio of cord blood to maternal blood.[79] The vitamin concentrations in cord blood are greater than but parallel to those in maternal blood.[79, 80, 81] Cord blood contains PLP, pyridoxamine phosphate and 4-PA in greatest quantities.[79] Indeed, of all water-soluble vitamins, vitamin B_6 has the greatest fetomaternal ratio.[76, 79] The intake of vitamin B_6 during the last trimester of pregnancy determines the nutritional state of the infant with respect to this vitamin.[79, 80] Although pregnancy is characterized by low dietary B_6 intake and by declining plasma PLP concentrations, no associated neonatal sequelae are observed.[12, 76, 82-85]

Needs of Full-Term Infants

The vitamin B_6 content of human milk reflects the vitamin B_6 nutritional status of the mother.[58, 86-92] The concentration of vitamin B_6 in human milk increases as maternal vitamin supplementation is increased. The concentration of vitamin B_6 is 140 µg/L (20 µg/100 kcal, range 15 to 30 µg/100 kcal) in milk obtained from mothers whose intake was below the RDA.[16, 86, 88, 90, 93] Mothers who consume between 2.5 and 5.9 mg/d of vitamin B_6 have milk concentrations that average 210 µg/L (30 µg/100 kcal, range 150 to 250 µg/L).[16, 86-88, 90, 91] The milk concentrations of mothers consuming 10 to 20 mg/d is 340 µg/L (50 µg/100 kcal, range 250 to 530 µg/L).[86, 87] The vitamin B_6 content of human milk may decline with prolonged lactation.[94]

The vitamin B_6/protein ratio in milk, generally used to assess vitamin B_6 status, may decline to levels as low as 7 µg/g in milk obtained from unsupplemented mothers.[86] However, a range of 8.5 to 30 µg/g was reported, depending upon the mother's intake of vitamin B_6.[16, 86-88, 90, 91] It seems prudent to recommend vitamin B_6 supplementation for lactating women. The range of vitamin B$_6$ contents of human and bovine milk, commercial formulas, juices and vitamin preparations for infants and toddlers are shown in Tables 1-4.

If the vitamin B$_6$ intake of a mother is adequate, the normal full-term infant has sufficient stores of the vitamin to meet its needs. Despite generally lower concentration of vitamin B$_6$ in human milk compared with standard formulas, breast-fed infants have adequate vitamin B$_6$ status.[86, 87, 95] Furthermore, available data suggest that formula-fed infants may not need the greater content of the vitamin and that formulas should match the vitamin B$_6$/protein ratio in human milk.[95] However, supplementing a mother's vitamin B$_6$ during lactation may result in greater plasma PLP concentrations in infants and increased rates of growth, compared with infants whose mothers receive lower intakes of the vitamin.[92] Further data are needed to address this apparently conflicting information.

Clinical vitamin B$_6$-deficiency, manifested by seizures, has been reported in formula-fed infants who were given an improperly sterilized milk, which partially destroyed the vitamin.[7, 87] The incidence of seizures was 0.3% when intakes of vitamin B$_6$ were 60 µg/d.[76] A dose of vitamin B$_6$, 260 µg/d, cured the seizure disorder but 300 µg/d normalized tryptophan metabolism.[76, 93] The best estimate for vitamin B$_6$ needs is given in Table 5.

No deficiency of vitamin B$_6$ is observed in full-term infants and children receiving 1,000 or 3,000 µg/d pyridoxine hydrochloride in TPN.[28] Infants also had adequate vitamin status when receiving parenteral vitamin B$_6$ at 110 µg/100 kcal.[26, 27] The recommended parenteral intake of vitamin B$_6$ in full-term infants, 1,000 µg/d, appears appropriate (Table 6).[27] Vitamin B$_6$ status appears appropriate in adults receiving water-soluble vitamins as part of total intravenous admixtures.[29]

Deficiency

In infants, dietary deprivation or malabsorption of vitamin B$_6$ results in hypochromic microcytic anemia, vomiting, diarrhea, failure to thrive, listlessness, hyperirritability, and seizures.[80, 87, 93] In adults, vitamin B$_6$ deficiency may result in depression, confusion,

peripheral neuritis, electroencephalograph abnormalities and seizures.[76, 80]

Several conditions are associated with abnormalities in vitamin B$_6$ metabolism that require pharmacologic doses of the vitamin for adequate function. These vitamin B$_6$-dependency syndromes include: pyridoxine-dependent seizures in the neonate, pyridoxine-responsive hypochromic microcytic anemia, xanthurenic aciduria, cystathioninuria, and homocystinuria. Additional vitamin B$_6$ may be necessary for infants receiving isoniazid and for breast-fed infants whose mothers receive isoniazid.[7] It has also been reported that theophylline depresses plasma PLP concentrations, which can be reversed by vitamin supplementation.[96] Children with hypophosphatemic rickets also may have biochemical evidence of vitamin B$_6$ deficiency.[97]

Quantitative assays for total vitamin B$_6$ generally had employed the microbiological assay of *Saccharomyces uvarum*.[86-89] Methods for assessing vitamin B$_6$ nutritional status include the tryptophan load test, measuring 4-PA excretion, the plasma PLP concentration, and measuring erythrocyte activity of aspartate aminotransferase (glutamic-oxalacetic transaminase) and alanine aminotransferase (glutamic-pyruvic transaminase).[75, 80] The erythrocyte glutamic-pyruvic transaminase index (EGPT) measures the enzyme activity before and after the addition of PLP. Normal vitamin B$_6$ status is indicated by an index of less than 1.25.[80, 88]

Toxicity

Doses of pyridoxine hydrochloride as high as 1.0 mg·kg^{-1}·d^{-1} are tolerated without ill effects in animals.[43] It appears that humans may be more vulnerable to high doses of pyridoxine than animals. A sensory neuropathy in adults ingesting megadoses of pyridoxine hydrochloride has been described.[98] Large doses of pyridoxine also may cause seizures in adults.[99]

Pantothenic Acid

In 1933, Williams[100] described an acid substance, part of the B complex, which was required for growth. Because the compound occurred widely in nature it was called pantothenic ("everywhere") acid.

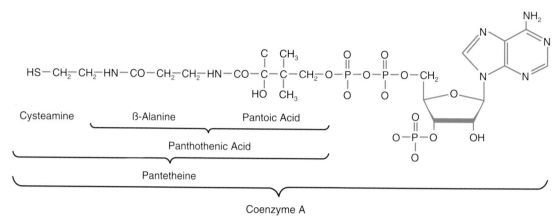

Figure 6: Pantothenic acid as part of coenzyme A.

It was not until 1947 that the biologic role of pantothenic acid was suggested, when Lipmann[101] reported that acetylation of sulfonamides required a coenzyme, coenzyme A, which was composed in part by pantothenic acid.

Physiology

The pantothenic acid molecule (Figure 6) consists of β-alanine joined to pantoic acid (2,4-dihydroxy-3,3-dimethylbutyric acid) by an amide bond. It serves as an integral part of coenzyme A, which functions in acyl group transfers in the synthesis of fatty acids, cholesterol, steroids, the oxidation of fatty acids, pyruvate, and α-ketoglutarate, and in other acetylation reactions.[5, 72, 102, 103]

Most pantothenic acid is ingested in the form of coenzyme A, which undergoes intestinal hydrolysis prior to absorption.[104] The vitamin is transported in the blood as pantothenic acid, then resynthesized to coenzyme A locally. Endogenous synthesis of the vitamin from pantoic acid and β-alanine is reported.[102] The plasma concentration of pantothenic acid in neonatal cord blood is several-fold greater than maternal blood.[102]

Needs of Full-Term Infants

The concentration of pantothenic acid in mature human milk is approximately 4 mg/L (0.6 mg/100 kcal, range 0.3 to 1.0 mg/100 kcal).[18, 68, 105, 106] Supplementing malnourished women or consuming extremely large quantities of the vitamin increases the amount of pantothenic acid in the milk.[58, 105, 106] In bovine milk, 30 to 35% of the vitamin is lost in processing.[105] The safe and adequate intake of pantothenic acid is given in Table 5. Infants receiving human milk or formula should ingest this amount during the first year of life.[5, 105]

The vitamin needs during TPN have been evaluated in a small number of pediatric patients.[26] Full-term infants and children who received 5 mg/d maintained stable plasma concentrations for 21 days. The recommendation for pantothenic acid in TPN, 5 mg/d, is appropriate for full-term infants and children (Table 6).

Deficiency

Because of the ubiquitous distribution of this vitamin, a clinical deficiency syndrome has not been reported.[103] The essential biologic role of pantothenic acid was delineated in animal experiments, but extraordinary circumstances were required to produce the deficiency in man. For example, experimental deficiency has been produced in volunteers fed the antagonist ω-methylpantothenic acid as part of a pantothenic acid-deficient diet.[103] Subjects developed "burning" feet, gastrointestinal disturbances, headache, insomnia, fatigue and muscle weakness. A deficiency of pantothenic acid also is observed in severe malnutrition. Pantothenic deficiency is considered to have caused the "burning feet syndrome" described in World War II prisoners in the Far East.[103]

Toxicity

Pantothenic acid is relatively nontoxic. High doses (100 to 20 g/d) have been reported to result in water retention and diarrhea.[43]

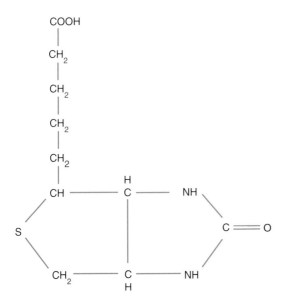

Figure 7: Biotin.

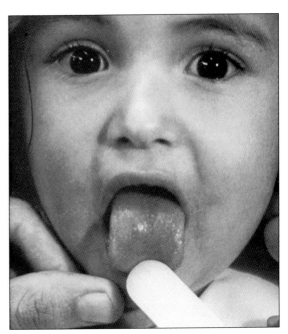

*Figure 8: Advanced chronic glossitis with marked papil-
lary atrophy typical of vitamin B complex deficiences.*

Biotin

*The discovery of biotin originated when Wildiers in 1901
recognized that yeasts required a growth factor other than
salts and sugars.[49] This growth factor ("bios") ultimately
proved to be composed of inositol, pantothenic acid, and a
third component which was crystallized in 1936.[49]*

It was later learned that the toxicity of raw eggs in
the diet is due to avidin, which is a biotin antagonist.
The function for which biotin is required, biochemical
carboxyl transfers, was not understood until it was
understood that the activity of the vitamin depended
on a covalent bond between biotin and its enzyme.[107]

Physiology

Biotin (Figure 7) functions as a coenzyme for carboxy-
lation, decarboxylation and transcarboxylation reactions. As such, it plays an important role in the
biosynthesis of amino and fatty acids and as a cofactor
in gluconeogenesis.

Small quantities of biotin are present in most plant
and animal foods. The major human source of biotin is
derived from intestinal bacteria. Biotin is absorbed by
passive diffusion and transported bound to plasma
proteins. Urinary excretion reflects dietary intake; fecal
excretion, generally unaffected by intake, indicates
enteric synthesis.[5, 108] Various biotin-dependent carboxylase deficiency states have been described. The

multiple carboxylase defect (pyruvate, propionyl coen-
zyme-A and methylcrotonyl CoA carboxylase) has
been shown to be biotin responsive.[72]

Needs of Full-Term Infants

The average biotin content of human milk during the
first week of lactation is 0.7 µg/L but in mature human
milk the content is 5.0 µg/L (0.7 µg/100 kcal, range 0.6
to 1.1 µg/100 kcal).[14, 18, 68, 108-110] Dietary supplementation of malnourished women will result in a rise in the
biotin content of the milk.[58] Cow milk is a rich source
of biotin.[111] The biotin content of human and bovine
milk, commercial formulas, and vitamin preparations
for infants and toddlers are shown in Tables 1, 2 and 4.

Recommended intakes for biotin have not been established. Urinary biotin excretion in infants increases in
the first days after birth and then declines until six
months when, possibly related to diet, it rises gradually
to adult values.[68] Biotin deficiency has not been reported
in infants fed either human milk or formulas despite a
wide range of intakes. The RDA for infants approximates the intake from human milk (Table 5).

Biotin deficiencies have been reported, however,
when the vitamin has been omitted from TPN solu-

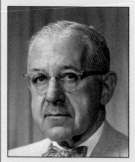

Paul Gyorgy M.D. received his degree from the University of Budapest in 1915. His pediatric training was at Heidelberg under Moro, a pupil of Escherich. After a period at Cambridge and the Babies and Children's Hospital of Cleveland, Gyorgy served as Pediatrician in Chief of the Hospital of the University of Pennsylvania from 1950 to 1957 and the Philadelphia General Hospital from 1957 to 1963. His research demonstrated the benefits of breast-feeding on infections; the beneficial effects of vitamin D supplementation; and partial elucidation of the vitamin B complex. In Heidelberg, he participated in the isolation of riboflavin (B$_2$) and biotin and at Cambridge and Cleveland he discovered and named pyridoxine (B$_6$). At Philadelphia he demonstrated that vitamin E deficiency is associated with susceptibility of red cells to hemolysis. J. Nutr. 109,17-23, 1979 (Photo courtesy of CNRC)

tions.[110, 112, 113] The vitamin needs during TPN have been investigated.[27] Full-term infants and children receiving 20 µg/d maintained stable, adequate plasma biotin concentrations for 21 days. Adequate serum biotin concentrations during 15 to 90 days of TPN also are reported in children receiving 30 to 90 µg/d.[28] The recommendation for biotin of 20 µg/d in TPN for full-term infants and children appears appropriate (Table 6).

Deficiency

In individuals fed normal diets, a deficiency of biotin is unlikely to occur. A deficiency state is observed, however, when gastrointestinal flora is suppressed or when biotin absorption is diminished, such as occurs in diets consisting of raw eggs.[108, 113] Symptoms of biotin deficiency include anorexia, nausea, glossitis, pallor, mental changes, alopecia and a fine maculosquamous dermatitis which becomes exfoliative.[72, 112, 113] Biotin deficiency has been reported in patients with short gut syndromes when the vitamin was omitted from TPN solutions.[110, 113] A young girl receiving TPN for six months reportedly developed a scaly dermatitis, alopecia, pallor, irritability, lethargy and markedly reduced

urinary excretion and plasma concentration of biotin.[113] Administration of biotin corrected the abnormalities. Biotin may enhance the treatment of seborrheic dermatitis, Leiner's disease, propionic acidemia and β-methylcrotonylglycinuria.[72, 110] Antibiotics reportedly may affect biotin status by decreasing enteric synthesis of the vitamin.[110] Biotin is commonly assayed by microbiological methods.

Toxicity

No cases of biotin toxicity have been reported.

Folate

A microcytic anemia usually associated with pregnancy was described in Hindu women in Bombay in the 1930s.[114] It was known then that the anemia could be treated with a yeast extract. The active compound in the extract was later found to be folic acid, which was isolated and identified as pteroylglutamic acid.[115] The name "folate" was used as a reference to a bacterial growth factor isolated from spinach and other "foliage."[116]

Physiology

Folate is the general term that describes compounds having nutritional and chemical properties similar to folic acid (pteroylglutamic acid, PGA), shown in Figure 9. The parent compound is a pteridine moiety joined to para-aminobenzoic acid. Reduction of the pyrazine ring to yield tetrahydrofolate, addition of multiple glutamyl residues and acquisition of one-carbon fragments result in activation of the vitamin. The coenzyme participates in the biosynthesis of purines and pyrimidines, in the metabolism of some amino acids and in the catabolism of histidine.[117, 118]

The vitamin is absorbed rapidly from the small intestine, primarily from the proximal third, although the entire small bowel has absorptive capacity.[119] Dietary folate occurs predominantly as polygltamate, usually as 5-methyl or 10-formyl pteroylpolyglutamate, which is hydrolyzed to the monoglutamate by the intestinal mucosa prior to absorption.[118] Zinc deficiency will decrease the conjugase activity, resulting in decreased folate uptake.[120] Folate then enters the portal circulation as the free,

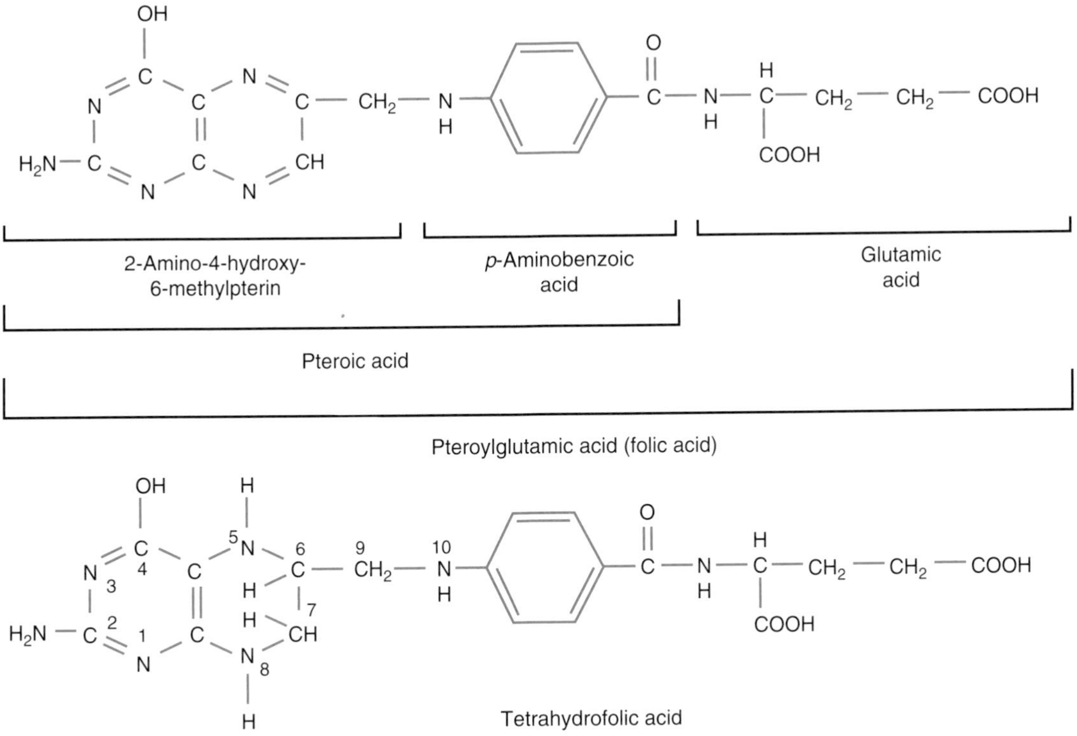

Figure 9: Folate.

monoglutamate derivative.[121] Absorption appears to be an active process that is enhanced by the presence of glucose.[122] The vitamin is inactivated by heat, canning and light exposure.[24]

Folate homeostasis is regulated, at least in part, by the enterohepatic cycle.[123] Normally, bile folate is reabsorbed efficiently, which results in a total body folate turnover of only 1% per day in adults.[117] Because the biliary folate content is large, enterohepatic recirculation results in a long half-life of the vitamin.[117, 121] Large quantities of the vitamin may be synthesized by colonic bacteria. Folate appears in serum in the free form and bound to low- and high-affinity carriers.[119] Transport into the tissues involves an active, carrier-mediated mechanism.[124] While urine may contain active folate and its metabolites, most folate excretion occurs in the feces via bile.[125]

Folate status is assessed by evaluating concentrations of the vitamin in sera and erythrocytes. Erythrocyte folate is less variable and is useful for assessing adequacy of long-term intake. Urinary excretion of FIGLU (formiminog-

lutamate), an intermediate in the metabolism of histidine to glutamic acid, is an indicator of folate deficiency. Mean red blood cell volume (MCV) and the degree of granulocyte segmentation also are used to assess status.

Needs of Full-Term Infants

The folate content of human milk increases after the first postpartum week from 5 to 10 µg/L to 20 to 40 µg/L at one month, and 50 to 100 µg/L at three months.[24, 88, 90, 118, 121, 126-128] Folate supplementation will increase the vitamin's concentration in the milk of malnourished women.[58, 90] Differences in folate concentrations between fore- and hindmilk have been reported.[126] The average folate contents of human and bovine milks are similar, approximately 50 µg/L (7 µg/100 kcal) (Tables 1-2). Commercially-prepared infant formulas contain a greater quantity of the vitamin (Tables 1-2). Folate is absent in multivitamin drops for infants, but is included in the chewable multivitamin tabs for children (Table 4).

The folate status of full-term infants fed commercial formula appears adequate.[128-130] Goat milk, containing 6 µg/L, is an inadequate source of folate.[118, 121] The Food and Agricultural Organization/World Health Organization (FAO/WHO) recommends a folate intake of 40 to 50 µg/d for infants in the first six months of life.[118] However, the US RDA of 25 µg/d, which averages 4.2 µg/kg/d during the first six months of life, provides a satisfactory folate intake.[5, 131] With respect to the content of folate in human milk, the Committee on Nutrition of the American Academy of Pediatrics' recommendation of 4 µg/100 kcal appears appropriate, and neither deficiency states nor low plasma folate concentrations have been reported in breast-fed full-term infants.[25, 127, 129, 130, 132] Indeed, a dose of 4 µg/100 kcal resulted in normal red cell morphology in a group of full-term infants.[128, 132]

Folate has been administered in TPN formulations to full-term infants in doses of 140 µg/d (15 µg/100 kcal).[26, 27] At those intakes, cord red blood cell folate concentrations remained unchanged for seven days, but were increased compared with cord blood concentrations when assessed at day 14 and 21. In children who received long-term parenteral nutrition, red cell folate concentrations remained stable for five months. Adequate serum and red cell folate concentrations during 15 to 90 days of TPN were reported in children receiving 200 to 600 µg/d.[28] An increase in folate concentration was observed from 0 to 90 days and with doses of 400 to 600 vs 200 µg/d.[28] The recommended parenteral folate intake in full-term infants and children of 140 µg/d appears appropriate.[27]

Deficiency

Nutritional folate deficiency is one of the most common hypovitaminoses in man.[118, 121, 122] Growth retardation, even in the absence of anemia, and abnor-

> *Sun Szo-mo (Tang Dynasty) was medical history's first dietary therapist. In his famous study of precious recipes, he wrote "A truly good physician first finds out the cause of the illness, and having found that, he first tries to cure it by food. Only when food fails, does he prescribe medication." In fact Dr. Sun diagnosed the vitamin deficiency disease beri-beri 1,000 years before it was identified by European doctors in 1642. Sun prescribed a strict dietary remedy that sounds remarkably modern: calf and lamb liver, wheat germ, almonds, wild pepper and other vitamin-packed edibles.*
>
> Daniel Reid, Eds Paul Zach,
> *The Magic of Chinese Medicine,*
> Taiwan APA Productions, 1984

malities in bone marrow, neurological status and small intestinal morphology have been described in folate deficiency.[133] In a population of infants who consumed boiled and pasteurized bovine milk, which has a low folate concentration, supplementation of the vitamin was shown to improve growth at four to six months of age, despite the absence of hematologic markers of deficiency.[134] Folate deficiency has been identified more commonly in small-for-gestational-age infants.[135] Deficiency states arise because of insufficient intake and/or poor absorption of the vitamin. Shojania[136] reported that neonates had faster plasma clearances of PGA compared with adults and concluded that tissue storage of folate was more efficient in the neonate. The fall in serum folate observed in the neonatal period reflects an increased need for folate for DNA and RNA synthesis.[136] Certain medications, e.g. phenobarbital and phenytoin, may increase the need for the vitamin through the induction of hepatic enzymes containing folate as a coenzyme. Requirements for folate increase during pregnancy, periods of intense hematopoiesis and growth.[24] Low plasma folate concentrations are encountered in vitamin B_{12} deficiency. Treatment with folate may improve the hematologic manifestations of vitamin B_{12} deficiency, but will not affect the progressive neurologic degeneration associated with that deficiency state. Iron deficiency may lead to decreased utilization of folate.[137] Folic acid therapy may inhibit zinc absorption.[138]

The hematological manifestations of folate deficiency include hypersegmentation of neutrophils (usually greater than 3.5 lobes), megaloblastosis and anemia.[118, 121, 135] The sequential changes due to a folate-deficient diet have been described in adults.[121] The earliest finding is a low serum folate concentration, observed after three weeks of deficient intake of the vitamin. Continued deficient intake results in hypersegmentation of neutrophils by five weeks. At 13 weeks, there is an increased urinary FIGLU excretion. A diminished erythrocyte folate concentration is noted by 17 weeks, and megaloblastosis and anemia are evidenced by 20 weeks of deficient intake.

From recent work, it appears that neural tube defects may be associated, at least in part, with a mother's folate deficiency prior to conception.[139] In 1976, Smithells reported significantly lower levels of red cell folate in mothers of babies with neural tube defects compared with levels in control mothers.[140] Women who take multivitamin preparations during the peri-conceptional period have a reduced risk of delivering an infant with a neural tube defect than women who do not take multivitamins.[141] It remains unclear whether a cause and effect relationship exists.[142]

Toxicity

Large doses of folic acid are encountered infrequently because the vitamin is not present in great quantity in over-the-counter preparations.[43] Folate may mask vitamin B_{12} deficiency and may depress the level of phenytoin.[43] Very large doses of folate may produce renal injury in animals.[121]

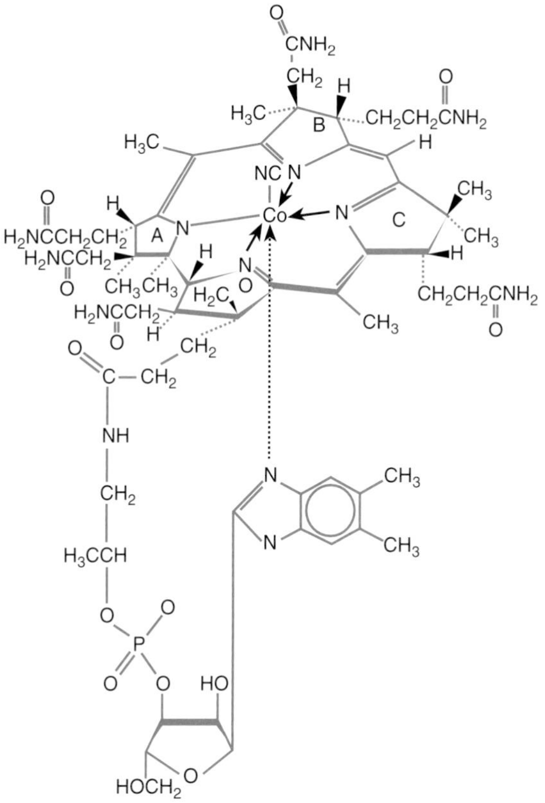

Vitamin B_{12}

The study of vitamin B_{12} began in 1822 with the first description of pernicious anemia by J.S. Combe.[143] Over a century later, Whipple, Minot and Murphy demonstrated that the previously fatal anemia could be successfully treated with large amounts of partially-cooked liver.[119, 144] Further unraveling of the puzzle was provided in 1929 by Castle,[145] who demonstrated an "intrinsic factor" present in gastric juice that could interact with an "extrinsic factor" in food to provide the anti-pernicious anemia substance, later identified as vitamin B_{12}. When the chemical was finally synthesized in 1947, it was called a B vitamin because of its water solubility and assigned the next available number, 12.[146]

Physiology

The structure of vitamin B_{12} is shown in Figure 10. The corrin ring is a macrocyclic ring formed by the linkage of four reduced pyrrol rings. In the case of vitamin B_{12}, the center of the ring is cobalt. Perpendicu-

Figure 10: Vitamin B_{12}.

lar to the ring is a nucleotide (5-6 dimethylbenzimidazole) linked to the ring by D-1-amino-2-propanol. "Cobalamin" is used to describe vitamin B_{12} regardless of the moiety attached to the cobalt. Cyanocobalamin is the stable compound synthesized in the laboratory. It is not found in significant amounts in food or in the human body and is not considered to be metabolically active. The placenta concentrates vitamin B_{12}, and newborn infants have two to three times the serum levels of their mothers.[12, 147, 148]

Upon ingestion, vitamin B_{12} is released from food at gastric pH. It is then complexed with salivary R binder, which has greater affinity than intrinsic factor.[148] At the alkaline pH of the upper small bowel, pancreatic enzymes digest the R binder and release vitamin B_{12}. Intrinsic factor then binds vitamin B_{12} to facilitate Ca-dependent absorption, at alkaline pH, across ileal mucosa. Within the mucosa, intrinsic factor is lost and a plasma transport protein is attached.[149] One to three percent of vitamin B_{12} is absorbed passively. An effective

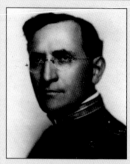

Joseph Goldberger M.D. (1874-1929) was a 1895 graduate of Bellevue Medical College. In 1899, he joined the US Public Health Service. In 1914, the Surgeon General asked Goldberger to investigate pellagra, a problem on which he focused for his remaining career. He visited the Methodist Orphan Asylum in Jackson, Mississippi. and found that 68 of 211 children but none of employees were afflicted with pellagra. Goldberger reasoned, "the explanation of the peculiar exemption ... will be found ... in a difference in the diet of the two groups of residents." He soon found that the younger infants received milk and were pellagra free. This was followed by a two-year experimental study in two Jackson orphanages in which a diet supplemented with milk and meat cured 72 cases but no recovery was observed in 32 children on a control diet. Goldberger soon demonstrated that dietary tryptophan accounted for the experimental results. J Nutr. 55:1-12, 1955 (Photo courtesy of NLM)

enterohepatic circulation of vitamin B_{12} accounts for its long half-life.[149] Intestinal bacteria may provide an additional source of vitamin B_{12}.[149] Resection of the terminal ileum, such as occurs commonly as a result of necrotizing enterocolitis, may impair vitamin B_{12} absorption.[150]

Vitamin B_{12} is active in metabolism in two forms: methylcobalamin and 5-deoxyadenosylcobalamin (coenzyme B_{12}).[119] The methylated version is involved in one-carbon transfers. In particular, vitamin B_{12} transfers a methyl group from tetrahydrofolate to homocysteine for the synthesis of methionine. Vitamin B_{12} is necessary for the regeneration of tetrahydrofolate. In vitamin B_{12} deficiency, folate may be trapped in its demethylated form, and as such it is unavailable for pyrimidine synthesis. The result is ineffective DNA synthesis, which is evident clinically as hypersegmentation of neutrophils and megaloblastic anemia. The sequential stages in the development of vitamin B_{12} deficiency have been described.[148]

Adenosylcobalamin participates in the reduction of purine and pyrimidine ribonucleotides to their corresponding deoxyribonucleotides necessary for DNA synthesis.[49] The adenosyl form also is necessary for converting methylmalonyl-coenzyme A to succinyl-CoA. In this role, vitamin B_{12} is a key factor in metabolizing fat, branched-chain amino acids, and carbohydrate.[119] A lack of vitamin B_{12} will result in an accumulation of methylmalonic acid, with subsequent excretion in the urine.

Needs of Full-Term Infant

The vitamin B_{12} content of human milk ranges from 1.2 µg/L at 1 week to 0.5 µg/L at six months of lactation.[16, 88, 90] The average concentration is 0.7 µg/L (0.1 µg/100 kcal, range 0.07 to 0.18 µg/100 kcal (Tables 1-2). Maternal supplementation with vitamin B_{12} tends to increase the vitamin content in the milk.[58, 88, 90] Breast-fed infants will receive adequate amounts of vitamin B_{12} if maternal serum (and, therefore, milk) vitamin B_{12} concentrations are normal. Unless the maternal diet is deficient, as would occur in the strict vegan or conditions exist which impair maternal vitamin absorption, the breast-fed infant will have an adequate vitamin B_{12} status. Oral doses as little as 0.1 µg/d, however, will correct or prevent a deficiency state in the breast-fed infant of a vegan.[149] The RDA of 0.3 µg/d (0.05 µg/kg/d) will provide a substantial margin of sufficiency during infancy.

Vitamin B_{12} status during TPN has been reported for full-term infants receiving 1.0 µg/d (0.1 µg/100 kcal.[26, 27] Those infants maintained vitamin B_{12} concentrations above reference controls, but these values tended to decline toward baseline cord blood values after 21 days of therapy. During the long-term administration of TPN in children, vitamin B_{12} levels remained above reference controls. Elevated serum vitamin B_{12} levels at 50 and 115 days of TPN are reported in children who received 2.5 to 7.5 µg/d.[28] The recommended intake of vitamin B_{12} in full-term infants and children of 1.0 µg/d from TPN possibly is excessive, and a dose of 0.75 µg/d may be more appropriate.[27]

Deficiency

Because cobalamin stores greatly exceed daily needs, deficiency of this vitamin is encountered rarely. Clinical circumstances producing vitamin B_{12} deficiency include lack of intrinsic factor (pernicious anemia, post-gastrectomy, destruction of gastric mucosa), small bowel bacterial overgrowth, specific intestinal mucosal defects (celiac disease, ileal resection), inborn errors of metabolism and drug interactions. Inadequate vitamin B_{12} intake can be caused by strict adherence to a vegan diet, i.e., a diet devoid of meat, poultry, fish, eggs and dairy products.[149, 151-153] In adults, the deficiency state is characterized by weakness, anemia, congestive heart failure, glossitis, lemon-colored skin and neurological conditions: paresthesias, degeneration of posterior and lateral columns of the spinal cord and peripheral neuritis.[151, 153]

Vitamin B_{12} deficiency is described in an exclusively breast-fed six-month-old male infant who presented to the hospital in a coma.[151] The mother of the infant was apparently healthy; she had eaten no animal products for eight years and took no vitamin supplements. Growth and development of the infant were appropriate until four months, when they appeared to regress. Hematologic findings included megaloblastic anemia, neutropenia, and thrombocytopenia. Urinary excretion of methylmalonic acid, glycine, methylcitric acid and homocystine were elevated. There was a dramatic response to intramuscular vitamin B_{12} administration. The mother had a normal hemogram, a low normal serum vitamin B_{12} concentration, and a moderate methylmalonic aciduria. Specker[153] reported elevated urinary methylmalonic acid concentrations in lactating vegan women and in their infants. The urinary excretion of methylmalonic acid declined following vitamin B_{12} therapy in infants and mothers.

Evidence of malabsorption of vitamin B_{12} is reported in six out of 14 children who had undergone ileal resection for necrotizing enterocolitis.[150] Although deficiency takes years to develop because of hepatic stores, it was recommended that vitamin B_{12} status should be evaluated in such children.

The most commonly used test for the adequacy of vitamin B_{12} is serum concentration.[145] Red cell concentrations are less reliable because they overlap between normal and deficient subjects and because they are low in folate and iron deficiency, despite ade-

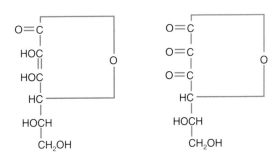

Figure 11: L-ascorbic acid and L-dehydroascorbic acid.

quate total body stores of vitamin B_{12}.[154] A functional test of vitamin B_{12} adequacy is the measurement of methylmalonic acid excretion with or without a loading dose of valine or isoleucine, but this test is less reliable and more complex.[145]

Toxicity

There are no reports of toxicity from large doses of vitamin B_{12}.

Vitamin C

Historically, vitamin C deficiency has been confused with or attributed to rickets and even to dental conditions.

In his Practical treatise upon dentition or breeding of teeth in children, Joseph Horlock[155] wrote in 1742 that "unfortunate infants have their swollen gums lanced to relieve what was supposed to be swelling due to mere dentition, when purple swelling over a tooth just coming was really due to the haemorrhage of infantile scurvy."

Physiology

The two principal forms of vitamin C, shown in Figure 11, are L-ascorbic acid and the oxidized form, dehydroascorbic acid. L-ascorbic acid, the biologically more active form of the vitamin, is an antioxidant which accelerates hydroxylation reactions in many biosynthetic processes.[156] It may provide electrons to enzymes that require prosthetic metal ions in a reduced form to achieve full activity, such as the hydroxylation of proline and lysine in collagen synthesis.[156, 157] Several functions of vitamin C-enhanced hydroxylase are known: the hydroxylation of lysine and methionine in carnitine biosynthesis, the catabolism of tyrosine, the synthesis of norepinephrine from dopamine and the conversion of tryptophan to 5-hydroxytryptophan in the biosynthesis of serotonin. Vitamin C is of particular importance to the preterm infant because it enhances the activity of the immature hepatic enzyme, *p*-hydroxyphenylpyruvic acid oxidase, which increases the catabolism of tyrosine.[156, 157, 158] Transient tyrosinemia resulting from vitamin C deficiency or high tyrosine and/or protein intakes was a common problem for preterm infants in the past.[25, 158, 159]

Vitamin C is involved in the synthesis of neurotransmitters. The human fetal brain contains four to eleven times the amount of vitamin C found in the adult brain.[160] The brain vitamin C content declines with increasing gestational age, but the content remains threefold greater than that in adults even after four weeks of age. The significance of the brain vitamin C concentration is unclear, but suggests that providing adequate vitamin C to the preterm infant may be important. The rise in serum vitamin C concentrations has been reported following the disruption of the blood brain barrier.[13, 161] As an antioxidant, vitamin C may be important to high-risk infants exposed to hyperoxic environments and mechanical ventilation.[13, 156, 157]

Placental transfer results in a greater concentration of vitamin C in the fetus and in cord blood than in the mother.[158] With optimal nutrition, the maternal/cord vitamin C ratio is 0.5. If the mother is vitamin C deficient, however, the ratio declines to 0.25.[162] The fetus, therefore, appears to be protected from maternal vitamin C deficiency.[13] Scurvy has been reported, however, in the offspring of mothers who were clinically vitamin C deficient.[12] There is a decline in maternal concentrations of the vitamin during pregnancy that is independent of nutritional status.[160, 162]

Vitamin C is absorbed in the upper small intestine and excreted in the urine primarily as oxalic acid. At moderate intakes, urinary excretion is the main source of elimination. At high intakes, the urinary excretion of the vitamin increases and with intakes

> Medicine that merely or mainly controls disease is no better than a farm in which nothing is done except to destroy the weeds.
> *Primary Health Care Pioneer,*
> *The Selected Works*
> *of Dr. Cicely D. Williams,*
> Naomi Baumslag, Editor,
> World Federation of Public
> Health Associations
> and UNICEF

above 3 g/d, the fecal excretion of the vitamin rises and protects against excessive intakes.[156, 163] Tissue concentrations are three to 10 times greater than those in plasma.[156] Because there is no storage of the vitamin, plasma and tissue concentrations are correlated positively.[156]

The availability of vitamin C is influenced by its physical characteristics. The vitamin C content of human milk is reduced 90% by pasteurization.[156, 164] The vitamin C content of pooled human milk is 50% lower than that of fresh milk.[164] Storage time, temperature, phototherapy and oxidation affect vitamin C concentrations.[13, 78] Reduced vitamin C concentrations are reported to follow exposure of milk to copper, iron and oxygen, and to febrile and gastrointestinal illnesses.[13, 158]

Needs of Full-Term Infants

The vitamin C concentration of human milk generally is stable during lactation, averaging 50 mg/L (8 mg/100 kcal, range 5 to 13 mg/100 kcal).[14-16, 88, 90, 165, 166] A 20% decline in milk concentration is reported after 6 to 25 months of lactation.[94, 167] When a lactating mother's diet is supplemented with vitamin C, an increase in milk concentration of the vitamin occurs only if her diet had been deficient in vitamin C.[58, 165] No effect of routine supplementation on milk vitamin C concentration is reported for American women.[16, 88, 90, 166]

Bovine milk contains a low concentration of vitamin C, probably because the calf is able to synthesize the vitamin.[157, 158, 164] The vitamin C contents of human and bovine milk, commercial formulas, juices and vitamin preparations for infants and toddlers are shown in Tables 1-4.

The vitamin C needs of full-term infants are obtained from estimates of the availability of the vitamin from human milk (Tables 1-2). Neonatal serum vitamin C concentrations decline during the first week and by five days are similar to maternal serum concentrations at delivery.[158] That low concentration is maintained in infants fed unsupplemented bovine milk.

Based on studies of urinary excretion and body saturation, formula-fed full-term infants require a minimum vitamin C supplement of approximately 10 mg/d to prevent scurvy.[156, 158] If supplemented with 20 mg/d, formula-fed full-term infants demonstrate serum concentrations similar to those of breast-fed infants.[158] Breast-fed full-term infants appear to be saturated with respect to their vitamin C needs.[158, 167] The vitamin C needs of the preterm infant may be similar to the full-term infant unless large quantities of tyrosine and/or protein (>5 g·kg^{-1}·d^{-1}) are administered.

An additional need for vitamin C is to enhance the absorption of iron.[168] Vitamin C reduces Fe^{3+} to the more soluble ion, Fe^{2+}. Ascorbic acid also binds to ionic iron to prevent it from binding to other dietary components which may be absorbed poorly. A molar ratio of ascorbic acid to iron ≥ 1.5 appears to facilitate iron absorption.[168] The high content of vitamin C in fruit juices for children may be an important means to ensure adequate iron absorption (Table 3).[22]

Plasma vitamin C concentrations have been reported for full-term infants receiving TPN.[26, 27] Full-term infants and children to eleven years of age who received 80 mg vitamin C daily maintained plasma concentrations of 1.1 mg/dL for 21 days. Based on serum vitamin C concentrations, borderline vitamin status was reported for children who received 80 mg/d for two to five months. Plasma vitamin C concentrations in those children were similar to those reported in vitamin C-sufficient adults receiving long-term TPN.[169] The parenteral intake of 80 mg/d appears appropriate for full-term infants and children (Table 6).[27]

Deficiency

A deficiency of vitamin C results in the clinical presentation of scurvy.

Scurvy, the first dietary deficiency disease to be recognized, was not a matter of concern for infants until the end of the nineteenth century, when the use of pasteurized milk and commercial formulas became prevalent. Infantile scurvy was observed in well-to-do families who had the means to purchase prepared infant formulas.

In 1938, Ingalls[164] described three cases in which scurvy was identified in preterm infants who died between 26 and 57 days of life. These infants were

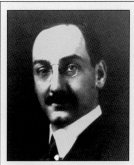

Alfred F. Hess M.D. graduated from the College of Physicians and Surgeons in 1901. He headed the pediatric service of the Beth Israel Hospital and the Home for Hebrew Infants where he conducted long term nutritional studies. Hess discovered that vitamin C is destroyed by heat processing and that this accounted for much of the scurvy of formula fed infants in that era. He proved that rickets was cured by cod liver oil. Hess demonstrated in 1927 that irradiated milk healed rickets. J. Nutr. 71:1-9, 1960 (Photo courtesy of NLM)

fed pooled, pasteurized human milk exclusively. He suggested that the daily dose of vitamin C for preterm infants should approximate the amount of this vitamin contained in unpasteurized human milk. Today, infantile scurvy is reported occasionally in urban settings where children are fed unsupplemented bovine milk exclusively for the first 6 to 12 months of life.[72]

The earliest clinical manifestation of scurvy in adults is petechial hemorrhages, which indicate increased capillary fragility.[13, 48, 158] A classic manifestation of scurvy in adults is wounds that fail to heal. In that situation, collagen fibrils and intercellular cement are deposited improperly, stopping bone growth. Infantile scurvy is manifested by irritability and tenderness, swelling and pseudoparalysis of the lower extremities. Enlargement of the costochondral junction (scorbutic rosary) is observed in scurvy and may be confused with rickets.[72] Characteristic radiologic abnormalities indicating a cessation of osteogenesis and marked bony changes, hyperkeratosis of hair follicles and mental status changes characterize the progression of the illness.[72, 170] Hemorrhagic manifestations in children include bleeding at the site of tooth eruption, bloody diarrhea, epistaxis, ocular bleeding and petechiae at pressure points. Anemia, secondary to decreased iron absorption or abnormal folate metabolism, is a common finding.[157] Sepsis and failure to thrive are characteristics of preterm infants reported with scurvy.[13]

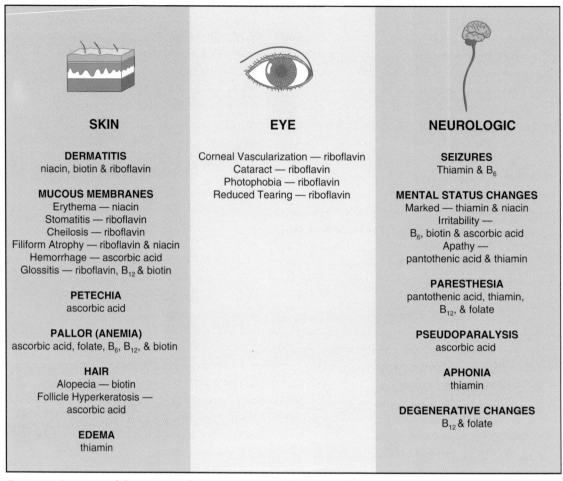

Figure 12: Summary of characteristic clinical presentations of water-soluble vitamin deficiencies. In general, the earliest manifestations involve either the skin, the eye or the central nervous system.

Plasma and leukocyte vitamin C concentrations reflect recent intake of the vitamin and are reported most often in assessing vitamin status.[156, 158] Acceptable plasma vitamin C values are >0.6 mg/dL; values below 0.2 mg/dL are observed in scurvy.[156, 169] Subclinical vitamin C deficiency is likely when the level of vitamin C in leucocytes is below 100 μg/g.[24]

Toxicity

Prolonged intakes of vitamin C in adults, >1.0 g/d, may cause oxaluria, uricosuria and acidification of the urine.[73] Renal calculi, therefore, may result from these changes. High doses also result in false positive tests for urinary glucose and occult blood in feces. Excessive doses of vitamin C may alter bactericidal functions of white blood cells and also provoke "rebound scurvy." Rebound scurvy has been reported in adults who reduce their high vitamin intakes abruptly.[43, 157, 163] The rebound phenomenon has been reported also in newborn infants of mothers who took large doses of the vitamin during pregnancy.[72, 73, 156] Potential problems with systemic acidosis may be encountered.[43, 171] The increased oxalic acid excretion would be detrimental in conditions such as congenital oxalosis/oxaluria, hyperuricemia and cystinuria.[43] Large doses of ascorbic acid may decrease the absorption of vitamin B_{12}, depress copper status, increase iron absorption to excessive amounts and exacerbate glucose-6-phosphate dehydrogenase deficiency.[43, 72, 171, 172]

Conclusion

When we consider the variability in the concentrations of vitamins in human milk, it is remarkable that the human milk-fed infant is protected from deficiencies of water-soluble vitamins.[173] Nevertheless, the best assessment of these needs appears to be based on those of the human milk-fed, full-term infant in whom deficiencies of water-soluble vitamins are rare. Deficiencies that arise in human milk-fed infants generally result from marked inadequacies in the mother's diet.

The water-soluble vitamin content of commercial formulas generally is greater than the content of vitamins in human milk. An upper limit for vitamin contents of formulas has been suggested to be five times the RDA.[174] Lower quantities, such as those at the RDA, generally provide an adequate status for the healthy infant and child.

A satisfactory status of water-soluble vitamins is observed in the full-term infant who is breast-fed or who receives commercially-prepared formula, and the toddler who receives a mixed diet. The toddler receiving a mixed diet including human milk or bovine milk and fruit juices will receive sufficient water-soluble vitamins. No additional water-soluble vitamin supplements are indicated in this population.

Figure 12 is organized to summarize the variety of presentations of water-soluble vitamin deficiency states. Now rare in the United States, deficiency states are reported in areas where malnutrition is prevalent or where unusual dietary restrictions are practiced. Thus, all infants and toddlers need water-soluble vitamins, which are found totally within their age-appropriate diets.

Case Histories

Case #1: A three-month-old breast-fed infant who had been thriving developed gastroenteritis and required hospitalization six days later for dehydration. At the time of hospitalization he was moribund, an arterial pH was 6.95. After fluid resuscitation, he showed signs of cerebral irritability and hypotonia sufficient to warrant mechanical ventilation. He developed cardiomegaly and seizures two days later. He was noted to have altered consciousness, episodes of "spasms," hepatomegaly, tachycardia, and peripheral edema. Cultures of blood, cerebrospinal fluid,

and urine were negative. His pH was 7.08 with an anion gap of 33 and both failed to correct with sodium bicarbonate. Thiamin 50 mg was given intravenously and within two hours the infant was awake and vigorous; within 36 hours he was extubated. He was continued on thiamin 5 mg/d and recovered unremarkably. Blood sampled before vitamin therapy demonstrated a low red cell transketolase activity 0.5 U/g Hgb (0.6 to 1.3 normal) and the TPP effect was 27% (normal <15%, severe beriberi >25%). The mother's transketolase was 0.8 and TPP effect was 18%. The mother, a 19-year-old, had no manifestations of thiamin deficiency. It was considered that maternal alcohol consumption was the likely etiology of her mild thiamin deficiency. This case demonstrates the development of cardiac beriberi ("shoshin" beriberi, "sho" meaning acute damage and "shin" meaning heart) in an infant of a mother with subclinical, borderline thiamin deficiency.[33]

Case #2: An eight-month-old male was admitted with a two-week history of screaming whenever he was handled. The birth history was unremarkable. The infant had only infrequent health care visits but was noted to be growing normally. He was fed evaporated milk without vitamin fortification and some cereal since birth. On examination, it was noted that he was pale and irritable but well-nourished. There was tenderness and decreased mobility of all limbs. A sepsis work-up was unremarkable. Skeletal X-rays revealed diffuse radiolucencies, epiphyseal changes and enlargement of the costochondral junctions. The serum ascorbic acid concentration was 0.14 mg/dL (normal >0.6 mg/dL).

The infant was treated with routine commercial formula (containing multivitamins that included vitamin C), and within five days had decreased tenderness and increased mobility of limbs. Within two weeks the skeletal survey showed healing of scurvy.[170]

Case #3: A 12-month-old girl presented with an eight-month history of short gut secondary to a volvulus. She was intolerant to feedings and required total parenteral nutrition. She had numerous complications and draining fistulae and required antibiotics almost continuously. Three months before evaluation, an erythematous rash was noted over the lower portion of the eyelids adjacent to the outer canthi. The rash spread, becoming more exfoliative, and exuded clear fluid. The rash was also observed at the angles of the mouth, around the nares, and in the perineal region. Topical antibiotics, glucocorticoids, and safflower oil were tried without benefit. Zinc supplements were provided in increasing dosages parenterally. The patient continued to worsen, she lost all body hair and developed a waxy pallor, irritability, lethargy and mild hypotonia.

Urinary organic acid excretion (specifically, methylcitrate, 3-hydroxyisovalerate, 3-methylcrotonylglycine) was increased. Plasma biotin concentrations were low. Biotin supplementation 1.0 mg/d for one week resulted in improvements in the rash and the irritability. The dose was increased to 10 mg. After two weeks, new hair growth was noted, the hypotonia had improved, and urinary organic acid excretion had normalized. Subsequently the biotin dose was tapered to 0.1 mg/d for maintenance. This was the original description of TPN-related biotin deficiency which occurred before biotin was added routinely to TPN solutions in pediatrics. It is important to note the prolonged usage of antibiotics which may have reduced any endogenous biotin synthesis.[113]

Historical Perspective...

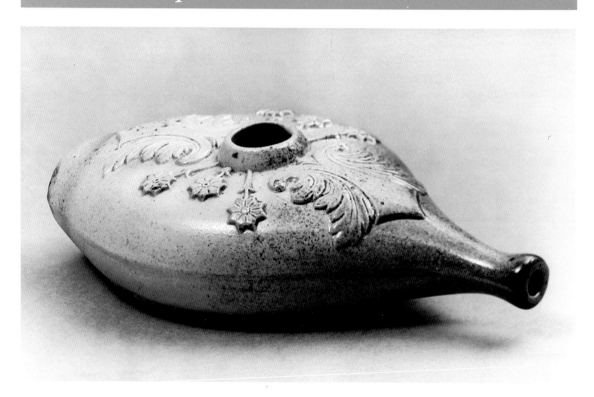

English feeding bottle, cream colored earthenware with shadings of burnt umber. Decorated, has opening for filling. Reverse side has a bas-relief of the young Queen Victoria.

References

1. King JC. Vitamin requirements during pregnancy. In: Campbell DM, Gillmer MDG, eds. *Nutrition in Pregnancy.* London: The Royal College of Obstetricians and Gynaecologists; 1983:33-45.

2. Dostalova L. Correlation of the vitamin status between mother and newborn during delivery. *Dev Pharmacol Ther.* 1982;4:45-57.

3. Baker H, Frank O, Thomson AD. Vitamin profiles of 174 mothers and newborns at parturition. *Am J Clin Nutr.* 1975;28:56-65.

4. Takaki K. Kakke', or Japanese beri-beri. *Lancet.* 1887;2: 189-190.

5. National Research Council (U.S), Subcommittee on the Tenth Edition of the RDAs. *Recommended Dietary Allowances.* Tenth ed. Washington, DC: National Academy Press; 1989.

6. Rindi G, Venura U. Thiamine intestinal transport. *Physiol Review.* 1972;52:821-827.

7. Moran JR, Greene HL. The B vitamins and vitamin C in human nutrition I. General considerations and "obligatory" B vitamins. *Am J Dis Child.* 1979;133: 192-199.

8. Gubler CJ. Thiamin. In: Machlin LJ, ed. *Handbook of Vitamins.* 2nd ed. New York: Marcel Dekker Inc; 1991: 233-282.

9. Davis RE, Icke GC. Clinical chemistry of thiamin. *Adv Clin Chem.* 1983;23:93-140.

10. Itokawa Y, Cooper JR. Ion movements and thiamin. II. Release of the vitamin from membrane fragments. *Biochim Biophys Acta.* 1970;196:274-284.

11. Heller S, Salkeld RM, Korner WF. Vitamin B1 status in pregnancy. *Am J Clin Nutr.* 1974;27:1221-1224.

12. Malone JI. Vitamin passage across the placenta. *Clin Perinatol.* 1975;2:295-307.

13. Schanler RJ, Nichols BL. The water soluble vitamins C, B1, B2, B6, and niacin. In: Tsang RC, ed. *Vitamin and Mineral Requirements in Preterm Infants.* New York: Marcel Dekker Inc; 1985:39-62.

14. Macy IG. Composition of human colostrum and milk. *Am J Dis Child.* 1949;78:589-603.

15. Adams CF. *Nutritive Value of American Foods.* Washington, DC: Agricultural Research Service; 1975.

16. Thomas MR, Sneed SM, Wei C. The effects of vitamin C, vitamin B6, vitamin B12, folic acid, riboflavin, and thiamin on the breast milk and maternal status of well-nourished women at 6 months postpartum. *Am J Clin Nutr.* 1980;33:2151-2156.

17. Knott EM, Kleiger SC, Torres-Bracamonte F. Factors affecting the thiamine content of breast milk. *J Nutr.* 1943;25:49-58.

18. Ford JE, Zechalko A, Murphy J, Brooke OG. Comparison of the B vitamin composition of milk from mothers of preterm and term babies. *Arch Dis Child.* 1983;58: 367-372.

19. Roderuck CE, Williams HH, Macy IG. Human milk studies. XXIII. Free and total thiamine contents of colostrum and mature human milk. *Am J Dis Child.* 1945;70:162-170.

20. Nail PA, Thomas MR, Eakin R. The effect of thiamin and riboflavin supplementation on the level of those vitamins in human breast milk and urine. *Am J Clin Nutr.* 1980;33:198-204.

21. Dostalova L, Salmenpera L, Vaclavinkova V, Heinz-Erian P, Schuep W. Vitamin concentrations in term milk of European mothers. In: Berger H, ed. *Vitamins and Minerals in Pregnancy and Lactation.* New York: Raven Press; 1988:275-298.

22. Pennington JAT. *Bowes & Church's Food Values of Portions Commonly Used.* 16th ed. Philadelphia: JB Lippincott Company; 1994.

23. Holt LE, Jr, Nemir RL, Snyderman SE, et al. The thiamine requirement of the normal infant. *J Nutr.* 1949; 37:53-66.

24. Wharton BA. *Nutrition and Feeding of Pre-term Infants.* Oxford: Blackwell Scientific Publications; 1987.

25. American Academy of Pediatrics, Committee on Nutrition. Nutritional needs of low-birth-weight infants. *Pediatrics.* 1985;75:976-986.

26. Moore MC, Greene HL, Phillips B, et al. Evaluation of a pediatrics multiple vitamin preparation for total parenteral nutrition in infants and children. I. Blood levels of water-soluble vitamins. *Pediatrics.* 1986;77: 530-538.

27. Greene HL, Hambidge KM, Schanler R, Tsang RC. Guidelines for the use of vitamins, trace elements, calcium, magnesium, and phosphorus in infants and children receiving total parenteral nutrition: report of the Subcommittee on Pediatric Parenteral Nutrient Requirements from the Committee on Clinical Practice Issues of The American Society for Clinical Nutrition. *Am J Clin Nutr.* 1988;48:1324-1342.

28. Marinier E, Gorski AM, Potier de Courcy G, et al.

Blood levels of water soluble vitamins in pediatric patients on total parenteral nutrition using a multiple vitamin preparation. *J Parent Ent Nutr.* 1989;13:176-184.

29. Shenkin A, Fraser WD, McLelland AJD, Fell GS, Garden OJ. Maintenance of vitamin and trace element status in intravenous nutrition using a complete nutritive mixture. *J Parent Ent Nutr.* 1987;11:238-242.

30. McCormick DB. Thiamin. In: Shils ME, Young VR, eds. *Modern Nutrition in Health and Disease.* Philadelphia: Lea and Febiger; 1988:355-361.

31. Goldsmith GC. Vitamin B complex. *Prog Food Nutr Sci.* 1975;1:559-609.

32. Rascoff H. Beriberi heart in a 4 month old infant. *J Am Med Assoc.* 1942;120:1292-1293.

33. Debuse PJ. Shoshin beriberi in an infant of a thiamine-deficient mother. *Acta Paediatr.* 1992;81:723-724.

34. Molony CJ, Parmelee AH. Convulsions in young infants as a result of pyridoxine (vitamin B6 deficiency). *J Amer Med Assoc.* 1954;154:405-406.

35. Wyatt DT, Noetzel MJ, Hillman RE. Infantile beriberi presenting as subacute necrotizing encephalomyelopathy. *J Pediatr.* 1987;110:888-891.

36. Van Gelder DW, Darby FU. Congenital and infantile beriberi. *J Pediatr.* 1944;25:226-235.

37. King EQ. Acute cardiac failure in the newborn due to thiamine deficiency. *Exp Med Surg.* 1967;25:173-177.

38. Cochrane WA, Collins-Williams C, Donohue WL. Superior hemorrhagic polioencephalitis (Wernicke's Disease occurring in an infant--probably due to thiamine deficiency from use of a soya bean product.) *Pediatrics.* 1961;28:771-777.

39. La Selve P, Demolin P, Holzapfel L, Blanc PL, Teyssier G, Robert D. Shoshin beriberi: an unusual complication of prolonged parenteral nutrition. *J Parent Ent Nutr.* 1986; 10:102-103.

40. Seear M, Lockitch G, Jacobson B, Quigley G, MacNab A. Thiamine, riboflavin, and pyridoxine deficiencies in a population of critically ill children. *J Pediatr.* 1992;121: 533-538.

41. Oriot D, Wood C, Gottesman R, Huault G. Severe lactic acidosis related to acute thiamine deficiency. *J Parent Ent Nutr.* 1991;15:105-109.

42. Wyatt DT, Nelson D, Hillman RE. Age-dependent changes in thiamin concentrations in whole blood and cerebrospinal fluid in infants and children. *Am J Clin Nutr.* 1991;53:530-536.

43. Alhadeff L, Gualtieri CT, Lipton M. Toxic effects of water soluble vitamins. *Nutr Rev.* 1984;42:33-40.

44. Emmett AD, Luros GO. Water-soluble vitamines. I. Are the antineuritic and the growth-promoting water-soluble B vitamines the same? *J Biol Chem.* 1920;43:265-280.

45. McCormick DB. Riboflavin. In: Shils ME, Young VR, eds. *Modern Nutrition in Health and Disease.* 7th ed. Philadelphia: Lea and Febiger; 1988:362-369.

46. Horwitt MK. Interpretations of requirements for thiamin, riboflavin, niacin- tryptophan, and vitamin E plus comments on balance studies and vitamin B6. *Am J Clin Nutr.* 1986;44:973-986.

47. Lust JE, Hagerman DD, Villee CA. The transport of riboflavin by the human placenta. *J Clin Invest.* 1954; 33:38-40.

48. Bates CJ, Liu DS, Fuller NJ, Lucas A. Susceptibility of riboflavin and vitamin A in breast milk to photodegradation and its implications for the use of banked breast milk in infant feeding. *Acta Paediatr Scand.* 1985;74:40-44.

49. Combs GF Jr. *The Vitamins: Fundamental Aspects in Nutrition and Health.* San Diego, CA: Academic Press Inc; 1992.

50. Chen MF, Boyce HW, Triplett L. Stability of the B vitamins in mixed parenteral nutrition solution. *J Parent Ent Nutr.* 1983;7:462-464.

51. Hovi L, Hekali R, Siimes MA. Evidence of riboflavin depletion in breast-fed newborns and its further acceleration during treatment of hyperbilirubinemia by phototherapy. *Acta Paediatr Scand.* 1979;68:567-570.

52. Sisson TR. Photodegradation of riboflavin in neonates. *Fed Proc.* 1987;46:1883-1885.

53. Ronnholm KAR. Need for riboflavin supplementation in small pre-terms fed with human milk. *Am J Clin Nutr.* 1986;43:1-6.

54. Lucas A, Bates C. Transient riboflavin depletion in pre-term infants. *Arch Dis Child.* 1984;59:837-841.

55. Cooperman JM, Lopez R. Riboflavin. In: Machlin LJ, ed. *Handbook of Vitamins.* 2nd ed. New York: Marcel Dekker Inc; 1991:283-310.

56. Roderuck CE, Coryell MN, Williams HH. Human milk studies: XXIV. Free and total riboflavin contents of colostrum and mature milk. *Am J Dis Child.* 1945;70: 171-175.

57. Hughes J, Sanders TAB. Riboflavin levels in the diet and breast milk of vegans and omnivores. *Proc Nutr Soc.* 1979;38:95A

58. Deodhar AD, Rajalakshmi R, Ramakrishnan CV. Studies on human lactation - Part III: Effect of dietary vitamin supplementation on vitamin contents of breast milk. *Acta Paediatr.* 1964;53:42-48.

59. Greene HL, Specker BL, Smith R, Murrell J, Swift R, Swift L. Plasma riboflavin concentrations in infants fed human milk versus formula: Comparison with values in rats made riboflavin deficient and human cord blood. *J Pediatr.* 1990;117:916-920.

60. Bates CJ, Prentice AM, Paul AA, Prentice A, Sutcliffe BA, Whitehead RG. Riboflavin status in infants born in rural Gambia, and the effect of a weaning food supplement. *Trans R Soc Trop Med Hyg.* 1982;76:253-258.

61. Lopez R, Cole HS, Montoya F, Cooperman JM. Riboflavin deficiency in a pediatric population of low socioeconomic status in New York City. *J Pediatr.* 1975; 105:420-422.

62. Fritz I, Said H, Harris C, Murrell J, Greene HL. A new sensitive assay for plasma riboflavin using high performance liquid chromatography. *J Amer Coll Nutr.* 1987;6:449.

63. Elvehjem CA, Madden RJ, Strong FM, Woolley DW. Relation of nicotinic acid and nicotinic acid amide to canine black tongue. *J Am Chem Soc.* 1937;59:1767-1768.

64. Sarett HP, Goldsmith GA. The effect of tryptophane on the excretion of nicotinic acid derivatives in humans. *J Biol Chem.* 1947;167:293-294.

65. Benton DA. Protein contents of the diet and requirements during the neonatal period. In: Lebenthal E, ed. *Textbook of Gastroenterology and Nutrition in Infancy.* New York: Raven Press; 1981:385-389.

66. Hankes LV. Nicotinic acid and nicotinamide. In: Machlin LJ, ed. *Handbook of Vitamins.* New York: Marcel Dekker Inc; 1984:329-377.

67. McCormick DB. Niacin. In: Shils ME, Young VR, eds. *Modern Nutrition in Health and Disease.* Philadelphia: Lea and Febiger; 1988:370-375.

68. Coryell MN, Harris ME, Miller S. Human milk studies XXII. Nicotinic acid, pantothenic acid and biotin contents of colostrum and mature human milk. *Am J Dis Child.* 1945;70:L50-L61.

69. Holt LE Jr. The adolescence of nutrition. *Arch Dis Child.* 1956;31:427-438.

70. Darby WJ, McNutt KW, Todhunter EN. Niacin. *Nutr Rev.* 1975;33:289-297.

71. Spivak JL, Jackson DL. Pellagra: an analysis of 18 patients and a review of the literature. *Johns Hopkins Med J.* 1977;140:295-309.

72. Moran JR, Greene HL. The B vitamins and vitamin C in human nutrition. II: 'Conditional' B vitamins and vitamin C. *Am J Dis Child.* 1979;133:308-314.

73. American Medical Association, Council on Scientific Affairs. Vitamin preparations as dietary supplements and therapeutic agents. *JAMA.* 1987;257:1929-1936.

74. Lumeng L, Li TK, Lui A. The interorgan transport and metabolism of vitamin B6. In: Reynolds RD, Leklem JE, eds. *Vitamin B6: Its Role in Health and Disease.* New York: Alan R Liss Inc; 1985:35-54.

75. Leklem JE. Vitamin B6: A status report. *J Nutr.* 1990; 1503-1507.

76. Bender DA. Vitamin B6 requirements and recommendations. *Eur J Clin Nutr.* 1989;43:289-309.

77. Fomon SJ. *Nutrition of Normal Infants.* St. Louis: Mosby-Year Book Inc; 1993.

78. Van Zoeren-Grobben D, Schrijver J, Van den Berg H, Berger HM. Human milk vitamin content after pasteurization, storage, or tube-feeding. *Arch Dis Child.* 1987;62:161-165.

79. Contractor SF, Shane B. Blood and urine levels of vitamin B6 in the mother and fetus before and after loading of the mother with vitamin B6. *Am J Obstet Gynec.* 1970; 107:635-640.

80. Driskell JA. Vitamin B6. In: Machlin LJ, ed. *Handbook of Vitamins.* New York: Marcel Dekker Inc; 1984:379-401.

81. Hamfelt A, Landgren E, Soderhjelm L. Plasma pyridoxal phosphate levels in newborn infants, their mothers and in the mothers' breast milk. *Upsala J Med Sci.* 1989;94:95-99.

82. Schuster K, Bailey LB, Mahan CS. Effect of maternal pyridoxine-HCI supplementation on the vitamin B6 status of mother and infant and on pregnancy outcome. *J Nutr.* 1984;114:977-988.

83. Reynolds RD, Polansky M, Moser PB. Analyzed vitamin B6 intakes of pregnant and postpartum lactating and nonlactating women. *J Am Diet Assoc.* 1984;84:1339-1344.

84. Black AE, Wiles SJ, Paul AA. The nutrient intakes of pregnant and lactating mothers of good socio-economic status in Cambridge, UK: some implications for recommended daily allowances of minor nutrients. *Brit J Nutr.* 1986;56:59-72.

85. Schuster K, Bailey LB, Dimperio D, Mahan CS. Morning sickness and vitamin B6 status of pregnant women. *Hum Nutr: Clin Nutr.* 1985;39:75-79.

86. Styslinger L, Kirksey A. Effects of different levels of vitamin B6 supplementation on vitamin B6 concentrations in human milk and vitamin B6 intakes of breast-fed infants. *Am J Clin Nutr.* 1985;41:21-31.

87. Borschel MW, Kirksey A, Hannemann RE. Effects of vitamin B6 intake on nutriture and growth of young infants. *Am J Clin Nutr.* 1986;43:7-15.

88. Thomas MR, Kawamoto J, Sneed SM, Eakin R. The effects of vitamin C, vitamin B6, and vitamin B12 supplementation on the breast milk and maternal status of well-nourished women. *Am J Clin Nutr.* 1979;32: 1679-1685.

89. Kirksey A, Udipi SA. Vitamin B6 in human pregnancy and lactation. In: Reynolds RD, Leklem JE, eds. *Vitamin B6: Its Role in Health and Disease.* New York: Alan R Liss; 1985:57-77.

90. Sneed SM, Zane C, Thomas MR. The effects of ascorbic acid, vitamin B6, vitamin B12, and folic acid supplementation on the breast milk and maternal nutritional status of low socioeconomic lactating women. *Am J Clin Nutr.* 1981;34:1338-1346.

91. West KD, Kirksey A. Influence of vitamin B6 intake on the content of the vitamin in human milk. *Am J Clin Nutr.* 1976;29:961-969.

92. Kang-Yoon SA, Kirksey A, Giacoia G, West K. Vitamin B6 status of breast-fed neonates: influence of pyridoxine supplementation on mothers and neonates. *Am J Clin Nutr.* 1992;56:548-558.

93. Bessey OA, Adam DJD, Hansen AE. Intake of vitamin B6 and infantile convulsions: A first approximation of requirements of pyridoxine in infants. *Pediatrics.* 1957; 20:33-44.

94. Karra MV, Udipi SA, Kirksey A, Roepke JLB. Changes in specific nutrients in breast milk during extended lactation. *Am J Clin Nutr.* 1986;43:495-503.

95. Heiskanen K, Salmenpera L, Perheentupa J, Siimes MA. Infant vitamin B6 status changes with age and with formula feeding. *Am J Clin Nutr.* 1994;60:907-910.

96. Ubbink JB, Delport R, Becker PJ, Bissbort S. Evidence of a theophylline-induced vitamin B6 deficiency caused by noncompetitive inhibition of pyridoxal kinase. *J Lab Clin Med.* 1989;113:15-22.

97. Reynolds RD, Lorenc RS, Wieczorek E, Pronicka E. Extremely low serum pyridoxal 5'-phosphate in children with familial hypophosphatemic rickets. *Am J Clin Nutr.* 1991;53:698-701.

98. Schaumburg H, Kaplan J, Windebank A, et al. Sensory neuropathy from pyridoxine abuse - A new megavitamin syndrome. *N Engl J Med.* 1983;309:445-448.

99. Snodgrass SR. Vitamin neurotoxicity. *Mol Neurobiol.* 1992;1:41-73.

100. Williams RJ, Lyman CM, Goodyear GH. "Pantothenic acid," a growth determinant of universal biological occurrence. *J Am Chem Soc.* 1933;55:2912-2927.

101. Lipmann F, Kaplan NO, Novelli GD, Tuttle LC, Guirard BM. Coenzyme for acetylation, a pantothenic acid derivative. *J Biol Chem.* 1947;167:869-879.

102. Gross SJ. Choline, pantothenic acid, and biotin. In: Tsang RC, ed. *Vitamin and Mineral Requirements in Preterm Infants.* New York: Marcel Dekker Inc; 1985: 191-201.

103. Fox HM. Pantothenic acid. In: Machlin LJ, ed. *Handbook of Vitamins.* New York: Marcel Dekker Inc; 1984:437-458.

104. Rose RC. Transport of ascorbic acid and other water-soluble vitamins. *Biochim Biophys Acta.* 1988;947:335-366.

105. Song WO, Chan GM, Wyse BW, Hansen RG. Effect of pantothenic acid status on the content of the vitamin in human milk. *Am J Clin Nutr.* 1984;40:317-324.

106. Johnston L, Vaughn L, Fox HM. Pantothenic acid content of human milk. *Am J Clin Nutr.* 1981;34:2205-2209.

107. McCormick DB. Biotin. In: Hegsted DM, Chichester CO, Darby WJ, McNutt KW, Stalvey RM, Stotz EH, eds. *Nutrition Review's Present Knowledge in Nutrition.* 4th ed. New York: Nutrition Foundation; 1976:217-225.

108. Roth KS. Biotin in clinical medicine-a review. *Am J Clin Nutr.* 1981;34:1967-1974.

109. Goldsmith SJ, Eitenmiller RR, Feeley RM, Barnhart HM, Maddox FC. Biotin content of human milk during early lactational stages. *Nutr Res.* 1982;2:579-583.

110. Bonjour JP. Biotin in man's nutrition and therapy-a review. *Int J Vitam Nutr Res.* 1977;47:107-118.

111. Bonjour J. Biotin. In: Machlin LJ, ed. *Handbook of Vitamins.* 2nd ed. New York: Marcel Dekker Inc; 1991: 393-427.

112. Hamil BM, Coryell M, Roderuck C, et al. Thiamine, riboflavin, nicotinic acid, pantothenic acid and biotin in the urine of newborn infants. *Am J Dis Child.* 1947; 74:434-446.

113. Mock DM, DeLorimer AA, Liebman WM, Sweetman L, Baker H. Biotin deficiency: an unusual complication of parenteral alimentation. *New Engl J Med.* 1981;304:820-823.

114. Wills L, Clutterbuck PW, Evans BDF. A new factor in the production and cure of macrocytic anaemias and its relation to other haemopoietic principles curative in pernicious anaemia. *Biochem J.* 1937;31:2136-2147.

115. Stokstad ELR. Some properties of a growth factor for Lactobacillus casei. *J Biol Chem.* 1943;149:573-574.

116. Mitchell HD, Snell EE, Williams RJ. The concentration of "folic acid". *J Am Chem Soc.* 1941;63:2284

117. Brody T. Folic acid. In: Machlin LJ, ed. *Handbook of Vitamins.* 2nd ed. New York: Marcel Dekker Inc; 1991: 453-489.

118. Davis RE. Clinical chemistry of folic acid. *Adv Clin Chem.* 1986;25:233-294.

119. Herbert VD, Colman N. Folic acid and vitamin B12. In: Shils ME, Young VR, eds. *Modern Nutrition in Health and Disease.* Philadelphia: Lea and Febiger; 1988: 388-416.

120. Tamura T, Shane B, Baer MT, King JC, Margen S, Stokstad ELR. Absorption of mono- and polyglutamyl folates in zinc-depleted man. *Am J Clin Nutr.* 1978;31: 1984-1987.

121. Herbert V. Recommended dietary intakes (RDI) of folate in humans. *Am J Clin Nutr.* 1987;45:661-670.

122. Gerson CD, Cohen N, Hepner GW, Brown N, Herbert V, Janowitz HD. Folic acid absorption in man: enhancing effect of glucose. *Gastroenterology.* 1971;61:224-227.

123. Hillman RS, McGuffin R, Campbell C. Alcohol interference with the folate enterohepatic cycle. *Trans Assoc Am Phys.* 1977;90:145-156.

124. Goldman ID. The characteristics of the membrane transport of amethopterin and the naturally occurring folates. *Ann NY Acad Sci.* 1971;186:400-422.

125. Herbert V, Das KC. The role of vitamin B12 and folic acid in hemato- and other cell-poiesis. *Vitamin Hormones.* 1976;34:1-30.

126. Brown CM, Smith AM, Picciano MF. Forms of human milk folacin and variation patterns. *J Pediatr Gastroenterol Nutr.* 1986;5:278-282.

127. Tamura T, Yoshimura Y, Arakawa T. Human milk folate and folate status in lactating mothers and their infants. *Am J Clin Nutr.* 1980;33:193-197.

128. Ek J, Magnus E. Plasma and red cell folate values and folate requirements in formula-fed term infants. *J Pediatr.* 1982;100:738-744.

129. Smith AM, Picciano MF, Deering RH. Folate intake and blood concentrations of term infants. *Am J Clin Nutr.* 1985;41:590-598.

130. Salmenpera L, Perheentupa J, Siimes MA. Folate nutrition is optimal in exclusively breast-fed infants but inadequate in some of their mothers and formula-fed infants. *J Pediatr Gastroenterol Nutr.* 1986;5:283-289.

131. Bailey LB. Evaluation of a new recommended dietary allowance for folate. *J Am Diet Assn.* 1992;92:463-468, 471.

132. Ek J, Magnus EM. Plasma and red blood cell folate in breast-fed infants. *Acta Pediatr Scand.* 1979;68:239-243.

133. Ek J. Folic acid and vitamin B12 requirements in premature infants. In: Tsang RC, ed. *Vitamin and Mineral Requirements in Preterm Infants.* New York: Marcel Dekker Inc; 1985:23-38.

134. Matoth Y, Zehavi E, Topper E, Klein T. Folate nutrition and growth in infancy. *Arch Dis Child.* 1979;54:699-702.

135. Strelling MK, Blackledge DG, Goodall HB. Diagnosis and management of folate deficiency in low birthweight infants. *Arch Dis Child.* 1979;54:271-277.

136. Shojania AM, Hornady G. Folate metabolism in newborns and during early infancy. *Pediatr Res.* 1970;4: 422-426.

137. Rodriguez MS. A conspectus of research on folacin requirements of man. *J Nutr.* 1978;108:1983-2075.

138. Newman V, Lyon RB, Anderson PO. Evaluation of prenatal vitamin-mineral supplements. *Clin Pharm.* 1987;6:770-777.

139. Edwards JH, Holmes-Siedle M, Lindenbaum RH. Vitamin supplementation and neural tube defects. *Lancet.* 1982;1:275-276.

140. Smithells RW, Shepard S, Schorah CJ. Vitamin deficiencies and neural tube defects. *Arch Dis Child.* 1976;51:944-950.

141. Mulinare J, Cordero JF, Erickson JD, Berry RJ. Periconceptional use of multivitamins and the occurrence of neural tube defects. *J Am Med Assoc.* 1988;260: 3141-3145.

142. Mills JL, Rhoads GG, Simpson JL, et al. The absence of a relation between the periconceptional use of vitamins and neural-tube defects. *N Engl J Med.* 1989;321:430-435.

143. Combe JS. History of a case of anemia. *Trans Med-Chirurg Soc Edinb.* 1821;1:194-204.

144. Minot GR, Murphy WP. Treatment of pernicious anemia by a special diet. *J Am Med Assoc.* 1926;87: 470-476.

145. Herbert V. Vitamin B12. In: Hegsted DM, Chichester CO, Darby WJ, McNutt KW, Stalvey RM, Stotz EH, eds. *Nutrition Review's Present Knowledge in Nutrition.* 4th ed. New York: Nutrition Foundation; 1976:191-203.

146. Rickes EL, Brink NG, Koniuszy FR. Crystalline vitamin B12. *Science.* 1948;107:396-397.

147. Bartels PC, Helleman PW, Soons JBJ. Investigation of red cell size-distribution histograms related to folate, vitamin B12 and iron state in the course of pregnancy. *Scand J Clin Lab Invest.* 1989;49:763-771.

148. Herbert V. The 1986 Herman Award Lecture. Nutrition science as a continually unfolding story: the folate and vitamin B12 paradigm. *Am J Clin Nutr.* 1987;46:387-402.

149. Herbert V. Recommended dietary intakes (RDI) of vitamin B12 in humans. *Am J Clin Nutr.* 1987;45:671-678.

150. Collins JE, Rolles CJ, Sutton H, Ackery D. B12 absorption after necrotizing enterocolitis. *Arch Dis Child.* 1984;59:731-734.

151. Higginbottom MC, Sweetman L, Nyhan WL. A syndrome of methylmalonic aciduria, homocystinuria, megaloblastic anemia and neurologic abnormalities in a vitamin B12-deficient breast-fed infant of a strict vegetarian. *New Engl J Med.* 1978;299:317-323.

152. Stollhoff K, Schulte FJ. Vitamin B12 and brain development. *Eur J Pediatr.* 1987;146:201-205.

153. Specker BL, Miller D, Norman EJ, Greene H, Hayes KC. Increased urinary methylmalonic acid excretion in breast-fed infants of vegetarian mothers and identification of an acceptable dietary source of vitamin B12. *Am J Clin Nutr.* 1988;47:89-92.

154. Harrison RJ. Vitamin B12 levels in erythrocytes in hypochromic anaemia. *J Clin Path.* 1971;24:698-700.

155. Lomax E. Difficulties in diagnosing infantile scurvy before 1878. *Med Hist.* 1986;30:70-80.

156. Olson JA, Hodges RE. Recommended dietary intakes (RDI) of vitamin C in humans. *Am J Clin Nutr.* 1987; 45:693-703.

157. Levine M. New concepts in the biology and biochemistry of ascorbic acid. *N Engl J Med.* 1986;314:892-902.

158. Irwin MI, Hutchins BK. A conspectus of research on vitamin C requirements of man.(2). *J Nutr.* 1976;106: 823-879.

159. Light IJ, Berry HK, Sutherland JM. Aminoacidemia of prematurity. *Am J Dis Child.* 1966;112:229-236.

160. Adlard BPF, De Souza SW, Moon S. Ascorbic acid in the fetal human brain. *Arch Dis Child.* 1974;49:278-282.

161. Arad ID, Eyal FG. High plasma ascorbic acid levels in pre-term neonates with intraventricular hemorrhage. *Am J Dis Child.* 1983;137:949-951.

162. Teel HM, Burke BS, Draper R. Vitamin C in human pregnancy and lactation. I. Studies during pregnancy. *Am J Dis Child.* 1938;56:1004-1010.

163. Jaffe GM. Vitamin C. In: Machlin LJ, ed. *Handbook of Vitamins.* New York: Marcel Dekker Inc; 1984:199-244.

164. Ingalls TH. Ascorbic acid requirements in early infancy. *N Engl J Med.* 1938;218:872-875.

165. Selleg I, King CG. The vitamin C content of human milk and its variation with diet. *J Nutr.* 1936;11:599-606.

166. Byerley LO, Kirksey A. Effects of different levels of vitamin C intake on the vitamin C concentration in human milk and the vitamin C intakes of breast-fed infants. *Am J Clin Nutr.* 1985;41:665-671.

167. Salmenpera L. Vitamin C nutrition during prolonged lactation: optimal in infants while marginal in some mothers. *Am J Clin.* 1984;40:1050-1056.

168. Fairweather-Tait S, Fox T, Wharf SG, Eagles J. The bioavailability of iron in different weaning foods and the enhancing effect of a fruit drink containing ascorbic acid. *Pediatr Res.* 1995;37:389-394.

169. Shils ME, Baker H, Frank O. Blood vitamin levels of long-term adult home total parenteral nutrition patients: the efficacy of the AMA-FDA parenteral multivitamin formulation. *J Parent Ent Nutr.* 1985;9: 179-188.

170. Grewar D. Scurvy and its prevention by vitamin C for-tified evaporated milk. *Can Med Assoc J.* 1959;80: 977-979.

171. Barness LA. Safety considerations with high ascorbic acid dosage. *Ann NY Acad Sci.* 1975;258:523-528.

172. Skekel A, Olivares M, Pizarro F, Chadud P, Lopez I, Amar M. Absorption of fortification iron from milk formulas in infants. *Am J Clin Nutr.* 1986;43:917-922.

173. Packard VS. Vitamins. In: Packard VS, ed. *Human Milk and Infant Formula.* New York: Academic Press; 1982:29-49.

174. McCormick DB. Water-soluble vitamins: Bases for suggested upper limits for infant formulas. *J Nutr.* 1989; 119:1818-1819.

Special Needs and Dangers of
Fat-soluble Vitamins A, E and K
Frank R. Greer M.D.

University of Wisconsin,
Madison, Wisconsin

Reviewed by Richard J. Schanler M.D., James W. Hansen M.D., Ph.D. and Steven J. Gross M.D.

Introduction

The fat-soluble vitamins, A, E and K, are all essential nutrients fitting the classic definition of a vitamin: an organic compound, present in very small quantities in natural foodstuffs, which are essential to normal metabolism and without which specific deficiency disease occurs. Vitamin D, historically considered to be a fat-soluble vitamin, is now considered a hormone and is discussed in Chapter 9.

Vitamins A, E and K are very important in infant nutrition. A deficiency of each vitamin has been associated with clinical disorders unique to infants. Pharmacological quantities of these nutrients have been used prophylactically and therapeutically in infants to treat these disorders, namely, bronchopulmonary dysplasia, retinopathy of prematurity, intraventricular hemorrhage and hemorrhagic disease of the newborn. A large body of literature has developed regarding the "protective effects" of these vitamins. As suggested by a recent reviewer, the use of these vitamins in pharmacological doses in the newborn resembles the tale of the Wizard of Oz.[1] In this fantasy, the wizard had no magical powers at all, but the belief that he did kept Dorothy and her friends following the yellow brick road.

This chapter will give an overview of the nutritional and therapeutic roles of these vitamins in infants. The gold standard for various vitamin requirements is based on the quantities ingested by exclusively breast-fed infants from healthy mothers. Unfortunately, a deficiency of vitamin K has been described for exclusively breast-fed infants. And, human milk may not provide the necessary requirements of these three vitamins for the rapidly-growing premature infant.

Historical Aspects

All three of these micronutrients were described and synthesized in the first half of the twentieth century, though their roles in nutrition, metabolism and disease continue to be ongoing areas of pediatric research.

Vitamin A

Vitamin A was the first of the fat-soluble vitamins to be discovered. Using one of the first rat colonies started solely for experimentation in nutrition in 1913, E. V. McCollum and his colleagues at the University of Wisconsin noted that diets containing butterfat or ether extracts of egg yolk improved growth in rats, compared with those containing lard and olive oil as a fat source. A growth-promoting factor was found in the "non-saponifiable fraction" of fat, which could be transferred into olive oil to support growth in rats. This growth-supporting substance was later named vitamin A.

Vitamin E

Discovered in 1922 by Evans and Bishop, "substance X" was described from work documenting that rats fed a diet of rancid lard could not reproduce. The name was changed to vitamin E in 1924, and a pure form of the vitamin was isolated from wheat-germ oil in 1936. A scientific name for the substance was decided by Evans and Calhoun (a professor of Greek at Berkeley) over dinner. When told by Evans that vitamin E permits an animal to bear offspring, Calhoun stated, "Well, 'childbirth' in Greek is tocos, and if it confers or brings childbirth, we will next employ the Greek verb phero. You have said that the term must have an ending consonant with its chemical–'ol', it being an

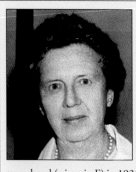

Gladys A. Emerson Ph.D. (1903-1984) received her advanced degree at Berkeley under Herbert Evans in 1932. Evans was a Hopkins M.D. graduate of 1908 who became Head of Anatomy at Berkeley in 1915. Emerson and Evans isolated pure tocopherol (vitamin E) in 1936. She worked at Merck Laboratories from 1942 until 1957 where she led in the synthesis of vitamin B_{12} and study of the metabolism of pyridoxine. Emerson then served as Chairman of Home Economics at UCLA until 1970. J. Nutr. 115,837-841,1985 (Photo courtesy of NLM)

alcohol; your substance is 'tocopherol,' and the pleasant task assigned me quickly is solved and not worth the delightful four-course dinner you have arranged."[2] In general, although vitamin E deficiency disease has been documented in many animal models, similar diseases attributed to vitamin E deficiency have not been described in humans, in whom there are unique and relatively few deficiency states. In fact, vitamin E has long been described as "a vitamin looking for a disease" and has a reputation as "the shady lady of human nutrition" for its reputed benefits in pharmacological doses for a range of diverse human disease states.

Vitamin K

While investigating cholesterol biosynthesis in 1929, Henrik Dam, a faculty member at the Biochemical Institute of the University of Copenhagen, discovered a hemorrhagic disease in chicks placed on fat-free diets. This disease in chicks was successfully treated with ether extracts of alfalfa. Though "K" was the first letter of the German word Koagulation, it was also by chance the first letter of the alphabet not in use at that time to describe an existing vitamin or vitamin-like activity. (We are left to wonder what happened to F, G, H, I and J.) The vitamin was initially isolated from alfalfa as a yellow oil (phylloquinone). Another form was isolated from putrefied fish meal,

which in contrast to the oil isolated from alfalfa, was a crystal (menaquinone).

Nomenclature

As is often the case, the nomenclature of these vitamins tends to be confusing at times and has continuously evolved as various biochemical forms of the vitamins have been described.

Vitamin A

The term vitamin A is a generic term for a group of closely related compounds, the basic constituent of which is all-trans retinol (see Figure 1). The alcohol group at the end of the carbon side chain extending from the ß-ionone ring can be oxidized to retinal (retinaldehyde) and then to retinoic acid. It can also be esterified with acyl-CoA fatty acids to form retinal esters, the most common one in animal tissue being retinal palmitate. Carotene is a yellow pigment found in plants, which is a precursor of retinol. One molecule of beta-carotene, the major plant carotenoid, is capable of yielding two molecules of vitamin A (See Figure 1). One IU of vitamin A is equal to 0.3 µg of all-trans-retinol or 0.6 µg of all-trans-ß-carotene. However, this nomenclature of vitamin A activity does not reflect biological activity after ingestion, as carotene is poorly absorbed. Therefore, in a somewhat confusing fashion, vitamin A activity is commonly expressed as retinol equivalents, one retinol equivalent being equal to 1 µg of all-trans-retinol, 6 µg of all-trans-ß-carotene, or 3.33 IU of vitamin A. (One µg of all-trans-retinol per retinol equivalent divided by 0.3 µg all-trans-retinol per one IU of vitamin A=3.33 IU of vitamin A per one retinol equivalent.)

Vitamin E

As with vitamin A, the term vitamin E is generic and refers to a group of eight compounds, four tocopherols and four tocotrienols with varying degrees of biological activity. The structure of the tocopherols consists of a complex ring with a long, saturated side chain (Figure 2), differing only in the position of the methyl groups on the ring. The most active of these compounds is alpha tocopherol, which accounts for greater than 90%

Vitamin A

Structure of Vitamin A

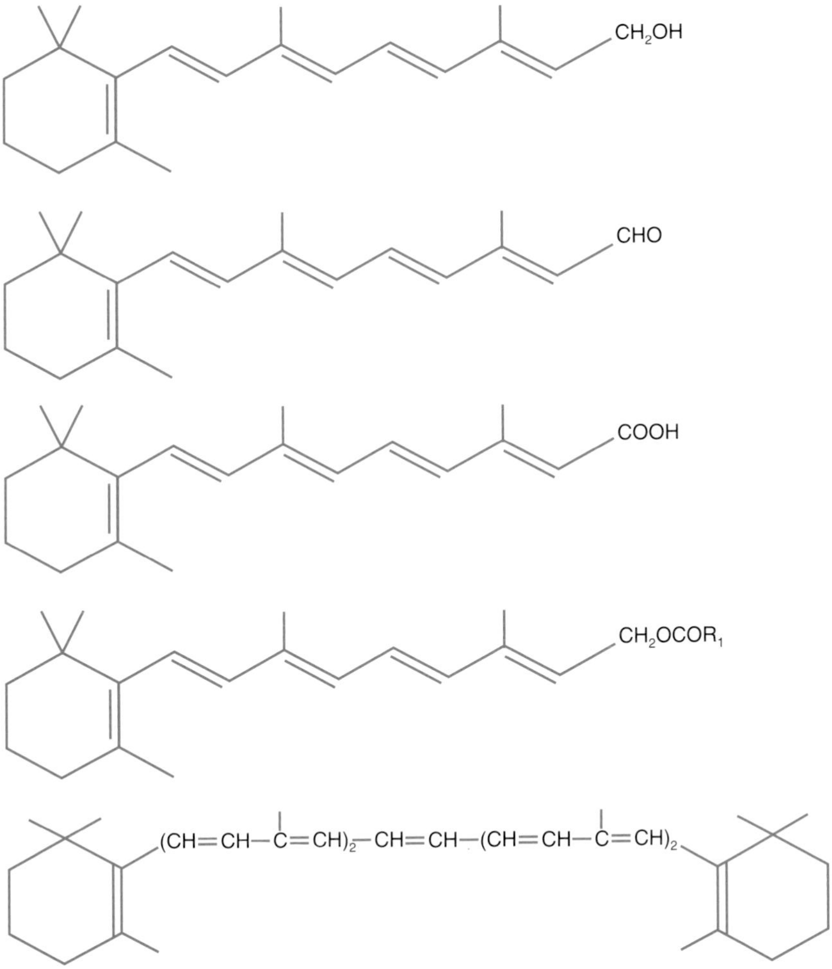

CH_2OH

all trans Retinol

CHO

Retinal (Retinaldehyde)

COOH

Retinoic Acid

CH_2OCOR_1

Retinyl Ester
R_1=fatty acid, i.e. palmitate

$(CH=CH-C=CH)_2-CH=CH-(CH=CH-C=CH)_2$

Beta-carotene

Figure 1: Structure of various forms of vitamin A important in nutrition.

of the vitamin E present in human tissues. The d stereoisomer of alpha tocopherol is the only naturally occurring form, though the most commonly used synthetic form contains both the d and l stereoisomers, l having 75% of the activity of the pure d form. The tocotrienols differ from the tocopherols in that they have three unsaturated bonds in the side chain and are of little importance in human nutrition. The only other vitamers of importance in infant nutrition are beta and gamma tocopherol. (Figure 2)

The naturally-occurring free alcohol of alpha tocopherol has a limited shelf life due to its interaction with oxygen to form the inactive tocopherol quinone form. Therefore, all commercially available forms of the vitamin are esterified to the acetate or succinate forms. Though resistant to oxidation, these forms are limited in biological activity until they are hydrolyzed by enzymes in the intestine and absorbed as free tocopherol.

Vitamin E activity can be expressed in international units. One IU is equal to the activity of 1 mg of d,

COMMON NAME   STRUCTURE   RELATIVE BIOLOGIC ACTIVITY TE*

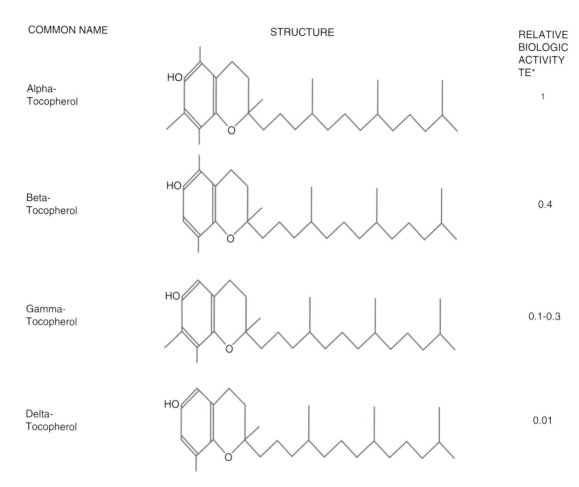

COMMON NAME	RELATIVE BIOLOGIC ACTIVITY TE*
Alpha-Tocopherol	1
Beta-Tocopherol	0.4
Gamma-Tocopherol	0.1-0.3
Delta-Tocopherol	0.01

*= Alpha-Tocopherol equivalents

Figure 2: Chemical structure and relative biological activities of tocopherols. Alpha-tocopherol is the most active vitamer. The three other tocopherols differ only in regard to the methyl substitutions on the benzene ring.

l-alpha-tocopherol acetate. A newer unit of expressing vitamin E activity is the alpha-tocopherol equivalent. Note that there is relatively little d-beta-tocopherol in the American diet, which has only 40% of the activity of d-alpha-tocopherol. However, d-gamma-tocopherol is abundant in the diet but has only 10% of the activity of d-alpha-tocopherol. Thus, bioactivity is not uniform among the forms of vitamin E. The ranking of vitamin E activity is alpha>beta>gamma>delta.

Vitamin K

Naturally occurring compounds with vitamin K activity occur in two forms (see Figure 3). The first of these,

phylloquinone or vitamin K_1, is synthesized by plants, and is used both for vitamin prophylaxis in the newborn and as a food additive (i.e., to infant formulas) in the United States. The second form, menaquinone, is actually a family of homologous compounds with unsaturated side chains differing only in the number of isoprenyl units. These are commonly referred to as the menaquinones. The relative potency of these two forms of vitamin K are unknown, nor is the role of menaquinone in human nutrition understood. Menaquinone-7 to menaquinone-13 are synthesized by bacteria. Menaquinone-7 has six additional isoprenyl units (Figure 3). Menaquinone 4 (not made by bacteria and not normally present in the human gastrointestinal tract) is used exclusively for vitamin K prophylaxis for infants in Japan. A third form of vitamin K is menadione, the synthetic form originally used for prophylaxis in newborns (Figure 3). However, it is highly protein-bound and was associated with adverse side effects in the newborn including hemolytic anemia, hyperbilirubinemia, kernicterus and even death.

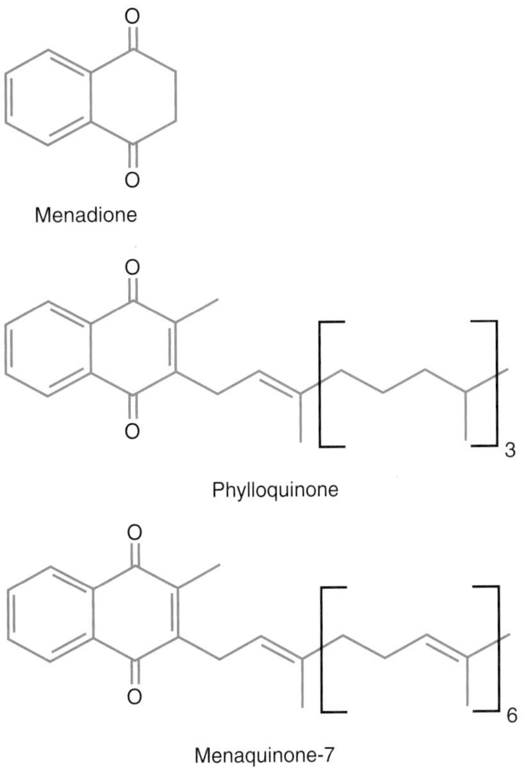

Function, Metabolism and Transport

Vitamins A, E and K have little in common when it comes to function and mechanism of action. Much more is known about vitamin A, whose function at the level of the cell nucleus is an exciting research area in the field of molecular biology. All of these vitamins are absorbed in the small intestine and require the presence of bile salts and pancreatic enzymes and the incorporation into chylomicrons for absorption. The placental transport from mother to fetus is limited for all three vitamins, particularly for vitamin K.

Vitamin A

Vitamin A, in addition to its role as a chromophore in the visual process (retina), is critical for a number of life processes including reproduction, cell metabolism, cell differentiation, hematopoiesis, bone development and pattern formation during embryogenesis. Ultimately, the retinoids elicit these effects through their ability to regulate gene expression at specific target sites in the nucleus of cells. Research on the mechanism of action of vitamin A has shown significant similarity to that of some hormones (steroids, thyroid, vitamin D), and has advanced the field of "hormone signaling." It now appears that the retinoid metabolites responsible for hormone-like signaling are all-trans retinoic acid and 9-cis retinoic acid. This signaling is mediated through specific nuclear receptors in cells of effector organs (Figure 4). Thus, because of retinoic acid's hydrophobic nature, it is able to penetrate the cell membrane and bind to nuclear receptors. Once activated, these nuclear receptors regulate gene expression by binding to short DNA segments near target genes (hormone-specific response elements), and they modulate transcription by mechanisms not well understood (Figure 4). Vitamin A receptors and their functions have recently been

Menadione

Phylloquinone

Menaquinone-7

Figure 3: Biologically active forms of vitamin K. Vitamin K$_1$ (phylloquinone) is the major dietary form. Vitamin K$_2$ (menaquinones) is synthesized by bacteria. Menadione, a synthetic compound, is not important in human nutrition.

reviewed in detail.[3] Carotenoids, like vitamin E, also function as antioxidants, important in moderating oxidant stress associated with such conditions as infection, cancer, and chronic lung disease.

Vitamin A metabolism is controlled by several elements, including the parenchymal and stellate cells of the liver involved in its processing and storage; a number of extracellular binding proteins that help to regulate tissue exposure to vitamin A despite huge fluctuations in dietary intake; and a group of intracellular binding proteins and enzymes that regulates intracellular storage, activation, and degradation. This matter has recently been extensively reviewed.[4, 5]

Ingested plant carotene or animal tissue retinal esters are converted to retinol in the proximal intestine, primarily after the action of hydrolases of the pancreas

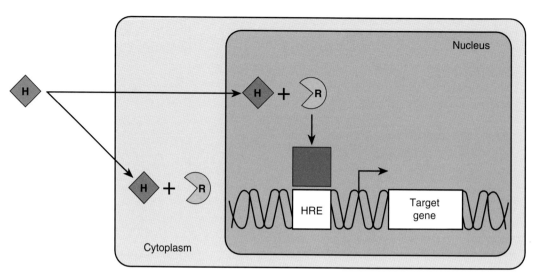

Figure 4: Nuclear hormone receptor signaling. Retinoic acid is known to function in a manner analogous to the other lipid-soluble hormones such as steroids, thyroid hormone and vitamin D. Because of its hydrophobic character, the hormone (H) is able to penetrate the cell membrane and bind to an intracellular receptor (R). Most steroid hormone receptors are in the cytoplasm and translocated to the nucleus after binding hormone. All other receptors, including those for thyroid hormone, vitamin D and retinoic acid, are nuclear proteins even in the absence of hormone. Unlike membrane receptor second messenger systems, in this pathway the ligand receptor complex becomes the signal to the nucleus where it directly interacts with hormone-specific response elements (HREs) in the target gene promoter and thereby elicits a transcriptional response. (From reference 3).

and intestinal brush border (Figure 5). Retinol in physiological concentrations is taken up into the enterocyte of the intestinal lumen, apparently by facilitated diffusion (carrier-mediated process). At pharmacological levels it can also be absorbed by passive diffusion. Published data suggest that the absorption of retinol from the intestine is less than 75% and is dependent on both the quantity and quality of dietary fat. Carotenoids are passively absorbed and have an absorption rate from 5 to 50%, with the absorption rate generally decreasing with increasing dietary intake, and dependent on the availability of fat and bile salts. The enzymatic mechanisms responsible for converting carotenoids to retinol are controversial but probably occur primarily within the enterocyte of the intestinal mucosa.

Retinol within the enterocytes exits the cells via the lymphatics after being reesterified with long-chain fatty acids and incorporated into chylomicrons (Figure 5). It is likely that specific intracellular binding proteins play an important role in facilitating metabolism of retinol and protecting the cells from excess free retinol, which can disrupt normal membrane structure and function. Chylomicrons are exocytosed into the intestinal lymph and move into the general circulation, where several processes occur–triacylglycerol hydrolysis, and apoliprotein exchange resulting in the formation of chylomicron remnants. Almost all retinyl esters present in the chylomicrons remain within chylomicron remnants, which are mainly cleared by the liver. Such remnant uptake may also occur in extrahepatic tissues (lung, leukocytes, adipose tissue, skeletal muscle and kidney) and this may be a way of delivering vitamin A to these tissues. In the newborn infant and particularly the preterm infant, vitamin A stores in the liver are relatively low and proportionately more of the total body vitamin A is stored in other tissues.

However, as the liver contains up to 90% of the body's vitamin A in older infants and children, most of the absorbed vitamin A is delivered to hepatic parenchymal cells after chylomicron remnants are

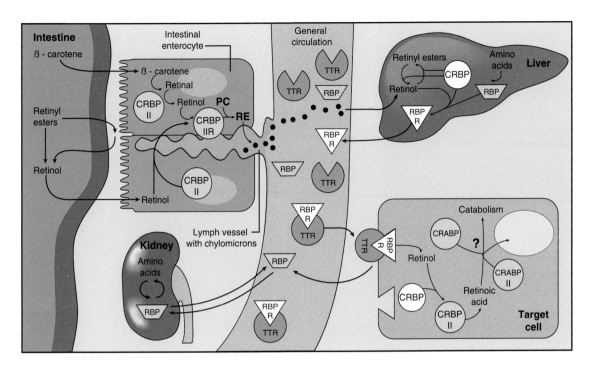

Figure 5: Vitamin A movement and metabolism in the body with possible participation of the cellular retinoid-binding proteins indicated. CRBP = cellular retinol binding protein; CRABP = cellular retinoic acid binding protein; RBB = retinol binding protein (circulating); TTR = transthyretin; RE = retinyl ester; R = retinol. (Adapted from Ong DE, 1994, reference 5.)

metabolized (Figure 5). The retinal esters are then hydrolyzed once again and transferred to the endoplastic reticulum where RBP (retinol binding protein) is found in high concentrations. Once bound to RBP, the complex is processed by the Golgi apparatus followed by secretion of the retinol-RBP from the parenchymal cells. This complex is then taken up by the perisinusoidal stellate cells in the liver, which contain 90 to 95% of the liver retinol (mostly as retinal palmitate). And 98% of the stellate cell vitamin A is in the form of retinyl esters packed together into cytoplasmic lipid droplets. This storage of retinyl esters in stellate cells, and the cells' ability to control mobilization of retinal palmitate, insures that the blood plasma retinol concentration remains close to 2 μmol/L, despite large fluctuations in vitamin A intake. The stellate cells may then secrete the retinol-RBP complex directly into the general circulation, or more likely back transfer to parenchymal cells takes place before release occurs.

RBP is a well described transport protein with a single retinal binding site, the synthesis of which is now known to occur both intrahepatically and extrahepatically. Most of the RBP secreted by the liver contains retinol in a 1:1 molar ratio and RBP is required for normal retinol secretion. In the general circulation, 95% of the RBP is associated with the transthyretin (prealbumin)- retinol complex and, except in the immediate postprandial state, essentially all of the plasma vitamin A is bound to RBP (Figure 5). This complex formed with transthyretin reduces glomerular filtration of retinol. The mechanism by which circulating retinol (complexed with RBP) is taken up by cells is not well described. In any event, the turnover of this complex in plasma is between 11 to 16 hours. After the complex delivers the retinol, RBP is excreted by the kidney. Many metabolites of retinol have been discovered in both blood and urine. Retinol can be reversibly oxidized to retinaldehyde, but further irreversible oxi-

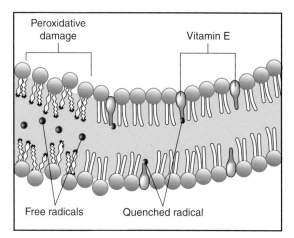

Figure 6: Biological role of vitamin E as a membrane antioxidant, protecting polyunsaturated fatty acids that are esterified in the phospholipid bilayer by halting the chain reactions that can lead to peroxidative damage. Adapted from Greer et al., 1991, reference 115.

dation yields retinoic acid. This is an important observation, as retinoic acid can support growth but not the visual function of retinol.

The placental transfer of vitamin A is an issue for the newborn infant. Pregnant mice and rats receiving a liberal supply of retinol show a wide difference between maternal and fetal retinol concentrations, suggesting, as with vitamin K (see below), that a relatively small proportion of the vitamin passes to the fetus.[6, 7] Transplacental transfer of retinol to the fetus is maintained regardless of maternal retinoid status; when maternal intake of retinol is restricted, the amount of retinol in fetal liver is similar to that of fetuses from mothers with ample retinol stores. Fetal RBP accumulates coincident with retinol accumulation and increases with the growth of the fetus during midgestation in the rat, suggesting transplacental transport of RBP-bound retinol. A later increase in fetal liver retinol with another rise in RBP is attributed to the onset of fetal RBP synthesis. The fact that fetal rat liver microsomes can actively synthesize retinyl ester leads to the suggestion that retinol is delivered to fetal liver as the RBP-retinol complex, and is esterified and stored as retinyl ester, as it is in the mature animal.

The mechanism and regulation of retinol transport from the maternal circulation to the fetus through the human placenta is not established. One study found a correlation between maternal and cord blood concentrations, but others demonstrated a lack of correlation between maternal and neonatal concentrations of retinol.[7, 8, 9] Cord retinol concentrations in concordant sex twins are as variable as the values in neonates born to different mothers.[9] From these findings it is suggested that at least in the last trimester, the human fetus participates in the regulation of retinol transport across the placenta.

Vitamin E

The primary role of vitamin E in humans is its ability to serve as an antioxidant in tissues, functioning in cell membranes as a free radical "scavenger." It acts by inhibiting the naturally occurring peroxidation of polyunsaturated fatty acids (PUFA) present in lipid layers of cell membranes, as it reacts more quickly with peroxyl radicals than do polyunsaturated fatty acids (Figure 6). Thus, it has the ability to scavenge free radicals that are generated both by the reduction of molecular oxygen and as a normal by-product of oxidative enzymes.[10, 11] Peroxidation begins when a hydrogen ion escapes from one of the carbons of a double bond, "unmasking" a highly reactive intermediate that can interact with free oxygen. The free radical formed interacts with another PUFA side chain and creates stable lipid hydroperoxides and more lipid free radicals. This process can potentially repeat as an endless chain reaction. Vitamin E is a chain-breaking antioxidant because of its ability to readily substitute for oxygen in this reaction by donating a stabilizing hydrogen ion to the "free radical" (Figure 6). This function appears to be particularly important in young, growing tissue in which forming normal membrane structures and maintaining their integrity are active biochemical processes. The different isomers of tocopherol have varying amounts of antioxidant and biological activity. Thus, gamma-tocopherol (a major form of dietary vitamin E in humans) has about one half the antioxidant activity but only one tenth the biological activity of alpha-tocopherol.

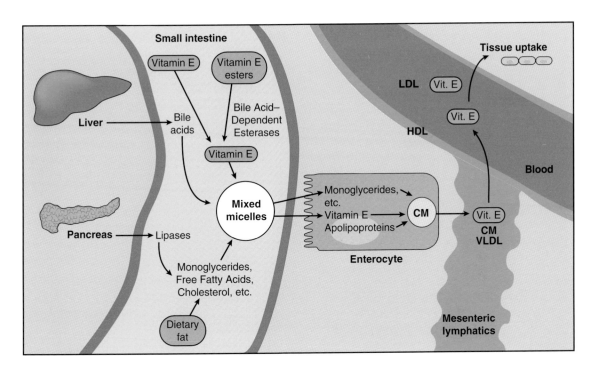

Figure 7: Processes involved in the intestinal absorption of vitamin E in humans. CM = chylomicron. Adapted from Hdydishi and Mino, 1987, reference 116.

Absorption of tocopherol occurs primarily in the mid-portion of the small intestine. Bile salts and pancreatic enzymes are necessary, as vitamin E must be solubilized into a lipid-bile micelle containing free fatty acids and monoglycerides, before secretion from the enterocytes.[12] Vitamin E esters must be hydrolyzed prior to absorption. Absorption into the enterocytes occurs by a nonsaturable, noncarrier-mediated, passive diffusion process, depicted in detail in Figure 7. The efficiency of absorption decreases as larger amounts of tocopherol are consumed.[13] In normal humans, an average absorption of at least 50% and perhaps as high as 70% can be assumed for normal dietary intake (0.4 to 1.0 mg in adults); however, this efficiency falls to less than 10% with pharmacological intakes as high as 200 mg. Decreased absorption of fat, as seen in premature neonates and children with steatorrhea, results in a parallel malabsorption of tocopherol.

Once absorbed, alpha and gamma tocopherols are incorporated into chylomicrons and very low density lipoproteins (VLDL), which are secreted into lymphatic vessels and into the venous circulation (Figure 7). No specific transport proteins in plasma have been identified, unlike vitamin A, though most circulating vitamin E is found in association with LDL and HDL in the fasting state. Vitamin E can pass from chylomicrons into tissues in two ways. Some tocopherol is released when circulating chylomicrons are metabolized by lipoprotein lipase and thus enter the tissue. After uptake of chylomicron remnants by the liver, tocopherol is resecreted into the circulation in association with lipoproteins. The mechanism of vitamin E transfer from plasma lipoproteins to tissues is unknown. Vitamin E is taken up by most tissues including liver, lung, heart, muscle, and adipose tissue. Fat accumulates tocopherol and can sequester it.[14] When the intake of vitamin E is high, the liver is the main site of storage, as with vitamin A. However, the total tocopherol pool of muscle and adipose tissue is much larger than the hepatic one, though tocopherol present in adipocytes is not readily available. Intracellularly, vitamin E compounds are concentrated wher-

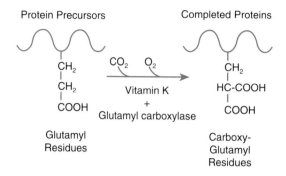

Figure 8: Vitamin K functions as a cofactor with the microsomal enzyme glutamyl carboxylase to convert glutamyl residues to gamma-carboxy-glutamic acid residues on precursor proteins (i.e., prothrombin).

ever there is abundant fatty acid, especially in the structures of the cell containing phospholipids (mitochondria, microsomes, and plasma membranes).

The metabolism and turnover of alpha-tocopherol have been studied only to a limited extent in humans and have not been adequately quantitated in any species. Regarding the metabolism of alpha-tocopherol, it is believed that once the alpha-tocopherol-oxyl radical is formed, then alpha-tocopherol can be regenerated, most likely by ascorbic acid. Very little vitamin E is recovered in urine, either intact or as a metabolite. Thus, vitamin E is not metabolized, but maintained in the body in the unoxidized state.[15] The major route of tocopherol excretion appears to be fecal elimination, possibly in association with bile secretion. This is especially true for gamma-tocopherol and for excess amounts of ingested vitamin E. When animals are fed a vitamin E-deficient diet, plasma and liver concentrations of alpha-tocopherol decrease rapidly. There seem to be two tocopherol pools present, at least in rats: a rapidly metabolized pool and a component that is retained for longer periods.[14] Depletion of tocopherol from adipose tissue and skeletal muscle is a slow process, and is presumably the source of the slowly metabolized pool.

Following an oral dose of 100 IU/kg of dl-alpha-tocopherol, normal infants have peak serum concentrations by six hours.[16] The plasma elimination half-life in the low-birthweight infant varies between two and four days.[17, 18, 19] Thus, accumulation may occur with repeated daily administration.

Although pregnancy is associated with high maternal concentrations of circulating vitamin E in proportion to rising plasma lipids, transplacental delivery of tocopherol to the fetus is limited. The ratio of maternal to fetal tocopherol concentration in blood is approximately 4:1, with the former concentration averaging 1.5 mg/dl and the latter 0.38 mg/dl.[20] Neonatal tissues have generally low concentrations of vitamin E and the low proportion of adipose tissue in premature infants further limits the total body vitamin E content. The vitamin E content of the fetus increases in late gestation along with the amount of adipose tissue. There is no information on the transport mechanisms for vitamin E from mother to fetus.

Vitamin K

Though it has been known for many years that vitamin K is important in the synthesis of the proteins important for coagulation, its mechanism of action was not determined until the 1970s. This was aided by the observation that the plasma of both animals and human subjects treated with coumadin anticoagulants contained a protein similar to prothrombin, but lacked its biological activity. This difference was subsequently shown to be due to the inability of the abnormal prothrombin to bind calcium ions.[21] In 1974, a previously unknown amino acid, gamma-carboxyglutamic acid ("gla") was isolated from bovine protein and shown to be missing from the plasma of animals anticoagulated with coumadin. This amino acid was subsequently shown to be the site of calcium binding in the prothrombin molecule. The precursor of prothrombin, or abnormal prothrombin, is a relatively small molecule containing 10 "glu" residues, which in the presence of vitamin K are converted (carboxylated) to "gla" residues (Figure 8). The conversion of the glutamyl residues ("glu") to gamma-carboxyglutamic acid ("gla") residues to create effective calcium binding sites requires the presence of the enzyme glutamyl carboxylase. Vitamin K is now known to be a necessary cofactor for the activity of this microsomal enzyme. This discovery of an amino acid that requires vitamin K for

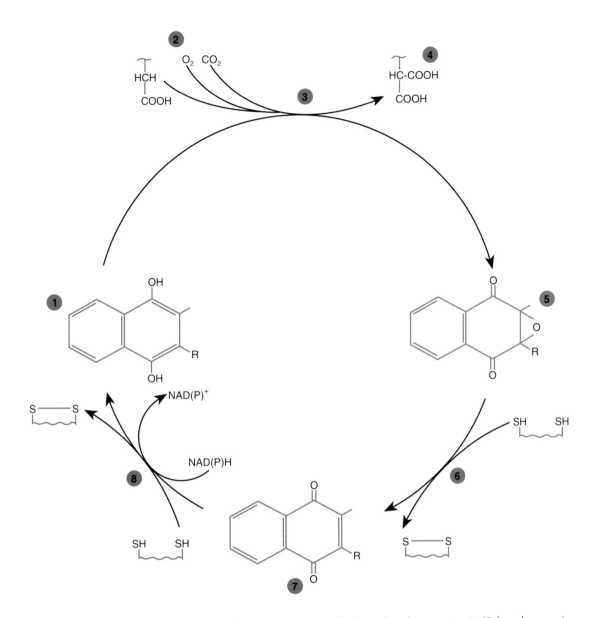

Figure 9: Metabolism of vitamin K_1 (1) in the liver. The conversion of a glutamyl residue on a vitamin K-dependent protein (2) to a gamma-carboxyglutamyl (gla) residue (4) by the enzyme glutamyl carboxylase (3), is dependent on the reduced vitamin K (1) and is coupled to the formation of vitamin K epoxide (5). The regeneration of vitamin K_1 from the epoxide form requires a dithio (–SH) dependent enzyme, epoxide reductase (6) to form the quinone form (7) of vitamin K and further reduction by a second dithiol dependent enzyme (8), quinone reductase, to the hydroquinone, vitamin K_1 (1). In this proposed vitamin K cycle, the two dithiol-dependent steps in vitamin K metabolism are blocked by the commonly used oral anticoagulants.

its synthesis has led to the identification of an entire family of vitamin K-dependent or "gla"-containing proteins in many tissues.

Though the exact role of vitamin K in the action of the vitamin K-dependent carboxylase is not known, it is apparent that during the conversion of glutamyl to gamma-carboxy-glutamyl residues on the vitamin K dependent peptides, vitamin K is converted to its 2, 3-epoxide form (Figure 9). Subsequently, the epoxide form of the vitamin is reduced to the quinone form by an epoxide reductase; it is reduced to the active coenzyme form, the hydroquinone, by various microsomal quinone reductases. It is hypothesized that the role of vitamin K is to abstract the hydrogen of a glutamyl residue as a proton from a vitamin K-dependent protein, leaving a carbanion which is attacked by free CO_2 to form gamma-carboxy-glutamic acid. Anticoagulants such as Warfarin (coumadin) apparently antagonize vitamin K action by inhibiting the epoxide reductase and quinone reductase activities of the liver (Figure 9). This action increases the concentration of vitamin K epoxide and results in an insufficient amount of the reduced form of vitamin K to promote the action of carboxylase in the liver and other tissues.

A multitude of vitamin K-dependent proteins have now been described, including proteins C, S, and Z, in plasma, as well as "gla"-containing proteins in kidney, spleen, lung, uterus, placenta, pancreas, thyroid, thymus, testes and bone. Carboxylase activity has been detected in most of these tissues as well. Two important bone "gla" proteins, osteocalcin and matrix gla-protein, have recently been amino acid sequenced. Several of these decarboxylated proteins have been proposed as markers for vitamin K subclinical deficiency, including decarboxylated prothrombin and osteocalcin.

Like vitamins A and E, vitamin K is absorbed from the small intestine into the lymphatic system, requiring the presence of both bile salts and pancreatic secretions.[22] Thus, phylloquinone (vitamin K1) is absorbed in association with chylomicrons. Specific carrier proteins are not known to exist, but in plasma it is associated with very low density low density and high density lipoproteins similar to vitamin E.[23, 24] Unlike vitamins A and E, however, vitamin K (menaquinone form) can be synthesized by colonic bacteria, though its absorption and role in human nutrition is controversial.

In rats, phylloquinone absorption appears to be by an energy-dependent process from the proximal por-tion of the small intestine.[25] In contrast, menaquinone absorption has been found to be a passive, non-carrier-mediated process from both the large and small intestines. There is little specific information about the intestinal absorption of vitamin K in man.

There is no specific information about vitamin K turnover in infants. It is apparent that vitamin K is stored largely in the liver and it is detected in the human fetus as early as ten weeks gestational age.[23] Though the primary form of vitamin K found in plasma is phylloquinone, menaquionones make up a significant amount of the vitamin K found in the adult human liver.[26] However, menaquinones are unde-tectable in the fetus, as well as in the infant during the first week of life.[23, 27, 28] Menaquinones increase in the liver of infants after birth from post mortem studies, but phylloquinone remains the predominant storage form.[23, 25, 26] In breast-fed infants, colonic flora is pre-dominantly lactobacillus, so a relative absence of menaquinones in these infants would not be a surprise. At the time of birth, the concentrations of phylloqui-none in the liver are 1.4 ng/g in preterm infants and 1.0 ng/g or less in term infants, values about 20% of the concentrations found in adult liver.[23] In another report, the phylloquinone content of infant liver was shown to increase dramatically after vitamin K pro-phylaxis (2 mg orally or parenterally) from <1 µg/g to 62-93 µg/g, but decreased very rapidly to as low as 2.9 µg/g five days after administration of vitamin K1.[29]

Vitamin K is not readily transported across the pla-centa from mother to fetus. Serum vitamin K concen-trations in cord blood are either undetectable or less than 50 pg/ml.[30-34] There is no maternal/fetal correla-tion. The concentration gradient across the placenta may be as high as 40:1, much higher than vitamins A and E.[23, 31, 33, 35] Large maternal doses of vitamin K, whether oral or parenteral, do not significantly affect this concentration gradient.[30, 31, 33, 36] Furthermore, maternal supplements of vitamin K prior to birth do not significantly affect the coagulation status of the newborn infant.[31, 33]

Compared with the other fat-soluble vitamins, why is vitamin K so low in the fetus and newborn infant? The answer to this question remains unknown. It has recently been reported that high or "normal" levels of phylloquinone may potentiate mutagenic or carcinogenic events in mice,[37, 38] as well as fetal sheep leukocytes.[39] From these observations it has been hypothesized that low plasma concentrations of phylloquinone may reduce the risk of mutagenic events during the period of rapid cell proliferation that occurs in the fetus and newborn. However, such potentiation has not been observed in human leukocytes following vitamin K administration.[40]

Assessment of Needs
Blood or Tissue Concentrations

For all three vitamins, laboratory assays are now available and sensitive enough to measure plasma concentrations in infants.

Retinol is associated with retinol binding protein in the peripheral circulation and, because the concentration of this protein stays relatively constant, plasma retinol is little affected by vitamin A intake. Thus, plasma vitamin A concentration is not useful as a measure of a vitamin A deficiency state. However, a relative dose-response test to small doses of vitamin A administered intravenously has been used to define a deficiency state of this vitamin. (See below).

For plasma vitamin E, tocopherol concentrations are generally measured by HPLC (high pressure liquid chromatography). This technique now differentiates alpha, beta and gamma isomers. An alpha tocopherol concentration of <0.6mg/dl is generally indicative of a deficiency state.[20, 41] However, because levels of this vitamin are greatly influenced by plasma lipids, tocopherol levels are generally reported in relation to total plasma lipid (the sum of plasma cholesterol and plasma triglycerides). This is an important concept, as in chronic cholestatic liver disease, the common finding of hyperlipoproteinemia may elevate serum vitamin E concentration into the normal range despite a deficiency state.[16, 42] Vitamin E:lipid molar ratios of <0.7 x 10⁻³ successfully predicted vitamin E deficiency in one study.[43]

> *Prevention and cure are not two weights to be balanced against each other, but essential elements that go to forge one weapon.*
> *Primary Health Care Pioneer*
> *The Selected works of*
> *Dr. Cicely D. Williams*
> Naomi Baumslag, Editor
> World Federation of
> Public Health Associations
> and UNICEF

For vitamin K, adult normal plasma concentrations are generally above 0.5 ng/ml. However, we have recently reported values generally less than 0.3 ng/ml in exclusively breast-fed infants during the first six months of life, who have no overt signs of vitamin K deficiency. Therefore, as with vitamin A, plasma concentrations of vitamin K are not sensitive enough to diagnose deficiency.

Assays of these vitamins in other tissues have been proposed to assess vitamin status. Liver and adipose tissue assays are not clinically practical for infant evaluation. Red cell tocopherol concentrations (generally 20% of plasma concentrations) can be measured in infants, but the variations of hematocrit and plasma lipid concentrations make interpretation of these values difficult. Tocopherol content of platelets has also been measured but this measurement requires too much blood to make this method practical in infants.

Functional Measures

Vitamin A status can be assessed by a relative dose-response test. If small doses of vitamin A are administered parenterally to infants in an adequate vitamin A nutritional state, there is a modest and short-lived (<5 hours) increase in serum vitamin A concentration. However, in subjects with poor vitamin A nutritional status, the increase in serum concentration is exaggerated and the return to baseline value is delayed. The difference between the fasting and five-hour concentrations divided by the fasting concentrations is referred to as the relative dose response.[44-46]

Vitamin E can be assessed with a red cell fragility (hemolysis) test. This assay measures in vitro hemolysis of red blood cell membranes in the presence of hydrogen peroxide. In general, a hemolysis rate of greater than 10% is a nonspecific measure of tocopherol deficiency.

Similarly, assays of prothrombin time or various vitamin K-dependent coagulation factors can be a functional assay for vitamin K deficiency. However, prothrombin time depends on visually observing the formation of a fibrin clot as the end point. The relationship between the concentration of prothrombin and the clotting time is nonlinear, requiring careful dilution curves to standardize activities. Thus, only in severe deficiency states is prothrombin time significantly increased. Furthermore, assessing coagulation factors in the newborn infant is complicated by the fact that "normal" plasma concentrations of these factors are 30 to 60% of adult concentrations and normal adult concentrations are not achieved until between two and 12 months of age, depending on the specific factor.[47]

Recent technological advances have more potential for diagnosing or predicting the vitamin K deficiency state. Partially carboxylated vitamin K-dependent proteins have now been described circulating in blood. The primary protein utilized for assessing vitamin K status at the present time is abnormal (partially carboxylated) prothrombin. While many terms have been used in the literature for this abnormal protein (des-gamma-carboxyprothrombin, hypocarboxyprothrombin, acarboxyprothrombin or PIVKA for protein induced in the absence of vitamin K), we will use PIVKA-II in this discussion. The designation "II" acknowledges the potential presence of other partially-carboxylated clotting factors which are vitamin K-dependent.

It should be noted that PIVKA-II is a heterogeneous molecule. It consists of a pool of partially-carboxylated prothrombin, as well as some completely des-gamma-carboxylated prothrombin.[48] The number of acarboxylated sites (up to ten) per individual prothrombin molecule and the specific sites involved remain an area of ongoing investigation. Likewise, the degree of physiological activity may vary with the number of des-gamma-carboxylated sites. A preparation lacking up to 20% of the gamma-carboxylated sites, primarily at the more carboxy-terminal sites on the molecule, has been demonstrated to have near normal physiological activity.[48]

Four methods have been described in the literature to measure PIVKA-II in the newborn and these have recently been reviewed in detail elsewhere.[49] However, only one of these methods is in widespread use at this time--specific antibody detection. The principle of this method is the preparation of a murine monoclonal antibody to PIVKA-II which is subsequently utilized in an enzyme-linked immunoabsorbent assay (ELISA). A number of such specific antibodies have now been described.[50-53] This methodology has been utilized for measurements in cord blood and infants through 12 weeks of age. Detection rates of PIVKA-II in cord blood have ranged from 10 to 50%.[52, 57] In a series of studies from the Netherlands in exclusively breast-feeding infants who received vitamin K at birth, PIVKA-II was detected in four of 262 infants at four weeks and 15 of 131 infants at 12 weeks of age.[58] When oral vitamin K was given weekly or daily in this same population, PIVKA-II was not detected in exclusively breast-fed infants at four and 12 weeks.[59, 60] Absolute quantitation by this method is difficult, but 1 arbitrary unit (AU) corresponds to approximately 1 µg of purified prothrombin. Healthy adults have PIVKA-II levels of less than 0.13 AU/ml.

Sources of Vitamins A, E and K for the Newborn Infant

As discussed above, "adequate" amounts of retinol cross the placenta to the fetus, especially in the last trimester. However, vitamin A stores in the newborn liver are relatively low compared with those of older infants and children. Mature human milk contains from 185 to 265 IU/dl of vitamin A, with retinal esters accounting for 94 to 96% of the total (Table 1). Colostrum contains even higher amounts. Infant formulas are fortified with vitamin A (Table 1), with the FDA (U.S. Food and Drug Administration) requiring a minimum of 165 IU/dl and a maximum of 500 IU/dl. Label claims are generally 200 IU/dl with a 40% over-age added. Intravenous forms of vitamin A are also available with a general recommendation of 70 to 100 µg retinol/kg/day.[61] It is of note, however, that intravenous administration of retinol is difficult because up to 75% of the dose may be lost on the intravenous tubing by the time it reaches the neonate.

As noted, vitamin E transport across the placenta is limited. As with vitamin A, the vitamin E content of colostrum is much higher than that of mature human milk. The vitamin E content of human milk and various formulas fed term infants are summarized in Table 1.

	Human Milk		Cow Milk Based Formula[1]			Soy Formula		
	Colostrum	Mature	Enfamil 20 cal/oz	SMA 20 cal/oz	Similac 20 cal/oz	Prosobee 20 cal/oz	Nursoy 20 cal/oz	Isomil 20 cal/oz
Vitamin A IU/dl	478-716[2]	185-265[3]	207	199	200	207	199	200
Vitamin E IU/dl	0.67-1.2[4]	0.45-0.83[4]	2.1	0.9	2.0	2.1	0.9	2.0
Vitamin K µg/dl[5]	0.06-0.09[6]	0.09-0.17[7]	5.7	5.4	5.4	10.2	10.2	10.00

[1]Formula values from published information available from formula companies.
[2]Values from Ajans, et al. 1965; Thomas, et al. 1981; Chappell, et al. 1985.
[3]Values from Gebre-Medhin, et al. 1979; Thomas, et al. 1981; Chappell, et al. 1985.
[4]Values from Jansson, et al. 1981; Harzen and Hang 1985; Dostalova, et al. 1988.
[5]Note additional vitamin K added to Soy formulas.
[6]Values from Canfield, et al. 1988; Greer, et al. 1991.
[7]Values from Canfield, et al. 1988; Greer, et al. 1991; Pietschning, et al. 1992.

Table 1: Vitamin A, E, K, content of human milk and example formulas.

The parenteral requirements of vitamin E remain somewhat controversial and are of course related to intravenous fat intake. The most widely used form of intravenous vitamins in the U.S. (MVI Pediatric, Armour Pharmaceuticals) contains 7 IU of alpha-tocopherol acetate per 5 ml vial. The recommended dose in the U.S. is 2.5 IU per kilogram of body weight.[61] The most widely used form of intravenous vitamin E in Europe (Vitalipid, Pharamacia) contains 1 IU per ml and ESPGAN (European Society for Pediatric Gastroenterology and Nutrition) recommends 1 IU per kg per day.

Unlike vitamins A and E, the vitamin K concentration in human milk is very low and remains low throughout lactation. It is apparent that it alone cannot meet the dietary requirements of vitamin K for the newborn infant. We have recently shown that in exclusively breast-fed infants through the first six months of life, daily vitamin K intakes averages only 10% of the recommended dietary allowance of 1 µg/kg/day.[69] In general, the concentration of phylloquinone in human milk is less than that of cow milk. Table 1 summarizes the recently reported values for human milk and formula. It would appear that on the balance, the vitamin K content of human milk is between 0.1 and 0.2 µg/dl. There are also large daily variations in human milk phylloquinone concentra-

tions in individual mothers, since the vitamin K content of milk is clearly affected by variations in dietary intake.

It is now common practice to supplement infant formulas with phylloquinone. At the present time, all commercial formulas available in the U.S. contain a minimum of 5 µg/dl. As expected, the vitamin K intake of formula-fed infants may be up to 100 times that of the exclusively breast-fed infants in the U.S.[69]

Another potential source of vitamin K for the newborn infant is the synthesis of menaquinones by the bacteria of the large intestine. However, for the exclusively breast-fed infant with an intestinal predominance of bifidobacteria that do not synthesize menaquinones, bacteria are a questionable source, as discussed above. On the contrary, bottle-fed infants have significantly greater numbers of intestinal bacteria that synthesize menaquinones, including Bacteroides fragilis, Esherichia coli, Clostridia, and Streptococcus faecalis. Menaquinones can act in vitro as a co-factor for the hepatic carboxylase.[72] We have reported that breast-fed infants have a near absence of menaquinones in the stools during the first week of life, as compared to formula-fed infants.[73] However, even for older formula-fed infants, there is no clear evidence that menaquinones synthesized in the large intestine are biologically available.

Deficiency

Of these three vitamins, vitamin A is the only one with a devastating worldwide pediatric deficiency state. It has been estimated that "90 to 100 million children worldwide are likely to be vitamin A-deficient with the consequence that their health and chance of survival are compromised."[74] The vast majority of these children are in Southeast Asia and the African subcontinent. Deficiency of vitamin A is not a problem among children in the United States, where intakes are very generous particularly in formula-fed infants. No cases have been reported for thirty years. Because vitamin A is important in cell differentiation and important to immune function, its deficiency increases the risk of infection from respiratory diseases, diarrhea and measles. In third world countries, recent studies have shown a significant reduction in mortality among infants and small children given vitamin A supplements. Vitamin A deficiency also has ocular manifestations. Night blindness is the earliest sign, which then progresses to xerosis (dryness and wrinkling) of the conjunctiva. Eventually, this may progress to corneal xerophthalmia. Approximately 250,000 children a year will become permanently blind from the resulting keratomalacia.

Vitamin E deficiency is much less of a problem in infants. A deficiency state was first described in premature infants in 1967, who presented at six to 11 weeks of age with anemia, elevated reticulocyte counts, and a marked increase in sensitivity of the erythrocytes to hemolysis in hydrogen peroxide (80 ± 14%).[75] All of these infants had low vitamin E concentrations (≤ 0.41 mg/dl), and symptoms resolved with vitamin E supplemental therapy. It was recognized at the time that this deficiency state was associated with the ingestion of formulas that were high in polyunsaturated fatty acids and relatively low in vitamin E. With the alteration of infant formulas used in this population, this hemolytic anemia has all but disappeared. In infants with chronic cholestasis and malabsorption (biliary atresia, cystic fibrosis, abetalipoproteinemia, etc.) vitamin E deficiency produces a progressive but reversible neurological deficit. This consists of peripheral neuropathy, cerebellar ataxia and posterior spinal column dysfunction.

Like vitamin A deficiency, vitamin K deficiency is a worldwide problem. Its deficiency in the newborn presenting as neonatal hemorrhage, is not a major concern in the United States and Canada, where nearly all newborn infants receive prophylactic vitamin K at birth. However, its use is still uncommon in many parts of the world today. The first large series of fifty infants with hemorrhagic disease of the newborn was published a century ago, and it was speculated that the disease was of an infectious etiology.[76] The treatment prescribed (fresh cow milk) was therapeutic for the infants in this report. In 1952, Dam et al published a study of over 33,000 infants in which they concluded that hypoprothrombinemia secondary to vitamin K deficiency occurred primarily in breast-fed infants in the first few days of life.[77] They also showed that it could be prevented by administering vitamin K to the infant shortly after delivery. This form of hemorrhagic disease in the newborn has subsequently been called "classic hemorrhagic disease." After this report, the American Academy of Pediatrics recommended that a large amount of synthetic vitamin K (5 mg) should be given intramuscularly to all newborn infants.[78] Following this recommendation, the first reports of kernicterus in premature infants associated with prophylactic vitamin K administration appeared in the literature.[79]

This was secondary to the hyperbilirubinemia of increased red cell hemolysis attributed to the water-soluble, highly protein-bound form of the vitamin (menadione) available at that time. Also, extremely large doses were given, up to 75 mg, to women in premature labor. These reports delayed the acceptance of vitamin K prophylaxis in the newborn. In 1961, the Committee on Nutrition of the American Academy of Pediatrics, after a careful review, recommended that vitamin K be given to all newborns as a single parenteral dose of 0.5-1.0 mg or an oral dose of 1.0-2.0 mg for prophylaxis of hemorrhagic disease.[80] Furthermore, vitamin K1, or phylloquinone, was now available and this fat-soluble form of the vitamin did not cause kernicterus, even when given in large doses (up to 10 mg). Subsequent reports from Cincinnati confirmed that classic hemorrhagic disease of the newborn was a disease of breast-feeding infants with an incidence as high as 1.7 per 100 among those who did not receive prophylactic vitamin K.[81, 82]

In the classic form of the disease, hemorrhage occurs between days two and ten of life and intracranial hemorrhage is uncommon. It is usually hallmarked by generalized ecchymosis or gastrointestinal bleeding. Bleeding from the circumcision site or umbilical cord stump is also common. It is easily treated with parenteral vitamin K without any permanent sequelae. A second form of the disease, late hemorrhagic disease of the newborn, is not so benign. The first series was not reported until 1966.[83] This disease occurs almost exclusively in breast-feeding infants who have not received vitamin K prophylaxis or who have gastrointestinal disorders associated with significant fat malabsorption (cystic fibrosis, biliary atresia, alpha-1-antitrypsin deficiency, etc). This is the most common form of the disease reported in the literature today, largely because of its devastating sequelae. In a recent review of 131 cases reported from 1970 to 1991, the mean age of onset was 5.6 ± 3.3 weeks.[84] There were 18 deaths (14%) and 82 (83%) cases of intracranial hemorrhage. Of the 113 survivors, 27 (24%) infants had permanent neurological sequelae. Fifty-five (42%) of the infants had significant liver disease/malabsorption at the time of diagnosis. One-hundred-and-eighteen infants (90%) were breast-fed. Eighty-nine infants received no vitamin K prophylaxis and 35 infants received oral prophylaxis. Only five infants were documented to have intramuscular prophylaxis, and all of these had significant liver disease.

A third form of hemorrhagic disease will be only briefly mentioned. This is relatively uncommon and usually associated with maternal anticonvulsant therapy (most commonly hydantoin or barbiturates) during pregnancy.[85, 86] In this disorder, bleeding occurs within 24 hours of birth. It may occur at any site; bleeding in the brain may be fatal. It can probably be prevented by administering very large quantities of

> *After a decline in sales of supplemental vitamins during the 1980's, there has been substantial increases during the 1990's. Do we really need to supplement the diets of infants and children?*
>
> Primary Health Care Pioneer
> The Selected works of
> Dr. Cicely D. Williams
> Naomi Baumslag, Editor
> World Federation of
> Public Health Associations
> and UNICEF

vitamin K to the mother prior to delivery. The exact mechanism of the effects of anticonvulsant therapy on vitamin K metabolism is unknown.

Is There a Need for Pharmacological Doses in Infants?

One of the great misadventures in neonatology was the use of very large doses of vitamin K (75 mg) for prophylaxis of hemorrhagic disease of the newborn in low-birthweight infants.[87] This produced hemolysis, exaggerated jaundice and even kernicterus in this population. Another misadventure occurred in the 1980s with the use of large doses of intravenous vitamin E (dl-alpha-tocopherol acetate in a polysorbate vehicle) in low-birthweight infants. A devastating toxic syndrome occurred, consisting of ascites, hepatomegaly, thrombocytopenia and renal failure. There were 38 deaths.[88] It was never clear whether the toxicity was secondary to vitamin E or the polysorbate vehicle, or both.

Despite these lessons from history, the use of pharmacological doses of these vitamins continues, especially in low-birthweight infants. Both vitamin K and vitamin E have been used in large doses to prevent or ameliorate intraventricular hemorrhage (IVH) in premature infants. Similarly, both vitamin A and vitamin E have been used to prevent bronchopulmonary dysplasia (BPD) in this same population. Large amounts of vitamin E have also been recommended to prevent retinopathy of prematurity (ROP).

The best studied of the treatments of neonatal disease with pharmacological quantities of vitamins has been that of vitamin E for ROP. Up to 100 mg/kg per day by mouth has been used. This subject has been reviewed many times.[89] Of the numerous trials, some reported no effect of vitamin E, some a significant decrease in severity but not incidence, and some a significant decrease in both incidence and severity of ROP. The most recent large trial of 755 infants[90] reported a significant decrease in the incidence of ROP in the treated group, but no significant decrease in the incidence of severe ROP. Similarly, because of its antioxidant effects, vitamin E has been studied for its potential to prevent bronchopulmonary dysplasia, with unsatisfactory results.[91] Vitamin E (20 mg/kg given intramuscularly three times in the first 48 hours of life) may also play a role in preventing or ameliorating IVH in very-low-birthweight infants, though it is less clear how the antioxidant effect of vitamin E would be as important here.[92, 93] However, as noted above, and as will be discussed under toxicity below, low-birthweight infants are potentially at risk from pharmacological doses of vitamin E.

Vitamin A has also been used in pharmacological doses (2000 IU/day intravenously) to prevent or ameliorate BPD, as in theory it is essential for promoting growth and orderly differentiation of regenerating bronchopulmonary epithelium.[94, 95] The results of the two studies published to date in very-low-birthweight infants have been contradictory, though there were differences in the two patient populations studied.[96] More information is needed before these large doses of vitamin A can be recommended routinely for premature infants at risk for developing BPD. All infants are at risk from toxicity associated with pharmacological doses of vitamin A.

Vitamin K has been used to prevent IVH in premature infants. As IVH may occur shortly after birth, most studies have looked at giving vitamin K to mothers during premature labor. As discussed above, it takes very large amounts of vitamin K (10-20 mg) to have any impact on cord phylloquinone concentration. Seven studies in the literature have examined the effects of maternal antenatal vitamin K administration on coagulation studies in premature infants.[31, 34, 97-101] In only one of these reports was maternal vitamin K administration found to significantly decrease the prothrombin time (PT) and partial thromboplastin time (PTT) in

> *The more a subject becomes specialized, the more it tends to pursue its own aggrandizement and perpetuation - sometimes irrespective of the general needs of the community, and the general resources of medical care.*
> *Primary Health Care Pioneer*
> *The Selected works of*
> Dr. Cicely D. Williams
> Naomi Baumslag, Editor
> World Federation of
> Public Health Associations
> and UNICEF

premature infants compared to controls.[99] Four of these studies reported the incidence of IVH.[31, 98, 99,101] Though two of four studies found a significantly decreased incidence of IVH in the vitamin K group, they were both complicated by the fact that the vitamin K groups also received more antenatal steroids[100] or phenobarbital[99] than the untreated groups. In another study, in which no differences were found, mothers receiving vitamin K all received phenobarbital as well.[101] However, in the study of Kazzi et al, in which only a few of 103 infants received antenatal steroids (and no antenatal phenobarbital was used), vitamin K was found to have no impact on IVH.[98] Thus, the balance of the evidence supports the fact that IVH in premature infants is not secondary to vitamin K deficiency.

Toxicity

Given the availability of synthetic retinol compounds, it is not surprising that toxic effects of vitamin A have been reported in children as well as adults. This subject has recently been reviewed in depth.[102] Though generally hundreds of thousands of IU are needed to produce toxicity in adults, much smaller amounts may produce toxicity in infants and children. Acute symptoms include irritability, nausea, vomiting, a bulging fontanel, fever and neurologic findings. Clinical signs of vitamin A intoxication include xerosis, dermatitis, alopecia, pseudoparesis and ataxia. Though most reports involve intakes of 100,000 IU per day or more, doses of 1,600 to 4,000 IU/kg per day in children have been reported to cause vitamin A toxicity.[102] Vitamin A is also teratogenic and this has become an important issue with the use of 13-cis-retinoic acid (a vitamin A derivative) in severe cases of cystic acne in women. Studies with pregnant animals clearly show that excessive amounts of vitamin A or one of its congeners, such as all-trans- retinoic acid or 13-cis-retinoic acid, result in dramatically

	Vitamin A (retinol equivalents, 1 µg÷1 equivalent)	Vitamin E (alpha-tocopherol equivalents, 1 µg÷1 equivalent)	Vitamin K (mg phylloquinone)
RDA	375 µg/kg/day	3	1 µg/kg/day
AAP Handbook	400 µg/kg/day	5-25	1 µg/kg/day
TPN	2300 (5ml of MVI Pediatric)	3-5	200 µg (5 ml MVI)
per gram PUFA		0.5	
prophylactic (birth)			0.5-1 mg IM

Table 2: Recommended intakes of vitamins A, E and K.

increased fetal death rates, and birth of offspring with characteristic defects. There is also a temporal association of high vitamin A intakes by pregnant women with babies born with defects characteristic of the effects of excessive vitamin A in animals. Likewise, the teratogenicity of 13-cis-retinoic acid has been established in epidemiological studies in humans.[102] Unfortunately, the lowest intake of vitamin A that has teratogenic potential in humans has not been established. However, many prenatal vitamin formulations contain 8,000 IU of vitamin A; this dose would seem to be safe given the many thousands of women taking these preparations.

In the previous section we have addressed the issue of the toxicity associated with vitamin K and vitamin E in the low-birthweight infant when various forms were given in pharmacological doses. There are other concerns about both of these vitamins. In trials in which vitamin E was used in large amounts to prevent ROP, BPD, or IVH, some investigators reported increased risks for sepsis and necrotizing enterocolitis.[90, 103] Likewise, even though vitamin E has been used to decrease the risk of IVH in premature infants, increased retinal hemorrhages have been reported in infants whose serum concentrations exceeded 6.0 mg/dl.[104] In general, adverse reactions to vitamin E in premature infants occur when serum concentrations are above 3.5 mg/dl, which usually does not occur unless intakes are greater than 100 mg/kg per day.[105] In 1985, after reviewing the use of large amounts of vitamin E in these patients, the American Academy of Pediatrics con-

cluded that "...prophylactic use of pharmacological vitamin E is experimental and cannot be recommended for routine use in infants weighing less that 1,500 g even if they require supplemental oxygen."[106]

Regarding vitamin K, the pharmacological dose (1-2 mg) given to newborns in Great Britain for prophylaxis of hemorrhagic disease has recently been associated with an increased incidence of childhood cancer.[107] In this study, a 1 mg dose of vitamin K given intramuscularly was associated with a relative risk ratio of 1.97 (95% confidence interval 1.04 to 2.84) for all forms of childhood cancer compared to oral or no newborn prophylaxis. From these data, the authors speculated that in a country such as Great Britain, with 700,000 annual deliveries, the routine use of intramuscular vitamin K would result in 980 extra cases of childhood cancer before the children reached ten years of age. However, five subsequent studies from Sweden, the United States, Denmark, Germany and Great Britain did not confirm the finding of the Golding study.[108, 109, 110, 111, 112] The American Academy of Pediatrics recently reviewed its position on the use of pharmacological doses of vitamin K in newborns and came to the conclusion that 1 mg intramuscularly or 2 mg orally should be continued in the newborn infant.[113]

Recommended Intakes
Vitamin A

The milk of well-nourished U.S. and European women contains 40 to 70 µg/dl of retinol and 20 to 40 µg/dl beta-carotene. In terms of retinol equivalents, beta-

Similarities
• All are generic designations for a family of compounds; Vitamins A & E are important antioxidants.
• Placental transfer - limited; maternal and fetal levels generally do not correlate.
• Absorbed from small intestine requiring bile salts and micellar formation; all are absorbed through the lymphatic system.
• Plasma transport; Vitamins E, K are transported by nonspecific proteins, i.e. LDL and HDL.
• All are stored in the liver; Vitamin E stored in other tissues (fat & muscle) exceeds that of the liver.
• There are deficiency states unique to neonates; Infant deficiency states of Vitamins A, K are worldwide problems.
• Pharmacological doses are used in newborns for prophylaxis and therapy.
• Pharmacological doses have resulted in neonatal disasters.
• Plasma levels not sufficient to assess needs; Vitamins A & E have functional methods of assessment.

Differences
• Vitamin A has specific cellular and circulating binding proteins.
• Vitamin K is extremely low in human milk at all stages, compared to A & E; deficiency state described in breast fed infants.
• Vitamin K can be synthesized by colonic bacteria.
• Vitamin K needs may be assessed by a circulating abnormal protein.

Table 3: Comparison of fat soluble vitamins (A, E, K).

carotene contributes only 10% of the vitamin A in milk.[114] Assuming a breast milk intake of 750 ml/day and a retinol concentration of 40 µg/dl, the intake of retinol would average at least 300 µg per day. Taking into account the variability of vitamin A in human milk, the present RDA for term infants is 375 µg per day of retinol.[114] However, it should be noted that standard formula contains approximately 90 µg/dl of retinol so that formula-fed infants consuming much more than 400 ml of formula would exceed the RDA. For intravenous usage, retinyl palmitate should be used, as relatively little of this compound is absorbed by the tubing. Using the standard preparation of multivitamins available for pediatric TPN solutions in the US, most infants will receive at least 375 µg of retinol a day. In Europe, the standard intravenous preparation (Vitainfrainfant, Pharmacia, dosed at 1 ml/kg/day up to 4 ml total volume) provides 100 µg/kg per day of retinol.

Vitamin E

Mature human milk contains 0.45 to 0.83 IU/dl of vitamin E (Table 1), which is 0.15 to 0.34 IU per gram of lipid, and 0.85 to 2.72 IU per gram of PUFA. For term infants between birth and six months, the present RDA is 3 IU of Vitamin E per day and increases to 4 IU per day beyond six months of age. Assuming an intake of 750 ml of human milk a day, a breast-feeding infant would receive 3.4 to 6.2 IU of vitamin E per day. No U.S. infant formula contains less that 0.9 IU vitamin E/dl, and most provide more than this (Table 1). With TPN solutions, infants should receive 3-5 IU of vitamin E per day, which is easily provided with M.V.I. Pediatric (Astra Pharmaceutical) containing 7 IU per 5 ml. In Europe, the standard pediatric intravenous preparation (VitaintraInfant, Pharmacia) does not contain vitamin E.

Vitamin K

For prophylactic purposes, full-term newborn infants should continue to receive 1 mg intramuscularly at birth. Formulas contain large amounts of vitamin K (at least 5 µg/dl). Human milk is low in vitamin K (less than 0.2 µg/dl, Table 1), but there are no general recommendations for vitamin K supplements to these infants or their mothers beyond the immediate newborn period. M.V.I. pediatric now contains 200 µg of vitamin K per 5 ml, which is adequate for TPN solutions as the RDA for vitamin K is only 1 µg/kg per day in infants and children.[112] The standard intravenous vitamin preparation used in Europe (VitaintraInfant, Pharmacia, dosed at 1 ml/kg/day up to a total volume of 4 ml) provides 50 µg/kg/day of vitamin K.

Summary

By way of conclusion, these three vitamins play important roles in infant nutrition. They share many similarities with one another, in addition to being fat-soluble vitamins. There are relatively few major differences beyond their structure and physiological effects. These differences and similarities are summarized in Table 3.

Case Histories

Case #1: A 7.0 kg female infant was admitted to the hospital at four and one-half months of age with hyperirritability and a recent onset of anorexia. The physical examination revealed a tense, bulging anterior cranial fontanel, and widened sutures. The skin was dry with desquamation of the palms and soles. No areas of skin tenderness were apparent. There was no jaundice or hepatosplenomegaly.

Past history revealed that this term infant weighed 3.6 kg at birth with no neonatal problems and was breast-feeding at the time of discharge from the hospital. At one month of age, the physician told the mother that the infant was not gaining weight appropriately and said something about being sure she gave the vitamin supplement. This discussion was interpreted by the parents to mean that the child was not receiving enough vitamins, and they started giving the supplement with every feeding instead of once a day. In addition, beginning at two and one-half months, the infant was given chicken liver daily in the form of a thick slurry, as the parents remembered

their grandparents talking about liver being a good source of vitamins.

Suspicious of vitamin A toxicity, the admitting physician ordered a total serum vitamin A concentration (retinol plus retinyl ester) as part of the initial workup. It was 150 µg/dl (normal is <30 µg/dl). The child was placed on a regular diet without vitamin supplements and the tense fontanel was treated with three spinal taps over a ten day period. Five weeks after presentation, the dry skin had improved, the fontanel was flat, and the serum vitamin A was down to 50 µg/dl.

Question: How would you estimate the vitamin A intake of this infant at two months of age?

Answer: Estimation of excess vitamin A given to infant: a. Vi-Daylin (1500 IU of vitamin A/ml) 5 ml/day x 1500 IU/ml x 0.3 µg retinol/IU x 60 days=135 mg (450,000 IU) b. Liver (250 µg/g) and assume one ounce consumption per day: 250 µg/gm x 30 gm x 60 days=450 mg (1,500,000 IU) c. Total (a plus b) extra retinol given over the two month period was approximately 585 mg. (1,950,000 IU). Intake of a breast-fed infant is normally about 375 µg per day (1250 IU).

Case #2: An 1,000-gram male infant was born at 28 weeks' gestation to a 24-year-old primigravida. He was diagnosed with severe respiratory distress syndrome which required ventilatory support for the first week of life. Although enteral feedings were begun on the sixth day of life, the infant had recurrent episodes of abdominal distention requiring frequent periods of withholding of these feedings. He received dextrose and electrolyte fluids intravenously, without intravenous vitamins. By six weeks of age the infant weighed 1,500 grams. Gavage feedings at this time were 3/4 strength of a standard formula at 150 ml/kg/day, without iron or vitamin supplements. Routine check of a hematocrit revealed a gradual decline from 48 to 24%. An astute house officer ordered the following tests prior to transfusion: reticulocyte count: 11.6%, platelet count: 400,000/mm.³ Blood smear: rare rbc fragments and moderate poikilocytosis. Serum tocopherol: 0.4 mg/dl (normal=>0.5 mg/dl). Serum tocopherol to total lipid ratio: 0.5 (normal>0.6)

Question: Should this infant be treated with supplemental vitamin E?

Answer: Yes. Infants who exhibit a vitamin E-dependent,

hemolytic anemia should receive supplemental tocopherol. Admittedly, this infant had a mild case. He was treated with a daily oral tocopherol dose of 25 units/kg. Repeat blood studies four weeks later demonstrated an increase in hematocrit to 30% in association with a decline in reticulocyte count to 3.5%, an increase in the serum concentration of vitamin E to 0.9 mg/dl and an increase in the ratio of serum vitamin E/total lipid to 0.8.

Comment: *Although vitamin E deficiency as the result of feeding a formula with an inappropriate content of tocopherol or a low vitamin E to PUFA ratio is a historical consideration, inadequate vitamin E intake secondary to poor tolerance of enteral feeds remains a possibility as in this case. Today, it is very likely that this deficiency would not have occurred, as this infant would have at least received intravenous supplements of vitamin E during the periods of feeding intolerance.*

Case #3: *A six-week-old female infant suddenly became lethargic and unresponsive after rolling off a couch onto a carpeted floor. The infant was full-term, appropriate for gestational age, and the product of an uncomplicated pregnancy, labor, and delivery. There was no history of maternal drug ingestion. The infant received 2 mg of vitamin K orally at the time of birth. In general, the child progressed well on exclusive breast-feeding without supplemental vitamins and no history of antibiotic therapy. Mild physiologic jaundice resolved by one week of age. On the day prior to presentation to the hospital emergency room, the child was described as active and feeding well. Initial physical examination revealed a comatose infant with a fixed and dilated right pupil, a bulging anterior cranial fontanel, abnormal posturing, slight scleral icterus, and hepatomegaly (5 cm below the costal margin). Initial laboratory studies included a hemoglobin of 12.0 gm/dl, white blood cell count of 10,300/mm³ with a normal morphological differential. Platelet count was 300,000/mm.³ Though the working diagnosis of emergency room personnel was child abuse, coagulation studies revealed a prothrombin time of greater than 50 seconds*

and partial thromboplastin time of greater than 120 seconds. Fibrinogen level was normal. Liver function studies revealed total serum bilirubin of 7.8 mg/dl with a direct fraction of 3.0 mg/dl. The serum glutamic oxaloacetic transaminase was 60 IU/ml (normal<40 IU/ml). A CT scan of the head revealed a 4x5 cm right parietal intracerebral hematoma.

The infant was treated with 15 ml/kg of fresh frozen plasma and 5 mg intramuscularly of vitamin K. Within 12 hours the blood clotting studies had normalized but the patient remained comatose. A subsequent workup revealed that this patient had cholestatic liver disease secondary to homozygous alpha-1-antitrypsin deficiency. After 10 days the infant was discharged on supplemental vitamins including vitamin K. Subsequent followup at six months of age revealed a normal neurologic examination.

Comment: *This apparently "healthy" full-term newborn infant developed vitamin K deficiency at six weeks of age, clinically manifested by an acute intracranial hemorrhage following relatively minor trauma. The etiology of this deficiency is undoubtedly related to the subsequent diagnosis of alpha-1-antitrypsin deficiency with cholestatic liver disease, interfering with vitamin K absorption. An initial diagnosis of child abuse is not unusual in these cases.*

Question: *What is the potential role of human milk feeding in this infant's bleeding disorder?*

Answer: *This infant was exclusively fed human milk, which is known to be very low in vitamin K. Historically, hemorrhagic disease of the newborn has been a disease of breast-fed infants. Many of these infants also are reported to have liver disease.*

Question: *Was the oral administration of vitamin K at birth an additional factor?*

Answer: *It is possible that the oral administration of vitamin K at birth contributed to the severity of the presentation, as the infant may not have retained all of the dose, or may not have effectively absorbed the dose. As there is little information on the half-life or hepatic storage of vitamin K in neonates, the relation of the initial dose of vitamin K to the outcome six weeks later is unclear.*

Historical Perspective...

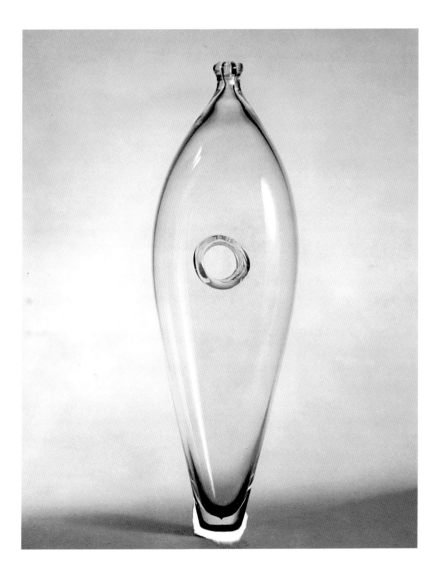

Glass feeding bottle, English, circa 1850.

Reference

1. Gorodischer R. Micronutrients and drug response: Vitamin A and vitamin E in the fetus and in the newborn. *Dev Pharmacol Ther.* 1990;15:166-172.

2. Evans HM. The pioneer history of vitamin E. *Vitamin Horm.* 1962;20:379-387.

3. Mangelsdorf DJ. Vitamin A Receptors. *Nutr Rev.* 1994; 52:S32-S44.

4. Blomhoff R. Transport and metabolism of Vitamin A. *Nutr Rev.* 1994;52:S13-S23.

5. Ong DE. Cellular transport and metabolism of vitamin A: Roles of the cellular retinoid-binding proteins. *Nutr Rev.* 1994;52:S24-S31.

6. Moore T. Vitamin A transport from mother to offspring in mice and rats. *Int J Vitam Nutr Res.* 1971;41:301-306.

7. Vobecky JS, Vobecky J, Shapcott D, Demers PP, Cloutier D, Blanchard R, Fisch C. Biochemical indices of nutritional status in maternal, cord, and early neonatal blood. *Am J Clin Nutr.* 1982;36:630-641.

8. Dostalova L. Correlation of the vitamin status between mother and newborn at delivery. *Dev Pharmacol Ther.* 1982;4:45-47.

9. Hustead VA, Gutcher GR, Anderson SA, Zachman RD. Relationship of vitamin A (retinol) status to lung disease in the preterm infants. *J Pediatr.* 1984;105:610-615.

10. Ehrenkranz RA. Vitamin E and the neonate. *Am J Dis Child.* 1980;134:1157-1166.

11. Tappel AL. Vitamin E as the biologic lipid antioxidant. *Vitam Horm.* 1962;20:493-501.

12. Machlin LJ. Vitamin E. In: Machlin LJ, ed. *Handbook of vitamins. Nutritional, biochemical and clinical aspects.* New York: Marcel Dekker; 1984:99-145.

13. Losowsky MS, Kelleher J, Walker BE. Intake and absorption of tocopherol. *Ann NY Acad Sci.* 1972;203: 212-222.

14. Bieri JG. Kinetics of tissue a-tocopherol depletion and repletion. *Ann NY Acad Sci.* 1972;203:181-191.

15. Kayden HJ, Traber MG. Absorption, lipoprotein transport, and regulation of plasma concentrations of vitamin E in humans. *J Lipid Res.* 1993;34:343-358.

16. Sokol RJ, Heubi JE, Iannaccone ST, Bove KE, Balistreri WF. Vitamin E deficiency with normal serum vitamin E concentrations in children with chronic cholestasis. *N Engl J Med.* 1984;310:1209-1212.

17. Colburn WA, Ehrenkranz RA. Pharmokinetics of a single intramuscular injection of vitamin E to premature neonates. *Pediatr Pharmacol.* 1983;3:7-14.

18. Bougle D, Boatroy MJ, Heng J, Vert P. Plasma kinetics of parenteral tocopherol in premature infants. *Dev Pharmacol Ther.* 1986;9:310-316.

19. Abbasi S, Jensen BK, Gerdes JS, Bhutani VK, Johnson L. Pharmokinetics of intravenous vitamin E in preterm infants. *Ann NY Acad Sci.* 1989;570:345-351.

20. Farrell PM. Vitamin E. In: Shils M, Young V, eds. *Modern Nutrition in Health and Disease.* Philadelphia: Lea and Ferbiger; 1988:340-354.

21. Esmon CT, Suttie JW, Jackson CM. The functional significance of vitamin K action. Difference in phospholipid binding between normal and abnormal prothrombin. *J Biol Chem.* 1975;250:4095-4099.

22. Blomstrand R, Forsgren L. Vitamin K$_1$^{3}H in man. Its intestinal absorption and transport in the thoracic lymph duct. *Int Z Vit Forschung.* 1968;38:45-64.

23. Shearer MJ, McCarthy PT, Crampton OE, Mattock MB. The assessment of human vitamin K status from tissue measurements. In: Suttie JW, ed. *Current Advances in Vitamin K Research.* New York: Elsevier; 1988:437-452.

24. Mattock M, Shearer MJ, Rahim S, Redmond S, ElGohari R, Barkhan P. The plasma transport of vitamin K1 (phylloquinone) in hyperlipoproteinaemia. *Clinical Science.* 1983;64:63P.

25. Hollander D, Rim E, Muralidhara KS. Vitamin K1 intestinal absorption *in vivo*: influence of luminal contents on transport. *Am J Physiol.* 1971;232:E69-E74.

26. Duello TJ, Matshiner JT. Characterization of vitamin K from human liver. *J Nutr.* 1972;102:331-335.

27. Shirahata A, Nakamura T, Ariyoshi N. Vitamin K1 and K2 contents in blood, stool, and liver tissues of neonates and young infants. In: Suzuki S, Hathaway WE, Bonnar J, Sutor AH, eds. *Perinatal Thrombosis and Hemostasis.* Tokyo: Springer-Verlag; 1991:214-223.

28. Kayata S, Kindberg C, Greer FR, Suttie JW. Vitamin K1 and K2 in infant human liver. *J Pediatr Gastro Nutr.* 1989;8:304-307.

29. Guillaumont M, Sann L, Leclercq M, Dostalova L, Vignal B, Frederich A. Changes in hepatic vitamin K1 levels after prophylactic administration to the newborn. *J Pediatr Gastro Nutr.* 1993;16:10-14.

30. Shearer MJ, Barkhan P, Rahim S, Stimmler L. Plasma vitamin KI in mothers and their newborn babies. *Lancet.* 1982;1:460-463.

31. Mandelbrot L, Guillaumont M, Leclercq M, Lefrére JJ, Gozin D, Daffos F, Forestier F. Placental transfer of vitamin KI and its implications in fetal hemostasis. *Thrombosis and Haemostasis.* 1988;60:39-43.

32. Hiraike H, Kimura M, Itokawa Y. Distribution of K vitamins (phylloquinone and menaquinones) in human placental and maternal and umbilical cord plasma. *Am J Obstet Gynecol.* 1988;158:564-569.

33. Widdershoven J, Lambert W, Motohara K, Monnens L, deLeenbeer A, Matsuda I, Endo F. Plasma concentrations of vitamin KI and PIVKA-II in bottle-fed and breast-fed infants with and without vitamin K prophylaxis at birth. *Eur J Pediatr.* 1988;148:139-142.

34. Yang Y-M, Simon N, Maertens P, Brigham S, Liu P. Maternal-fetal transport of vitamin KI and its effect on coagulation in premature infants. *J Pediatr.* 1989;115:1009-1013.

35. Pietersma-de Bruyn ALJM, van Haard PMM, Beunis MHJ, Hamulyák K, Kuijpers JC. Vitamin KI levels and coagulation factors in healthy term newborns till 4 week after birth. *Haemostatis.* 1990;20:8-14.

36. Tamura R, Takasaki K, Yanaihara T, Maruyama M, Nakagama T. Effect of vitamin K administration in the mother on prevention of vitamin K deficiency in the neonate. *Acta Obstet Gynaecol Jpn.* 1986;38:880-886.

37. Israels LG, Walls GA, Ollman DJ, Friesen E, Israels ED. Vitamin K as a regulator of benzo(a) pyrene metabolism, mutagenesis, and carcinogenesis. *J Clin Invest.* 1983;71:1130-1140.

38. Israels LG, Ollman DJ, Israels ED. Vitamin KI as a modulator of benzo(a)pyrene metabolism as measured by in vitro metabolite formation and *in vivo* ANA - adduct formation. *Int J Biochem.* 1985;17:1263-1266.

39. Israels LG, Ollman DJ, Israels ED. Vitamin KI increases sister chromatid exchange in vitro in human leukocytes and *in vivo* in fetal sheep cells: A possible role for "vitamin K deficiency" in the fetus. *Pediatr Res.* 1987;22:405-408.

40. Cornelissen EAM, Smeets D, Merkx G, DeAbreu R, Kollee L, Monnens L. Analysis of chromosome aberrations and sister chromatid exchanges in peripheral blood lymphocytes of newborns after vitamin K prophylaxis at

birth. *Pediatr Res.* 1991;30:550-553.

41. Mino M, Kitagawa M, Nagagawa S. Red blood cell tocopherol concentrations in a normal population of Japanese children and premature infants in relation to the assessment of vitamin E status. *Am J Clin Nutr.* 1985;41:631-638.

42. Sabesin SM. Cholestatic lipoproteins - their pathogenesis and significance. *Gastroenterology.* 1982;83:704-709.

43. Thurnham DI, Davies JQ, Crump BJ, Situnayake AD, Davis M. The use of different lipids to express serum tocopherol-lipid ratios for the measurement of vitamin status. *An Clin Biochem.* 1986;23:514-520.

44. Flores H, Campos F, Araujo CRC, Underwood BA. Assessment of marginal vitamin A deficiency in Brazilian children using the relative dose response procedure. *Am J Clin Nutr.* 1984;40:1281-1289.

45. Underwood BA. Hypovitaminosis A: International Programmatic Issues. *J Nutr.* 1994;124:S1467-S1472.

46. Amedee-Manesme O, Anderson D, Olson JA. Relation of the relative dose response to liver concentrations of vitamin A in generally well-nourished surgical patients. *Am J Clin Nutr.* 1984;39:898-902.

47. Andrew M, Paes B, Milner R, Johnston M, Mitchell L, Tollefsen D, Powers P. Development of the human coagulation system in the full-term infant. *Blood.* 1987;70:165-172.

48. Liska DJ, Suttie JW. Location of gamma-carboxyglutamyl residues in partially carboxylated prothrombin preparations. *Biochemistry.* 1988;27:8636-8641.

49. Von Kries R, Greer FR, Suttie JW. Assessment of vitamin K status of the newborn infant. *J Pediatr Gastro Nutr.* 1993;16:231-238.

50. Amiral J, Grosley M, Plassart V, Mimilla F, Chambrette B. Development of a monoclonal immunoassay for the direct measurement of decarboxyprothrombin of plasma. *Thrombosis and Haemostasis.* (Abstract). 1991;65:648.

51. Belle M, Brebant R, Guinet R, Leclercq M. Detection of human plasmatic des-gamma-carboxyprothrombins by enzyme-linked immunosorbent assay using a new monoclonal antibody. In Press.

52. Bovill EG, Soll RF, Lynch M, Landesman M, Freie M, Church W, McAuliffe T, Davidson K, Sadowski J. Vitamin KI metabolism and the production of

des-carboxy prothrombin and protein C in the term and premature neonate. *Blood.* 1993;81:77-83.

53. Motahara K, Endo F, Matsuda I. Effect of vitamin K administration on acarboxyprothrombin (PIVKA-II) levels in newborns. *Lancet II.* 1985;242-244.

54. Motohara K, Takayi S, Endo F, Kiyota Y, Matsuda I. Oral supplementation of vitamin K for pregnant women and effects on levels of plasma vitamin K and PIVKA-II in the neonate. *J Pediatr Gastro Nutr.* 1990;11:32-36.

55. Von Kries R, Shearer MJ, Widdershoven J, Motohara K, Umbach G, Göbel U. Des-gamma-carboxyprothrombin (PIVKA-II) and plasma vitamin K1 in newborns and their mothers. *Thrombosis and Haemostasis.* 1992;68: 383-387.

56. Cox A, McCarthy PT, Harrington DJ, Shearer MJ. Human vitamin K status assessment: value of plasma des-gamma-carboxyprothrombin and vitamin K1. *Int J Vit Nutr Res.* 1997; In press.

57. Greer FR, Marshall SP, Severson R, Smith DA, Shearer MJ, Pace DG, Joubert PH. A new mixed-micellar preparation for oral vitamin K prophylaxis: comparison with an intramuscular formulation in breast-fed infants. *Lancet.* In press.

58. Cornelissen E, Kollée L, DeAbreu R, Van Baal JM, Motohara K, Verbruggen B, Monnens LAH. Effects of oral and intramuscular vitamin K prophylaxis on vitamin K1, PIVKA-II and clotting factors in breast-fed infants. Archives of Disease in Childhood 1992;67:1250-1254.

59. Cornelissen E, Kollee L, van Lith T, Motohara K, Monnens LAH. Evaluation of a daily dose of 25 µg vitamin K1 to prevent Vitamin K deficiency in breast-fed infants. *J Pediatr Gastro Nutr.* 1993;16:301-305.

60. Cornelissen E, Kollée L, DeAbreu RM, Motohara K, Monnens LAH. Prevention of vitamin K deficiency in infancy by weekly administration of vitamin K. *Acta Pediatr.* 1993;82:656-659.

61. Committee on Nutrition, American Academy of Pediatrics. *Pediatric Nutrition Handbook.* Third edition. 1993.

62. Ajans ZA, Sarrif A, Husbands M. Influence of vitamin A on human colostrum and early milk. *Am J Clin Nutr.* 1965;17:139-142

63. Thomas MR, Pearsons MH, Demkowicz M. Vitamin A and vitamin E concentrations of the milk from mothers of pre-term infants and milk of mothers of full term infants. *Acta Vitaminol Enzymol.* 1981;3:135-144.

64. Chappell JE, Clandinin FT. Vitamin A and E content of human milk at early stages of lactation. *Early Hum Dev.* 1985;11:157-167.

65. Gebre-Medhin M, Vahlquist A, Hovander Y, Uppsäll L, Vahlquist B. Breast milk composition in Ethiopian and Swedish mothers. 1. Vitamin A and ß-carotene. *Am J Clin Nutr.* 1976;29:441-451.

66. Jansson L, Akesson B, Hoomberg L. Vitamin E and fatty acid composition of human milk. *Am J Clin Nutr.* 1981;34:8-13.

67. Harzer G, Haug M. Correlation of human milk vitamin E with different lipids. In: Schaub J, ed. *Composition and physiological properties of human milk.* Amsterdam: Elsevier; 1985:247-254.

68. Dostalova L, Salmenperä L, Vaclavinkova V, Heinz-Erian P, Schüep W. Vitamin concentration in term milk of European mothers. In: Berger H, ed. *Vitamins and minerals in pregnancy and lactation.* New York: Raven Press Ltd; 1988:275-298.

69. Greer FR, Marshall S, Cherry J, Suttie JW. Vitamin K status of lactating mothers, human milk and breast-feeding infants. *Pediatrics.* 1991;88:751-756.

70. Canfield LM, Hopkinson JM. State of the art vitamin K in human milk. *J Pediatr Gastro Nutr.* 1989;8:430-441.

71. Pietschning B, Haschke F, Vanura H, Shearer M, Veitl V, Kellner S, Schuster E. Vitamin K in breast milk: no influence of maternal dietary intake. *Eur J Clin Nutr.* 1992;47:209-215.

72. Vermeer C, Hamulyák K. Pathophysiology of vitamin K-deficiency and oral anticoagulants. *Thrombosis and Haemostasis.* 1991;66:153-159.

73. Greer FR, Mummah-Schendel LL, Marshall S, Suttie JW. Vitamin K1 (phylloquinone) and vitamin K2 (menaquinone) status in newborn infants during the first week of life. *Pediatrics.* 1988;81:137-140.

74. Underwood BA. Vitamin A in animal and human nutrition. In: Sporn MB, Roberts AB, Goodman DS. *The retinoids.* Vol 1. New York: Academic Press; 1984: 281-392.

75. Oski FA, Barness LA. Vitamin E deficiency: a previously unrecognized cause of hemolytic anemia in the premature infant. *J Pediatr.* 1967;70:211-220.

76. Townsend CW. The haemorrhágic disease of the newborn. *Arch Pediatr.* 1894;11:559-565.

77. Dam H, Dyggve H, Larsen H, Plum P. The relation of vitamin K deficiency to hemorrhagic disease of the newborn. *Adv Pediatr.* 1952;5:129-153.

78. American Academy Pediatrics. *Standards and Recommendations for Hospital Care of Newborn Infants.* 1954;92.

79. Allison AC. Danger of vitamin K to newborn. *Lancet.* 1955;1:669 (Letter).

80. Committee on Nutrition, American Academy of Pediatrics. Vitamin K compounds and their water-soluble analogues: Use in therapy and prophylaxis in pediatrics. *Pediatrics.* 1961;28:501-507.

81. Sutherland JM, Glueck HI, Gleser G. Hemorrhagic disease of the newborn. *Am J Dis Child.* 1967;113:524-533.

82. Keenan WJ, Jewett T, Glueck H. Role of feeding and vitamin K in hypoprothrombinemia of the newborn. *Am J Dis Child.* 1971;121:271-277.

83. Goldman HJ, Deposito F. Hypoprothrombinemic bleeding in young infants. *Am J Dis Child.* 1966;111: 430-432.

84. Loughnan PM, McDougall PN. Epidemiology of late onset haemorrhagic disease: a pooled data analysis. *J Paediatr Child Health.* 1993;29:177-181.

85. Mountain KR, Hirsch J, Gallus AS. Neonatal coagulation defect due to anticonvulsant drug treatment in pregnancy. *Lancet.* 1970;1:265-268.

86. Srinivasan G, Seeler RA, Tiruvury A, Pildes RS. Maternal anticonvulsant therapy and hemorrhagic disease of the newborn. *Obstet Gynecol.* 1982;59:250-252.

87. Odell GB. Therapeutic misadventures in neonatal care. In: Gluck L, ed. *Modern Perinatal Medicine.* St. Louis: Year Book Medical Publishers Inc; 1974:232.

88. Martone WJ, Williams WW, Mortensen ML, Gaynes RP, White JW, Lorch V, Murphy D, Sinha SN, Frank DJ, Kosmetatos N, Bodenstein CJ, Roberts RJ. Illness with fatalities in premature infants: Association with an intravenous vitamin E preparation, E-Ferol. *Pediatrics.* 1986;78:591-600.

89. Muller DPR. Vitamin E therapy in retinopathy of prematurity. *Eye.* 1992;6:221-225.

90. Johnson L, Quinn GE, Abbasi S, Otis C, Goldstein D, Sacks L, Porat R, Fong E. Delivoria-Papadopoulos M,

Peckham G, Schaffer DB, Bowen FW. Effect of sustained pharmacologic vitamin E levels on incidence and severity of retinopathy of prematurity: a controlled clinical trial. *J Pediatr.* 1989;114:827-838.

91. Ehrenkranz RA, Ablow RC, Warshaw JB. Effect of vitamin E on the development of oxygen-induced lung injury in neonates. *Ann NY Acad Sci.* 1982;393:452-465.

92. Poland R. Vitamin E for prevention of perinatal intracranial hemorrhage. *Pediatrics.* 1990;85:865-867.

93. Chiswick M, Gladman G, Sinha S, Toner N, Davies J. Vitamin E supplementation and periventricular hemorrhage in the newborn. *Am J Clin Nutr.* 1991;53: S370-S372.

94. Shenai JP, Kennedy KA, Chytil F, Stahlman MT. Clinical trial of vitamin A supplementation in infants susceptible to bronchopulmonary dysplasia. *J Pediatr.* 1987;111:269-277.

95. Pearson E, Bose C, Snidow T, Ranson L, Young T, Bose G, Stiles A. Trial of vitamin A supplementation in very low birth weight infants at risk for bronchopulmonary dysplasia. *J Pediatr.* 1992;121:420-427.

96. Shenai JP, Rush MG, Stahlman MT, Chytil F. Vitamin A supplementation and bronchopulmonary dysplasia - revisited. *J Pediatr.* 1992;121:399-401.

97. Dickson RC, Stubbs TM, Lazarchick J. Antenatal vitamin K therapy of the low-birth-weight infants. *Am J Obstet Gynecol.* 1994;170:85-89.

98. Kazzi NJ, Ilagan NB, Liang KC, Kazzi GM, Poland RL, Grietsell LA, Fugii Y, Brans YW. Maternal administration of vitamin K does not improve the coagulation profile of preterm infants. *Pediatrics.* 1989;84:1045-1050.

99. Morales WJ, Angel JL, O'Brien WF, Knuppel RA, Marsalisi F. The use of antenatal vitamin K in the prevention of early neonatal intraventricular hemorrhage. *Am J Obstet Gynecol.* 1988;159:774-779.

100. Pomerance JJ, Teal JG, Gogolock JF, Brown S, Stewart ME. Maternally administered antenatal vitamin K1: effect on neonatal prothrombin activity, partial thromboplastin time, and intraventricular hemorrhage. *Obstet Gynecol.* 1987;70:235-241.

101. Thorp JA, Parriott J, Ferrette-Smith D, Meyer BA, Cohen GR, Johnson J. Antepartum vitamin K and phenobarbital for preventing intraventricular hemorrhage in the premature newborn: A randomized, double-blind, placebo-controlled trial. *Obstet Gynecol.* 1994;83:70-76.

102. Hathcock JM, Hattan DG, Jenkins MY, McDonald JT, Sundaresan RP, Wilkening VL. Evaluation of vitamin A toxicity. *Am J Clin Nutr.* 1990;52:183-202.

103. Finer NN, Peters KL, Hayek Z, Merkel CL. Vitamin E and necrotizing enterocolitis. *Pediatrics.* 1984;73:387-393.

104. Rosenbaum AL, Phelps DL, Isenberg SJ, Leake RD, Dorey F. Retinal hemorrhage in retinopathy of prematurity associated with tocopherol treatment. *Ophthalmology.* 1985;92:1012-1014.

105. Neal PR, Erickson P, Baenziger JC, Olson J, Lemons JA. Serum vitamin E levels in the very low birth weight infant during oral supplementation. *Pediatrics.* 1986;77: 636-640.

106. Committee on Nutrition, American Academy of Pediatrics. Nutritional needs for low-birth-weight infants. *Pediatrics.* 1985;75:976-986.

107. Golding J, Greenwood R, Birmingham K, Mott M. Childhood cancer, intramuscular vitamin K, and pethidine given during labour. *BMJ.* 1992;305:341-346.

108. Ekelund H, Finnstrom O, Gunnarskog J, Källen B, Larsson Y. Administration of vitamin K to newborn infants and childhood cancer. *BMJ.* 1993;307:89-91.

109. Klebanoff MA, Read JS, Mills JL, Shiono PH. The risk of childhood cancer after neonatal exposure to vitamin K. *N Engl J Med.* 1989;329:905-908.

110. Olsen JH, Hertz H, Blinkenberg K, Verder H. Vitamin K regimens and incidence of childhood cancer in Denmark. *BJM.* 1994;308:895-896.

111. Von Kries R, Göbel U, Hachmeister A, Kaletsh U, Michaelis J. Vitamin K and childhood cancer: A population based case-control study in Lower Saxony, Germany. *BMJ.* 1996;313:199-203.

112. Ansell P, Ball D, Roman E. Childhood leukemia and intramuscular vitamin K. Findings from a case control study. *BMJ.* 1996;313:204-205.

113. Vitamin K Ad Hoc Task Force. Controversies concerning vitamin K and the newborn. American Academy of Pediatrics. *Pediatrics.* 1993;91:1001-1003.

114. Subcommittee on the Tenth Edition of the RDAs Food and Nutrition Board Commission on Life Sciences National Research Council. *Recommended Dietary Allowances.* 10th Edition. Washington, DC: National Academy Press; 1989.

115. Greer FR, Zachman RE, Farrell PM. Neonatal vitamin metabolism--fat-soluble. In: Cowett RM, ed. *Principles of Perinatal-Neonatal Metabolism.* New York: Springer Verlag; 1991:531-558.

116. Hdydishi O, Mino M, eds. *Clinical and Nutritional Aspects of Vitamin E.* New York: Elsevier; 1987:169-181 .

Inborn Errors of Metabolism

Helen K. Berry[1]
Nancy D. Leslie[2]

Professor Emerita of Pediatrics,[1] Division of Human Genetics,[2]
Children's Hospital Medical Center,
Cincinnati, Ohio

Reviewed by A. Wesley Burks M.D., James W. Hansen M.D., Ph.D. and Rebecca S. Wappner M.D.

Introduction

Inborn errors of intermediary metabolism typically result from mutations in the genes coding for enzymes of catabolism. These enzymes may participate in the processing of ingested substances such as amino acids or sugars, the removal of waste chemicals or the conversion of stored energy to usable energy. Human metabolism is like an automatic assembly line in a chemical factory. Substances arrive at specific points where they must be picked up and either converted to another substance or transported to another section of the factory. The workers in the factory are enzymes: proteins whose job is to make the necessary conversions rapidly and efficiently. These proteins are so specific they control a single type of reaction. The synthesis of each enzyme is controlled by a specific gene. Like any assembly line, hitches occur. The worker is absent or defective and cannot carry out its catalytic function. The gene has made a mistake, giving out the wrong message or no message; a metabolic block occurs. Most of theses metabolic errors are transmitted from generation to generation as autosomal recessive traits.

In 1900, approximately 150 infants died for every 1,000 live births; it was estimated that five of the 150 deaths were related to genetic defects. Today, infant mortality has been reduced by 90%. Yet, five of the current 10 deaths per 1,000 live births still have a genetically related cause. Though genetic diseases are individually rare, collectively they are significant, accounting for 25 to 35% of all infant deaths and a high proportion of infant morbidity.

Increasing costs of health care direct attention to programs that aim at preventing death or long-term physical and/or mental handicaps associated with genetic diseases. Newborn screening programs play a vital role in early diagnosis, allowing preventive therapy for a number of these biochemical genetic disorders. However, only a few of the known 1,500 to 2,000 metabolic disorders are included in newborn screening batteries. Other disorders are associated with severe illnesses very early in life and many affected infants may die with their condition undiagnosed. Physicians should be highly suspicious when confronted with an acutely ill infant, usually irritable or lethargic, with seizures, sepsis, hypotonia, jaundice, tachypnea, vomiting, unusual odor or family history of sibling deaths.

Much of our knowledge of metabolic pathways has come from study of these naturally occurring defects. It has become apparent that many inborn errors show clinical, biochemical and genetic heterogeneity. Newborn screening programs were quick to identify "variant" disease forms, producing milder or perhaps no morbidity. Direct study of mutations in the genes coding for the defective enzyme has opened a new dimension to the study of inborn errors. In some cases, mutation analysis can predict response to therapy or stratify patients so that study of therapeutic options can proceed in a more controlled fashion.

A term baby discharged at 20 hours of age on breast-feeding returned to the birth hospital at 48 hours for refusal to feed. The mother had nursed three previous children and noted the baby's poor suck. On evaluation the baby looked dehydrated, was 15% below birth weight and was tachypneic. Her glucose was normal; her pH was 7.11 with a large base deficit. Her electrolytes showed a depressed HCO_3^- with an anion gap of 35. Her urine was positive for ketones.

Comment

The initial diagnosis of this baby was dehydration related to inadequate breast-feeding, but the evolution was too rapid and the acidosis too profound. The presence of ketonuria is a red flag. Although babies can and do make ketones during transition, they are rarely ketonuric on dipstick. The baby had methyl malonic acidemia. With earlier discharge from the birth hospital, this type of baby will present more and more often to the doctor's office or community emergency room. A high degree of suspicion is needed for correct diagnosis and aggressive intervention.

The PKU Story

"All the observations made on the patients with phenylketonuria are consistent with the hypothesis that the effects of some detrimental substance on the central nervous system have been overcome by the use of the phenylalanine-restricted diet. It seems probably that such diets should be initiated at a very early age in order to prevent irreversible damage to the central nervous system."

Armstrong and Tyler, 1955.

In 1934, Folling discovered that phenylpyruvic acid was excreted in certain cases of mental deficiency.[1] Adding ferric chloride to these patients' urine produced an unusual blue-green color, and Folling identified the source of the color. He noted the familial incidence of phenylketonuria (PKU) in the first patients he described. Later he found that blood from these individuals contained increased amounts of phenylalanine.[2]

Studies by Penrose[3] and others[4, 5] showed that phenylketonuria is inherited as a simple autosomal recessive trait. In 1953, Jervis demonstrated that the enzymatic system for conversion of phenylalanine to tyrosine is absent in PKU.[6]

Conversion of phenylalanine to tyrosine occurs in hepatocytes and is catalyzed by phenylalanine hydroxylase, its cofactor, tetrahydrobiopeterin (BH_4), and a second enzyme, dihydropteridine reductase (DHPR), which keeps the cofactor in its active (tetra hydro) form. Although elevations of blood phenylalanine (hyperphenylalaninemia) may result from a defect in any component of the system, mutations in the phenylalanine hydroxylase gene are responsible for 99% of the cases of hyperphenylalaninemia.

The term hyperphenylalaninemia encompasses a wide range of clinical and biochemical symptoms. PKU refers to elevation of blood phenylalanine resulting from partial or complete deficiency of phenylalanine hydroxylase. Once the gene for phenylalanine hydroxylase was cloned[7] and mutation screening of affected individuals was carried out,[8] genetic heterogeneity was seen as the explanation. Phenylalanine hydroxylase maps to 12q22-q24 in the human genome,[9] and more than 70 mutations have been described.[10]

In normal individuals, as much as three-quarters the phenylalanine in the diet is converted to tyrosine, with the remainder used for protein synthesis, minor amounts for decarboxylation to phenylethylamine or excretion unchanged in the urine.[11] When the pathway to tyrosine is blocked, phenylalanine accumulates in body fluids and tissues, and the major alternative pathway, transamination to phenylpyruvic acid, becomes significant. There is a progressive increase in production of phenylpyruvic acid and its metabolites, phenyllactic and o-hydroxyphenylacetic acids, as blood phenylalanine rises.

Diagnosis

With few exceptions, prior to 1962 the only instance in which phenylketonuria was recognized early in infancy occurred when a child was born into a family in which an older sibling had been identified as having PKU. There are no symptoms in the infant with PKU. Blood phenylalanine concentration, normal in cord blood, rises soon after birth. Within 24 hours, phenylalanine increases into the range of four to six mg/dL.[12] Urine screening programs, so effective in detecting PKU in the mentally retarded population, were ineffective when applied to infants, since phenylpyruvic acid was not excreted in urine of affected infants until as late as six weeks of age.[13] The development of a simple procedure for measuring phenylalanine in dried blood spots, known as the Guthrie test, opened the way for testing infants for phenylketonuria prior to discharge from the newborn nursery.[14] Screening soon after birth for PKU has now become accepted medical practice in most states of the states of the U.S. and many developed countries of the world. Following identification of presumptive positive infants by screening, diagnostic investigation should be carried out with a minimum of delay so that treatment can begin as soon as possible, preferably by three weeks of age.[15] The classical phenotype of PKU is usually defined as blood phenylalanine elevation greater than 1,200 micromole/L (20 mg/dL).[16]

Preventive Therapy

In late 1950, two groups of workers, Armstrong and colleagues[17] in the United States, and Woolf and coworkers[18] in London, independently and almost simultaneously began using diets low in phenylalanine, though their results were not published until later. Armstrong and co-workers fed mixtures of L-amino acids to patients with phenylketonuria in place of protein and succeeded in reducing phenylalanine levels with marked clinical improvement. The London group used charcoal-treated protein hydrolysates as a phenylalanine-free amino acid mixture. Woolf described the diet preparation to Bickel, who was caring for a two-year-old patient recently found to have phenylketonuria. Bickel prepared the diet, gave it to his patient and, in 1953, published the first report describing marked clinical improvement in a patient fed a phenylalanine-restricted diet.[19] It soon became clear that while certain aspects of behavior were improved by using the phenylalanine-restricted diets, mental damage was not reversible. To be effective, treatment had to be started early in life.[20] Clinical interest quickened and attention centered on the younger patient. By 1958, commercial low-phenylalanine products became available; these were nutritionally adequate except for their deficiency in phenylalanine.

Dietary Changes - Dietary Needs

The treatment of phenylketonuria consists of providing a nutritionally balanced diet containing enough phenylalanine to meet the needs of a growing child without exceeding his capacity to utilize it. Dietary intake of phenylalanine is limited by replacing protein-rich foods with low-phenylalanine or phenylalanine-free protein substitutes. The requirement for phenylalanine, an

Age	Phenylalanine (mg/kg)	Protein (gm/kg)	Energy (cal/kg)
0-3 mo	40-70	2.5-3.5	120
4-6 mo	30-50	2.5-3.2	110
7-12 mo	30-40	2.5-3.0	105
1-3 yr	20-40	2.0-2.5	100
4-6 yr	15-35	1.5-2.0	90
7-10 yr	10-25	1.0-1.5	70
11-15 yr	10-25	1.0-1.5	45-55
15-18 yr	5-15	1.0-1.3	40-45
Adult	5-10	1.0-1.3	40

Table 1: Recommended daily intakes of nutrients for children with phenylketonuria.

essential amino acid, is provided by including small amounts of natural low-protein foods. The objective of treatment is to reduce serum phenylalanine from concentrations above 20 mg/dL to a range between 3 and 6 mg/dL. Studies of patients with PKU have provided approximate requirements for age ranges between infancy and adulthood (Table 1). The need for phenylalanine (per kilogram body weight) is greatest during infancy and diminishes significantly with age, so that by school age a child needs less than half as much and the adult about 10% of the infant requirement. This means that the total requirement for a given child may remain relatively constant, in the range of 200 to 500 mg/day from one to 11 years of age.[21] Tyrosine becomes an essential amino acid in subjects with phenylketonuria; estimated daily requirements for infants are 250 to 350 mg/kg.[21] Protein requirement is provided by a semi-synthetic diet derived either from a modified protein hydrolysate or from a mixture of L-amino acids. Restriction of phenylalanine intake by restriction of protein intake is not effective.[22] Needs for carbohydrate, fat (including essential fatty acids), minerals and vitamins are met by the special dietary products and by supplements of natural foods. Composition of formulas for treatment of PKU and of human milk are shown in

Excerpt From A Letter To Helen Berry
Radcliffe Infirmary, Oxford
27 March 1961

I am writing to ask for your help in a problem we have met in this country concerning the treatment of phenylketonurics during the first year of life. In the majority of cases these children do well physically and mentally; however, in a considerable minority the children develop a severe fiery rash, particularly in the diaper region, which is unresponsive to conventional treatment and tends to extend into the intertriginous folds. The child ceases gaining weight and developmental progress is also arrested; the child is miserable, apathetic and sometimes has anorexia and vomiting. This has in extreme cases proceeded to death. In other cases the condition has been cured dramatically by giving them cow's milk, either instead of or as well as the low-phenylalanine diet. We have never observed this in a child over one year of age. The skin changes resemble those described for deficiency of essential fatty acids, but we have been able to show that fatty acids are not responsible. It is obviously a deficiency of some kind, and my guess would be that it is phenylalanine that is too low in the diet. If you have never come across this condition it would be helpful to know just what your own infants are being fed.

L.I. Woolf

the Appendix. The recommendation for protein should be met from the chosen low-phenylalanine formula.

These formulas should never be used for normal infants. A diagnosis of phenylketonuria must be confirmed before administration; close biochemical monitoring of phenylalanine and other plasma amino acids is essential. Other precautions for managing the diet include provision of daily monitoring of blood phenylalanine concentrations until phenylalanine decreases to treatment range and stabilizes; weekly monitoring until four years of age, with monthly monitoring thereafter; tyrosine intake sufficient to maintain plasma tyrosine concentrations within normal limits of 50 to 100 micromol/L; adjustment of phenylalanine

intake when blood phenylalanine concentrations rise or fall outside the therapeutic range; frequent measurements of weight and height; periodic assessment of other nutritional parameters.[15] Pre-term infants with phenylketonuria present special problems. Additional protein and energy may be needed for "catch-up" growth, and the phenylalanine requirement may be greater than 90 mg/kg/day, depending on growth rate. Shortland et al reported that phenylalanine intake of 100 mg/kg/day and tyrosine of 270 to 290 mg/kg/day were required for a 1,560 gm infant with PKU to achieve catch-up growth of 20 gm/kg/day.[23]

Use of amino acid-restricted diets provides examples of the necessary balance among nutrients that make up normal diets. Tissue catabolism occurs if a baby with PKU reduces intake of a low-phenylalanine formula so that there is insufficient nitrogen in the diet, or if an amino acid, including phenylalanine, is not present in sufficient amounts to meet requirements for that amino acid. This releases phenylalanine along with the deficient nutrient. Hence, there may be a paradoxical rise in serum phenylalanine concentration as a consequence. Similarly, if insufficient calories are provided, protein sources may be utilized for energy, again resulting in increase in serum phenylalanine.

The first signs of an amino acid deficiency are refusal to eat, followed by failure to gain weight or weight loss. Woolf was correct in deducing the cause of the symptoms outlined above. During early years of treatment other reports appeared of similar clinical symptoms in children on phenylalanine-restricted diets, including deaths from overtreatment.[24] Other adverse effects included changes in red blood cell precursors and anemia, corrected by addition of phenylalanine to the diet,[25, 26] bone changes[27, 28] and mental retardation.[29, 30, 31, 32]

How Are We Doing

Clinical symptoms described by early investigators included, in addition to severe mental retardation, agitated behavior, EEG abnormalities, seizures, diminished pigmentation, eczema, hypertonicity, inability to walk or talk and erratic and aggressive behavior.[33] Because of widespread and efficient newborn screening programs, followed by early treatment with a diet low in phenylalanine, these symptoms are no longer seen in affected individuals.[34] Benefits of early treatment are well established: children with PKU attend ordinary schools and have general ability within the normal range, though mean intelligence quotients are about half a standard deviation lower than those of unaffected siblings.[29, 32, 35-38] Many reports suggest that terminating the low-phenylalanine diet in most patients is accompanied by deterioration in intellectual and neuropsychological functioning.[35-38] Outcome is closely associated with blood phenylalanine control at all ages.[39]

Post-mortem material from patients with untreated phenylketonuria has shown reduced myelination, reduction of lipid content of brain white matter, and deficient cerebrosides in white matter lipid.[40, 41] Abnormalities in magnetic resonance imaging of brain white matter,[42] neurologic deterioration[43] and an abnormal EEG[44] can be detected in early-treated as well as untreated adolescents and adults with PKU.

Phenylalanine is probably responsible for the neurotoxic effects observed in phenylketonuria. Although the exact mechanism remains unclear, phenylalanine's effects on synthesis of myelin and other brain proteins, as well as its interference with neurotransmitter production, are involved.

A breast-fed baby presented at nine days of age following a positive newborn screening test for PKU. The phenylalanine level in blood collected at 48 hours of age was 6 mg/dL by the Guthrie test. Phenylalanine measured quantitatively at nine days was 15 mg/dL. The baby was started on a low-phenylalanine formula supplemented first by breast milk, then by small amounts of cow milk-based formula. At three years of age, his average phenylalanine is 4 mg/dL on a prescribed intake of phenylalanine typical for classical PKU.

Comment

This baby did not meet the criteria for classical PKU at diagnosis, since serum phenylalanine prior to treatment was only 15 mg/dL. In retrospect, this was probably due to the relatively low protein content of breast milk compared to conventional formula. As time passed, it became apparent that his excellent phenylalanine control was not due to residual phenylalanine hydroxylase

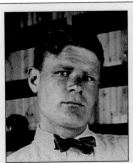

L. Emmett Holt, Jr., M.D. (1895-1975) trained in pediatrics under Howland. Beginning in 1944, Holt carried out studies of amino acid requirements in adults and infants at the New York Medical Center. Quantitative requirements for each of the essential amino acids were determined for young infants. It was discovered that histidine, non-essential in the adult, was essential in the infant. These studies were extended to infants with phenylketonuria and histidinemia. Holt was the first to apply stable isotopes in the study of amino acid requirements. Snyderman, S.E. *Amino Acid Requirements in History of Pediatrics 1850-1950* ed by B.L. Nichols, A Ballabriga and N. Kretchmer Raven Press, NY. 1991, 211-218. (Photo courtesy of NLM)

activity but to meticulous adherence to the prescribed diet. Since some whole protein is required for infants with PKU it is possible to use breast milk as a source. Unfortunately, the necessity to mix formula and adhere to a prescribed amount of phenylalanine removes much of the convenience and spontaneity of nursing and our families have not had a great deal of success with it.

Maternal PKU

The harmful effects of PKU are not limited to those who inherit the disease directly. Retrospective surveys indicated that maternal phenylalanine concentrations >20 mg/dl during pregnancy were associated with an increased frequency of fetal complications, including intrauterine growth retardation, microcephaly, mental retardation and a high incidence of heart defects.[45] The best chance for a pregnant woman with PKU to have a healthy baby is for strict dietary control of phenylalanine concentration, from preconception throughout the pregnancy. Offspring of mothers whose phenylalanine levels are above 600 micromol/L (10mg/dL) are at risk for damage.[46, 47]

A 24-year old married woman with PKU, diagnosed by newborn screen and treated with a phenylalanine-restricted diet, came for preconceptional counseling. She had remained on her diet into adulthood but followed a

*"relaxed" phenylalanine intake, maintaining phenylala-
nine levels in the 15 to 17 mg/dL range. After counseling
about the possible effects of maternal PKU on the fetus and
the need for very strict phenylalanine control, requiring
much more vigilance than she was currently practicing, she
began a strict diet, designed to maintain her serum phenylalanine around 4 to 5 mg/dL. She achieved her phenylalanine goal, conceived, and maintained serum phenylalanine
in the 2 to 6 mg/dL range on weekly
specimens throughout the pregnancy.
Serial ultrasound examination of the
fetus showed normal growth and no
evidence of cardiac disease. She delivered at term and her baby had no dys-
morphic features, no cardiac disease
and had growth parameters all at the
25th to 50th percentiles for age.*

Comment

Pregnancy is a time of high motivation and it is impressive that some
women with below average IQs have
succeeded in the very burdensome
dietary restriction needed to optimize chances for a healthy baby. The
final answer on subtle school problems in the offspring of women with
PKU is not in yet, but it is clear that
anything less than scrupulous dietary
control portends a poor outcome for
the baby. This is a different scenario
than in maternal diabetes, where
both mother and fetus are at risk from casual control.
The risk of poor phenylalanine control is borne solely
by the baby. The results are encouraging, but demonstrate a need for alternative treatment strategies for
PKU, even in view of the success of newborn screening
and diet in preventing mental retardation in affected
children.

Galactosemia

Classic galactosemia is a defect in carbohydrate metabolism in which galactose, a component of the milk
sugar, lactose, cannot be converted to glucose, the
form in which it is utilized by the body.

*I had been working on improv-
ing the physical (organoleptic)
properties of semi-synthetic diets.
Diets are a mainstay of treatment for inborn errors of metabolism which modifies the
environment of the homozygous
affected proband – a form of
treatment named euphenic by
Joshua Lederberg. Donough
O'Brien commented to me after
my publication of an article in
the NEJM: "Sorry to hear about
the attack of organoleptics so
soon after you had recovered
from euphenia."*

Charles R. Scriver,
OC, MDCM, FRS
The McGill University -
Montreal Children's
Research Institute
Montreal, Quebec, Canada

Galactosemia was first described by von Reus in
1908.[48] Mason and Turner provided the first detailed
description of the syndrome.[49] Their patient failed to
gain weight, had hepatosplenomegaly, jaundice, albu-
minuria and mellituria. The urinary sugar was galactose; the infant improved markedly on a lactose-free
formula. Schwarz and associates[50] demonstrated that
red cells also metabolize galactose and that red cells of
affected persons accumulate galac-
tose-1-phosphate after ingestion of
milk or galactose. These observations suggested that the enzyme
defect was in subsequent metabolism of galactose-1-phosphate. The
biochemical defect was shown to be
a marked deficiency in galactose-1-
phosphate uridyl transferase
(GALT), the enzyme catalyzing the
second step in the pathway.[51]
Although the liver is the major site
of galactose-glucose interconversion,
the transferase enzyme is expressed
in all tissues. Enzyme activity in circulating erythrocytes provides an
accessible source of activity for
screening or quantitation.

Galactosemia is inherited as an
autosomal recessive trait. The
human transferase gene has been
cloned and sequenced by Leslie et
al[52] and a number of mutations
identified.[53]

The galactosemic infant may appear normal at birth,
but symptoms begin after exposure to galactose.
Almost all infants will exhibit failure to thrive and prolonged jaundice. Feeding difficulties, vomiting and
diarrhea are common. Early coagulopathy may produce a picture similar to necrotizing enterocolitis.
Cataracts may be present but will often be missed
unless specifically looked for. There is a high frequency
of neonatal deaths due to *E. coli* sepsis.[54]

Diagnosis

Symptomatic infants with galactosemia may have
indirect hyperbilirubinemia and hypoglycemia. Urine

may have reducing substances present if collected soon after presentation, but urine galactose quickly disappears after galactose is withdrawn from the diet. Generalized aminoaciduria will be present, but does not distinguish galactosemia from other metabolic liver diseases such as tyrosinemia. The most reliable diagnostic tool is assay of erythrocytes for transferase activity.[55] Patients with classical galactosemia have no detectable activity; heterozygous parents have no clinical symptoms but have approximately half the normal transferase activity.[56] Rare patients with clinical symptoms have variant forms of the enzyme with measurable activity in the range of 10 to 20% of normal.[57] Demonstration of accumulation of galactose-1-phosphate in red cells reinforces the diagnosis and is useful in monitoring the progress of treatment.[58]

Screening for galactosemia, carried out on all newborns in 43 in states/territories of the United States[59] and in many other countries,[60] has greatly reduced the mortality and morbidity associated with the disease. Caution must be exercised in interpreting results in infants who are transfused to ameliorate hyperbilirubinemia. Transfusion of red cells may raise the transferase level into the measurable range but will not completely normalize GALT activity. Tests carried out on dried blood spots collected from infants prior to hospital discharge reveal transferase deficiency[61] or metabolite accumulation.[62, 63] Babies with galactosemia may be symptomatic before the results of screening are available. A suspicious test for galactosemia in an infant whose spitting up disappears after a switch from cow milk-based formula to soy-based formula should identify infants requiring follow-up testing. Prenatal diagnosis can be made by assay of the transferase enzyme in chorionic villi or cultured amniotic fluid cells, and by galactitol estimations in amniotic fluid.[64]

Preventive Therapy

Galactose ingestion by affected infants can be fatal; removal of the offending carbohydrate from the diet brings about dramatic recovery. Early suspicion and withdrawal of galactose from the diet may prevent progression to frank cirrhosis. Exchange transfusion may be an appropriate emergency measure in the jaundiced and toxic galactosemic baby.[65]

Dietary Changes - Dietary Needs

The prescribed treatment for galactosemia is immediate removal from the diet of foods that contain lactose and other oligosaccharides incorporating galactose. The goal is then to provide sufficient energy and nutrients for normal growth and development. Nutrient requirements of children with galactosemia are the same as for unaffected children.

Compositions of commercially available products that are suitable for infants with galactosemia are shown in the Appendix. Foods to which lactose or milk solids are added should be strictly avoided. This information can be difficult to obtain. Careful attention to labels showing additives can prevent inadvertent feeding of lactose and galactose. Antibiotics and other medications that have lactose as filler or sweetener must be avoided. The effectiveness of restricting dietary galactose can be monitored by measuring galactose-1-phosphate in erythrocytes and urinary galactitol excretion.

Galactose restriction during pregnancy in heterozygous women has been advised, although there is no evidence of benefit from the restriction.[66] Even when maternal lactose intake is restricted, affected infants accumulate galactose-1-phosphate in cord blood.[66, 67] Pregnancy in women with classical galactosemia is rare, since many will have ovarian failure. A homozygous woman during pregnancy showed increased galactose-1-phosphate in red cells, increased urinary galactitol and large amounts of lactose, in spite of a galactose-free diet throughout.[68] Galactose in the mother arose from de novo synthesis of lactose.

How Are We Doing

Early diagnosis and prompt treatment by feeding a lactose-galactose free diet prevents or reverses the initial clinical complications. However, the long-term response to dietary intervention in galactosemia has not been uniformly satisfactory in preventing intellectual and language deficits. Komrower found below-average intelligence in early-diagnosed and well-treated patients.[69] Fishler et al found intellectual function within normal range in children identified and treated prior to one month of age (mean IQ 95) or between one and three months (mean IQ 91).[70] Visual-perceptual difficulties and problems with social adjustment were described by both investigators. Waisbren et al found significantly lower verbal than performance score in a group of seven early-treated patients with galactosemia, identified initially through newborn screening.[71] All the children had delays or early speech difficulties and subsequent language disorders. Gitzelmann and Steinmann confirmed that early-treated patients made reasonable though suboptimal progress, were prone to speech defects and had visual-perceptual deficits in spite of strict early treatment.[72] Central nervous system dysfunction and intellectual deficits have been confirmed in large retrospective studies.[73, 74] In these studies there was no significant relation between IQ and age of initiating treatment. Female patients with galactosemia have a high incidence of acquired ovarian failure in spite of dietary galactose restriction.[75]

Intrauterine effects of galactosemia may account for the low birthweight and cataracts found in infants with galactosemia, and the problems in mental development, speech, and ovarian function may originate prenatally.

The long-term outcome of galactosemic patients is cause for concern. Initial assumptions that dietary intervention would result in correction of the problems proved erroneous. Many questions need to be answered to plan a strategy for improving outcome. In defense, many lives have been saved by lactose restriction during the last 50 years.

> *There are many other things to be considered besides defects in proteins.*
> *Primary Health Care Pioneer*
> *The Selected Works of*
> *Dr. Cicely D. Williams*
> Naomi Baumslag, Editor
> World Federation of
> Public Health Associations
> and UNICEF

A two-day-old term infant was transferred to the regional neonatal intensive care unit for suspected necrotizing enterocolitis. The baby had no birth asphyxia and had been in the normal nursery until the second day when vomiting, bloody diarrhea and abdominal distention began. She was evaluated, treated for sepsis and given intravenous fluids. After several days she was fed a cow milk-based formula and once again developed diarrhea. A switch to a soy-based formula led to resolution of symptoms. On the eighth day of life, the newborn screen report was returned, highly suspicious for galactosemia.

Comment

This baby had many of the symptoms of NEC, but none of the typical risk factors. Her symptoms resolved quickly after withdrawing lactose. Without a high degree of clinical suspicion or the newborn screening test, she would have remained without symptoms on soy formula until later consequences of undiagnosed galactosemia occurred. She had cataracts on slit lamp exam, but they were not noted until the newborn screen result returned.

Maple Syrup Urine Disease

This inborn error of metabolism derived its interesting name from the odor of the urine, which is reminiscent of maple syrup. In 1954, Menkes, Hurst and Craig,[76] in a paper entitled "New syndrome: progressive familial infantile cerebral dysfunction associated with unusual urinary substances," described a family in which four siblings died in the newborn period. Dancis and others found increased amounts of leucine, isoleucine and valine were present in blood and urine of an affected child, together with keto acids derived from these amino acids.[77] In a subsequent study of the same child, the hydroxy acids were identified.[78] The disease as first described occurred in early infancy and most cases the infants died before four weeks of age.

Maple syrup urine disease (MSUD) is the prototype of disorders of organic acid metabolism, which have the common feature of presenting as a metabolic emergency in the newborn. The symptoms and signs are not unlike those of neonatal sepsis in that metabolic acidosis is present and there is central nervous system dysfunction. The CNS dysfunction is out of proportion to the observed acidosis.

MSUD is a spectrum of diseases resulting from different mutations that impair the mitochondrial branched-chain alpha-keto acid dehydrogenase complex. The initial transamination of the branched-chain amino acids (BCAA), valine, isoleucine and leucine, proceeds normally to yield the corresponding alpha-keto acids; the second step, oxidative decarboxylation of the keto acids,

Age	ILE (mg/kg)	LEU (mg/kg)	VAL (mg/kg)	Protein (gm/kg)	Energy (kcal/kg)
0-3 mo	60-70	90-110	70-85	2.5-3.5	120
4-6 mo	40-60	65-90	50-70	2.5-3.5	110
7-12 mo	30-40	50-65	40-50	2.5-3.0	105
1-3 yr	20-35	35-50	25-35	2.0-2.5	100
Total/Day					
Age	mg	mg	mg	g	kcal
4-6 yr	240-300	350-500	280-380	35	1700
7-10 yr	240-400	400-600	280-450	40	2400

Table 2: Recommended daily intakes of nutrients for children with Maple Syrup Urine Disease. (Adapted from Berry[19] and Elsas and Acosta.[20])

is defective.[79] The consequence of the defect is accumulation of BCAA and their corresponding keto acids in blood, cerebrospinal fluid and urine. In general there is no detectable activity of the branched-chain keto acid dehydrogenase complex in the classic form of MSUD. Variant forms have been described with reduced levels of decarboxylase activity compared to normal.

Diagnosis

Infants with classical MSUD are normal at birth; BCAA concentrations in cord blood are also normal, but rise during the first 24 hours to diagnostic levels.[80, 81] By the fourth to fifth day, affected infants become listless, refuse to eat and vomit.[82] This progresses to loss of reflexes, alternating hypertonicity and hypotonicity, convulsions and irregular respiration. Untreated infants are first lethargic, then comatose. Milder variants may have clinical symptoms only after a protein load or febrile illness. Tests for MSUD, included in a number of large-scale newborn screening programs, reveal an incidence of 1 in 200,000 to 300,000.[83] In spite of its rarity in the general population, an incidence of 1 in 176 newborns is found in the inbred Mennonite community of Lancaster, Pennsylvania.[84] Early diagnosis of classical MSUD is most likely to be based on recognitions of early clinical signs and symptoms. If diagnosis is delayed beyond one to two weeks of age, those who

survive the acute neonatal period show severe mental retardation and cerebral palsy. When the patient presents with clinical symptoms, the urine 2,4-dinitrophenylhydrazine (DNPH) test for keto acids is useful for preliminary screening. Diagnosis is confirmed by quantitative amino acid analysis and urinary organic acid determinations, followed by demonstrating deficiency in decarboxylation of BCAA in leukocytes or cultured skin fibroblasts.[85] Measuring alpha-keto acid decarboxylase activity in cultured amniotic fluid cells, or direct analysis of tissue from chorionic villus biopsy, can be used for prenatal diagnosis.[86, 87]

Preventive Therapy

Emergency treatment may be required for infants with acute symptoms; peritoneal dialysis[88] or hemodialysis[89] produce dramatic, temporary improvement. Use of BCAA-free formula given by nasogastric tube or parenteral nutrition hastens resolution of metabolic decompensation.[90] Acute episodes may be triggered by infections, vaccinations, surgery or a sudden increase in protein intake. Death can occur.[91, 92] Supportive insulin therapy may be helpful in critically ill patients.[93] Emergency measures and a restricted diet may be necessary during acute episodes in patients with variant MSUD, similar to that used in patients with the classical form. Long-term treatment is based on dietary restriction of BCAA.

Precipitate	Time to Appe	Action to Take	Ketone
Trace	60 sec	None	- (Neg)
Slight	30-45 sec	Watch Patient	- Repeat test in 12 hrs
Moderate	30 sec	Increase fluids Decrease BCAA Repeat in 6 hrs	+/- (Trace)
Strong	10 sec	Omit BCAA Repeat every 12 hrs until DNPH is **Slight** and Ketone is **Neg**	+++

Table 3: Interpretation of Dinitrophenyhlhydrazine (DNPH) and Ketone tests. (*Ketostix, Ames Division, Miles Laboratory, Elkhart, IN.)*

Dietary Changes - Dietary Needs

The dietary management of MSUD is complicated because the intake of three essential amino acids, leucine, isoleucine and valine must be carefully regulated. Enough of each of these amino acids must be included in the diet to meet needs for growth. Excess of any one of the three will permit the reappearance of symptoms and signs of MSUD. Similarly, deficiency of any one of the three can bring about tissue catabolism with consequent accumulation of the other two.

Snyderman et al devised the first diets for treatment of MSUD that consisted of mixtures of crystalline L-amino acids, omitting leucine, isoleucine and valine.[82] Vitamins, minerals, fat and carbohydrate were added, and the requirements for BCAA were provided by small amounts of natural foods in the form of milk, gelatin and low-protein fruits and vegetables. Commercial special medical foods have been developed based on these principles. The nutritive composition of commercially available dietary products free of branched-chain amino acids for treating children with MSUD are shown in the Appendix.

The selected formula should be prescribed to furnish 2.5 to 3.0 g/kg protein equivalent. The requirements for BCAA (Table 2) are met from a natural protein source.[94, 95] Infant formula or, for older children, low-protein foods, are added once plasma BCAA are close to normal range. In our experience, it is preferred that the RDA for protein come from the amino-acid modified formula. The isoleucine and valine content in natural food, especially cow's milk, is low relative to leucine, and supplementing these as free L-amino acids may be necessary. A trial of thiamine (50 to 300mg/day) is advisable, though infants with the classic form of MSUD are rarely responsive.[96]

Plasma amino acid concentrations should be measured at least weekly during the first months of life. The objective is to maintain BCAA in the range of two to three times normal values. Home management is aided by daily monitoring of urinary keto acids using the 2,4-dinitrophenylhydrazine reaction. Keto acid excretion is estimated by the time interval at which yellow turbidity appeared after adding the reagent to urine (Table 3).

How Are We Doing

The long-term outcome of classic MSUD is uncertain; both mental retardation and cerebral palsy are common. A summary of outcome following treatment in more than 150 patients with classic MSUD indicated that approximately one-fifth of the classic MSUD patients died; one-third had IQ scores >90; and one-third had IQ scores between 70 and 90.[85] Verbal scores were consistently higher than performance scores. Important influences on intellectual and neurologic outcome in children with MSUD were the length of time after birth they were exposed to elevated branched-chain amino and keto acid concentrations, and the long-term biochemical control.[95] A delay in diagnosis of more than 10 to 14 days was associated with neurologic signs. A relaxed treatment protocol, allowing concentrations of branched-chain amino and keto acids to rise to five to six times normal means (rather than the recommended two to three times normal), was followed for approximately ten years.[96] Chronic mild to moderate elevations were associated with dysmyelinating changes in brain, demonstrating the need for continued strict adherence to dietary modifications.

The basis for the cerebral dysfunction in patients with MSUD has not been determined. Among the theories proposed for pathogenesis are decreased energy sources for the brain, decreased neurotransmitters and interruption of myelin production. Keto-iso-caproic acid, derived from leucine is thought to be the principal neurotoxic metabolite.[96]

Patients with MSUD present complications in diagnosis, treatment and long-term management. Childhood illnesses, minor in a normal child, can become major crises. Careful attention to formula intakes may abort some crises, but careful monitoring is necessary to assure that improvement is taking place. Dietary treatment has been life-saving for affected children. Nevertheless, many children with MSUD have severe handicaps, both physically and neurologically. Preventive approaches should continue to focus on early diagnosis and treatment, genetic counseling and prenatal monitoring.

A nine-day-old baby born to Mennonite parents presented with a two-day history of poor feeding. In the emergency room the baby was hypertonic and poorly responsive to physical examination and needle sticks. Poor ventilatory effort prompted endotracheal intubation and ventilatory support. No improvement in clinical status was seen after two days of intravenous fluids containing 5% dextrose and antibiotics. At eleven days of age, results of quantitative amino acid analysis of the baby's serum, drawn at admission, were finished in the reference laboratory, showing a picture diagnostic of MSUD. The infant was treated with nasogastric administration of a formula free of branched-chain amino acids, supplemented by valine and isoleucine. Extra calories were provided by glucose and intravenous lipids given through a centrally placed venous catheter. The leucine level decreased to nearly normal levels in three days, and the neurologic status improved.

Comment

Several points can be made from this case. First, and most obvious, not all illness in babies is due to sepsis. Second, populations that are highly inbred have a higher incidence of recessive disorders in general, and a higher degree of clinical suspicion should be invoked when presented with a sick infant from one of these groups. In Mennonites from two counties in Pennsylvania the prevalence of MSUD is about 1:176 newborns. (See reference 84.) Third, when suspicion is high, a phone call to the reference lab can often result in your specimen being analyzed on a priority basis, so the answer is returned faster. Last, the induction of an anabolic state is of great importance in reversing the critical status in MSUD and other inborn errors. Infusion of 5% dextrose is not sufficient; high rates of glucose infusion, supplemented by insulin if necessary, and specific metabolic formulas can be highly effective.

Historical Perspective...

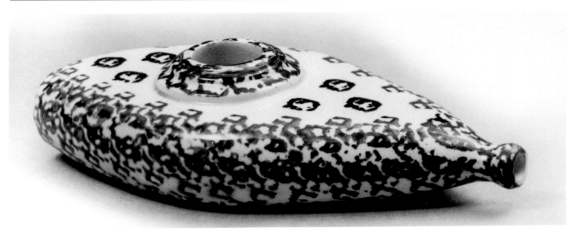

English feeding bottle, blue transfer decoration, circa 1800.

References

1. Folling A. Uber Ausscheidung von Phenylbrenztraubasure in den Harn als Stoffwechselanomalie in Verbindung mit Imbezillitat. *Z Physiol Chem.* 1934;227:169-176.

2. Folling A. Uber das vorkommen von L-Phenylalanine in Harn und Blut bei Imbeczillitas phenylpyruvica. *Z Physiol Chem.* 1938;254:115-116.

3. Penrose LS. Inheritance of phenylpyruvic amentia (phenylketonuria). *Lancet.* 1935;2:192-194.

4. Jervis GA. The genetics of phenylpyruvic oligophrenia. (a contribution to the study of the influence of heredity on mental defect.) *J Ment Sci.* 1939;85:719-762.

5. Monroe TA. Phenylketonuria. Data on forty-seven British families. *Ann Eugenics.* 1947;14:60-88.

6. Jervis GA. Phenylpyruvic oligophrenia: deficiency of phenylalanine oxidizing system. *Proc Soc Exp Biol Med.* 1953;82:514-515.

7. DiLella AG, Kwok SCM, Ledley FD, Marvit J, Woo SLC. Molecular structure and polymorphic map of human phenylalanine hydroxylase gene. *Biochemistry.* 1986;25:742-749.

8. Okano Y, Eisensmith RC, Guttler F, et al. Molecular basis of phenotypic heterogeneity in phenylketonuria. *N Engl J Med.* 1991;324:1232-1238.

9. Lidsky AS, Law ML, Morse HG, et al. Regional mapping of phenylketonuria hydroxylase gene and the phenylketonuria locus in the human genome. *Proc Natl Acad Sci USA.* 1985;82:6221-6225.

10. Eisensmith RC, Woo SLC. Molecular basis of phenylketonuria: Mutations and polymorphisms in the phenylalanine hydroxylase gene. *Human Mutat.* 1992;1:13-23.

11. Salter M, Knowles RG, Pogson CI. Quantification of the importance of individual steps in the control of aromatic amino acid metabolism. *Biochem J.* 1986;234:635.

12. Berry HK, Porter LJ. Newborn Screening for Phenylketonuria. *Pediatrics.* 1982;70:505-506.

13. Berry HK, Umbarger B, Sutherland B. Testing of newborn siblings in phenylketonuric families. *JAMA.* 1964;189:641.

14. Guthrie RA, Susi A. A simple phenylalanine method of detection of phenylketonuria in large populations of newborn infants. *Pediatrics.* 1963;32:338-343.

15. Medical Research Council Working Party on Phenylketonuria. Recommendations on the dietary management of phenylketonuria. *Brit Med J.* 1993;306:115-119.

16. Berry HK. Hyperphenylalaninemias and tyrosinemias. *Clin Perinatol.* 1976;3:15-40.

17. Armstrong MD, Tyler FH. Studies on Phenylketonuria. 1. Restrice Phenylalanine Intake in Phenylketonuria. *J Clin Invest.* 1955;34:565-580.

18. Woolf LI, Griffiths R, Moncrieff A. Treatment of phenylketonuria with a diet low in phenylalanine. *Brit Med J.* 1955;1:57-64.

19. Bickel H, Gerrard J, Hickmans EM. Influence of phenylalanine intake on phenylketonuria. *Lancet.* 1953;11:812-813.

20. Knox WE, An evaluation of the treatment of phenylketonuria with diets low in phenylalanine. *Pediatrics.* 1960;16:1-11.

21. Elsas LJ, Acosta PB. Nutrition support of inherited metabolic disease. In: Shils ME, Young VR, eds. *Modern Nutrition in Health and Disease.* Seventh ed. Philadelphia: Lea & Febiger; 1988.

22. Berry HK, Sutherland BS, Guest GM. Chemical and clinical observations during treatment of children with phenylketonuria. *Pediatrics.* 1965;21:929.

23. Shortland D, Smith I, Frances DEM, et al. Amino acid and protein requirements in a preterm infant with classic phenylketonuria. *Arch Dis Child.* 1985;60:262-265.

24. Rubin MI. Deficiency syndromes or hypophenylalaninemias. In: Cohen BE, Rubin MI, Szeinberg A, eds. *International Symposium on Phenylketonuria and Allied Disorders.* Tel Aviv: Translators' Pool; 1971;166-199.

25. Sherman JD, Greenfield JB, Ingall D. Reversible bone marrow vacuolizations in phenylketonuria. *N Engl J Med.* 1964;270:810-814.

26. Rouse BM. Phenylalanine deficiency syndrome. *J Pediatr.* 1966;69:246-249.

27. Feinberg SB, Fisch RO. Roentgenologic findings in growing long bones in phenylketonuria: a preliminary study. *Radiology.* 1962;78:394-398.

28. Murdock MM, Holman GN. Roentgenologic bone changes in phenylketonuria. *Am J Dis Child.* 1964;107:523-532.

29. Hackney IM, Hanley WB, Davidson W, Lindsao L. Phenylketonuria: mental development, behavior and termination of low phenylalanine diet. *J Pediatr.* 1968; 72:646-655.

30. Hudson FP, Mordaunt VL, Leahy I. Evaluation of treatment begun in first three months of life in 184 cases of phenylketonuria. *Arch Dis Child.* 1970;45:5-12.

31. Hanley WB, Lindsao L, Davidson W, et al. Malnutrition with early treatment of phenylketonuria. *Pediatr Res.* 1970;4:318-327.

32. Smith I, Beasley MG, Ades AE. Effect on intelligence of relaxing the low phenylalanine diet in phenylketonuria. *Arch Dis Child.* 1990;65:311-316.

33. Knox WE. Phenylketonuria. In: Stanbury JB, Fredrickson DS, Wyngaarden JB, eds. *The Metabolic Basis of Inherited Disease.* New York: McGraw-Hill Book Co; 1960:331.

34. Scriver CR, Kaufman S, Eisensmith RC, Woo SLC. The hyperphenylalaninemias. In: Scriver CR, Beaudet AL, Sly WS, Valle D, eds. *The Metabolic and Molecular Bases of Inherited Disease.* Vol I, Seventh ed. New York: McGraw Hill Book Co; 1995:27;1043.

35. Smith I, Lobascher ME, Stevenson JE, Wolff OH, Schmidt H, Grubel-Kaiser S, Bickel H. Effect of stopping low-phenylalanine diet on intellectual progress of children with phenylketonuria. *Brit Med J.* 1978;11:723-726.

36. Brunner RL, Jordan MK, Berry HK. Early-treated phenylketonuria: neuropsychologic consequences. *J Pediatr.* 1983;102:831-835.

37. Seashore MR, Friedman E, Novelly RA, Bapat V. Loss of intellectual function in children with phenylketonuria after relaxation of dietary phenylalanine restriction. *Pediatrics.* 1985;75:226-232.

38. Ris MD, Williams Se, Hunt MM, et al. Early-treated phenylketonuria: Adult neuropsychologic outcome. *J Pediatr.* 1994;124:388-392.

39. Smith I, Beasley M, Ades EA. Intelligence and quality of dietary treatment in phenylketonuria. *Arch Dis Child.* 1990;65:472-478.

40. Crome L, Pare CMB. Phenylketonuria-a review and a report of the pathological findings in four cases. *J Mental Sci.* 1960;106:862-883.

41. Crome L, Tymms V, Woolf LI. A chemical investigation of the defects of myelination in phenylketonuria. *J Neurol Neurosurg Psychiat.* 1962;25:148.

42. Bick U, Fahrendorf G, Ludolph AC, et al. Disturbed myelination in patients with untreated hyperphenylalaninemia: evaluation with magnetic resonance imaging. *Eur J Pediatr.* 1991;150:185-189.

43. Thompson AF, Smith I, Brenton D, et al. Neurological deterioration in young adults with phenylketonuria. *Lancet.* 1990;336:602-605.

44. Pietz J, Benninger C, Schmidt H, et al. Long-term development of intelligence (IQ) and EEG in 34 children with phenylketonuria treated early. *Eur J Pediatr.* 1988; 147:361-367.

45. Lenke RR, Levy HK. Maternal phenylketonuria and hyperphenylalaninemia: an international survey of the outcome of untreated and treated pregnancies. *N Engl J Med.* 1993;303:1202-1208.

46. Koch R, Levy HL, Matalon R, et al. The North American Collaborative Study of maternal phenylketonuria: status report 1993. *Am J Dis Child.* 1993;147:1224-1230.

47. Levy HL, Matalon R, Kamath S. *Maternal PKU Collaborative Study: Midwest region newsletter.* January, 1995.

48. von Reus A. Zuckerausscheidung im Sauglingsalter. *Wien Med Wchnschr.* 1908;58:799-803.

49. Mason HH, Turner ME. Chronic galactosemia: report of a case with studies on carbohydrates. *Am J Dis Child.* 1935;50:359-374.

50. Schwarz V, Golberg L, Komrower GM, Holzel A. Some disturbances of erythrocyte metabolism in galactosemia. *Biochem J.* 1956;62:34-40.

51. Isselbacher KJ, Anderson EP, Kurahashi K, Kalkar HM. Congenital galactosemia, a single enzymatic block in galactose metabolism. *Science.* 1956;123:635-636.

52. Levy HK, Sepe SJ, Shish Ve, et al. Sepsis due to Escherichia coli in neonates with galactosemia. *N Engl J Med.* 1977;197:823.

53. Anderson EP, Kalckar HM, Kurahashi K, Isselbacher KJ. A specific enzymatic assay for the diagnosis of congenital galactosemia. *J Lab Clin Med.* 1957;50:569.

54. Donnell GN, Bergren WR, Bretthaurer MS, Hansen RG. The enzymatic expression of heterozygosity in families of children with galactosemia. *Pediatrics.* 1960;25:572.

55. Segal S, Rogers S, Holtzapple PG. Liver galactose-1-phosphate uridyl transferase. Activity in normal and galactosemic subjects. *J Clin Invest.* 1971;50:500-506.

56. Donnell GN, Bergren WR, Perry G, Koch R. Galactose-1-phosphate in galactosemia. *Pediatrics.* 1963;31:802-810.

57. Leslie ND, Immerman EB, Flach JE, et al. The human galactose-1-phosphate uridyl transferase gene. *Genomics.* 1992;14:474.

58. Segal S, Berry GT. Disorders of Galactose Metabolism. In: Scriver CR, Beaudet AL, Sly WS, Valle D, eds. *The Metabolic and Moelcular Bases of Interited Disease.* Vol I, Seventh ed. New York: McGraw-Hill Book Co; 1995: chap 25.

59. Newborn Screening Committee, the Council of Regional Networks for Genetic Services (CORN). *National Newborn Screening Report-1991.* New York; CORN: July, 1964.

60. Levy HL. Screening fof galactosemia. In: Burman D, Hotlon JB, Pennock CA, eds. *Inherited Disorders of Carbohydrate Metabolism.* Lancaster: MTP Press; 1980:133.

61. Beutler E, Baluda MD. A simple spot screening test for galactosemia. *J Lab Clin Med.* 1966;68:137-141.

62. Paigen K, Pacholec F, Levy HL. A new method of screening for inherited disorders of galactose metabolism. *J Lab Clin Med.* 1982;99:895.

63. Hill G, O'Reilly D, Robertson EA. A simple screening test for galactosemia based on accumulation of galactose and galactose-1-phosphate. In: Naruse H, Irie M, eds. *Neonatal Screening. Proceedings of the internationals ymposium of neonatal screening for inborn errors of metabolism.* Amsterdam/Oxford/Princeton: Excerpta Medica; 1983:252.

64. Holton JB, Allen JT, Gillett MG. Prenatal diagnosis of disorders of galactose metabolism. *J Inherit Metab Dis.* 1989;12(Suppl 1):202-206.

65. Haworth JC, Coodin FJ. Liver failure in galactosemia successfully treated by exchange blood transfusion. *Can J Med Assoc.* 1971;105:301-312.

66. Irons M, Levy HL, Pueschel S, Castree K. Accumulation of galactose-1-phosphate in the galactosemic fetus despite maternal milk avoaidance. *J Pediatr.* 1985;107: 261-263.

67. Donnell GN, Koch R, Fishler K, Mg WG. Clinical aspects of galactosemia. In: Burman D, Holton JB, Pennock CA, eds. *Inherited Disorders of Carbohydrate Metabolism.* Lancaster: MTP Press; 1980:103-115.

68. Brivet M, Raymond JP, Konopka P, et al. Effect of lactation in a mother with galactosemia. *J Pediatr.* 1989; 115:280-282.

69. Komrower GM, Lee DH. Long-term follow-up of galactosaemia. *Arch Dis Child.* 1970;45:367-373.

70. Fishler K, Koch R, Donnell GN, Wenz E. Developmental aspects of galactosemia from infancy to childhood. *Clin Pediatr.* 1980;19:38-44.

71. Waisbren SE, Norman TR, Schnell RR, Levy HL. Speech and language deficits in early treated children with galactosemia. *J Pediatr.* 1983;102:75-77.

72. Gitzelmann R, Steinmann B. Galactosemia: how does long-term treatment change the outcome? *Enzyme.* 1984; 32:37-46.

73. Waggoner DD, Buist NRM, Donnell GN. Long-term prognosis in galactosemia: results of a survey of 350 cases. *J Inherit Metab Dis.* 1991;13:802-818.

74. Schweitzer S, Shin Y, Jakobs C, Brodehl J. Long-term outcome in 134 patients with galactosaemia. *Eur J Pediatr.* 1993;152:36.

75. Kaufman FR, Kogut MD, Donnell GN, et al. Hypergonadotropic hypogonadism in female patients with galactosemia. *N Engl J Med.* 1981;304:994-998.

76. Menkes JH, Hurst PL, Craig JM. New syndrome: progressive familial infantile cerebral dysfunction associated with unusual urinary substances. *Pediatrics.* 1954;14:462-467.

77. Dancis J, Levitz M, Westall RG. Maple syrup urine disease: branched chain keto-aciduria. *Pediatrics.* 1960; 25:72-79.

78. Patrick AD. Maple Syrup Urine Disease: *Arch Dis Child.* 1961;36:269-272.

79. Dancis J, Hutzler J, Levitz M. The diagnosis of maple syrup rine disease (branched-chain ketoaciduria) by the in-vitro study of the peripheral leukocyte. *Pediatrics.* 1963;32:234-238.

80. DiGeorge AM, Rezvani I, Garibaldi LR, Schwartz M. Prospective study of maple-syrup-urine disease for the first four days of life. *N Engl J Med.* 1982;307:1492-1495.

81. Wendel U, Lombeck I, Bremer JH. Maple-syrup-urine disease. *N Engl J Med.* 1983;308:1100-1101.

82. Snyderman SE, Norton PM, Roitman E, Holt LE Jr. Maple syrup urine disease, with particular reference to dietotherapy. *Pediatrics.* 1964;34:454-472.

83. Collaborative study on the frequency of inborn errors of metabolism. *Humangenetic.* 1975;30:273-286.

84. Marshall L, diGeorge A. Maple syrup urine disease in the Old Order Mennonites (Abstract). *Am J Hum Genet.* 1981;33:138.

85. Chuang DT, Shih VE. Disorders of branched chain amino acid and keto acid metabolism In: Scriver CR, Beaudet AL, Sly WS, Valle D, eds. *The Metabolic and Molecular Bases of Inherited Disease.* Vol. I, Seventh ed. New York: McGraw-Hill Book Co; 1995:Chap 34.

86. Wendel U, Rudiger HW, Passarge E, Mikkelsen M. Maple syrup urine disease: rapid prenatal diagnosis by enzyme assay. *Humangenetic.* 1973;19:127-128.

87. Kleijer WJ, Horsman D, Mancini GM, et al. First-trimester diagnosis of maple syrup urine disease on intact chorionic villi. *N Engl J Med.* 1985;313:1608.

88. Wendel U, Becker K, Przyrembel H, et al. Peritoneal dialysis in maple-syrup urine disease: studies on branched-chain amino and keto acids. *Eur J Pediatr.* 1980;134:57-63.

89. Rutledge SL, Hvens PL, Haymond MW, et al. Neonatal hemodialysis: effective therapy for the encephalopathy of inborn errors of metabolism. *J Pediatr.* 1990;116:125-128.

90. Berry GT, Heidenreich R, Kaplan P, et al. Branched-chain amino acid-free parenteral nutrition in the treatment of acute metabolic decompensation in patients with maple syrup urine disease. *N Engl J Med.* 1991;324:175-179.

91. Riviello JJ Jr, Rezvani I, DiGeorge AM, Foley CM. Cerebral edema causing death in children with maple syrup urine disease. *J Pediatr.* 1991;119:42-45.

92. Levin MI, Scheimann A, Lewis RA, Beaudet AL. Cerebral edema in maple syrup urine disease. *J Pediatr.* 1993;122:167.

93. Wendel U, Langenbeck U, Lombeck I, Bremer HJ. Maple syrup urine disease - therapeutic use of insulin in catabolic states. *Eur J Pediatr.* 1982;139:172-175.

94. Berry HK. Special and therapeutic formulas for inborn errors of metabolism. In: Tsang RC, Nichols BL,eds. *Nutrition During Infancy.* Chap 21. Philadelphia: Hanley & Belfus Inc; 1988.

95. Elsas LJ, Acosta PB. Nutrition support of inherited metabolic diseases. In: Shils Me, Young VR, eds. *Modern Nutrition in Health and Disease.* Seventh ed. Philadelphia: Lea & Febiger; 1988:chap 63.

96. Fernhoff PM, Lubitz D, Danner DJ, et al. Thianmine response in maple syrup urine disease. *Pediatr Res.* 1985; 19:1011-1016.

97. Kaplan P, Mazur A, Field M, et al. Intellectual outcome in children with maple syrup urine disease. *J Pediatr.* 1991;119:46-50.

98. Treacy E, Clow CL, Reade TR, et al. Maple syrup urine disease: interrelations between branched-chain amino-, oxo- and hydroxy acids; implications for treatment; associations with CNS dysmyelination. *J Inherit Metab Dis.* 1992;15:121-135.

Recognizing and Managing Food Allergy

Stacie M. Jones M.D. and A. Wesley Burks M.D.

Department of Pediatrics,
University of Arkansas for Medical Sciences,
Little Rock, Arkansas

Reviewed by Helen K. Berry and Erkki Savidahti

Introduction

Adverse food reactions encompass a wide variety of reactions to food and food additives (Table 1). An adverse food reaction is a general term that can apply to any untoward response following the ingestion of a food or food additive.[1] These adverse reactions may be divided into two categories, food allergy (hypersensitivity) and food intolerance.

Food allergy or food hypersensitivity is an immunologic reaction resulting from the ingestion of a food or food additive. Most commonly, this reaction is a Type I, an immediate hypersensitivity reaction that is mediated by immunoglobulin E (IgE). Less frequentley these reactions can involve other non-IgE-mediated immunologic reactions. Food hypersensitivity occurs only in a very limited patient population and usually in response to a limited number of foods or food additives.

Food intolerance involves a much broader category of adverse reactions, and is non-immunologic in nature. The reactions are typically due to an abnormal physiologic response to one or possibly many foods or food additives. Food intolerance may be manifested as metabolic reactions (i.e., lactose intolerance); food toxicity (i.e., Staphylococcal food poisoning or histamine release from scromboid fish poisoning); pharmacologic properties of foods or food additives (i.e., caffeine in coffee or monosodium glutamate as a food additive); and idiosyncratic responses.

Both food hypersensitivity and food intolerance reactions occur in children less than two years of age. The importance of being able to distinguish between these two categories of adverse food reactions cannot be overstated. This distinction is important for establishing a proper diagnosis and for providing appropriate treatment.

Prevalence

While the true prevalence of food allergy is unknown, consumer surveys indicate that the public perception of the prevalence of food allergy is high.[2,3] As much as 33% of the general population believe that they, or members of their family, are allergic to at least one food.[2] The current medical literature indicates that the actual prevalence of food allergy appears involve be less than 1% of the population. Bock prospectively studied 480 children from birth until their third birthday. He noted that 133 of these children were thought to have food allergy by history, but only 8% had confirmed evidence during oral food challenge.[4] A Danish group studying 1,759 infants during the first year of life reported a 2.2% incidence of cow milk allergy alone.[5] Several well-designed studies have shown that most of these reported food allergic reactions occur during the first two years of life. Because of the discrepancies between the general public's perception and the actual incidence of food allergy, the medical community often faces a difficult task when diagnosing, educating and treating a food-allergic child.

Common Food Allergens

Foods are composed of proteins, carbohydrates and lipids. Food allergens are primarily composed of water-soluble glycoproteins with molecular weights ranging from 10,000 to 60,000 daltons.[6] These glycoproteins are largely resistant to treatment with acids, heat or proteases, thereby retaining their allergenic potential in almost all conditions.

A very small number of foods account for the most of food allergic reactions. In children, the most common food allergens are proteins found in milk,

Adverse food reaction	any untoward response following the ingestion of a food or food additive
Food allergy (hypersensitivity)	an immunologic reaction resulting from the ingestion of a food or food additive
Food intolerance	an abnormal physiologic response to an ingested food or food additive that is non-immunologic in nature

Table 1: Definition of terms.

egg, peanuts, soybeans, tree nuts, fish, shellfish and wheat (Table 2).

Cow Milk

Cow milk is generally the first foreign protein encountered by infants and is one of the most common allergens in the first year of life. Cow milk is composed of at least 20 different proteins which may cause antibody production.[7] Milk proteins are divided into two major fractions: casein and whey.[7] Casein comprises 76 to 86% of the cow milk protein and has five basic fractions.[8] Whey is primarily comprised of β-lactoglobulin, α-lactalbumin and bovine serum albumin with very small quantities of other proteins.[8] Routine pasteurization is not adequate to denature these proteins. Extreme heat processing may denature some of the milk proteins, but may only serve to change the allergenicity of others.[7]

Immunoblotting techniques have shown extensive cross-reactivity among milk proteins from cows, goats and sheep.[9] Clein found that at least 50% of individuals allergic to cow milk were also allergic to goat milk.[10]

Chicken Egg

Chicken egg is a common food allergen, especially in children younger than two years of age. Egg white possesses more allergenic potential than egg yolk.[11] Ovalbumin, ovomucoid and ovotransferrin are the major proteins in egg white.[12-15] These egg proteins remain unchanged after cooking, therefore retaining their allergenic properties in both raw and cooked form.[16] Egg-allergic children have IgE antibodies that cross-react with egg proteins from different bird species.[16]

Peanuts

Peanuts are members of the legume family. Peanuts are one of the most allergenic foods in children and adults and account for a large proportion of reported fatal and near-fatal anaphylactic reactions to ingested food antigens. Unlike milk, egg and soy sensitivity in children, peanut sensitivity is typically not lost over time and frequently remains a life-long allergy. Peanut proteins are classified as albumin and globulin, with globulins divided as arachin and conarachin.[17] Two major allergens have recently been described, Ara h 1 and Ara h 2, with molecular weights of 17,000 and 63,500 daltons, respectively.[18, 19] Peanut protein is found in many products, including flour and processed nuts, and retains its allergenicity despite extensive processing.[20] In one study, processed peanut oil could be safely ingested by 10 peanut-allergic individuals.[21] After processing, peanut oil contains no detectable peanut protein; however, in patients with severe anaphylaxis, peanut oil should still be avoided as an extra safety measure (i.e., in case of incidental contamination of the oil).

Soybeans

Soybeans, like peanuts, are members of the legume family and are commonly found in many commercially-prepared foods. Soybean proteins can cause food allergic reactions in children but rarely in adults. Four major protein fractions have been identified in soybeans, none showing more allergenicity than others.[22] Although extensive in vivo cross-reactivity can be seen among soybean allergic individuals when tested with other legumes, clinical cross-reactivity to more than one legume is rare.[23] Due to extensive processing, soybean oil, like peanut oil, has been shown to be safe in soybean-allergic patients.[24]

Tree Nuts

Tree nuts appear to be major food allergens in adults but less commonly in children. Like peanuts, these allergens frequently produce more severe, life-long reactions. Nuts commonly implicated include almonds, Brazil nuts, cashews, filberts (hazelnuts), hickory nuts, pecans, pine nuts, pistachios and walnuts. *In vivo* cross-reactivity is common among the tree nuts, but the clinical significance of these reactions is unknown.[25] Although tree nuts and peanuts come from different botanical families, patients with peanut allergy should avoid ingestion of tree nuts and vice versa. In processing tree nuts, some companies use peanuts as fillers and flavorings; therefore, these products can be contaminated with peanut protein, which would pose a risk to the peanut allergic patient.

Fish

Fish represent another group that contains allergens causing allergic food reactions in both children and adults.[26] Gad c 1 or Allergen M from codfish has been extensively studied and is known to be a major food allergen.[27] It is a heat-stable, protease-resistant glycoprotein found in the myogen fraction of the white meat of fish. In a study of pediatric and adult patients with fish allergy, predominant IgE binding was to a 12.5 kD protein in catfish, cod and snapper. This protein is similar to Gad c 1.[28] Immunologic cross-reactivity has been shown among multiple fish species.[28, 29, 30] In a study of 11 patients who were clinically allergic to fish, all had multiple prick skin test reactivity and *in vitro* cross-reactivity on immunoblotting to numerous fish species. In this group, positive oral challenges occurred only to one fish 63% of the patients, to two fish species in 9% and to three fish species in 18%.[29] In a follow-up study, this same group demonstrated that unlike most other food antigens, fish proteins are more labile when heated or lyophilized. In blinded food challenges, none of 18 patients with known IgE-mediated food allergy to fresh cooked tuna or salmon reacted when given canned tuna or salmon. This study also showed decreased specific binding to the protein fractions on immunoblot analysis when comparing fresh fish with the comparable canned variety.[31] These findings indicated that preparation of fish led to destruction of the responsible allergens. These findings also underscore the fact that skin test positivity may not correlate with clinical reactivity.

Seafood

Seafoods are common allergens in adults but relatively uncommon in children. These allergens include mol-

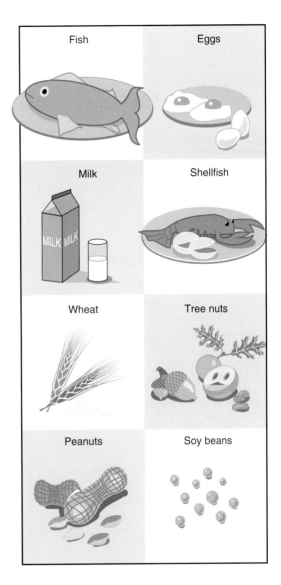

Table 2: Common allergens.

lusks (snails, mussels, oysters, scallops, clams, squid and octopus), and crustacea (shrimp, lobsters and crabs). Shrimp allergens have been extensively studied and contain multiple allergenic fractions.[32, 33] Pen a 1 is considered the most important allergen and is a protein derived from tropomyosin.[34] Like other allergen groups, extensive *in vitro* cross-reactivity has been demonstrated among various seafoods; however, no challenge studies are available to correlate these findings with clinical symptoms.[35] Like only a few other

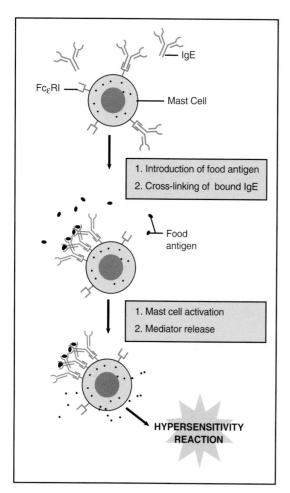

Figure 1: Example of a food allergen triggering a cutaneous reaction. Food allergens [*] transported through small fissures in the skin or via the circulation bind to IgE on mast cells and Langerhans cells, triggering an immune response. These cells secrete cytokines and other mediators that enhance the immune reaction. These substances serve to recruit other cell types into action in the circulation and at the target tissue site, thus perpetuating the immune reaction. Cells involved include keratinocytes (Ker), Langerhans cells (LC), mast cells (MC), T helper lymphocytes (TH), eosinophils (Eos), monocytes (Mono), macrophages (MØ) and basophils (Baso). Cytokines produced include IL-1, IL-3, IL-4, IL-5, IL-6, IL-8, IL-10, IL-13, TNF and GM-CSF. Mediators secreted include histomine, tryptase, prostagladin D$_2$ (PGD$_2$), platelet-activating factor (PAF), major basic protein (MBP), eosinophilic cationic protein (ECP), eosinophil-derived neurotoxin (EDN), eosinophil peroxidase (EPO) and others. (Adapted from Sampson, HA. Acta Derm Venerol 1992;176S:34-37.)

food allergens (i.e., peanuts, tree nuts and fish), seafood allergy tends to be life long and is frequently associated with more severe clinical symptoms.

Wheat

Wheat and other cereal grains stet the last major category of food allergens in children. Reactions to cereal grains are uncommon but do occur. Grains are made up of several fractions including gliadins, globulins, glutens and albumins.[36] Several investigators have shown elevated wheat-specific antibodies and multiple radioallergosorbent test (RAST) and prick skin test (PST) positivity in patients with cereal grain allergy.[36, 37] In a recent study of 145 children with histories and/or PSTs suggestive of food allergy to one or more cereal grains, only 21% had symptomatic reactivity by food challenge; 80% were reactive to only one grain. Among patients with clinical reactivity to grains, immunologic cross-reactivity was demonstrated to multiple protein fractions among six grains tested (wheat, rye, oat, barley, rice and corn). This cross-reactivity was seen both in positive skin tests and immunoblot analyses.[37] These findings indicate that eliminating all cereal grains from the diet based on clinical reactivity to one grain is unwarranted.

Immunopathophysiology

Children with food hypersensitivity demonstrate a myriad of clinical signs and symptoms. To fully appreciate the spectrum of clinical disease and to institute appropriate therapy, a thorough understanding of the underlying immunopathology is needed. IgE-mediated disease is by far the most commonly encountered food hypersensitivity. Much information is available regarding the mechanisms of IgE-mediated disease processes. Non-IgE-mediated disease is less common and more obscure, both clinically and with regard to the pathophysiologic mechanisms of disease.

IgE-Mediated Food Hypersensitivity

A lack of development or a breakdown in oral tolerance may result in a variety of hypersensitivity reactions following the ingestion of a food allergen. The best defined food-allergic reactions are thought to be IgE-mediated or Type I immediate hypersensitivity reactions. In a genetically susceptible individual, a breakdown in oral tolerance results in the excessive production of food-specific IgE antibodies. These food-specific antibodies bind high affinity $Fc_\varepsilon I$ receptors on mast cells and basophils and low affinity $Fc_\varepsilon II$ receptors on macrophages, monocytes, lymphocytes, eosinophils and platelets. After a food allergen is ingested, it may be transported by the circulation to the gastrointestinal tract, skin, respiratory tract and other organs to produce hypersensitivity reactions (Figure 1). The allergen binds the food-specific IgE antibodies and IgE receptors to stimulate release of mediators on mast cells and basophils. These mediators include histamine, tryptase, prostaglandins and leukotrienes. They produce immediate hypersensitivity by promoting local vasodilatation, smooth muscle contraction and mucous secretion.[38] The activated mast cells release various cytokines that also play a part in cell recruitment and perpetuation of the IgE-mediated late-phase response. The first four to eight hours of the immune response is heralded by infiltration primarily of neutrophils and eosinophils into the inflammatory site. These cells are activated and release various mediators, including platelet-activating factor, peroxidases and eosinophilic granule proteins (major basic protein, eosinophilic cationic protein, eosinophil-derived neurotoxin and eosinophil peroxidase). During the next 24 to 48 hours, lymphocytes and monocytes infiltrate the area, releasing numerous cytokines to produce a more chronic inflammatory response.[39] With repeated allergen ingestion, mononuclear cells are stimulated to release histamine-releasing factor (HRF), a cytokine that interacts with surface-bound IgE on basophils, and possibly mast cells, to increase their releasibility. The "spontaneous" release of HRF *in vitro* has been associated with increased cutaneous irritability in children with atopic dermatitis[40] and with increased bronchial hyperreactivity in asthmatics.[41]

Many clinical symptoms have been associated with IgE-mediated allergic reactions. These symptoms include cutaneous, respiratory, gastrointestinal and generalized anaphylaxis. A rise in plasma histamine has been associated with the above symptoms after blinded food challenges.[42] Elevated serum tryptase levels have

been found in patients following anaphylaxis.[43] Increased stool and serum PGE_2 and PGF_2 have been seen after food challenges causing diarrhea.[44]

Non-IgE-Mediated Food Hypersensitivity

Although anecdotal reports can be found that implicate non-IgE-mediated mechanisms in the food allergic response, little scientific support can be found in the medical literature that they cause of significant food allergic reactions. Type II (antigen antibody-dependent cytotoxicity) hypersensitivity reactions have only been implicated in one report that suggested antibody-dependent thrombocytopenia following milk ingestion.[45] Type III (antigen-antibody complex-mediated) hypersensitivity reactions have been studied by several investigators. Food antigen-antibody complexes form in both normal individuals and individuals with food allergy. One to three hours following the ingestion of milk, normal children have IgG, IgM and IgA-specific antibodies to B-lactoglobulin.[46] Although patients with food allergy have increased levels of food-specific IgG and IgE, little evidence exists for food allergen-induced immune complex-mediated disease.[47-49] Type IV (cell-mediated) hypersensitivity has been implicated in many food allergic disorders where symptoms do not appear until several hours after food ingestion. Lymphocyte proliferation can be seen *in vitro* in patients having adverse symptoms following the ingestion of milk or soy,[50] but some degree of proliferation can also be seen in normal individuals.[51] Extensive investigation is currently ongoing in an attempt to clarify this issue of cell-mediated involvement in these adverse food responses.

Clinical Manifestations

The clinical manifestations of food hypersensitivity generally fall into two categories, IgE-mediated and non-IgE-mediated reactions. The importance of making the appropriate distinctions between the two groups cannot be overstated. These distinctions must be understood and applied to each food-allergic patient in order to provide adequate diagnosis, treatment, and prognostic counseling. For example, it is important to recognize that an IgE-mediated reaction to wheat will likely be "outgrown" (following a period

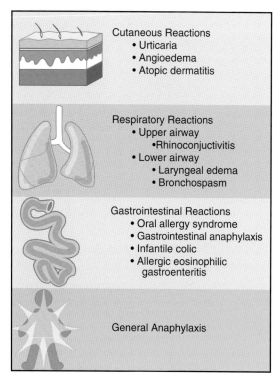

Table 3: Clinical manifestations of IgE-mediated food hypersensitivity.

on a full elimination diet), whereas a non-IgE-mediated reaction to wheat secondary to celiac disease will be lifelong.

IgE-mediated Reactions
Cutaneous Reactions
Cutaneous hypersensitivity reactions are the most common and most easily recognized manifestations of food allergy reactions, especially in the young child. The ingestion of food allergens can lead to immediate skin manifestations or aggravation of more chronic skin conditions. Skin manifestations are the most widely studied areas of food hypersensitivity.

Acute urticaria and angioedema are the most commonly encountered cutaneous manifestations of food hypersensitivity reactions.[52] These reactions are easily recognized by parents and medical personnel alike. Because the reaction is immediate, these responses frequently provide the cause and effect relationship needed to recognize the allergen. The most commonly ingested foods causing these reactions in children

include milk, eggs, peanuts and tree nuts. Contact with other foods including meats, vegetables and fruits may also cause acute urticaria. Food allergy is rarely a cause of chronic urticaria or angioedema (i.e., lasting longer than six weeks).[53]

The most common chronic cutaneous manifestation of food hypersensitivity is atopic dermatitis. Atopic dermatitis (AD) is a chronic, eczematous skin disorder that usually begins in early infancy and has a typical age-related distribution (Figure 2).[54] This skin disorder is characterized by extreme pruritus, chronically relapsing course, and association with asthma and allergic rhinitis.[55] A variety of factors are known to exacerbate AD, including irritants, heat, humidity, emotional stress, infections and allergens. The pathogenic role of food allergens in the development of AD has been the subject of much investigative debate. In a study of children with atopic dermatitis seen in allergy and dermatology clinics, investigators found that one-third of patients had at least one double-blind, placebo-controlled food challenge (DBPCFC) positive to common food allergens.[56] A single ingestion of a food allergen is unlikely to cause an eczematous lesion, but repeated ingestion of the allergen can result in the chronic changes seen in AD.

In 1992, Sampson reported his findings after studying 320 patients with AD for evidence of food hypersensitivity.[57] These patients ranged in age from six months to 25 years. They were highly atopic, with 45% having both asthma and allergic rhinitis, and 95% with a positive family history for atopy. Only 23% of patients had AD alone. Double-blind, placebo-controlled food challenges provoked a variety of symptoms within minutes to two hours. Cutaneous reactions were seen in 75% of positive reactions, but symptoms were confined to the skin alone in 30% of positive challenges. Skin symptoms usually consisted of a markedly pruritic, erythematous, morbilliform rash that developed at the patients' predilection sites for eczema. Urticarial lesions were rarely seen on initial challenge, but were commonly seen on follow-up challenge after the offending food allergen had been restricted from the diet for one to two years. In the initial positive challenges, gastrointestinal symptoms developed in 41% of patients (nausea, abdominal cramping, vomiting and/or diarrhea); upper respiratory symptoms

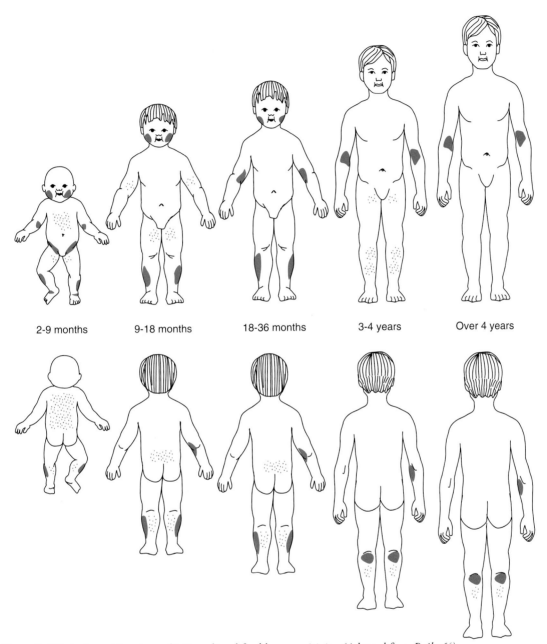

2-9 months   9-18 months   18-36 months   3-4 years   Over 4 years

Figure 2: Clinical manifestations of IgE-mediated food hypersensitivity. (Adapted from Rajka.[54])

developed in 33% (throat itching or tightness, hoarseness and dry hacking cough); and wheezing developed in 10%. Egg, milk and peanut accounted for over two-thirds of the positive DBPCFCs.

During positive DBPCFCs, both immediate and late-phase reactions have been documented.[39, 40, 42, 58-60] The hallmark skin response is the pruritic, erythema-tous, morbilliform rash that typically develops within a few minutes and lasts for 30 to 120 minutes following food allergen ingestion. This reaction is believed to be secondary to an IgE-mediated cutaneous mast cell activation; this is evidenced by a rise in plasma hista-mine concentration[42] and a lack of evidence for imme-diate basophil activation.[40] Evidence also exists that

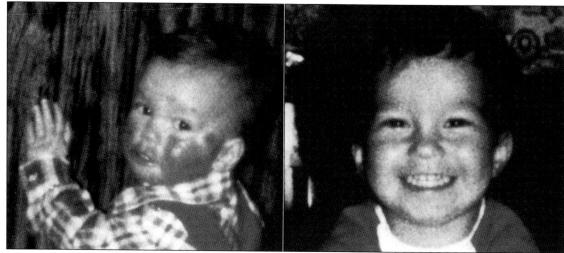

Figure 3: Young child with diagnosis of atopic dermatitis and food hypersensitivity. (Left) Prior to challenge and dietary elimination of food allergen. (Right) After challenge and on a full dietary elimination of the offending food allergen. (Courtesy of Dr. Hugh Sampson, Johns Hopkins University.)

suggests an IgE-mediated late phase reaction following a positive DBPCFC. Approximately four to eight hours following a positive food challenge, diffuse pruritus and, occasionally, an erythematous macular rash will develop. Sampson has seen a significant rise in circulating neutrophils and a fall in circulating eosinophils during this time period.[57] Eosinophils were further examined in a few patients and noted to shift from a "normodense" profile before challenge to a "hypodense" profile after a positive challenge, indicating an activated state. Skin biopsies obtained from these sites 8 to 14 hours following a positive challenge revealed an infiltration of eosinophils into lesional sites, with deposit of major basic protein in the dermis.[39] Biopsy specimens of more chronic skin lesion show a shift in cellular infiltrates to include primarily monocytes and lymphocytes.

In food-allergic patients, the chronic ingestion of food allergens has been associated with spontaneous *in vitro* release of a cytokine, histamine-releasing factor (HRF), from mononuclear cells.[40] The generation of HRF was associated with increased spontaneous basophil histamine release *in vitro*, increased basophil releasability *in vitro*, and increased cutaneous hyperirritability to a variety of minor external stimuli. HRF was found to activate basophils through surface-bound IgE. Once patients were placed on appropriate allergen elimination

diets for six to nine months, the spontaneous release of HRF, spontaneous basophil histamine release and basophil releasability decreased to normal levels. In addition, cutaneous hyperirritability diminished.

On prospective evaluation of 113 patients with atopic dermatitis, investigators found that those patients with previously positive DBPCFC who maintained an appropriate allergen elimination diet experienced a markedly greater improvement in their eczematous rash than those patients not maintaining an elimination diet or in those with AD not related to food hypersensitivity[58] (Figure 3). In a series evaluating patients after one to two years of complete allergen avoidance diet, one third of symptomatic food allergies were lost at follow-up challenge.[61] Loss of food hypersensitivity varied among foods. A follow-up challenge to milk, egg, wheat and peanut were more commonly positive, whereas a follow-up challenge to soy was commonly negative. Most children who tended to "outgrow" their clinical reactivity were likely to do so during the first one to three years of allergen avoidance. Prick skin tests were commonly noted to be positive, even once clinical reactivity was lost.[61]

Respiratory Reactions

Both upper and lower respiratory tract symptoms may develop within minutes to two hours following ingestion of a food allergen. Symptoms typical of rhinoconjunctivitis (tearing, pruritus and conjunctival injection of eyes; nasal congestion, pruritus, rhinorrhea and sneezing) are commonly seen during food allergy reactions; however, upper airway symptoms alone are uncommon.[52] Nasal histamine release during positive food challenges have been reported, suggesting the role of nasal mast cells in the immediate phase allergic response.[62]

Lower airway symptoms seen during food allergic reactions include coughing, laryngeal edema (hoarseness, throat itching and/or tightness) and wheezing.[63] In a study of 140 asthmatic children, 6% had wheezing induced by food challenge.[64] Another study screened 300 asthmatic adults and children for evidence of food allergy; 25 had either history, skin tests or radioallergosorbent tests (RASTs) suggestive of food-induced symptoms. Twenty (2% of total) had documented wheezing provoked by food challenge.[65]

Evidence for bronchial hyperreactivity in both large and small airways has been demonstrated through spirometry during positive food challenge.[63, 66] James, et al., evaluated spirometry and methacholine inhalation challenges before and after DBPCFC in 26 asthmatics with food hypersensitivity. Significant increases in airway reactivity (i.e., two-fold or greater change in the provocative dose causing a 20% fall in forced expiratory volume in one second [PD20 FEV1]) were seen in seven of 12 patients who experienced chest symptoms during positive challenge.[66]

Although ingesting food allergens is rarely the case of chronic asthma, the diagnosis should be considered in those patients who have positive skin tests or RASTs to food allergens. Since multiple triggers can contribute to asthma and isolated bronchospasm, food-induced disease can only be confidently diagnosed following a strict elimination diet and subsequent blinded challenge.

Gastrointestinal Reactions

IgE-mediated mechanisms are responsible for a variety of gastrointestinal disorders induced by food allergen exposure. These disorders include the oral allergy syndrome, gastrointestinal anaphylaxis, infantile colic and a subset of allergic eosinophilic gastroenteritis.

The oral allergy syndrome is considered a type of contact dermatitis confined almost exclusively to the oropharynx. It is characterized by itching and swelling of the lips, tongue, palate and/or throat immediately following contact with a food allergen. These symptoms typically resolve rapidly and spontaneously once allergen contact is eliminated. This syndrome is most commonly seen in patients with allergic rhinitis and aeroallergen sensitivity, especially ragweed and birch pollen, after ingesting of certain fruits and/or vegetables.[67] Patients with birch sensitivity may have symptoms after ingesting raw potatoes, carrots, celery, apples and hazelnuts.[68,69] Likewise, patients with ragweed sensitivity may experience symptoms after ingesting bananas or melons (cantaloupe, watermelon, honeydew).[70, 71] The diagnosis of this syndrome can be made after a suggestive history and positive prick skin tests to the implicated fruits or vegetables.[72] Skin tests must be performed frequently using fresh fruits or vegetables instead of commercial extracts for a reliable response. This is done by first pricking into the fresh food with the skin device, then pricking the patient's skin.

Gastrointestinal anaphylaxis is the IgE-mediated form of gastrointestinal (GI) reaction caused by ingestion of a food allergen. These reactions occur within minutes to two hours of allergen ingestion and accompany other immediate-type reactions in other target

> *'Twas a Sage said it, and the Saying's good,*
> *The Mother's Milk's the only wholesome Food.*
> *Large Meals upon the Sucking Babe bestow,*
> *And freely let the Snowy Fountains flow...*
> *Life's fed with Life itself, and Blood with Blood.*
> *From Hers it circles thro' its little Veins,*
> *And growing Strength in ev'ry Part maintains.*
> *Have you not heard it in the Cradle cry,*
> *And seen the ready Nurse to feed it, fly?*
> *How soon it Laughs to see the swelling Breast,*
> *Seizes the Nipple, and returns to Rest?*
>
> *Pediatrics of the Past*
> An anthology complied and edited by
> John Ruhrah, M.D., 1925
> Paul B. Hoeber, Inc.,
> Publishers, New York, NY

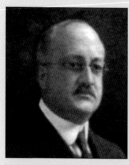

John Ruhräh M.D.

(1872-1935) received his medical degree from the College of Physicians and Surgeons, Baltimore, in 1894. He became Professor of Pediatrics at the University of Maryland in 1916. Ruhräh introduced the use of soy formulas in 1909. A historian, Ruhräh published *Pediatrics of the Past* in 1925. His chapter on Pediatric Poems contains many early descriptions of infant feeding practices in rhyme. Ruhräh's own poem on infant feeding, which is found in the preface of this book, ends, "a hundred years will soon go by/And I predict no one will know/What makes the baby gain and grow." Pediatric Profiles editor B. S. Veeder, Mosby St. Louis, 1957, 149-154 (Photo courtesy of Med.& Chirurg. Faculty of MD)

organs, such as the skin or respiratory tract.[73] Typical symptoms include abdominal pain or cramping, nausea, vomiting and/or diarrhea. The best animal model of IgE-mediated gastrointestinal food hypersensitivity is the rodent. The ingestion of a food allergen will induce the following immediate changes in the rat GI tract: sharp increase in gastric acid production in the stomach, delayed gastric emptying and mast cell degranulation with a rise in intraluminal histamine and serum rat mast cell protein II (RMCP II). These findings are seen immediately in a sensitized rat after feeding with an appropriate allergen.[74] After prolonged feeding of the allergen, RMCP II levels continued to be elevated, but to a much lesser degree than initially seen.[75] As a correlate in children with atopic dermatitis and food allergy, the frequent ingestion of a food allergen appears to induce partial desensitization of GI mast cells, resulting in less pronounced symptoms.[73] These diminished responses often make it difficult to diagnose a patient with food allergy manifested as gastrointestinal symptoms. By strictly avoiding the suspected allergen for up to two weeks, a child will frequently develop symptoms such as vomiting during a challenge even when vomiting was not seen during chronic ingestion of the allergen. The prolonged avoidance period serves to "unmask" the symptoms, allowing for more precise definition of the problem.

Infantile colic is a poorly defined syndrome that typically develops in infants between age two and four weeks and resolves during the third or fourth month of life. The syndrome is characterized by inconsolable crying, abdominal pain and cramping, excessive gas and abdominal bloating. Infantile colic affects the lives of 20% of families with infants less than four months of age.[76] Many psychosocial and dietary causes have been implicated, but none have been defined as the true, single etiologic agent. Because no standardized criteria exist to define the syndrome, a causal factor is frequently difficult to establish. The role of cow milk has been suggested as an etiologic agent for many years.[77] In an uncontrolled Swedish trial, investigators found that 13 of 19 breast-fed infants with colic improved when cow milk was illiminated from the mother's diet.[78] Lothe and associates studied 60 colicky infants in a blinded, cross-over trial. Twenty-nine percent improved on both milk and soy formulas, 18% improved only on soy formula, and 53% improved only after feeding with a casein hydrolysate formula.[79] These studies underscore the importance of recognizing cow's milk intolerance in some infants with colic. It is estimated that only 10 to 15% of infantile colic is actually caused by a true IgE-mediated food allergy.[80]

The diagnosis of food-induced infantile colic can be made by several brief trials of hypoallergenic formula (i.e., Alimentum, Nutramigen). The symptoms should resolve after two to three days and return when regular formula or breast-feeding is resumed. The symptoms are generally short-lived, so challenges can be performed every three to four months.

Allergic eosinophilic gastroenteritis is a disease characterized by peripheral eosinophilia, eosinophilic infiltration of the bowel wall, and a variety of clinical symptoms. A subset of patients (10 to 15%) with this disorder will have symptoms resulting from an IgE-mediated food allergy mechanism. The disorder is characterized by post-prandial nausea and vomiting, abdominal pain or cramping, diarrhea, weight loss (adults) and failure to thrive (children).[81] In addition, evidence of food aversion with refusal to eat may be seen in young children. Children may present with findings such as chronic vomiting or reflux that may be suggestive of pyloric stenosis or even more serious conditions.

Some children have even undergone unnecessary Nissan fundoplication without resolution of symptoms.

The stomach and small intestine are the most common sites of involvement in allergic eosinophilic gastroenteritis, but the esophagus and large intestine can also be involved.[82] The most striking histologic findings are eosinophilic infiltration and edema that can involve the mucosal, muscular or serosal layers.[83] Most patients with IgE-mediated disease have the mucosal form of the disease. In addition, these patients may have elevated serum IgE levels,[84] peripheral eosinophilia, iron deficiency anemia (usually due to fecal blood loss), hypoalbuminemia (due to protein-losing enteropathy or malabsorption) and multiple positive prick skin tests to a variety of foods and aeroallergens.[85] Stools are frequently positive for occult blood and for Charcot-Leyden crystals, presumably due to extruded mucosal eosinophils. Abnormal D-xylose absorption tests, indicative of mucosal disease and malabsorption, may also be positive. The diagnosis relies on maintaining of a high index of clinical suspicion coupled with an appropriate history and demonstration of eosinophilic infiltration on bowel biopsy. An extended elimination diet and/or elemental formula feedings for up to 12 weeks may be necessary before symptoms completely resolve and bowel biopsies normalize.

Generalized Anaphylaxis

In addition to the IgE-mediated cutaneous, respiratory, and gastrointestinal symptoms already discussed, patients with food allergies may experience additional symptoms typical of anaphylaxis. These symptoms are cardiovascular in nature and include cardiac dysrhythmias, hypotension, and vascular collapse. Two recent series by Yunginger and Sampson have addressed the fatal and near-fatal anaphylactic food reactions seen in adults and children, respectively.[86, 87] In both series patients with known food allergies unknowingly ingested a food allergen which provoked life-threatening anaphylaxis. In Sampson's study of 13 children between ages two and 17 years, the responsible foods were peanuts, tree nuts, eggs and milk. Six of the 13 patients died having had onset of their symptoms within three to 30 minutes of allergen ingestion, but

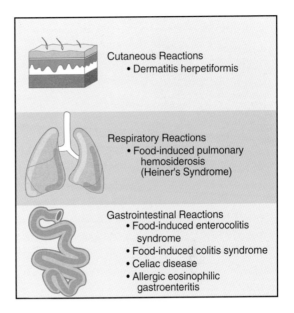

Table 4: Clinical manifestations of non-IgE-mediated food hypersensitivity.

only two received epinephrine within the first hour. Of the seven patients who survived, all had symptoms within five minutes of allergen ingestion, and six of the seven received epinephrine within 30 minutes. Approximately half of the patients experienced a biphasic response with initial mild oral and cutaneous symptoms followed by catastrophic cardiovascular symptoms within 15 minutes to two hours later. Despite medical attention, three patients experienced severe vascular and respiratory collapse requiring prolonged ventilatory and vasopressor support.[87] These findings underscore the importance of strict allergen avoidance, prompt use of epinephrine in emergency situations following accidental allergen ingestion and the necessity of prolonged patient observation in a medical facility following an allergen ingestion.

Non-IgE-mediated Reactions (Table 4)

Food-induced enterocolitis syndrome is a disorder that is most commonly seen in infants between one week and two months of age. The usual presentation is an infant with protracted, often blood-streaked diarrhea, vomiting and growth failure.[88] Symptoms can be severe enough to cause dehydration and a "shock-like" appearance. At presentation infants are

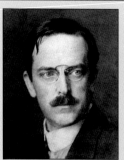

Clemens von Pirquet M.D. (1874-1929) trained in pediatrics under Heubner and Escherich. Pirquet began a career of immunological research in 1902 and introduced the concept of allergy to describe the hypersensitivity occurring in serum sickness in 1906. Pirquet was appointed the first Professor of Pediatrics at Hopkins in 1908. He left the U.S. in 1911 to assume Escherich's chair in Vienna. In Vienna, he constructed some of the first standards for normal growth, which were used by Stuart in constructing the first percentile growth charts. Pirquet reasoned that sitting height reflected energy expenditure and developed the nem (three nutritional equivalents of milk = 2 kCal) system of infant feeding based upon sitting height. This system was widely used in the relief efforts after World War I. *Clemens von Pirquet: His Life and Work.* Wagner, R. Johns Hopkins Press, Baltimore. 1968 (Photo courtesy of NLM)

frequently evaluated for sepsis due to their acutely ill appearance. Further historical evaluation typically points to cow milk and/or soy protein as the cause. Increased fecal leukocytes and occult blood will frequently be present. Malabsorption is evident from the presence of stool- reducing substances, hypoproteinemia and reduced D-xylose test. Small bowel biopsies reveal flattened villi, mucosal edema, and the presence of inflammatory cells including lymphocytes, eosinophils and mast cells. A food challenge with the offending antigen generally results in protracted vomiting and/or diarrhea within minutes to several hours, occasionally leading to shock.[89]

The immunopathogenesis of this disorder remains essentially unknown. Serum titers of the offending antigen may rise in response to allergen challenge.[50] An increase in IgM and IgA-containing plasma cells have been reported in jejunal biopsies.[90, 91] More recently, IgE-mediated activation of local gastrointestinal mast cells has been implicated.[92, 93] Further work must be done to more specifically define the immunologic factors involved in this syndrome.

Diagnosis is based on clinical history, elimination diet and oral food challenge. Prick skin tests and RASTs are negative in this disorder. Eliminating of the offending

allergen will result in improvement or resolution of symptoms within 72 hours. Commonly both milk and soy proteins are involved; therefore, administration of a casein hydrolysate formula is the best choice for complete allergen elimination. Oral food challenges can be performed in those patients with unclear diagnoses following a trial on an elimination diet. Challenges must be performed in a medical facility due to the potential severity of the reactions. Challenge consists of administering a total of 0.6g/kg body weight of the suspected food protein.[88] Challenge should begin with a test dose and proceed until the total dose is given over a one hour period. Symptoms may develop immediately or within four to eight hours after allergen ingestion. Three of the following five criteria are necessary to define a positive challenge: 1) symptoms of vomiting and/or diarrhea; 2) a 3,500/mm³ rise in the absolute neutrophil count between pre-challenge and six to eight hour post-challenge; 3) the appearance of blood in the stool; 4) the appearance of fecal leukocytes and/or mucous; and 5) the appearance of Charcot-Leyden crystals or eosinophilic debris in the stool via Hansel's stain. Patients typically have resolution of their enterocolitis symptoms by 18 to 24 months of age.

Food-induced colitis syndrome is a disorder typically seen in the first few months of life. The usual presentation is that of a normal, healthy-appearing infant with recurrent gross or occult blood in the stools. Patients may have normally-formed stools or mild diarrhea, but in contrast to those infants with enterocolitis syndrome, those with colitis are not generally ill-appearing. The causal antigens are typically milk and/or soy proteins.[94] Gastrointestinal lesions are confined to the large intestine and consist of mucosal edema, with eosinophilic infiltration of the lamina propria and epithelium.[95]

Eliminating the offending allergen leads to resolution of symptoms within 72 hours, but mucosal lesions may take up to one month to resolve. Patients generally respond well to a casein hydrolysate formula, and symptoms most often disappear within 12 to 24 months of dietary restriction.

Celiac disease, or gluten-sensitive enteropathy, is a malabsorption disorder that may present during the first one to two years of life following the introduction of cereal grains to the diet. Typical symptoms include diarrhea, steatorrhea, abdominal distention, flatulence, weight loss, and occasionally, nausea and vomiting.[96] Oral ulcers and other extra-intestinal manifestations secondary to malabsorption are not uncommon. These symptoms are associated with total villous atrophy and extensive cellular infiltrate on small bowel biopsy. The cause of this disease. Sensitivity to gliadin, the alcohol-soluble portion of gluten found in wheat, barley, oat and rye.

The immunopathogenesis of this disorder remains unclear. On biopsy specimen, small bowel infiltrates consist of primarily CD8+ cytotoxic/suppressor lymphocytes.[97] IgM and IgA-containing B lymphocytes are increased in the lamina propria; serum IgA antibodies are increased and IgM antibodies frequently decreased.[98, 99] Gluten-specific IgA antibodies are present in over 80% of adults and children with untreated celiac disease.[100] Based on animal models of celiac disease it has recently been suggested that there is a type IV, cell-mediated mechanism of immune dysfunction; however, definitive studies remain to be performed.[101, 102]

The diagnosis of celiac disease typically requires an appropriate history coupled with small bowel biopsy findings of villous atrophy and inflammatory infiltrate. Diagnosis is confirmed when symptoms and biopsy abnormalities resolve after six to twelve weeks on a gluten-free diet.[103] Serum IgA antigliadin and antiendomysial antibodies are usually present and aid in the diagnosis.[104, 105] Gluten-containing foods must be eliminated to maintain control of symptoms and to avoid the increased risk of malignancy.[106]

Allergic eosinophilic gastroenteritis is a disorder that has been discussed previously as an IgE-mediated disease. However, only a subset of patients with this disorder have an IgE-mediated mechanism; other mechanisms that cause disease activity are unknown at present.

Food-induced pulmonary hemosiderosis (Heiner's syndrome) is a rare syndrome that occurs in infants.[107] It involves recurrent episodes of pneumonia associated with pulmonary infiltrates, hemosiderosis, gastrointestinal blood loss, iron-deficiency anemia and failure to thrive. Hemosiderin-laden macrophages may be found on lung biopsy or in early morning gastric aspirates. This syndrome is associated with hypersensitivity primarily cow milk protein, and rarely to egg or pork protein, but the non-IgE-mediated immunologic mechanism is otherwise unknown.[108] Peripheral eosinophilia and demonstration of multiple cow milk precipitins in serum can be found. Due to the presence of milk-specific IgG antibodies and *in vivo* lymphocyte proliferation to milk protein, antigen-antibody complexes and lymphocyte-mediated hypersensitivity reactions to milk are postulated in the immunopathogenesis. The diagnosis is generally made by demonstrating milk precipitins in the serum and by improvement of symptoms when the implicated food allergen, most commonly milk is eliminated from the diet.

Dermatitis herpetiformis is a highly pruritic skin rash that is often mistaken for atopic dermatitis. Typically this disease is characterized by a chronic, pruritic, papulovesicular rash over the extensor surfaces and buttocks. This disorder is associated with gluten-sensitive enteropathy, which occurs in up to 85% of patients with dermatitis herpetiformis.[109] Deposition of IgA can be seen in the dermoepithelial junction of both involved and uninvolved skin. IgA may form complexes with complement to activate those pathways causing increased inflammation. Although many patients with dermatitis herpetiformis

> *I know very well in how unbeaten and almost unknown a Path I am treating; for sick Children, and especially Infants, give no other Light into the Knowledge of the Diseases, than what we are able to discover from their uneasy Cries, and the uncertain Tokens of their Crossness; for which Reason, several Physicians of the first Rank have openly declared to me, that they will go unwillingly to take care of the Diseases of children, especially such as are newly born, as if they were to unravel some strange Mystery, or cure some incurable Disease.*
>
> Walter Harris, M.D.
> Fellow of the College of Physicians at London and Professor of Chirurgery
> *Pediatrics of the Past*
> John Ruhräh, M.D., Editor
> Paul B. Hoeber, Inc,
> New York, publisher

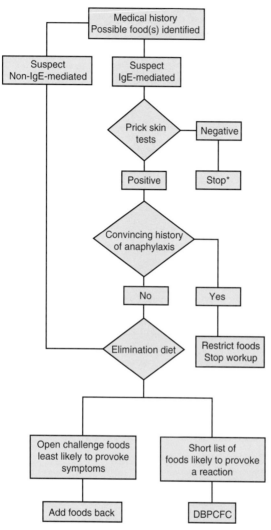

*Figure 4: Steps in the diagnosis of food hypersensitivity. *Unless non-IgE-mediated food reaction is possible. (Modified from James, Jm. Pediatr. Allergy Immune. 1992; 3;67-73.)*

have associated enteropathy demonstrated on biopsy, most have little or no gastrointestinal symptoms.[110]

Diagnosing this disorder depends on the presence of typical skin lesions, IgA deposits on skin biopsy, and resolution of symptoms with administration of dapsone or other sulfones. Eliminating gluten from the diet will result in resolution of skin symptoms and normalization of intestinal biopsy findings over time. In general, the full spectrum of this disorder is milder than celiac disease.

Diagnosing Food Allergy

As in any medical disorder, the initial steps for diagnosing a child with food allergy begin with a careful medical history and physical examination (Figure 4). The true value of the medical history relies on accurate recall of symptoms and time course of events, as well as the physician's ability to remain unbiased during the interview process. The history may be very useful in acute, more life-threatening events such as anaphylaxis, but in less overt instances the medical history has been found to correlate with true allergic reactions (as diagnosed by blinded food challenge) less than 50% of the time.[111,112] As noted in Table 5, several points from the medical history are important in establishing that a food allergic reaction occurred: 1) the food suspected to provoke the reaction, 2) the quantity of the suspected food ingested, 3) the length of time between ingestion of the food and the development of symptoms, 4) a description of the symptoms provoked, 5) whether similar symptoms developed on other occasions when the food was ingested, 6) if other factors (e.g., exercise) occurred in relation to the food ingestion and/or symptoms, and 7) length of time since the last reaction to the food occurred. In chronic disorders, such as atopic dermatitis, the history may not be a reliable indicator of the offending food allergen. The physical examination, although not diagnostic, is important to help rule out other disorders that mimic food allergy (e.g., dermatitis herpetiformis).

Once a food allergic reaction is suspected, a number of methods have been used to better define the etiologic agent(s) involved (Table 6). These methods include diet diary, elimination diet, allergy prick skin tests, radioallergosorbent tests (RAST), basophil histamine release, intestinal mast cell histamine release, intestinal biopsy and double-blind, placebo-controlled food challenges. A diet diary is a useful tool in conjunction with the medical history to obtain dietary and symptoms information. This diary is best used prospectively to obtain information, since it relies only on patient or parent compliance in record keeping, not on patient or parent memory. Patients and/or parents are asked to keep a chronologic record of all food intake over a specific time and asked to record any adverse symptoms experienced during that period.

This record can then be reviewed on subsequent visits to help establish information relating to the adverse events. Like the medical history, the diet diary is not diagnostic it will only provide clues to the diagnosis.

An elimination diet is commonly used both in diagnosing and managing adverse food reactions. Based on the medical history, dietary information, and possibly *in vivo* tests (i.e., skin tests), a suspected food allergen(s) can be identified and eliminated from the child's diet. This elimination should be strict and occur for a period of two weeks before other assessment is performed. The success of an elimination diet depends on several factors: 1) correct identification of the allergen or allergens involved, 2) the patient's ability to maintain a diet free of the offending food, and 3) the assumption that no other factors will provoke similar symptoms during the elimination period. Due to the diffficulty in meeting all of the above criteria, elimination diets are rarely diagnostic, especially in chronic conditions such as atopic dermatitis or asthma.

Allergy prick skin tests (PST) are highly reproducible[113] and very useful in screening patients for IgE-mediated food allergies. May and Bock provided guidelines that are useful in establishing positive PSTs.[111] A prick or a puncture is performed using a standardized, glycerinated commercial food allergen extract, a positive (histamine) control and a negative (saline) control. A wheal (excluding surrounding erythema) of at least 3mm greater than the negative control is considered positive, and those less than 3mm are considered negative. Using the above criteria, Sampson evaluated 40 children with AD with blinded food challenges to establish the reliability of PST in predicting food allergic reactions. Skin tests were noted to have an excellent negative predictive accuracy of 82 to 100% but a poor, and highly variable, positive predictive accuracy of 25 to 75% when DBPCFC were used as the "gold standard" for diagnosis.[114] Other investigators have confirmed these findings and reported greater than 95% negative predictive value and poor positive predictive value. Based on these findings, PSTs are an excellent means of excluding IgE-mediated food hypersensitivity, but provide little help in firmly establishing a diagnosis. Positive PSTs are most commonly used in conjunction with the

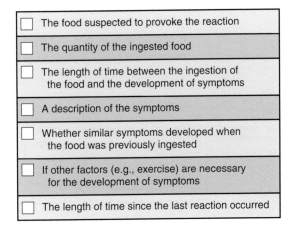

☐	The food suspected to provoke the reaction
☐	The quantity of the ingested food
☐	The length of time between the ingestion of the food and the development of symptoms
☐	A description of the symptoms
☐	Whether similar symptoms developed when the food was previously ingested
☐	If other factors (e.g., exercise) are necessary for the development of symptoms
☐	The length of time since the last reaction occurred

Table 5: Details of medical history.

medical history and diet diary to establish a plan for diet elimination or food challenge. Intradermal skin tests are more sensitive than prick tests, but are much less specific in assessing food allergy.[115] The higher false positive reactions and increased risk of systemic reactions seen with some intradermal food testing limits its practical use. Some exceptions to the above statements on PST include: 1) sensitivity to some fruits and vegetables may not be detected with commercial extracts and require prick testing with "fresh" produce to elicit a reaction,[72] 2) children less than one year of age may have IgE-mediated food allergy, but negative or very small skin tests, and children less than two years of age may have smaller overall skin wheal diameters,[116] and 3) a positive skin test in isolation that provokes a serious, systemic anaphylactic reaction may be considered diagnostic.

Radioallergosorbent tests (RASTs) and similar *in vitro* assays are used to identify food-specific antibodies in serum. Although frequently used to screen for food allergies, RASTs are considered less reliable than PST. Sampson found that like PST, RAST had an excellent negative predictive accuracy approaching 100%, but a positive predictive accuracy of 0 to 57% when compared to DBPCFC.[114] If the higher end of positivity of food-specific IgE antibodies are used from high-quality laboratories, the information provided can be similar to PSTs.

Basophil histamine release has been shown to be important in patients with atopic dermatitis and food hypersensitivity. Basophil histamine release assays are primarily used in research and academic settings.

☐	Diet diary
☐	Elimination diet
☐	Prick skin test
☐	Radioallergosorbent tests (RAST)
☐	Basophil histamine release
☐	Intestinal mast cell histamine release
☐	Double-blind, placebo-controlled food challenge (DBPCFC)

Table 6: Diagnostic methods for determining food allergies.

Commercially available assays have been developed for use in screening for food allergy, but currently these assays provide no more predictive power than prick skin tests and are much more cumbersome and costly to obtain.

Intestinal mast cell histamine release is primarily a research procedure that is performed on intestinal mast cells from biopsy specimens. Histamine release is measured after adding food antigens to the intestinal mast cells. The procedure correlates closely with symptoms of the gastrointestinal tract after challenge but not with other symptoms provoked by challenge.[92]

The double-blind, placebo-controlled food challenge (DBPCFC) has been considered the "gold standard" for diagnosing food hypersensitivity.[119] During the past decade, this test has been used by many investigators to diagnose food allergy in both children and adults.[56, 112, 120-122] Foods thought to be unlikely to provoke a food allergic reaction or those foods correlated with negative history or negative skin tests may be screened with open or single-blind challenge.[120] Several considerations should be met before conducting a food challenge: 1) suspected foods should be eliminated from the diet for one to two weeks prior to challenge; 2) antihistamines should be discontinued long enough to establish a positive histamine skin test (usually five to seven days but longer periods may be required for the long-acting preparations); 3) other medications (e.g., oral corticosteroids) should be reduced to levels that will not mask symptoms (i.e., discontinue use two to four weeks

before challenge); 4) asthmatic patients must have evidence of enough pulmonary reserve to withstand an acute reaction if provoked (i.e., forced expiratory volume in one second [FEV_1]>70%); and 5) emergency medical equipment to treat symptoms of anaphylaxis must be available.

The food challenge is conducted with the patient in a fasting state. The food protein is in the form of a lyophilized powder disguised in a capsule or liquid form. The initial dose is given below that expected to provoke symptoms (usually 125 mg to 500 mg). The dose is then doubled every 15 to 60 minutes until approximately ten grams of challenge protein have been given. If the blinded portion of the challenge is tolerated, an open challenge must be given under observation to confirm the accuracy of the DBPCFC.[123]

The DBPCFC should be a paired challenge with each blinded challenge protein coupled to a placebo.[119, 124] The order of administration should be blinded to the investigators and should be determined by an uninvolved third party, such as a dietitian. A standardized scoring system should be used to assess symptoms at regular intervals during the testing period. An objective scoring system prevents introduction of observer bias and provides for a more reliable and unequivocal challenge setting. Patients undergoing challenge must be observed for a time period following the challenge. This period depends on the type of disorder suspected. For IgE-mediated reactions, two to four hours following the challenge is adequate. For food-induced enterocolitis or colitis syndrome the observation period is typically for four to eight hours post-challenge. The DBPCFC should be performed in a clinic or hospital setting where trained medical personnel are present.[125] Emergency medical equipment should be present in case anaphylaxis occurs.

For many non-IgE-mediated food reactions, there are no diagnostic tests of value and the medical history becomes of even greater importance. In patients with food-induced enterocolitis or colitis syndrome, symptoms may resolve completely on an appropriate elimination diet. These patients can be challenged in a blinded or an open fashion with the implicated food at a total dose of 0.6 grams of food protein/kg body weight given over one hour.[88] Observation must be continued for four to eight hours due to the frequent delay in onset of symptoms. Emergency equipment must be available for these challenges as well. In particular, fluid resuscitation may be necessary. In the enterocolitis syndrome, peripheral neutrophil counts can be followed for four to six hours post-challenge to assess whether an increase has occurred. Stools can be followed for occult blood, PMNs and eosinophils.

Endoscopy and biopsy are required to diagnose malabsorption syndromes and allergic eosinophilic gastroenteritis.[83, 103] Ideally, biopsy specimens should be obtained when the patient is ingesting the suspected food and when on a prolonged elimination diet. Histologic appearance should be different during the two periods with normalization of architecture and reduction of cellular infiltrates seen after elimination diet. In celiac disease an additional biopsy is required after reintroduction of the gluten-containing food. Quantitation of IgA anti-gliadin and endomysial antibodies are useful screening tests in celiac disease.[104, 105] In dermatitis herpetiformis, demonstration of junctional IgA deposition is diagnostic. Diagnosis of Heiner's syndrome depends on the demonstration of milk precipitins and peripheral eosinophilia.[108]

Treatment

The successful treatment of children with food hypersensitivity involves several steps. The two most important aspects of treatment are good education and the institution of an appropriate elimination diet. Medical therapy is used as an adjunct to the above aspects to provide further care to the patient in the case of an "accidental" contact with the food allergen. Medical therapy is primarily supportive and cannot take the place of a strict elimination diet.

Education

Once a child is diagnosed with a food allergy, treatment begins by educating the parents, grandparents, siblings, other care providers and schools or daycare centers. These individuals should be taught to read labels appropriately and given educational material to help them detect potential sources of hidden food allergens. This strategy however, depends on the proper labeling of food by the food industry. Several cases of severe

adverse food reactions have been due to improper labeling of foods.[126] In addition, caregivers should be taught to recognize and treat adverse food reactions. Emphasis should be placed on prompt treatment, especially in more severe anaphylactic reactions. As mentioned previously, in a study of children with fatal and near-fatal anaphylaxis following food allergen ingestion, those patients with fatal reactions either had a delay in treatment or no epinephrine treatment administered.[87]

Support groups and "hotlines" are available to provide good information on food-allergy. The best source of support and information for the family with a food allergic child is the Food Allergy Network (4744 Holly Avenue, Fairfax, VA 22030). This organization provides a newsletter with up-to-date information on food allergies.

Elimination diet

Once the diagnosis of food allergy has been established, the only proven, successful therapy is complete elimination of the responsible food allergen from the diet. Elimination diets should be confined to foods documented to cause adverse reactions. Cases of severe malnutrition as a result of unnecessary dietary elimination have been reported.[127, 128] Broad restriction diets based on history, PST or RAST results should not be used to define a prolonged elimination diet. Restriction of all members of a botanical family or food group has been shown to be unwarranted and potentially dangerous in most circumstances.[23, 31, 37] Strict elimination of a documented food allergen(s) will typically provide relief of immediate symptoms, and prolonged elimination for one to three years will generally lead to resolution of the food allergy. Studies on both children and adults indicate that the exceptions to this rule are seen in patients with allergies to peanuts, tree nuts, fish and shellfish which are typically life-long and do not resolve permanently on an elimination diet.[25, 61, 129]

Once the allergen is determined, a strict elimination diet is required to resolve symptoms and possibly develop a tolerance. In most cases of IgE-mediated food allergy, eliminating only one or two foods is required. Some children will require elimination of both milk and soy protein thereby requiring formula supplementation with a casein hydrolysate formula (i.e., Nutramigen or Alimentum). Partially hydrolyzed

☐ **Mild Reaction**
Involving skin only
1) Oral antihistamines (i.e., Diphenhydramine) 2) Subcutaneous epinephrine (1:1000) for   progression of symptoms** 3) Close observation
☐ **Moderate Reaction**
Involving skin and/or respiratory and/or GI systems

1) Oral or intravenous antihistamines
    (i.e., Diphenhydramine)
2) Inhale beta-agonist therapy
3) Subcutaneous epinephrine (1:1000) for
    progression of symptoms **
4) Intravenous fluid support
    (Intravenous fluid support is the only therapy
    recommended for non-IgE-mediated GI reactions)
5) Close observation

☐ **Severe Reaction**
Involving skin/all systems

1) Subcutaneous epinephrine (1:1000) as
    first line drug**
2) Intravenous antihistamines
    (i.e., Diphenhydramine)
3) Inhaled beta-agonist therapy
4) Oxygen support
5) Intravenous fluid support
6) Intravenous corticosteroids
7) Close observation

** Epinephrine remains the drug of choice for all
life-threating or severe IgE-mediated reactions and may
be life-sustaining.

*Table 7: Steps to follow during an adverse food
reaction.*

formulas (i.e., Carnation Good Start) are inadequate
dietary supplements for children allergic to milk, due
to the presence of intact milk proteins. In more atypi-
cal patients (i.e., those with allergic eosinophilic gastroenteritis), dietary restriction of multiple foods may
be necessary to gain control of symptoms. In addition,
these children will frequently be intolerant of even
fully hydrolyzed formulas. Reintroduction of foods
may be slow and supplementation with an elemental
formula made of amino acids without intact poteins
(i.e., Neocate or Vivonex) may be necessary.

In non-IgE-mediated food hypersensitivity, an
appropriate elimination diet must also be strictly fol-

lowed to resolve symptoms. In enterocolitis and colitis
syndromes, milk protein is the most common cause of
symptoms. However, as many as 50% of children will
show clinical reactivity to both milk and soy protein;
therefore, the elimination of both of these proteins and
formula supplementation with a casein hydrolysate
(i.e., Nutramigen or Alimentum) is frequently
required. Rarely these children will have reactivity to
even these extensively hydrolyzed formulas and require
supplementation with an elemental amino acid formula (i.e., Neocate). In celiac disease, dietary elimination of all gliadin-containing products is required;
therefore, these patients represent one group in which
an entire food group (i.e., cereal grains) must be eliminated from the diet.

In hopes of preventing food hypersensitivity, some
clinicians and parents advocate the use of soy formulas
in infants at high risk for atopic disease. This practice is
unwarranted based on the fact that sensitivity to soy
protein is a common culprit in food hypersensitivity
reactions. The use of a casein hydrolysate formula in
high risk infants is more appropriate and supported by
numerous studies evaluating allergen prophylaxis.

All patients on dietary restriction should have periodic nutritional evaluations to ensure proper caloric
intake and vitamin and mineral balance.[130] Dietary
supplementation with deficient vitamins and/or minerals may be necessary to maintain the recommended
daily allowances of these substances (e.g., calcium supplementation in children with dietary restriction of
milk protein). Periodic nutritional evaluations can also
be helpful in assessing growth and development in
these children.[130]

Medical therapy

Medical therapy is designed to be supportive rather
than prophylactic or curative (Table 7). Several medications have been used in an attempt to protect
patients with food hypersensitivity. These medications
include antihistamines, corticosteroids, prostaglandin
synthetase inhibitors and cromolyn sodium.[131]
Although these drugs may modify or "mask" symptoms, none totally ameliorate the disease and many
have untoward side effects. In a double-blind, crossover trial evaluating the effect of cromolyn on symp-

toms during food challenge in ten patients with atopic dermatitis and food allergy, cromolyn demonstrated no benefit in treatment of food hypersensitivity.[132] Anecdotal reports supporting the role of immunotherapy in food hypersensitivity have appeared. A recent double-blind, controlled trial of "rush" immunotherapy in peanut-allergic patients was conducted. These patients were placed on a "rush" or accelerated desensitization protocol in which the peanut allergen was given in rapid doses over hours to days, rather than in standard fashion over weeks to months. The results demonstrated efficacy in three patients, but the rate of adverse systemic reactions was almost three times higher than standard immunotherapy.[133] The study was halted prematurely due to a patient death. This study emphasized the high risk of administering immunotherapy for food allergens. Sublingual neutralization and subcutaneous provocation therapies have been advocated by some physicians, but well controlled studies have not been able to produce reliable data and most demonstrate a lack of efficacy for these treatments.[134]

Supportive therapy should be administered during an adverse food reaction. This may consist of oral or intravenous antihistamines, intravenous corticosteriods, intravenous fluid, beta-agonists aerosols and subcutaneous epinephrine (1:1,000). For life-threatening or severe anaphylaxis, epinephrine remains the drug of choice and may be life-sustaining. Patients with food hypersensitivity and their families should be well equipped with auto-injectable epinephrine (e.g., EPIPEN® or EPIPEN JR.®) at all times and should be educated with regard to its use in emergency situations. Additional therapy may be required to manage more chronic problems of asthma, allergic rhinitis and atopic dermatitis.

Natural History

It is generally believed that most children become tolerant or "outgrow" their food allergies within the first few years of life. In a prospective study in Denmark that evaluated milk allergy in children through their third birthdays, most children lost their allergy by age three years.[5] In another prospective study of 75 children with food allergy, approximately one-third of children lost their clinical reactivity after one to two years of full dietary allergen restriction.[61] Skin tests and RAST results frequently remained positive even after clinical reactivity was lost, thereby emphasizing the poor positive predictive value of these tests. One of the most important factors in the development of tolerance was the degree to which dietary restriction was kept. Those with full restriction appeared to lose reactivity sooner than those that were poorly compliant with dietary elimination. In addition, the particular food involved in the food hypersensitivity was important for outcome, i.e. patients with fish, shellfish or peanut allergies rarely lost reactivity.

Less information is available for non-IgE-mediated food reactions. Anecdotal reports indicate that children with enterocolitis and colitis syndromes caused by foods tend to "outgrow" their reactivity during the same time frame as seen with IgE-mediated food allergies. Celiac disease is most commonly a life-long sensitivity, requiring elimination of gluten-containing foods from the diet for life.

Prophylaxis

Through the years, much attention has been focused on the role of restricting the mother's diet during pregnancy and lactation in preventing food allergy. One well-designed study followed 212 Swedish women from mid-pregnancy. Of these mothers, 108 were placed on restriction diets eliminating cow milk and eggs, and 104 continued on their normal diets. No difference was seen among the infants for development of atopic disease, serum IgE, or PST, leading the authors to conclude that dietary allergen elimination during pregnancy has no protective effect on the development of allergy.[135] Many groups have studied the potential protective effect of maternal dietary restriction during lactation, especially as it relates to infants from highly atopic families. As a result of these studies, most investigators report some protective effect of allergen elimination during lactation.[136-144] The most recent well-designed study was from Zeiger and colleagues. This group prospectively followed a group of 288 children from birth to four years. Their prophylactic group consisted of maternal avoidance of cow milk, eggs and peanuts during the third trimester and during lactation; infant use of a casein hydrolysate formula for supplementation or weaning; avoidance of all solid foods for six months in infants; cow milk, corn, soy, citrus and wheat avoidance for 12 months; and egg, peanut and fish avoidance for 24 months. After four years of age, the "overall" prevalence of food allergy and AD remained lower in the prophylactic group, but no change was seen in asthma, allergic rhinitis, or positive inhalant PST.[143, 144] These studies all indicate some benefit from the use of allergen-avoidance diets (both the mothers during lactation and in allergen introduction in infants) in high-risk groups to prevent the development of food allergy-associated AD.

Animal studies suggest that introducing multiple foods early in life increases the likelihood of inducing food hypersensitivity.[145] Studies in children have shown a direct correlation between the number of solid foods introduced during the first four months of life and the prevalence of AD at age two years.[136] These studies and others indicate that delayed solid food allergen introduction until four to six months of life reduces the risk of atopic disease in some children.

Summary

In children less than two years of age, food antigens represent the most commonly encountered foreign proteins that confront the body and its immune system. In most children, tolerance develops to ingested food proteins and no adverse reactions occur. In 2 to 8% of the general population, tolerance will not develop and the immune system will mount a response to these foreign substances. Most of these responses will be IgE-mediated food allergy or hypersensitivity reactions and will include cutaneous, respiratory, and/or gastrointestinal symptoms. A subset of these reactions will involve more generalized anaphylaxis and will be life-threatening.

Although much information is known about the immunopathology of food hypersensitivity disorders, the picture is far from complete. Rigorous scientific trials are ongoing in attempts to establish pathogenesis and develop new diagnostic and treatment protocols. At present prompt, recognition, appropriate diagnosis, allergen elimination and patient/parent education are vital to successfully managing of food-allergic children.

Case Histories

Case #1: S.R. is a white male who presented at age seven months with a history of chronic eczema. An erythematous facial rash began at three weeks of age and progressed to the extensor surfaces of the extremities by age eight weeks. By five months of age the rash was associated with intense pruritus, especially when breast-feeding followed maternal egg ingestion. There were no other medical illnesses recognized. Family history was significant for a mother with allergic rhinitis and asthma. On evaluation at seven months of age, the physical exam was normal except for a dry, crusting, erythematous maculopapular rash on the cheeks, post-auricular regions and popliteal fossae. A diagnosis of atopic dermatitis was made and an allergy evaluation revealed positive prick skin tests to egg, milk and wheat. Oral food challenges were performed to egg, milk and wheat and were positive only to egg. A full restriction diet was instituted, including maternal dietary restriction of egg during lactation, elimination of egg protein-containing foods and formula supplementation with a milk formula after cessation of breast-feeding. The rash cleared and the patient was symptom-free on the egg restriction diet. On rechallenge one year later, the patient was able to ingest egg without further symptoms or evidence of rash.

Discussion: This case represents a typical scenario of an IgE-mediated food hypersensitivity. The important features were suggested in the clinical course and family history. The value of elimination diet and food challenge is reiterated by the fact that the history and skin tests suggested three possible allergens, but confirmation of only one was obtained during food challenge. The importance of a strict elimination diet is shown by restriction of both the child's and the lactating mother's diet. Lastly, the development of tolerance to the food allergen was seen due to the family's diligence in dietary restriction.

Case #2: Z.C. is a black female who presented to the emergency room at eight weeks of age with vomiting, diarrhea, fever, pallor, lethargy and hypotension. This child had been breast-fed for two weeks, then switched to a milk protein formula. Loose stools and post-prandial emesis began within two days of starting the formula. At six weeks of age, the infant was evaluated for failure to thrive and pyloric stenosis, but no etiology was found.

Formula was changed to a soy protein formula with continuation of symptoms. The patient then presented to the emergency room with the above symptoms approximately two hours after a formula feeding. Intravenous fluids were started and a septic work-up performed. Patient was transferred to the intensive care unit and was treated with intravenous hydration and antibiotics. The infant made a quick recovery and oral feeds with Pedialyte were restarted 24 hours after admission. Formula was advanced on day two of admission. Within six to eight hours of starting soy formula the infant had another episode of vomiting, fever and hypotension requiring fluid resuscitation. Allergy evaluation revealed negative prick skin tests to milk and soy. Stool samples were positive for occult blood. A diagnosis of milk and soy protein-induced enterocolitis syndrome was suspected. The infant was placed on Nutramigen and the family instructed on the dietary elimination of milk and soy proteins. All symptoms resolved and the patient was discharged to home with a negative work-up for sepsis. One month later a single blind challenge to milk and soy were per-

formed under close medical supervision. Vomiting occured within two to four hours of ingestion of both milk and soy, a rise in absolute neutrophil count of 3,800/mm was seen four hours post-challenge, and stools were hemoccult positive for blood. All of these findings confirmed the diagnosis of food-induced enterocolitis syndrome. Milk and soy proteins were eliminated until age 18 months. At rechallenge, both proteins were well tolerated and elimination diet was halted.

Discussion: *This case represents a fairly typical, although dramatic, scenario of food-induced enterocolitis syndrome. This syndrome is non-IgE-mediated. The important initial clues to the diagnosis are in the history and clinical course. The immunologic hallmark of the disease is the occurence of negative allergy testing to specific allergens (i.e., skin tests or RAST) with the association of occult or frank blood in the stools and elevated neutrophil counts following specific protein ingestion. Once again, an appropriate restriction diet of the causative proteins was crucial to this infant's survival and good clinical outcome.*

Historical Perspective...

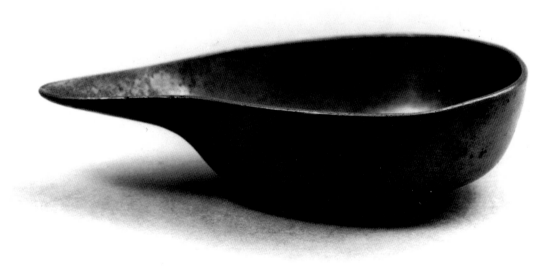

English pewter pap boat, circa 1780.

References

1. Anderson JA, Sogn DD, eds. Adverse reactions to foods. American Academy of Allergy and Immunology/NIAID: 1984. NIH Pub No. 84-2442:1-6.

2. Sloan AE, Powers ME. A perspective on popular perceptions of adverse reactions to foods. *J Allergy Clin Immunol.* 1986;78:127-133.

3. Schreiber RA, Walker WA. Food allergy: facts or fiction. *Mayo Clin Proc.* 1989;64:1381-1402.

4. Bock SA. Prospective appraisal of complaints of adverse reaction to foods in children during the first 3 years of life. *Pediatrics.* 1987;79:683-688.

5. Host A, Halken S. A prospective study of cow's milk allergy in Danish infants during the first 3 years of life. *Allergy.* 1990;45:587-596.

6. Lemanske RF, Taylor SL. Standardized extracts, foods. *Clin Rev Allergy.* 1987;5:23-36.

7. Bleumink E, Young E. Identification of the atopic allergen in cow's milk. *Int Arch Allergy.* 1968;34:521-543.

8. Swaisgood HE. Chemistry of milk protein. In: Fox PF, ed. *Developments in Dairy Chemistry..* London: Applied Science Publishers Ltd; 1982:1-59.

9. Sampson HA. Adverse reactions to foods. In: Middleton RE, Reed CE, Ellis EF, et al, eds. *Allergy: principles and practice.* St. Louis: CV Mosby; 1993: 1665-1666.

10. Clein NW. Cow's milk allergy in infants and children. *Int Arch Allergy Appl Immunol.* 1958;13:245-256.

11. Anet J, Back JF, Baker RS, et al. Allergens in the white and yolk of hen's egg. *Int Arch Allergy Appl Immunol* 1985;77:364-371.

12. Langeland T. A clinical and immunological study of allergy to hen's egg white. III. Allergens in hen's egg white studied by crossed radio-immunoelectrophoresis. *Allergy.* 1982;37:521-530.

13. Hoffman DR. Immunochemical identification of the allergens in egg white. *J Allergy Clin Immunol.* 1983;71: 481-486.

14. Langeland T, Harbitz O. A clinical and immunological study of allergy to hen's egg white. V. Purification and identification of a major allergen (antigen 22) in hen's egg white. *Allergy.* 1983;38:131-139.

15. Holen E, Elsayed S. Characterization of four major allergens of hen egg white by IEF/SDS-PAGE combined with electrophoretic transfer and IgE-immunoautoradiography. *Int Arch Allergy Appl Immunol.* 1990;91:136-141.

16. Langeland T. A clinical and immunological study of allergy to hen's egg white. VI. Occurrence of proteins cross-reacting with allergens in hen's egg white as studied in egg white from turkey, duck, goose, seagull, and in hen egg yolk, and hen and chicken sera and flesh. *Allergy.* 1983;38:399-412.

17. Bush RK, Taylor SL, Nordlee JA. Peanut sensitivity. *Allergy Proc.* 1989;10:261-264.

18. Burks AW, Williams LW, Helm RM, et al. Identification of a major peanut allergen, Ara h I, in patients with atopic dermatitis and positive peanut allergen. *J Allergy Clin Immunol.* 1991;88:172-179.

19. Burks AW, Williams LW, Connaughton C, et al. Identification and characterization of a second major peanut allergen, Ara h II, utilizing the sera of patients with atopic dermatitis and positive peanut challenge. *J Allergy Clin Immunol.* 1992;90:962-969.

20. Nordlee JA, Taylor SL, Jones RT, et al. Allergenicity of various peanut products as determined by RAST inhibition. *J Allergy Clin Immunol.* 1981;68:372-375.

21. Taylor SL, Busse WW, Sachs MI, et al. Peanut oil is not allergenic to peanut-sensitive individuals. *J Allergy Clin Immunol.* 1981;68:372-375.

22. Burks AW, Brooks JR, Sampson HA. Allergenicity of major component proteins of soybean determined by ELISA and immunoblotting in children with atopic dermatitis and positive soy challenges. *J Allergy Clin Immunol.* 1988;81:1135-1142.

23. Bernhisel-Broadbent J, Sampson HA. Cross-allergenicity in the legume botanical family in children with food hypersensitivity. *J Allergy Clin Immunol.* 1989;83: 435-440.

24. Bush RK, Taylor SL. Nordlee JA, et al. Soybean oil is not allergenic to soybean-sensitive individuals. *J Allergy Clin Immunol.* 1985;76:242-245.

25. Bock SA, Atkins FM. The natural history of peanut. *J Allergy Clin Immunol.* 1989;83:900-904.

26. Aas K. Studies of hypersensitivity to fish. A clinical study. *Int Arch Allergy Appl Immunol.* 1966;29:346-363.

27. Ilsayed S, Bennich H. The primary structure of allergen M from cod. *Scand J Immunol.* 1975;4:203-208.

28. James JM, Helm RM, Burks AW, et al. Comparison of pediatric and adult IgE antibody binding to fish proteins. *Clin Exp Allergy.* (submitted).

29. Bernhisel-Broadbent J, Sampson HA. Fish hypersensitivity. I. Laboratory studies and oral challenges in fish allergic patients. *J Allergy Clin Immunol.* 1992;89:730-737.

30. Pascual C, Esteban MM, Crespo JF. Fish allergy: Evaluation of the importance of cross-reactivity. *J Pediatr.* 1992;121:S29-S34.

31. Bernhisel-Broadbent J, Sampson HA. Fish hypersensitivity. II. Clinical relevance of altered fish allergenicity secondary to various preparation methods. *J Allergy Clin Immunol.* 1992;90:622-629.

32. Lehrer SB, McCants ML, Salvaggio JE. Identification of crustacea allergens by crossed radioimmunoelectrophoresis. *Int Arch Allergy Appl Immunol.* 1985;77:192-194.

33. Lehrer SB, Ibanez MD, McCants ML, et al. Characterization of water-soluble shrimp allergens released during boiling. *J Allergy Clin Immunol.* 1990;85:1005-1013.

34. Daul CB, Slattery M, Lehrer SB. Shared antigenic/allergenic epitopes between shrimp Pen a I and fruit fly extract. *J Allergy Clin Immunology.* 1993;91:341.

35. Waring NP, Daul CB, deShazo RD, et al. Hypersensitivity reactions to ingested crustacea: Clinical evaluation and diagnostic studies in shrimp-sensitive individuals. *J Allergy Clin Immunol.* 1985;76:440-445.

36. Sutton R, Hill DJ, Baldo BA, et al. Immunoglobulin E antibodies to ingested cereal flour components: Studies with sera from subjects with asthma and eczema. *Clin Allergy.* 1982;12:63-74.

37. Jones SM, Magnolfi CF, Cooke SK, Sampson HA. Immunologic cross-reactivity among cereal grains and grasses in children with food hypersensitivity. *J Allergy Clin Immunol.* 1995;96:341-351.

38. Holgate ST, Robinson C, Church MK. Mediators of immediate hypersensitivity. In: Middleton RE, Reed CE, Ellis EF, et al, eds. *Allergy: principles and practice.* St. Louis: CV Mosby, 1993:267-301.

39. Sampson HA. The role of food allergy and mediator release in atopic dermatitis. *J Allergy Clin Immunol.* 1988;81:635-645.

40. Sampson HA, Broadbent KR, Bernhisel-Broadbent J. Spontaneous release of histamine from basophils and histamine-releasing factor in patients with atopic dermatitis and food hypersensitivity. *N Engl J Med.* 1989;321:228-232.

41. Alam R, Kuna P, Rozniecki J, et al. The magnitude of the spontaneous production of histamine-releasing factor by lymphocytes in vitro correlates with the state of bronchial hypersensitivity in patients with asthma. *J Allergy Clin Immunol.* 1987;79:103-108.

42. Sampson HA, Jolie PL. Increased plasma histamine concentrations after food challenges in children with atopic dermatitis. *N Engl J Med.* 1984;11:372-376.

43. Schwartz LB, Yuninger JW, Miller J, et al. Time course of appearance and disappearance of human tryptase in the circulation after anaphylaxis. *J Clin Invest.* 1989;83:1551-1555.

44. Buissert PD, Youlten EJF, Heinzelmann DL, et al. Prostaglandin synthesis inhibitors in prophylaxis of food intolerance. *Lancet.* 1978;1:906-908.

45. Cafrey EA, Sladen GE, Isaacs PET, et al. Thrombocytopenia caused by cow's milk (letter). *Lancet.* 1981;2:316.

46. Paganelli R, Levinsky RJ, Brostoff J, et al. Immune complexes containing food proteins in normal and atopic subjects after oral challenges and effect of sodium cromoglycate on antigen absorption. *Lancet.* 1979;1:1270-1272.

47. Falth-Magnusson K, Kjellman NIM, Magnusson KE. Antibodies IgG, IgA, and IgM to food antigens during the first 18 months of life in relation to feeding and development of atopic disease. *J Allergy Clin Immunol.* 1988;81;743-749.

48. Kemeny DM, Urbanek R, Amlot PL, Ciclitira PJ, et al. Sub-class of IgG in allergic disease I. IgG subclass antibodies in immediate and non-immediate food allergy. *Clin Allergy.* 1986;16:571-581.

49. Paganelli R, Quiti I, D'Offizi GP, et al. Immune-complexes in food allergy: a critical reappraisal. *Ann Allergy.* 1987;59:157-161.

50. McDonald PJ, Goldblum RM, Van Sickle GJ, et al. Food protein induced enterocolitis: Altered antibody response to ingested antigen. *Pediatr Res.* 1984;18:751-785.

51. May CD, Alberto R. In vitro responses of leukocytes to food proteins in allergic and normal children:

Lymphocyte stimulation and histamine release. *Clin Allergy.* 1972;2:335-344.

52. Bock SA, Atkins FM. Patterns of food hypersensitivity during sixteen years of double-blind placebo-controlled oral food challenges. *J Pediatr.* 1990;117:561-567.

53. Champion RH, Roberts SO, Carpenter RG, et al. Urticaria and angioedema: a review of 554 patients. *Br J Dermatol.* 1969;81:588-597.

54. Rajka G. Clinical aspects. In: Rajka G, ed. *Essential Aspects of Atopic Dermatitis.* Berlin, Germany: Springer-Verlag; 1989:7-12.

55. Blaylock WK. Atopic dermatitis: Diagnosis and pathobiology. *J Allergy CLin Immunol.* 1976;57:62-79.

56. Burks AW, Mallory SB, Williams LW, et al. Atopic dermatitis: Clinical relevance of food hypersensitivity reactions. *J Pediatr.* 1988;113:447-451.

57. Sampson HA. The immunopathogenic role of food hypersensitivity in atopic dermatitis. *Acta Derm Venereol.* 1992;176:34-37.

58. Sampson HA, McCaskill CM. Food hypersnesitivity and atopic dermatitis: Evaluation of 113 patients. *J Pediatr.* 1985;107:669-675.

59. Leiferman KM, Ackerman SJ, Sampson HA, et al. Dermal deposition of eosinophil granule major basic protein in atopic dermatitis. Comparison with onchocerciasis. *N Engl J Med.* 1986;313:282-285.

60. Charlesworth EN, Kagey-Sobotka A, Norman PS, et al. Cutaneous late-phase response in food-allergic children and adolescents with atopic dermatitis. *Clin Exp Allergy.* 23:391-397.

61. Sampson HA, Scanlon SM. Natural history of food hypersensitivity in children with atopic dermatitis. *J Pediatr.* 1989;115:23-27.

62. Silber GM, Sampson HA. Nasal mediator release following double-blind placebo-controlled oral food challenges. *J Allergy Clin Immunol.* 1988;81:185.

63. James JM, Bernhisel-Broadbent J, Sampson HA. Respiratory reactions provoked by double-blind food challenges in children. *Am J Respir Crit Care Med.* 1994; 149:59-64.

64. Novembre E, De Martino M, Vierucci A. Foods and respiratory allergy. *J Allergy Clin Immunol.* 1988;81: 1059-1065.

65. Onorato J, Merland N, Terral C, et al. Placebo-

controlled double-blind food challenge in asthma. *J Allergy Clin Immunol.* 1986;78:1139-1146.

66. James JM, Eigenmann PA, Eggleston PA, Sampson HA. Airway reactivity changes in asthmatic patients undergoing blinded food challenges. *Am J Respir Crit Care Med.* 1996;153:597-603.

67. Amelot PL, Kemeny DM, Zachary C, et al. Oral allergy syndrome: Symptoms of IgE-mediated hypersensitivity to foods. *Clin Allergy.* 1987;17:33-42.

68. Dreborg S, Roucard T. Allergy to apple, carrot, and potato in children with birch-pollen allergy. *Allergy.* 1983;38:167-172.

69. Calkhoven PG, Aalberse M, Koshte VL, et al. Cross-reactivity among birch pollen, vegetables and fruits as detected by IgE antibodies is due to at least three distinct cross-reactive structures. *Allergy.* 1987;42:383-390.

70. Anderson LB, Dreyfuss EM, Logan J, et al. Melon and banana sensitivity coincident with ragweed pollinosis. *J Allergy Clin Immunol.* 1970;45:310-319.

71. Enberg RN, Leickly FE, McCullough J, et al. Watermelon and ragweed share allergens. *J Allergy Clin Immunol.* 1987;79:867-875.

72. Ortaloni C, Ispano M, Pastorello EA, et al. Comparison of results of skin prick tests (with fresh foods and commercial food extracts) and RAST in 100 patients with oral allergy syndrome. *J Allergy Clin Immunol.* 1989; 83:683-690.

73. Sampson HA. Food allergy. *J Allergy Clin Immunol.* 1989; 84:1062-1067.

74. Patrick RB, Diamant SC, Gall DG. Motility effects of intestinal anaphylaxis in the rat. *Am J Physiol.* 1988;255: G505-G511.

75. Turner MW, Barnett GE, Strobel S. Mucosal mast cell activation patterns in the rat following repeated feeding of antigen. *Clin Exp Allergy.* 1990;20:421-427.

76. Hide DW, Guyer DM. Prevalence of infant colic. *Arch Dis Child.* 1982;57:559-560.

77. Jakobsson I, Lindberg T. Cow's milk as a cause of infantile colic in breast-fed infants. *Lancet.* 1978;2:437-439.

78. Jakobsson I, Lindberg T. Cow's milk proteins cause infantile colic in breast-fed infants: a double blind crossover study. *Pediatrics.* 1983;71:2-6.

79. Lothe L, Lindberg T, Jakobsson I. Cow's milk formula as a cause of infantile colic: a double blind study. *Pediatrics.* 1982;70:7-10.

80. Sampson HA. Infantile colic and food allergy: Fact or fiction? *J Pediatr.* 1989;115:583-584.

81. Min KU. Eosinophilic gastroenteritis. In: Metcalfe DD, Sampson HA, Simon RA, eds. *Food Allergy: Adverse Reactions to Foods and Food Additives.* Cambridge, MA: Blackwell Scientific Publications; 1991:167-168.

82. Katz AJ, Goldman H, Grand RJ. Gastric mucosal biopsies in eosinophilic (allergic) gastroenteritis. *Gastroenterology.* 1977;73:705-709.

83. Johnstone JM, Morson BS. Eosinophilic gastroenteritis. *Histopathology.* 1978;2:335-348.

84. Caldwell JH, Tennenbaum JI, Bronstein HA. Serum IgE in eosinophilic gastroenteritis: response to intestinal challenge in two cases. *N Engl J Med.* 1975;292:1388-1390.

85. Waldman TA, Wochner RD, Laster RD, et al. Allergic gastroenteropathy: A cause of excessive gastrointestinal protein loss. *N Engl J Med.* 1967;276:761-769.

86. Yunginger JW, Sweeney KG, Sturner WQ, et al. Fatal food-induced anaphylaxis. *JAMA.* 1988;260:1450-1452.

87. Sampson HA, Mendelson L, Rosen JP. Fatal and near-fatal anaphylactic reactions to food in children and adolescents. *N Engl J Med.* 1992;327:380-384.

88. Powell GK. Milk and soy induced enterocolitis of infancy: Clinical features and standardization of challenge. *J Pediatr.* 1978;93:553-560.

89. Goldman AS, Anderson DW, Sellers WA, et al. Milk allergy. I. Oral challenge with milk and isolated milk proteins in allergic children. *Pediatrics.* 1963;32:425-443.

90. Perkkio M, Savilahti E, Kuitunen P. Morphometric and immunohistochemical study of jejunal biopsies from children with intestinal soy allergy. *Eur J Pediatr.* 1981; 137:63-69.

91. Pearson JR, Kingston D, Shiner M. Antibody production to milk proteins in the jejunal mucosa of children with cow's milk protein intolerance. *Pediatr Res.* 1983;17: 406-412.

92. Selkekk BH. A comparison between in vitro jejunal mast cell degranulation and intragastric challenge in patients with suspected food intolerance. *Scand J Gastroenterol.* 1985;20:299-303.

93. Nolte H, Schiotz PO, Kruse A, et al. Comparison of intestinal mast cell and basophil histamine release in children with food allergic reactions. *Allergy.* 1989;44: 554-565.

94. Gryboski JD. Gastrointestinal milk allergy in infants. *Pediatrics.* 1967;40:354-362.

95. Goldman H, Proujansky R. Allergic proctitis and gastroenteritis in children. *Am J Surg Pathol.* 1986;10: 75-86.

96. O'Mahony S, Ferguson A. Gluten-sensitive enteropathy (celiac disease). In: Metcalfe DD, Sampson HA, Simon RA, eds. *Food Allergy: Adverse Reactions to Foods and Food Additives.* Cambridge, MA: Blackwell Scientific Publications; 1991:189-192.

97. Selby WS, Janossy G, Bofill M, et al. Lymphocyte subpopulations in the human small intestine. The findings in normal mucosa and in the mucosa of patients with adult coeliac disease. *Clin Exp Immunol.* 1983;52:219-228.

98. Baklein K, Brandtzaeg P, Fausa O. Immunoglobulins in jejunal mucosa and serum from patients with adult coeliac disease. *Scand J Gastroenterol.* 1977;12:149-159.

99. Asquith P, Thompson RA, Cooke WT. Serum immunoglobulins in adult coeliac disease. *Lancet.* 1969; 2:129-131.

100. Scott H, Fausa V, Ed J, Brandtzaeg P. Immune response patterns in coeliac disease: Serum antibodies to dietary antigens measured by an enzyme linked immunosorbent assay. *Clin Exp Immunol.* 1984;57:25-32.

101. Ferguson A. Models of immunologically driven small intestinal damage. In: Marsh MN, ed. *Immunopathology of the small intestine.* Chichester: John Wiley and Sons; 1987:225-252.

102. Marsh MN. Studies of intestinal lymphoid tissue. XI. The immunopathology of cell-mediated reactions in gluten sensitivity and other enteropathies. *Scanning Microsc.* 1988;2:1663-1684.

103. McNeish AS, Harms HK, Rey T, et al. The diagnosis of coeliac disease. *Arch Dis Child.* 1979;54:783-786.

104. Tucker NT, Barghuthy FS, Prihoda TJ, et al. Antigliadin antibodies detected by enzyme-linked immunosorbent assay as a marker of childhood celiac disease. *J Pediatr.* 1988;113:286-289.

105. Kumar V, Lerner A, Valeski JE, et al. Endomysial antibodies in the diagnosis of celiac disease and the effect of gluten on antibody titers. *Immunol Invest.* 1989;18:533-544.

106. Holmes GKT, Prior P, Lane MR, et al. Malignancy in

coeliac disease: Effect of a gluten free diet. *Gut.* 1989; 30:333-338.

107. Heiner DC, Sears JW. Chronic respiratory disease associated with multiple circulating precipitins to cow's milk. *Am J Dis Child.* 1960;100:500-502.

108. Lee SK, Kniker WT, Cook CD, et al. Cow's milk-induced pulmonary disease in children. *Adv Pediatr.* 1978;25:39-57.

109. Hall RP. The pathogenesis of dermatitis herpetiformis: Recent advances. *J Am Acad Dermatol.* 1987;16:1129-1144.

110. Katz SI, Hall RP, Lawley TJ, et al. Dermatitis herpetiformis: The skin and the gut. *Ann Intern Med.* 1980;93:857-874.

111. Bock SA, Lee WY, Remigio LK, et al. Studies of hypersensitivity reactions to foods in infants and children. *J Allergy Clin Immunol.* 1978;62:327-334.

112. Sampson HA. Role of immediate food hypersensitivity in the pathogenesis of atopic dermatitis. *J Allergy Clin Immunol.* 1983;71:473-480.

113. Taudorf E, Malling HJ, Laursen LC, et al.Reproducibility of histamine prick test. *Allergy.* 1985;40:344-349.

114. Sampson HA, Albergo R. Comparison of results of skin tests, RAST, and double-blind placebo-controlled food challenges in children with atopic dermatitis. *J Allergy Clin Immunol.* 1984;74:26-33.

115. Bock SA, Buckley J, Houst A, May CD. Proper use of skin tests with food extracts in diagnosis of food hypersensitivity. *Clin Allergy.* 1978;8:559-564.

116. Menardo JL, Bousquet J, Rodiere M, et al. Skin test reactivity in infancy. *J Allergy Clin Immunol.* 1985;74: 646-651.

117. Pollard HM, Stuart GJ. Experimental reproduction of gastric allergy in human beings with controlled observations on the mucosa. *J Allergy.* 1942;13:467-473.

118. Reimann HJ, Lewin J. Gastric mucosal reactions in patients with food allergy. *Am J Gastroenterol.* 1988;83: 1212-1219.

119. Sampson HA. Immunologically mediated food allergy: The importance of food challenge procedures. *Ann Allergy.* 1988;60:262-269.

120. Bock SA, Sampson HA, Atkins FM, et al. Double-blind, placebo-controlled food challenge (DBPCFC) as an office procedure: A manual. *J Allergy Clin Immunol.* 1988;82:986-997.

121. Bernstein M, Day JH, Welsh A. Double-blind food challenge in the diagnosis of food sensitivity in the adult. *J Allergy Clin Immunol.* 1982;70:205-210.

122. Atkins FM, Steinberg SS, Metcalfe DD. Evaluation of immediate adverse reactions to foods in adult patients. I. Correlation of demographic, laboratory, and prick skin test data with response to controlled oral food challenge. *J Allergy Clin Immunol.* 1985;75:348-355.

123. Leinhas JL, McCaskill CC, Sampson HA. Food allergy challenges: Guidelines and implications. *J Am Dietetic Assoc.* 1987;87:608.

124. Metcalfe DD, Sampson HA. Workshop on experimental methodology for clinical studies of adverse reactions to foods and food additives. *J Allergy Clin Immunol.* 1990; 86:421-442.

125. Executive Committee of the Academy of Allergy and Immunology. Personnel and equipment to treat systemic reactions caused by immunotherapy with allergic extracts [Position statement]. *J Allergy Clin Immunol.* 1986;77: 271-273.

126. Gern J, Sampson HA. Allergic reactions to milk-contaminated "nondiary" products. *N Engl J Med.* 1991; 324:976-979.

127. Bierman CS, Shapiro GG, Christie DL, et al. Eczema, rickets, and food allergy. *J Allergy Clin Immunol.* 1978; 61:119-127.

128. David TJ, Waddington E, Stanton RHJ. Nutritional hazards of elimination diets in children with atopic dermatitis. *Arch Dis Child.* 1984;59:323-325.

129. Bock SA. The natural history of food sensitivity. *J Allergy Clin Immunol.* 1982;69:173-177.

130. Koerner CB, Sampson HA. Diets and nutrition. In: Metcalfe DD, Sampson HA, Simon RA, eds. *Food Allergy: Adverse Reactions to Foods and Food Additives.* Cambridge, MA: Blackwell Scientific Publications; 1991: 332-354.

131. Sogn DD. Medications and their use in the treatment of adverse reactions to foods. *J Allergy Clin Immunol.* 1986;78:238-243.

132. Burks AW, Sampson HA. Double-blind placebo-controlled trial of oral cromolyn in children with atopic dermatitis and documented food hypersensitivity. *J Allergy Clin Immunol.* 1988;81:417-423.

133. Oppenheimer JJ, Nelson HS, Bock SA, et al. Treatment

of peanut allergy with rush immunotherapy. *J Allergy Clin Immunol.* 1992;90:256-262.

134. Jewett DL, Gein G, Greenberg MH. A double-blind study of symptom provocation to determine food sensitivity. *N Engl J Med.* 1990;323:429-433.

135. Falth-Magnusson K, Kjellman NIM. Development of atopic disease in babies whose mothers were receiving exclusion diet during pregnancy-A randomized study. *J Allergy Clin Immunol.* 1987;80:869-875.

136. Kajosaari M, Saarinen U. Prophylaxis of atopic disease by six months total solid food elimination. *Acta Paediatr Scand.* 1983;72:411-414.

137. Matthew D, Taylor B, Norman A, et al. Prevention of eczema. *Lancet.* 1977;1:321-324.

138. Cant A, Bailes J, Marsden R, et al. Effect of maternal dietary exclusion on breast-fed infants with eczema: Two controlled studies. *Br Med J.* 1986;293:231-233.

139. Chandra R, Puri S, Hamed A. Influence of maternal diet during lactation and use of formula feeds on development of atopic eczema in high risk infants. *Br Med J.* 1989;299:228-230.

140. Hattevig G, Kjellman B, Sigurs N, et al. Effect of maternal avoidance of eggs, cow's milk and fish during lactation upon allergic manifestations in infants. *Clin Exp Allergy.* 1989;19:27-32.

141. Sigurs N, Hattevig G, Kjellman B. Maternal avoidance of eggs, cow's milk, and fish during lactation: Effect on allergic manifestations, skin-prick tests, and specific IgE antibodies in children at age 4 years. *Pediatrics.* 1992;89: 735-739.

142. Zeiger RS, Heller S, Mellon MH, et al. Effect of combined maternal and infant food-allergen avoidance on development of atopy in early infancy: A randomized study. *J Allergy Clin Immunol.* 1989;84:72-89.

143. Zeiger RS, Heller S, Mellon MH, et al. Genetic and environmental factors affecting the development of atopy through age 4 in children of atopic parents: A prospective randomized study of food allergen avoidance. *Pediatr Allergy Immunol.* 1992;3:110-127.

144. Hanson DG, Vaz NM, Maia LCS, et al. Inhibition of specific immune response by feeding protein antigens. III. Evidence against maintenance of tolerance to ovalbumin by orally induced antibodies. *J Immunol.* 1979;123:2337-2343.

145. Fergusson DM, Horwood LJ, Beautrias AL, et al. Eczema and infant diet. *Clin Allergy.* 1981;11:325-331.

Rationale for Breast-feeding

Richard J. Schanler M.D.[1,2]

Nancy F. Butte Ph.D.[2]

Section of Neonatology[1] and
USDA/ARS Children's Nutrition Research Center,[2]
Department of Pediatrics,
Baylor College of Medicine, Houston, TX

"On teleologic grounds, it is reasonable to suppose that the milk of each species is well adapted to the particular needs of that species."[1]

Introduction

The Committees on Nutrition of the American Academy of Pediatrics and the Canadian Paediatric Society have strongly recommended breast-feeding for full-term infants.[1,2] Human milk is recommended as the exclusive nutrient source for feeding full-term infants during the first six months after birth, and its continued use with the addition of solid foods is advised for at least the first year.[1,2] The recommendation to feed human milk arises from its acknowledged benefits with respect to infant nutrition, gastrointestinal function, host defense and psychological well-being. Favorable outcomes of breast-feeding are reported both for infants and mothers. The unique species-specificity of human milk should be considered in any discussion of the merits of breast-feeding. This chapter will focus on the rationale for breast-feeding by describing human milk composition and the effect of maternal diet; the specific nutritional and nonnutritional factors that facilitate superior nutrient absorption, host defense and gastrointestinal function; and the functional outcomes of breast-feeding for infants and mothers.

Epidemiology of Breast-feeding in the United States

The rates of breast-feeding in the United States have fluctuated throughout this century. The incidence and duration of breast-feeding declined in the 1950s and 1960s, but increased in the early 1980s (Figures 1-2). The rates have declined since then. Some of the variability in rates of breast-feeding can be accounted for by such factors as race and ethnicity, maternal age and maternal education. There are marked differences in rates of breast-feeding within geographic regions of the United States. Figures 1-2 and Table 1 depict the data accumulated each year by the Ross Mothers' Survey (Ross Laboratories, Columbus, OH) from new mothers in the United States. The respondent mothers are telephoned when their infants are six months of age and are asked how they fed their infants in the hospital and at five to six months. As the survey has a 54% response rate, biases are acknowledged.[3] The data, therefore, may under-represent the indigent and those mothers in the lowest socioeconomic group who may not have responded to the survey.[3] Nevertheless, the data are the best available, and aid in predicting trends and areas where specific interventions should be targeted.[3]

Milk Composition
Nutritional Aspects

It is important to understand the unique specificity of the components of human milk. Many factors have dual roles: one as a nutrient source or to facilitate nutrient absorption, and the other to promote host defense or gastrointestinal function. Human milk is remarkable for the variability of its composition.[4] This variability may serve to improve nutrient composition in a way that is specifically adapted to the needs of the infant.[4]

Protein (Nitrogen)

In the first few weeks after birth, the total nitrogen content of the milk of women who deliver preterm infants (preterm milk) is greater than that of the milk of

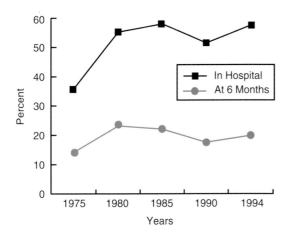

Figure 1: Percentage of infants breast-fed in the hospital and at five to six months in the United States (Ross Mothers' Survey, Ross Laboratories, Columbus, OH).

women delivering full-term infants (term milk).[5-8] Usually after the first few weeks of lactation, the total nitrogen content in both milks declines similarly to the level in what is called mature milk.[7, 8] Approximately 20% of the total nitrogen is in the form of nonprotein nitrogen-containing compounds such as free amino acids and urea in contrast to bovine milk, which has 5% nonprotein nitrogen.[9, 10] There is debate as to how much of these nonprotein nitrogen-containing compounds contribute to nitrogen utilization.[11, 12] The rate of absorption of nonprotein nitrogen, determined by stable isotope methods, has been estimated at 13 to 43%.[11, 12]

The protein quality, or the proportion of whey and casein proteins, of human milk differs from that of bovine milk (30% casein and 70% whey vs 82% casein and 18% whey, respectively).[10] The caseins are a group of proteins with low solubility in acid media. Whey proteins remain in solution after acid precipitation. Generally, the soluble proteins in the whey fraction are more easily digested and tend to facilitate more rapid gastric emptying.[13] The whey protein fraction provides lower concentrations of phenylalanine, tyrosine and methionine and higher concentrations of taurine than the casein fraction of milk.[14-17] The pattern of amino acids in the plasma of breast-fed infants is used as a reference in infant nutrition, thus avoiding potentially toxic imbalances in the levels of various amino acids.[18, 19]

The type of proteins contained in the whey fraction differs between human and bovine milks. The major human whey protein is α-lactalbumin, a protein involved in the mammary gland synthesis of lactose, and a nutritional protein for the infant. *Lactoferrin, lysozyme, and secretory immunoglobulin A (sIgA) are specific human whey proteins involved in host defense.[20-22] Because these host defense proteins resist proteolytic digestion, they are capable of a first line of defense by lining the gastrointestinal tract.* The three host defense proteins essentially are absent in bovine milk, where the major whey protein is β-lactoglobulin.[10]

Lipid

The lipid system in human milk, responsible for providing approximately 50% of the calories in the milk, is structured to facilitate superior fat digestion and absorption.[4, 23] The lipid system is composed of an organized milk fat globule, a pattern of fatty acids (high in palmitic 16:0, oleic 18:1 and the essential fatty acids; linoleic 18:2ω-6, and linolenic 18:3ω-3) characteristically distributed on the triglyceride molecule (16:0 at the 2-position of the molecule), and bile salt-stimulated lipase.[24, 25] As the lipase is heat-labile, it is important to recognize that the superior fat absorption from human milk is reported only when unprocessed milk is fed.[24] Most manufacturers of infant formulas have attempted to modify their fat blends to mimic the fat absorption in human milk. Thus, the mixture of fatty acids in formulas differs from that in human milk. Generally, to achieve similar proportions of fat absorption as observed from human milk, formulas have a greater quantity of medium chain-length fatty acids than human milk.

Of the macronutrients in human milk, fat is the most variable in content.[26] The fat content rises slightly throughout lactation, changes over the course of one day, increases within-feed, and varies from mother to mother.[27] The interindividual variation tracks through lactation and is not affected by diet, but may be affected by maternal body composition.[28, 29]

The pattern of fatty acids in human milk also is unique in its composition of very long-chain fatty acids. Arachidonic acid (20:4ω-6) and docosahexaenoic

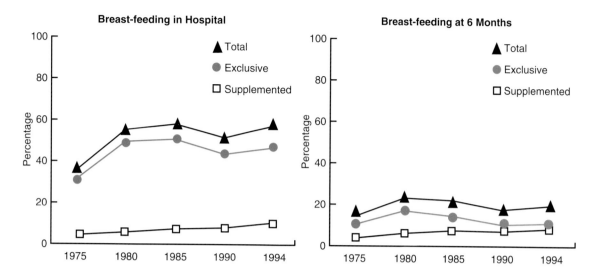

Figure 2: Percentage of infants breast-fed in the United States (Ross Laboratories).

acid (22:6ω-3), which are derivatives of linoleic and linolenic acids, respectively, are found in human but not bovine milk. Arachidonic and docosahexaenoic acids functionally have been associated with cognition, growth and vision.[30-32]

Carbohydrate

The carbohydrate composition of human milk is important as a nutritional source of lactose and for the presence of oligosaccharides. Although studies in full-term infants demonstrate that feces contain a small proportion of unabsorbed lactose, its presence is assumed to be a normal physiological effect of feeding human milk.[33, 34] A softer stool consistency, more non-pathogenic bacterial fecal flora and improved absorption of minerals have been attributed to the presence of small quantities of unabsorbed lactose from human milk feeding.[35, 36] Oligosaccharides are carbohydrate polymers and glycoproteins (also including mucins) important in the host defense of the infant.[37]

Mineral and Trace Elements

The concentration of calcium and phosphorus in human milk is significantly lower than in bovine milk and infant formula. The content of these macrominerals is relatively constant through lactation. The macrominerals in human milk are more bioavailable than those in infant formula because of the manner in which they are packaged. In human milk, the minerals are bound to digestible proteins and are also present in complexed and ionized states which are readily bioavailable.[38]

The concentrations of iron, zinc and copper decline through lactation.[39, 40] Nonetheless, the concentrations of copper and zinc appear adequate to meet the infant's nutritional needs through lactation. The concentration of iron, however, may not meet the infant's needs after six months of breast-feeding.[40, 41] Most authorities agree that an iron supplement initiated at that time is indicated to prevent subsequent iron deficiency anemia.

Vitamins

Maternal vitamin status may affect the content of vitamins in the milk. Generally, maternal vitamin deficiency may result in low concentrations in milk that increase in response to dietary supplementation. This is more common for water-soluble than fat-soluble vitamins (see below).

Vitamin K deficiency may be a concern in the breast-fed infant. Bacterial flora are responsible for providing adequate vitamin K. The intestinal flora of

	In-Hospital			At 5-6 Months		
	1986	1990	1994	1986	1990	1994
All infants	56.9	51.5	57.4	23.1	19.0	21.3
Primiparous	57.9	52.5	59.7	19.8	16.2	19.4
Multiparous	55.9	50.6	55.3	26.8	21.8	22.8
Grade School	33.6	31.6	38.8	13.3	11.3	15.5
High School	48.1	41.3	47.7	16.6	12.8	14.9
Non-College	47.2	41.0	47.4	16.4	12.7	14.9
College	74.7	69.8	72.9	35.4	30.0	31.2
Employed Full-Time	55.4	51.3	58.6	11.6	10.5	14.1
Employed Part-Time	64.4	59.1	62.5	26.6	22.5	24.2
Total Employed	58.7	54.1	59.9	17.0	14.7	17.5
Not Employed	55.9	49.7	55.3	27.1	22.3	24.1
Less than $10,000	32.6	30.5	39.9	9.2	8.3	10.9
$10,000-$14,999	51.5	43.7	50.5	18.7	13.3	15.9
$15,000-$24,999	61.2	52.6	57.3	25.6	19.0	20.3
$25,000 +	70.3	66.0	68.6	31.4	27.1	28.4
Less than 20 years	34.3	30.0	39.9	7.4	6.3	8.4
20-24 years	52.5	44.0	51.2	16.8	12.1	15.0
25-29 years	63.6	57.3	61.5	27.1	21.2	23.2
30-34 years	68.2	64.2	66.3	35.6	30.0	29.5
35 + years	65.1	65.4	67.7	36.2	34.9	34.6
LBW <5 lb 8 oz	39.8	36.5	44.3	12.4	10.4	12.1
New England	59.9	53.2	58.4	25.9	21.8	22.0
Middle Atlantic	51.7	46.4	51.9	22.5	17.8	19.9
East North Central	52.5	47.1	52.9	21.2	17.4	18.9
West North Central	60.3	54.0	59.6	23.4	19.4	20.1
South Atlantic	48.7	44.2	52.5	18.1	15.0	18.3
East South Central	38.7	36.3	42.3	13.7	11.4	13.4
West South Central	51.3	45.7	51.9	16.7	13.9	16.3
Mountain	76.9	68.9	73.6	35.0	29.2	31.1
Pacific	75.6	69.0	72.7	34.2	27.5	30.5
WIC	38.0	33.7	44.3	11.6	8.9	12.6
Non-WIC	66.1	62.9	68.8	28.7	25.4	28.6
Pediatricians	57.9	52.5	58.2	23.6	19.4	21.6
General Practitioners	55.8	49.1	55.2	22.5	18.2	20.4
Black	27.1	23.0	33.2	8.4	6.8	10.3
White	63.1	57.6	62.3	26.5	22.1	23.9
Hispanic	51.9	48.0	57.8	17.7	14.2	18.9

Table 1: Percentage of infants breast-fed in the hospital and at five to six months in the United States, according to demographic factors (Ross Mothers' Survey, Ross Laboratories, Columbus, OH).

the breast-fed infant make less menaquinone and the content of vitamin K in human milk is low. Infant formula contains vitamin K. Therefore, to meet initial vitamin K needs, a single dose of vitamin K is given at birth to all newborns.[42]

Non-nutritional Factors
Nucleotides
Although they can be synthesized endogenously, it appears that exogenous nucleotides may have a role in a variety of metabolic functions.[43] Nucleotides consist of either a purine (uracil, cytosine, thymine) or pyrimidine (adenine, guanine, hypoxanthine, xanthine) base and a pentose sugar (ribose or deoxyribose) joined by mono-, di-, or triphosphate esters. As such, they serve as immediate precursors of RNA (ATP, GTP, CTP, UTP) and DNA (dATP, dGTP, dCTP, dTTP) synthesis. Nucleotides represent 2 to 5% of the nonprotein nitrogen in human milk.[44] Numerous functions have been attributed to dietary nucleotides. These include effects on lymphoid, intestinal, and hepatic tissues and in lipid metabolism.[43, 44] Exogenous nucleotides[44] have a positive effect on the growth of *Bifidobacteria* in stool flora.

Gastrointestinal
Many hormones (cortisol, somatomedin-C, insulin-like growth factors, insulin, thyroid hormone), growth factors (epidermal growth factor, nerve growth factor), and gastrointestinal mediators (neurotensin, motilin) present in human milk may affect gastrointestinal function and/or body composition. Epidermal growth factor (EGF) is a polypeptide that stimulates DNA synthesis, protein synthesis, and cellular proliferation in intestinal cells.[45] EGF resists proteolytic digestion and is found in the intestinal lumen of suckling animals. Nerve growth factor may play a role in the innervation of the intestinal tract. The hormonal components in milk may affect intestinal growth and mucosal function. Free amino acids may exert dual roles in infants. Taurine may be trophic for intestinal growth and glutamine may be a fuel for the small intestine.[45]

Host Defense
A variety of heterogeneous agents that possess antimicrobial activity are found in human milk.[20, 22, 37, 46]

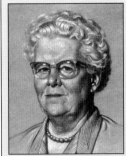

Edith B. Jackson, M.D. (1895-1977) was a Hopkins graduate who trained in pediatrics at Bellevue Hospital. She joined the faculty at Yale where she assisted chairman Edwards Park, a Howland trainee, with the testing of vitamin D for prevention of rickets. From 1930 to 1936 Jackson trained with Sigmund Freud in Vienna. She returned to Yale to direct the Psychiatric Services for Children at New Haven Hospital under chairman Grover Powers, another Howland trainee. Jackson created a "rooming-in" unit where the family was allowed to participate in the delivery and care of newborn. The rooming-in experience provided " a stimulus to breast feeding...an implement to improved baby care, and...a method of education of the mother in the responsibilities and techniques of raising a baby." By mid-century, residents trained in this unit became Chairmen of half of the Pediatric Departments in the U.S. and family centered care soon became the national norm. Silberman, S. L., Pioneering in family-centered maternity and infant care: Edith B. Jackson and the Yale rooming-in research project. Bull His Med 1990; 64:262-287 (Drawing courtesy of CNRC)

Many of these agents persist through lactation and are resistant to the digestive enzymes in the infant's gastrointestinal tract. The antimicrobial activities generally are found at mucosal surfaces, such as those of the gastrointestinal, respiratory and urinary tracts.

Specific factors such as lactoferrin, lysozyme and sIgA comprise the whey fraction of human milk protein, generally resist proteolytic degradation, and line mucosal surfaces, preventing microbial attachment and inhibiting microbial activity.[20-22, 47] Lactoferrin has antimicrobial activity when not conjugated to iron (apolactoferrin). It may function with other host defense proteins to effect microbial killing. Lysozyme is active against bacteria by cleaving cell walls. Plasma cells synthesize sIgA against specific antigens. The enteromammary and bronchomammary immune systems summarize the important part of the protective nature of human milk.[48, 49] In each system, the mother produces sIgA antibody when exposed to a foreign antigen via either her respiratory or gastrointestinal

Component, units/L	Human milk	Bovine milk
Energy, kcal	680	680
Protein, g	10	33
%Whey/Casein	72/28	18/82
Fat, g	39	38
%MCT/LCT	2/98	8/92
Carbohydrate, g	72	47
%Lactose	100	100
Calcium, mg	280	1200
Phosphorus, mg	140	920
Magnesium, mg	35	120
Sodium, mg	180	480
Potassium, mg	525	1570
Chloride, mg	420	1020
Zinc, μg	1200	3500
Copper, μg	250	100
Iron, μg	300	460
Vitamin A, IU	2230	1000
Vitamin D, IU	22	24
Vitamin E, IU	2.3	0.9
Vitamin K, μg	2.1	4.9
Thiamin (vitamin B1), μg	210	300
Riboflavin (vitamin B2), μg	350	1750
Pyridoxine (vitamin B6), μg	93	470
Niacin, mg	1.5	0.8
Biotin, μg	4	35
Pantothenic acid, mg	1.8	3.5
Folic Acid, μg	85	50
Vitamin B12, μg	1	4
Ascorbic acid, mg	40	17

Table 2: Composition of mature human milk and bovine milk. (Adapted from references 3, 42, 206-209.)

tract. The plasma cells traverse the lymphatic system and are secreted at mucosal surfaces, including that of the mammary gland. Ingesting milk, therefore, provides the infant with passive sIgA antibody against the offending antigen. The systems are active in infants against a variety of antigens.[20, 48, 49]

The products of lipid hydrolysis, free fatty acids and monoglycerides, may exhibit anti-microbial activity against a variety of pathogens.[50] These lipid end products may prevent attachment and infection with viruses and protozoa, such as *Giardia*. The activity of human milk bile-salt-stimulated lipase also may affect host defense.

The class of carbohydrates including the oligosaccharides and glucoconjugates of protein affect intestinal bacterial flora and facilitate the growth of *Lactobacillus species*. These agents also mimic bacterial epithelial receptors in the respiratory tract, and in doing so, prevent pathogenic agents from attaching to the epithelial lining of mucosal surfaces. A variety of oligosaccharides and glycoproteins act as receptor analogues for multiple antimicrobial agents.[37]

White blood cells (90% of which are neutrophils and macrophages) in human milk contribute to the antimicrobial activity through phagocytosis and intracellular killing.[21] The lymphocytes in human milk may contribute to cytokine production (T-cells) or IgA production (B-cells).[21, 46]

In summary, the composition of human milk is a complex mixture of compounds with several roles in nutrition, gastrointestinal function, and host defense. The components are in a dynamic state, occasionally affected by maternal diet and well-being, and appear uniquely suited to the human infant. A representation of the composition of mature human milk is difficult because of the dynamic nature of the nutrients, but for comparative purposes, the tabulation of mature human milk and bovine milk composition is given in Table 2.

Milk Volume

Milk volume has been measured conventionally by the test-weighing technique, that is, weighing the infant before and after each feeding for at least 24 hours. In industrialized societies, mean milk volumes reported for healthy, exclusively breast-fed infants range from about 750 to 800 g/d, but milk intakes for an individual infant may be as low as 450 g/d or as high as 1,200 g/d.[3] The volume of milk consumed has been

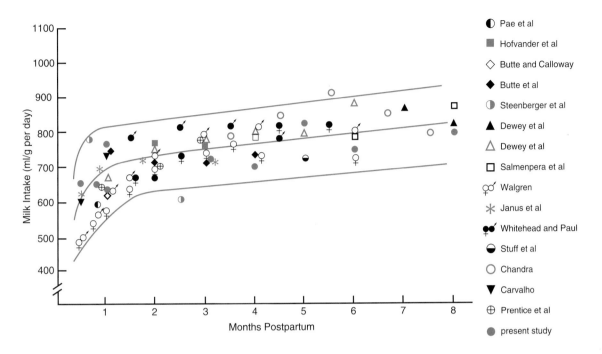

Figure 3: Twenty-four hour milk intakes of exclusively breast-fed infants measured by the test-weighing technique. (Reproduced with permission from Neville MC, R Keller, J Seacat, V Lutes, M Neifert, C Casey, J Allen, P Archer, 1988. Studies in human lactation: milk volumes in lactating women during the onset of lactation and full lactation. Am J Clin Nutr 48:1375-86.)

shown consistently to be influenced by the infant's current weight, weight gain, birth weight and gender.[6,51-53] The effects of birth weight and gender, however, are accounted for by the infant's current weight.

In underprivileged populations, human milk intakes (mean values ranging from 525 to 885 g/d)[54-59] are similar to or less than those reported for industrialized populations. Interpretation of many studies that report lower milk intakes is confounded by unmeasured or undocumented food supplementation.[60]

The pattern of human milk intake during the first eight months of life is displayed in Figure 3.[53] Milk intakes are low on the first two days, increase markedly on days three and four, and then gradually increase to levels seen in full lactation. At the beginning of lactation, many women produce more milk than the infant consumes. Even in established lactation, evidence from wet nurses[61] and mothers nursing twins or triplets[62] supports the view that infant demand, rather than maternal lactation capacity, determines milk intake.

Addition of milk substitutes or solid foods is associated with a decline in human milk intake. Instead of acting as supplements, milk substitutes and solid foods have been shown to displace human milk.[63,64] Because the timing of weaning varies, milk intakes reported for older breast-fed infants tend to be more variable. Mean (range) milk intakes of a cohort of healthy infants were 769 (335 to 1,144), 637 (205 to 1,185), and 445 (27 to 1,154) g/d recorded at six, nine, and 12 months of age, respectively.[3]

Maternal factors that influence milk volume have been investigated in a number of studies. Age, parity, current weight, body mass index, body fat, and weight gain during pregnancy have not been shown to influence milk production in well-nourished women.[29, 51, 52] Smoking has been shown to have a deleterious effect on milk intake in full-term Chilean infants[65] and on milk production rates in U.S. mothers who expressed milk for their preterm infants.[66] The inhibitory effect of smoking may be related to lower basal prolactin levels in smokers.[67] Combined estrogen/progestin oral contraceptives have a moderate inhibitory effect on milk yield, whereas Norplant® implants and vaginal rings containing the natural hormone progesterone have no effect on milk yield or breast-feeding duration.[68]

Effect of Maternal Nutrition on Milk Production

Evidence from diverse populations indicates that the capacity to produce milk of sufficient quantity and quality to support the growth of infants is satisfactory, even when the mother's dietary supply of nutrients is limited.[3] The additional nutritional needs imposed by lactation do not require drastic alterations in diet. Around the world, vastly diverse diets support adequate milk production. On the other hand, a chronically deficient diet resulting in depletion of maternal nutrient stores may adversely affect milk composition.

With the exception of extreme dietary deprivation, maternal energy intake seems to have only a weak or indirect effect on milk volume. A weak correlation between dietary energy intake and milk volume has been reported during early lactation.[29,69] Short-term diet restriction to 1,500 kcal/d for one week did not compromise milk production rates; however, there was some suggestion that diets with less than 1,500 kcal/d compromised subsequent milk production.[70] A 20-hour fast did not alter milk secretion rates,[71] neither did a ten-week weight reduction program that achieved a 538-kcal deficit affect milk volume or composition.[72]

There is no consistent evidence that diet affects the concentration of milk protein, even in malnourished populations.[73-75] Total nitrogen, nonprotein nitrogen (NPN) and amino acids in the milk of poorly nourished and well-nourished mothers did not differ.[73, 76] The effects of protein supplementation on milk protein concentration are less consistent. Increasing protein intake from 46 to 134 g/d increased total nitrogen and NPN concentration in milk in Swedish mothers.[77] Alterations in specific milk components, i.e., lactoferrin and α-lactalbumin, have been noted, but inconsistently.[73, 75, 78]

> *The composition of preterm human milk: teleological or coincidental?*
> Gilberta R. Pereira M.D.
> Children's Hospital
> of Philadelphia
> Philadelphia, Pennsylvania

The types of fatty acids in human milk are influenced primarily by the type and proportion of fat in the diet.[79] The fraction of milk lipids derived from endogenous fat synthesis within the mammary gland is increased by a low-fat diet. A reduction in dietary fat from 40 to 10% of total calories caused an increase in the milk content of short-chain saturated fatty acids.[80] The fatty acid composition of milk is also influenced by the consumption of partially hydrogenated fats and oils.[81] Vegetarians have been shown to have a higher concentration of linoleic acid in their milk.[82] There is no evidence that the cholesterol or phospholipid content of human milk is altered by diet.[79]

In general, the fat-soluble vitamins are susceptible to the vitamin status of the mother, and the water-soluble vitamins in milk are more responsive to maternal diet. Maternal vitamin A deficiency is associated with decreased levels of vitamin A in milk.[83, 84] Milk vitamin D is directly affected by maternal vitamin D status. Vitamin D concentrations were undetectable in the presence of vitamin D deficiency and responded to supplementation and ultraviolet light.[85] Pharmacologic doses of ergocalciferol (2,500 g) can result in toxic levels of vitamin D in milk.[86] The vitamin K concentration in human milk also is responsive to supplementation.[87]

Although influenced by maternal intake, a regulatory mechanism prevents elevation of milk vitamin C beyond approximately 160 mg/L.[88, 89] Milk thiamin can be increased to a ceiling of approximately 200 g/L.[90] In beriberi, the thiamin content of human milk declines. Milk niacin and B_6 depend largely on maternal intake and respond to supplementation.[91, 92] Although folate is preferentially secreted into milk at the expense of the mother's folate stores, milk concentrations can decline with severe folate deficiency. Milk folate increased rapidly after folate supplementation in lactating women with megaloblastic anemia.[93] In well-nourished American women, the vitamin B_{12} in human milk was not correlated with dietary B_{12} or use of B_{12} supplements.[94] Milk vitamin B_{12} content, however, is lower in complete vegetarian women, malnourished women, and those with latent pernicious anemia due secondarily to hypothyroidism.[95] The vegan mother, who eats no meat products, is at risk of vitamin B_{12} deficiency; her infant may be at risk of vitamin B_{12} deficiency, and may show signs of deficiency before the mother.[96] Maternal vitamin supplementation will provide vitamin sufficiency.[97]

Milk concentrations of calcium, phosphorus and magnesium, which are tightly regulated in the plasma, are not susceptible to dietary perturbations.[3] Iron and copper in human milk are independent of nutrient status.[98-100] Zinc supplementation (15 mg/d for seven months) did not affect milk zinc concentration in well-nourished women.[101] Selenium concentration in milk is directly related to plasma levels, when the latter are less than 100 g/L.[102] The mammary gland accumulates iodine, resulting in milk concentrations that vary widely with diet.[103]

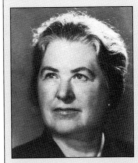

Icie G. Macy Hoobler Ph.D.
(1891-1984) graduated from Yale University in 1920 where her mentor, L. B. Mendel introduced her to the exciting era of essential nutrient discovery. Her thesis was on cottonseed flour. She joined the Merrill-Palmer School for Motherhood and Child Development in Detroit in 1923 where she opened a nutrition research laboratory. Macy's research focused on maternal metabolism during reproduction; composition and secretion of human milk; and body composition of normal growth. She married B. R. Hoobler in 1936, a pediatrician, who had collaborated at Cornell Medical School with Howland in the study of nitrogen balances of infants. J. Nutr. 114, 1351-1362,1984 (Photo courtesy of Wayne State U.)

Benefits of Breast-feeding for the Infant
Body Composition
Although lower concentrations of calcium and phosphorus are observed in human milk compared with formula, measures of bone mineralization are similar between human milk- or formula-fed full-term infants during the first year of life.[104-107]

Gastrointestinal Function
Gastric emptying is faster after feeding human milk than bovine milk-derived formula.[13] The clinical impression is that large gastric residual volumes are reported less frequently in preterm infants fed human milk. Many factors in human milk may stimulate gastrointestinal growth and motility, and enhance maturity of the gastrointestinal tract.

Morbidity
Numerous studies conducted in developing countries delineate the protective effects of breast-feeding. In developing areas, the incidence of gastroenteritis and respiratory disease and overall morbidity and mortality are lower in breast-fed infants than in infants fed milk substitutes.[108, 109] In developed countries such as the United States, breast-fed infants have lower rates of

diarrhea, lower respiratory tract illness, acute and recurrent otitis media, and urinary tract infection.[110-112] Not only is the attack rate lower, but the duration and severity of illness appear to be lessened in the breast-fed infant.[113]

In developed countries, there are fewer incidents of gastroenteritis in breast-fed infants.[108, 114] The incidence of diarrheal disease in infants breast-fed for 12 months was one-half that of formula-fed infants.[113] When adjusting for potentially confounding variables such as number of siblings and day care attendance, the same differences were observed. Infants who were breast-fed for at least 13 weeks were found to have a significantly lower incidence of gastroenteritis (vomiting or diarrhea as a discrete illness lasting 48 hours or more) to one year of age than infants who were fed formula from birth.[115] These observations were significant even when controlled for confounding variables such as social class, maternal age and smoking. As socioeconomic status is linked closely to morbidity, it is important to examine its effect in breast-fed infants. The protective effects of breast-feeding appear as strong, and the degree of morbidity decreased, even in affluent populations in the United States.[113]

Respiratory illnesses are reduced in frequency and/or duration in breast-fed infants.[114-117] The incidence of wheezing is less and overall lower respiratory tract infection is decreased.[114, 117] The incidence of otitis media and recurrent otitis media was reduced in infants breast-fed for four or more months.[118, 119] This protective effect was observed even when the data were controlled for confounding variables such as family history of allergy, family size, use of day care and smoking. Not only was the incidence of otitis media reduced in infants breast-fed for one year, but the duration of each episode was reduced significantly compared with formula-fed infants.[113]

A case-controlled study reported that the incidence of urinary tract infection was reduced in breast-fed infants.[120] The study matched groups for hospitalization, age, gender, social class, birth order and smoking status of the mother.[120] A mechanism for this protection has been suggested. Oligosaccharide excretion in the urine has been shown to prevent bacterial adhesion to urinary epithelial cells.[121] Other reports suggest that the host defense proteins, lactoferrin and sIgA, are excreted in the urine of human milk-fed preterm infants.[122]

Preterm infants have a lower incidence of necrotizing enterocolitis (NEC) when fed human milk compared with formula.[123] The lower incidence of NEC is observed even if the supply of mother's milk is low and formula is used as a supplement. Thus, both partial and exclusive use of mother's milk appears to protect the preterm infant from this devastating condition. Although the mechanism for protection from NEC is unclear, feeding IgA-IgG preparations appears to reduce its incidence.[124] These data suggest that by lining the gastrointestinal tract with host defense proteins, the infant is protected from this inflammatory condition.

The incidence of sepsis and a variety of other neonatal infections is reduced in preterm infants receiving human milk.[125, 126] Early feeding of colostrum also appears to reduce the incidence of infection in low birthweight infants compared with those fed formula.[127]

Chronic Disease

Perhaps the most intriguing data are those suggesting a lower incidence of chronic disorders in children who were breast-fed as infants. There may be protective effects against Crohn's disease, lymphoma, specific genotypes of type I juvenile diabetes mellitus and certain allergic conditions.[128-130] There are conflicting data regarding the protection against allergy afforded by breast-feeding.[131] In some reports where no protection was observed, maternal diet may not have excluded the potentially offending antigens. In other reports, breast-feeding appears to be protective against food allergies.[22, 37] Atopic dermatitis may be lessened in infants whose mothers follow a restricted diet. A lower incidence of atopic conditions is reported in breast-fed infants with a family history of atopy.[132]

There may be a relationship between breast-feeding and the development of type I insulin dependent diabetes mellitus (IDDM).[130] IDDM was more likely when breast-feeding was less than three months and bovine milk proteins were introduced before four months of age.[130] Elevated concentrations of specific IgG antibody to bovine serum albumin that cross-reacts with ß-cell-specific surface protein have been identified in children with IDDM.[133] It is estimated that up to 30% of type I IDDM could be prevented by removing bovine milk from the diet for the first three months.[130]

In summary, a large quantity of data is being collected that demonstrates the markedly protective effects of breast-feeding, in the developed world as well as in the developing world.

Neurobehavioral Aspects

Maternal-infant bonding is enhanced during breast-feeding. In addition, improved long-term cognitive and motor abilities in full-term infants have been directly correlated with the duration of breast-feeding. Even when adjusted for socioeconomic status and parent education significant increments were observed at three, four, and five years of age in a limited set of cognitive test scores that paralleled the duration of breast-feeding.[134] Improved long-term cognitive development in preterm infants has also been correlated with the receipt of human milk during their hospitalization.[135, 136] A series of studies indicated that human milk-fed, full-term and preterm infants have improved visual function compared with infants not receiving these fatty acids in their diet.[30 32, 137, 138]

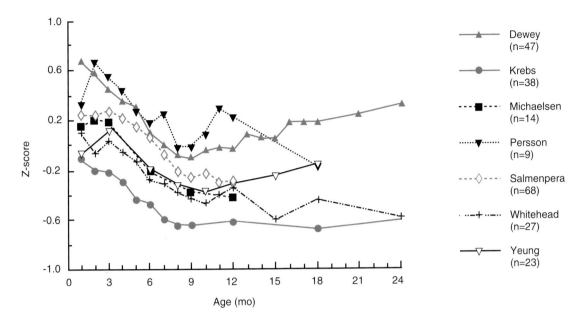

Figure 4: Mean NCHS weight-for-age Z-score of infants breast-fed for at least 12 months, reproduced with permission from World Health Organization.[145]

Growth Patterns of Breast-fed Infants

There is substantial evidence that the growth patterns of healthy breast-fed infants are distinct from formula-fed infants who conform more closely to the National Center for Health Statistics (NCHS) growth reference.[139-144] Breast-fed infants grow faster in the first two months and slower thereafter when compared with the NCHS reference. The slower growth of breast-fed infants is more evident in weight than height. Deviation from the NCHS curves is explained in part by the fact that the curves were based on predominantly formula-fed infants enrolled in the Fels Longitudinal Study from 1929 to 1975. Relative to the NCHS growth reference, the growth of breast-fed infants may be deemed unsatisfactory and may lead to early food supplementation and cessation of breast-feeding, which would increase the risk of infection and decrease contraceptive protection.

To address this issue, the World Health Organization recently assembled a working group to compile growth data of infants fed according to current WHO recommendations, which advocate exclusive breast-feeding for at least four months and partial breast-feeding for the remainder of the first year or possibly longer.[145] Seven longitudinal data sets met the technical prerequisites for inclusion in the analysis.[51,141,143,144,146-148] Relative to the NCHS reference, the weight-for-age curves displayed a consistently downward trend after the first two to three months, declining to a mean value of approximately -0.5 Z-score at 12 months (Figure 4). The mean length-for-age Z-scores also declined throughout the first year, averaging -0.29 at 12 months for the pooled sample (Figure 5). Weight-for-length Z-scores were higher than the NCHS reference for the first six to eight months, but declined in later infancy, averaging -0.32 at 12 months (Figure 6). The decline in weight and length Z-scores was related to the duration of breast-feeding. Infants not given formula or other milks were heavier during the first three months, and lighter and shorter at 12 months. Infants given supplementary solid foods at four to five months were lighter prior to four months than infants supplemented later. Infants supplemented after eight months were lighter and leaner throughout the first 12 months.

The growth pattern of breast-fed infants differed from that of formula-fed U.S. and European infants studied contemporaneously.[145] The weight-for-age,

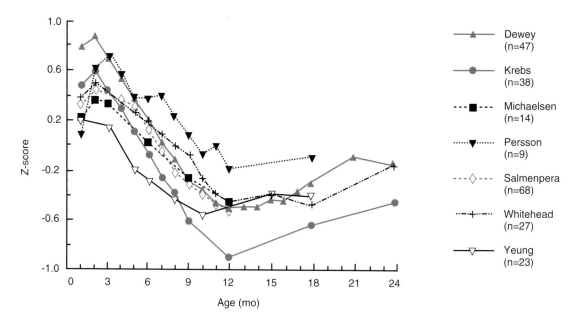

Figure 5: Mean NCHS length-for-age Z-score of infants breast-fed for at least 12 months, reproduced with permission from the World Health Organization.[145]

length-for-age and weight-for-length Z-scores were greater than zero for the first eight months, but close to zero at nine to 12 months. In contrast to breast-fed infants, the formula-fed infants did not display the downward growth trend during the second six months of life.

The causes of the distinct growth patterns of breast-fed and formula-fed infants are partially understood. Lower growth velocities observed in breast-fed infants are associated with lower nutrient intakes.[6, 51, 52] The lower energy intakes of breast-fed infants persist after the introduction of solids.[63, 149] Since these lower intakes do not seem attributable to inadequate lactation, regulation of infant appetite or weaning practices may differ between feeding groups. Slower growth velocity in breast-fed infants is not associated with obvious deleterious functional consequences. A U.S. study showed no association between energy intake and morbidity, or achievement of developmental milestones in infants fed breast milk through the first year of life.[64] Awareness of these distinct growth patterns should factor into the clinician's evaluation of infant growth and minimize the risk of prematurely introducing complementary foods to breast-fed infants.

Jaundice in Breast-fed Infants

Jaundice due to unconjugated hyperbilirubinemia has been associated with breast-feeding in terms of two entities, one manifesting during the first week and the other usually peaking after the first week of age.[150, 151] In the first week after birth, jaundice in a breast-fed infant may be related to inadequate milk intake and poor lactation performance. The treatment is aimed at decreasing the enterohepatic recirculation of bilirubin by increasing milk intake through an increase in the frequency of breast-feeding. By increasing the frequency of breast-feeding, the milk supply will increase and jaundice will decline.[152] If hyperbilirubinemia is advanced and milk production is low, formula may be given to the infant after each breast-feeding, while a manual or mechanical method for milk expression is used by the mother to stimulate milk production. Alternatively, a supplemental nursing system (SNS, Medela, McHenry, IL) may be used to encourage frequent breast-feeding and to allow the infant to receive larger volumes of milk. The SNS is a device made up of a reservoir or container of milk connected to a small soft catheter that is inserted into the infant's mouth while at the breast. While suckling, milk from the SNS flows into the infant's mouth by gravity.

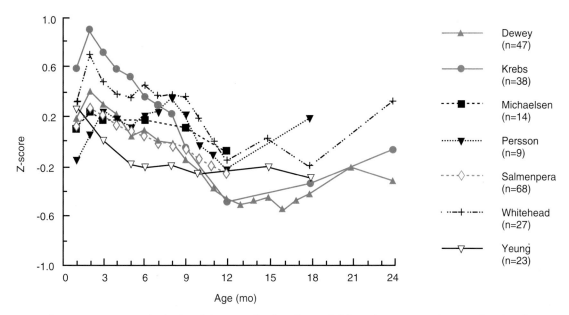

Figure 6: Mean NCHS weight-for-length Z-score of infants breast-fed for at least 12 months, reproduced with permission from the World Health Organization.[145]

This may be avoided by appropriate lactation counseling early after delivery and appropriate follow-up of infants after hospital discharge.

The classical entity "breast milk jaundice" usually begins insidiously and peaks after the first week of age. Despite adequate maternal lactation performance and infant milk intake and growth, the infant remains jaundiced. This is thought to be related either to one or more factors in human milk, or to a combination of specific milk factors and a susceptible infant.[153] It is believed that the presence of these factors stimulates the enterohepatic recirculation of bilirubin. In extreme circumstances, usually when the serum bilirubin concentration exceeds 20 mg/dl, the hyperbilirubinemia can be reduced by interrupting breast-feeding for two to four days. If this course is chosen, the mother must be encouraged to maintain her milk supply with a manual or mechanical method while the infant receives commercial formula. When breast-feeding resumes, the serum bilirubin may rise slightly, but once the cycle is interrupted, the recurrence of jaundice is unlikely. This entity is unrelated to maternal lactation performance. The infants appear healthy and well-nourished.

Benefits of Breast-feeding to the Mother

Recovery from childbirth is accelerated by the oxytocin's action on uterine involution.[154] Although breast-feeding should not be considered a reliable means of contraception, it prolongs the period of postpartum anovulation.[155] Menstruation resumes between 34 and 65 weeks postpartum, and ovulation between 30 and 40 weeks postpartum. Frequency, intensity and timing of feeds affect the endocrinologic responses that modulate ovulatory status.[156]

Studies examining whether breast-feeding promotes postpartum weight loss are conflicting,[157-163] in part because of varying classifications of breast-feeding and inclusion of women on weight-reduction diets. In a study of 1,423 Swedish women, a measure of lactation intensity and duration was only weakly correlated with weight loss.[158] Prolonged breast-feeding may confer some advantage in terms of weight loss. Compared with nonlactating women, weight loss of lactating women was greater from one to 12 months postpartum, but not from 12 to 24 months postpartum.[157] Currently, there is no evidence that breast-feeding prevents subsequent development of obesity.

Bone demineralization occurs during lactation, with compensatory remineralization after weaning.[164-167]

Lactation has been shown to confer a protective effect against osteoporosis and bone fracture in later life,[168-171] but this has not been confirmed in all studies.[172-174]

A protective effect of breast-feeding against breast cancer has been found in some studies,[175-185] but not in others.[180-185] In a recent multicenter study of 14,000 premenopausal and postmenopausal women, cancer risk was lower in premenopausal women.[179] Breast-feeding and the duration of breast-feeding were associated with a reduction in cancer risk in the premenopausal women. The effects were even greater in premenopausal women who had a cumulative total of 24 months of breast-feeding or who were 20 years or younger when they first lactated.

Transmission of Infection via Breast-feeding

In general, it is unwarranted to consider breast-feeding a means of transmitting disease to the healthy, full-term infant. Only in exceptional circumstances is breast-feeding contraindicated. Conventional attitudes, however, may differ. It is appropriate to recommend breast-feeding to the mother who has mastitis and is undergoing treatment for the condition. Maternal herpes infections localized to the perineal area or the oral mucosa do not pose a risk to the breast-fed infant.[186] Maternal herpetic lesions localized to the areola, however, do pose a risk and the infant should not be breast-fed while these lesions remain. Cytomegalovirus excretion is common in human milk when the mothers are seropositive for cytomegalovirus.[187] In the full-term infant, this is not a concern with respect to breast-feeding. Maternal rubella or maternal rubella immunization does not increase the risk of disease in the breast-fed infant.[186, 188] To date, most authorities approve of breast-feeding for mothers exposed to and infected with the hepatitis viruses. In the era prior to hepatitis B immunization, hepatitis B surface-antigen-positive mothers were advised to breast-feed their infants.[189] No increase in hepatitis B was reported from this recommendation. Although mothers with active miliary tuberculosis should not breast-feed, mothers who are seroconverters or receiving antituberculosis therapy may breast-feed their infants.

The data for human immunodeficiency virus are of concern.[186, 190-192] Although transplacental transmission may occur in 30% of cases when the mother is seropositive during pregnancy, the data for lactation are less clear. The virus has been isolated from human milk and there are suggestions of transmission of HIV from breast-feeding. There are reports, however, that human milk protects the recipient infant from HIV. Until more data are accumulated, the guidelines from the Centers For Disease Control in Atlanta suggest that mothers who are seropositive for HIV should not breast-feed. The World Health Organization advises that because the transmission of HIV in milk is uncertain, breast-feeding should be encouraged, especially in developing countries. In that recommendation, the risk/benefit ratio of not breast-feeding was greater in developing countries than the risk of transmission of HIV.

The data regarding potential transmission of disease via breast-feeding have been summarized in the 1994 Red Book (23rd Edition), Report of the Committee on Infectious Diseases of the American Academy of Pediatrics.

Xenobiotics

A number of drugs may be secreted into human milk, but only a few are thought to be contraindications to breast-feeding.[193] These include chemotherapeutic agents, radioactive isotopes, drugs of abuse, lithium, ergotamine and drugs that suppress lactation. In addition, anticonvulsants, antihistamines, sulfa drugs and salicylates may have effects on some breast-feeding infants. Potential exposures from environmental agents also should be considered. Caffeine may enter milk, but maternal consumption of one or two caffeine-containing beverages per day may not be associated with significant manifestations in the infant.[3] The use of alcohol is controversial.[3] Some studies have indicated that alcohol may affect the infant's behavior adversely. Some changes on developmental tests at one year also have been attributed to the maternal ingestion of alcohol. Cigarette smoking may affect milk volume.[66]

Secretion of medications into milk is affected by dose schedule and duration, feeding pattern of the infant, and the infant's total diet and age. The timing of breast-feeding should avoid peak blood concentrations of selected medications. For some medications, the stage of lactation (age of the infant) will determine the safety of the agent. Sulfa drugs would not be indicated in the first month of lactation, but may pose no concern to the infant who is several months of age. The mother should be encouraged to discuss any medication with her physician.

Dietary Supplements for Breast-fed Infants

Under normal conditions, an infant should not be bottle-fed for the first two weeks, after which time lactation usually is well established. Infants may be confused by a rubber nipple or pacifier, which require different tongue and jaw motions. Furthermore, if the appetite or the sucking response is partially satiated by water or formula, the infant will take less from the breast, causing diminished milk production which may lead to lactation failure. Sterile water and glucose water supplements may exacerbate hyperbilirubinemia because they prevent adequate milk (calorie) intake.[194] It must be realized that unconjugated (indirect) bilirubin is not water-soluble, must be eliminated in the feces and is not excreted in the urine.[42]

Under usual circumstances, the healthy, breast-fed, full-term infant requires little in the way of vitamin and mineral supplements. All infants, however, require vitamin K at birth. Because of differences in milk content and fecal flora, when compared with the infant fed formula, the breast-fed infant must rely on this vitamin K supplement to normalize the prolonged prothrombin time observed at birth.[42] The vitamin D concentration in human milk may be insufficient to prevent rickets, especially in dark-skinned infants.[195] Infants may need a vitamin D supplement, especially if exposed to minimum amounts of sunlight.[106,107,196] Iron absorption from human milk is excellent, but because the concentration of iron declines during lac-

"Programming" is the process whereby a stimulus of insult at a critical stage of development could result in a permanent or long lasting effect on the structure or function of the organism. Many early events during critical windows have life-long effects. The question is whether early intervention can operate in this programming way. Extensive evidence in animals and new evidence in humans suggests that it can. This has important public health implications, and raises the issue that we can no longer think about infant feeding simply in terms of meeting nutrient needs — we must think about long term biological effects on early nutrition on later outcomes.

Alan Lucas, M.D.
Dunn Nutritional Laboratory
Cambridge, United Kingdom

tation, the breast-fed infant requires an iron supplement after six months of age.[40] In summary, the only supplement definitely needed by a breast-fed infant is iron, and this supplement is needed only after six months of age.

Collection and Storage of Human Milk

An important property of breast-feeding is the relative freedom from bacterial contamination of human milk.[197] However, contamination can be a problem with artificially collected and stored human milk. Standards have been published by the Human Milk Banking Association of North America.[198, 199] Human milk banks processing pooled milk from multiple donors must use pasteurization methods to avoid disease transmission.[186] Because maternal T lymphocytes may be absorbed intact through the gastrointestinal tract of newborn infants, the possibility raises theoretical questions about the safety of feeding "fresh" (unfrozen or unheated) human milk from a woman other than the infant's own mother.

General techniques for ensuring cleanliness during milk expression begin with good hand washing using soap and water. Electric breast pumps generally are more effective than manual pumps or manual expression.[200] Hand pumps of the bicycle-horn variety may cause breast trauma, contamination of milk, and should not be used. Collection kits should be rinsed, then cleaned with hot soapy water and dried in the air. Dishwasher cleaning also is adequate. Glass or hard plastic containers should be used for milk storage. Bacteriologic testing may not be necessary for milk collected to feed a mother's own infant, unless poor collection technique is suspected. Milk to be fed within 48 hours of collec-

WHO/UNICEF Ten Steps to Successful Breast-feeding
1. Written breast-feeding policy should be available.
2. Health care staff should be trained to implement the policy.
3. Educate pregnant women in prenatal classes and visits.
4. Initiate breast-feeding within 1/2 hour of birth.
5. Demonstrate how to breast-feed and maintain lactation.
6. Use only breast milk, unless medically not indicated.
7. Practice rooming-in 24 hours/day.
8. Encourage breast-feeding on demand.
9. Give no artificial nipples or pacifiers.
10. Facilitate the development of breast-feeding support groups.

Table 3: Overview of WHO/UNICEF ten steps to successful breastfeeding. (Adapted from references 203, 205.)

tion can be refrigerated without significant bacterial proliferation.[200]

Freezing is the preferred method of storing milk that will not be fed within 48 hours.[200] Single milk expressions should be packaged separately for freezing. Unlike heat treatment, freezing preserves many of the nutritional and immunologic benefits of human milk. When frozen appropriately, milk can be stored for as long as three to six months. Milk should be thawed rapidly, usually by holding the container under running tepid (not hot) water. Milk should never be microwaved. After milk is thawed, it should not be refrozen. Thawed milk should be used completely within 24 hours, or discarded.

Experienced personnel should maintain quality control of in-hospital breast pumps and methods of milk fortification, and should ensure appropriate methods of delivering milk to the infant.[200] To ensure the best delivery of fat when continuous infusions are used, the feeding syringe should be oriented with the tip upright, the syringe emptied completely after each use, and the shortest amount of tubing used.[201]

Hospital Lactation Programs

Because the initial hospital experience may affect the ultimate outcome of breast-feeding, programs have been designed to facilitate maternal decisions to breast-feed. Model programs promote a philosophy of maternal and infant care that advocates breast-feeding in a normal physiologic manner.[202] In 1991, UNICEF and WHO began an international campaign, The Baby Friendly Hospital Initiative, to promote breast-feeding.[203-205] The WHO/UNICEF ten steps program is outlined in Table 3. The guidelines are useful for hospitals to consider when developing their own programs.

References

1. Nutrition Committee of the Canadian Paediatric Society, Committee on Nutrition of the American Academy of Pediatrics. Breast-Feeding. *Pediatrics.* 1978;62:591-601.

2. American Academy of Pediatrics, Committee on Nutrition. Encouraging breast-feeding. *Pediatrics.* 1980; 65:657-658.

3. Institute of Medicine, Subcommittee on Nutrition During Lactation. *Nutrition During Lactation.* Washington, D.C. National Academy Press: 1991.

4. American Academy of Pediatrics, Committee on Nutrition. Nutrition and lactation. *Pediatrics.* 1981;68: 435-443.

5. Atkinson SA, Bryan MH, Anderson GH. Human milk: Difference in nitrogen concentration in milk from mothers of term and premature infants. *J Pediatr.* 1978; 93:67-69.

6. Butte NF, Garza C, Johnson CA, Smith EO, Nichols BL. Longitudinal changes in milk composition of mothers delivering preterm and term infants. *Early Hum Dev.* 1984;9:153-162.

7. Schanler RJ, Oh W. Composition of breast milk obtained from mothers of premature infants as compared to breast milk obtained from donors. *J Pediatr.* 1980;96:679-68l.

8. Gross SJ, David RJ, Bauman L, Tomarelli RM. Nutritional composition of milk produced by mothers delivering preterm. *J Pediatr.* 1980;96:641-644.

9. Carlson SE. Human milk nonprotein nitrogen: occurrence and possible functions. In: Barness LA, ed. *Advances In Pediatrics.* Chicago: Year Book Medical Publishers Inc; 1985:43-70.

10. Hambraeus L. Proprietary milk versus human breast milk in infant feeding, a critical appraisal from the nutritional point of view. *Pediatr Clin N Am.* 1977;24: 17-35.

11. Heine W, Tiess M, Wutzke KD. [15]N tracer investigations of the physiological availability of urea nitrogen in mother's milk. *Acta Paediatr Scand.* 1986;75:439-443.

12. Fomon SJ, Bier DM, Matthews DE, et al. Bioavailability of dietary urea nitrogen in the breast-fed infant. *J Pediatr.* 1988;113:515-517.

13. Billeaud C, Guillet J, Sandler B. Gastric emptying in infants with or without gastro-oesophageal reflux according to the type of milk. *Eur J Clin Nutr.* 1990;44: 577-583.

14. Rassin DK, Gaull GE, Raiha NCR, Heinonen K. Milk protein quantity and quality in low-birth-weight infants. IV. Effects on tyrosine and phenylalanine in plasma and urine. *J Pediatr.* 1977;90:356-360.

15. Gaull GE, Rassin DK, Raiha NCR, Heinonen K. Milk protein quantity and quality in low-birthweight infants. III. Effects on sulfur amino acids in plasma and urine. *J Pediatr.* 1977;90:348-355.

16. Jarvenpaa AL, Raiha NC, Rassin DK. Feeding the low-birth-weight infant: I. Taurine and cholesterol supplementation of formula does not affect growth and metabolism. *Pediatrics.* 1983;71:171-178.

17. Jarvenpaa AL, Rassin DK, Raiha NCR, Gaull GE. Milk protein quantity and quality in the term infant. II. Effects on acidic and neutral amino acids. *Pediatrics.* 1982;70:221-230.

18. Lindblad BS, Alfven G, Zetterstrom R. Plasma free amino acid concentrations of breast-fed infants. *Acta Paediatr Scand.* 1978;67:659-663.

19. Rassin DK. Amino acid responses in neonatal nutrition and their implications for the central nervous system. In: Barness L, ed. *Protein Requirements in the Term Infant.* Princeton: Excerpta Medica; 1988:3-9.

20. Goldman AS, Chheda S, Keeney SE, Schmalsteig FC, Schanler RJ. Immunologic protection of the premature newborn by human milk. *Semin Perinatol.* 1994;18:495-501.

21. Lonnerdal B. Biochemistry and physiological function of human milk proteins. *Am J Clin Nutr.* 1985;42:1299-1317.

22. Hanson LA, Ahlstedt S, Andersson B, et al. Protective factors in milk and the development of the immune system. *Pediatrics.* 1985;75 (Suppl):172-176.

23. Hernell O, Blackberg L. Human milk bile salt-stimulated lipase: functional and molecular aspects. *J Pediatr.* 1994; 125:S56-S61.

24. Jensen RG, Hagerty MM, McMahon KE. Lipids of human milk and infant formulas: a review. *Am J Clin Nutr.* 1978;31:990-1016.

25. Jensen RG, Jensen GL. Specialty lipids for infant nutrition. I. Milks and formulas. *J Pediatr Gastroenterol Nutr.* 1992; 15:232-245.

26. Butte NF, Garza C, Smith EO. Variability of macronutrient concentrations in human milk. *Eur J Clin Nutr.* 1988;42:345-349.

27. Neville MC, Keller RP, Seacat J, Casey CE, Allen JC,

Archer P. Studies on human lactation. I. Within-feed and between-breast variation in selected components of human milk. *Am J Clin Nutr.* 1984;40:635-646.

28. Nommsen LA, Lovelady CA, Heinig MJ, Lonnerdal B, Dewey KG. Determinants of energy, protein, lipid, and lactose concentrations in human milk during the first 12 months of lactation: the DARLING study. *Am J Clin Nutr.* 1991;53:457-465.

29. Butte NF, Garza C, Stuff JE, Smith EO, Nichols BL. Effect of maternal diet and body composition on lactational performance. *Am J Clin Nutr.* 1984;39:296-306.

30. Uauy R, Hoffman DR. Essential fatty acid requirements for normal eye and brain development. *Semin Perinatol.* 1991;15:449-455.

31. Innis SM. Human milk and formula fatty acids. *J Pediatr.* 1992;120:S56-S61.

32. Carlson SE, Werkman SH, Rhodes PG, Tolley EA. Visual-acuity development in healthy preterm infants: effect of marine-oil supplementation. *Am J Clin Nutr.* 1993;58:35-42.

33. Whyte RK, Homer R, Pennock CA. Faecal excretion of oligosaccharides and other carbohydrates in normal neonates. *Arch Dis Child.* 1978;53:913-915.

34. MacLean WC, Fink BB. Lactose malabsorption by premature infants: magnitude and clinical significance. *J Pediatr.* 1980;97:383-388.

35. Ziegler EE, Fomon SJ. Lactose enhances mineral absorption in infancy. *J Pediatr Gastroenterol Nutr.* 1983; 2:288-294.

36. Schanler RJ. Suitability of human milk for the low birthweight infant. *Clin Perinatol.* 1995;22:207-222.

37. Hanson LA, Adlerberth I, Carlsson B, et al. Host defense of the neonate and the intestinal flora. *Acta Paediatr Scand. (Suppl).* 1989;351:122-125.

38. Neville MC, Watters CD. Secretion of calcium into milk: a review. *J Dairy Sci.* 1983;66:371-380.

39. Casey CE, Hambidge KM, Neville MC. Studies in human lactation: zinc, copper, manganese, and chromium in human milk in the first month of lactation. *Am J Clin Nutr.* 1985;41:1193-1200.

40. Dallman PR, Siimes MA, Stekel A. Iron deficiency in infancy and childhood. *Am J Clin Nutr.* 1980;33:86-118.

41. Saarinen UM. Need for iron supplementation in infants on prolonged breast-feeding. *J Pediatr.* 1978;93:177-180.

42. Greer FR, Suttie JW. Vitamin K and the newborn. In: Tsang RC, Nichols BL, eds. *Nutrition During Infancy.* Philadelphia: Hanley & Belfus; 1988:289-297.

43. Carver JD, Walker WA. The role of nucleotides in human nutrition. *Nutr Biochem.* 1995;6:58-72.

44. Uauy R, Quan R, Gil A. Role of nucleotides in intestinal development and repair: implications for infant nutrition. *J Nutr.* 1994;124:S1436-S1441.

45. Sheard NF, Walker WA. The role of breast milk in the development of the gastrointestinal tract. *Nutr Rev.* 1988;46:1-8.

46. Goldman AS, Sharpe LW, Goldblum RM. Anti-inflammatory properties of human milk. *Acta Paediatr Scand.* 1986;75:689-695.

47. Goldman AS, Smith CW. Host resistance factors in human milk. *J Pediatr.* 1973;82:1082-1090.

48. Kleinman RE, Walker WA. The enteromammary immune system. *Dig Dis Sci.* 1979;24:876-882.

49. Fishaut M, Murphy D, Neifert M, McIntosh K, Ogra PL. Bronchomammary axis in the immune response to respiratory syncytial virus. *J Pediatr.* 1981;99:186-191.

50. Isaacs CE, Kashyap S, Heird WC, Thormar H. Antiviral and antibacterial lipids in human milk and infant formula feeds. *Arch Dis Child.* 1990;65:861-864.

51. Michaelsen KF, Larsen PS, Thomsen BL, Samuelson G. Weight, length, head circumference, and growth velocity in a longitudinal study of Danish infants. *Dan Med Bull.* 1994;41:577-585.

52. Dewey KG, Heinig MJ, Nommsen LA, Lonnerdal B. Maternal vs infant factors related to breast milk intake and residual milk volume: the DARLING study. *Pediatrics.* 1991;87:829-837.

53. Neville MC, Keller R, Seacat J, et al. Studies in human lactation: milk volumes in lactating women during the onset of lactation and full lactation. *Am J Clin Nutr.* 1988;48:1375-1386.

54. Hennart P, Vis HL. Breast-feeding and postpartum amenorrhoea in Central Africa. *J Trop Pediatr.* 1980;26: 177-183.

55. van Steenbergen WM, Kusin JA, Kardjati, de With C. Energy supplementation in the last trimester of pregnancy in East Java, Indonesia: effect on breast-milk output. *Am J Clin Nutr.* 1989;50:274-279.

56. Brown KH, Ahmed AN, Robertson AD, Giashuddin AM.

Lactational capacity of marginally nourished mothers: relationships between maternal nutritional status and quantity and proximate composition of milk. *Pediatrics.* 1986;78:909-919.

57. Imong SM, Jackson DA, Wongsawasdii L, et al. Predictors of breast milk intake in rural Northern Thailand. *J Pediatr Gastroenterol Nutr.* 1989;8:359-370.

58. Creed de Kanashiro H, Brown KH, Lopez de Romana G, Lopez T, Black RE. Consumption of food and nutrients by infants in Huascar (Lima) Peru. *Am J Clin Nutr.* 1990;52:995-1004.

59. Orr-Ewing AK, Heywood PF, Coward WA. Longitudinal measurements of breast milk output by a ^2H_2O tracer technique in rural Papua New Guinean women. *Hum Nutr Clin Nutr.* 1986;40C:451-467.

60. World Health Organization. The quantity and quality of breast milk. Geneva: WHO, 1985.

61. Macy IG, Hunscher HA, Donelson E, Nims B. Human milk flow. *J Dis Child.* 1930;39:1186-1204.

62. Saint L, Maggiore P, Hartmann PE. Yield and nutrient content of milk in eight women breast-feeding twins and one woman breast-feeding triplets. *Br J Nutr.* 1986; 56:87-95.

63. Stuff JE, Nichols BL. Nutrient intake and growth performance of older infants fed human milk. *J Pediatr.* 1989;116:959-968.

64. Dewey KG, Heinig MJ, Nommsen LA, Lonnerdal B. Adequacy of energy intake among breast-fed infants in the DARLING study: relationships to growth velocity, morbidity, and activity levels. *J Pediatr.* 1991;119:538-547.

65. Vio F, Salazar G, Infante C. Smoking during pregnancy and lactation and its effect on breast-milk volume. *Am J Clin Nutr.* 1991;54:1011-1016.

66. Hopkinson JM, Schanler RJ, Fraley JK, Garza C. Milk production by mothers of premature infants: influence of cigarette smoking. *Pediatrics.* 1992;90:934-938.

67. Andersen AN, Lund-Andersen C, Larsen JF, et al. Suppressed prolactin but normal neurophysin levels in cigarette smoking breast-feeding women. *Clin Endocrinol.* 1982;17:363-368.

68. Winikoff B, Semeraro P, Zimmerman M. *Contraception during breast-feeding: a clinician's handbook.* New York: Population Council Publishers; 1988.

69. Prentice A, Paul A, Black A, Cole T, Whitehead R.

Cross-cultural differences in lactational performance. In: Hamosh M, Goldman AS, eds. *Human Lactation 2: Maternal and Environmental Factors.* New York: Plenum Press; 1986:13-44.

70. Strode MA, Dewey KG, Lonnerdal B. Effects of short-term caloric restriction on lactational performance of well-nourished women. *Acta Paediatr Scand.* 1986;75: 222-229.

71. Neville M, Oliva-Rasbach J. Is maternal milk production limiting for infant growth during the first year of life in breast-fed infants? In: Goldman AS, Atkinson SA, Hanson LA, eds. *Human Lactation 3: The Effects of Human Milk on the Recipient Infant.* New York: Plenum Press; 1987:123-133.

72. Dusdieker LB, Hemingway DL, Stumbo PJ. Is milk production impaired by dieting during lactation? *Am J Clin Nutr.* 1994;59:833-840.

73. Lonnerdal B, Forsum E, Gebre-Medhin M, Hambraeus L. Breast milk composition in Ethiopian and Swedish mothers. II. Lactose, nitrogen, and protein contents. *Am J Clin Nutr.* 1976;29:1134-1141.

74. Villalpando SF, Butte NF, Wong WW, et al. Lactation performance of rural Mesoamerindians. *Eur J Clin Nutr.* 1992;46:337-348.

75. Sanchez-Pozo A, Lopez-Morles J, Izquierdo A, Martinez-Valverde A, Gil A. Protein composition of human milk in relation to mother's weight and socioeconomic status. *Hum Nutr Clin Nutr.* 1987;41C:115-125.

76. Svanberg U, Gebre-Medhin M, Ljunqvist B, Olsson M. Breast milk composition in Ethiopian and Swedish mothers. III. Amino acids and other nitrogenous substances. *Am J Clin Nutr.* 1977;30:499-507.

77. Forsum E, Lonnerdal B. Effect of protein intake on protein and nitrogen composition of breast milk. *Am J Clin Nutr.* 1980;33:1809-1813.

78. Miranda R, Sarvia NG, Ackerman R, Murphy N, Berman S, McMurray DN. Effect of maternal nutritional status on immunological substances in human colostrum and milk. *Am J Clin Nutr.* 1983;37:632-640.

79. Jensen RG. *The Lipids of Human Milk.* Boca Raton: CRC Press; 1989.

80. Hachey DL, Silber GH, Wong WW, Garza C. Human lactation II: endogenous fatty acid synthesis by the mammary gland. *Pediatrics.* 1989;25:63-68.

81. Chappell JE, Francis T, Clandinin MT. Vitamin A and E content of human milk at early stages of lactation. *Early Hum Dev.* 1985;11:157-167.

82. Sanders THB, Ellis TR, Dickerson JWT. Studies of vegans: the fatty acid composition of plasma choline-phosphoglycerides, erythrocytes, adipose tissue, breast milk and some indicators of susceptibility to ischemic heart disease in vegans and omnivore controls. *Am J Clin Nutr.* 1978;31:805

83. Butte NF, Calloway DH. Evaluation of lactational performance of Navajo women. *Am J Clin Nutr.* 1981; 34:2210-2215.

84. Gebre-Medhin M, Vahlquist A, Hofvander Y, Uppsall L, Vahlquist B. Breast milk composition in Ethiopian and Swedish mothers. I. Vitamin A and β-carotene. *Am J Clin Nutr.* 1976;29:441-451.

85. Hollis BW, Lambert PW, Horst RL. Factors affecting the antirachitic sterol content of native milk. In: Holick MF, Gray TK, Anast CS, eds. *Perinatal Calcium and Phosphorous Metabolism.* Amsterdam: Elsevier; 1983:157-182.

86. Greer FR, McCormick A, Loker J. Changes in fat concentration of human milk during delivery by intermittent bolus and continuous mechanical pump infusion. *J Pediatr.* 1984;105:745-749.

87. von Kries R, Shearer M, McCarthy PT, Haug M, Harzer G, Gobel U. Vitamin K1 content of maternal milk: influence of the stage of lactation, lipid composition, and vitamin K1 supplements given to the mother. *Pediatr Res.* 1987;22:513-517.

88. Bates CJ, Prentice AM, Prentice A, Lamb WH, Whitehead RG. The effect of vitamin C supplementation on lactating women in Keneba, a West African rural community. *Int J Vitam Nutr Res.* 1983;53:68-76.

89. Byerley LO, Kirksey A. Effects of different levels of vitamin C intake on the vitamin C concentration in human milk and the vitamin C intakes of breast-fed infants. *Am J Clin Nutr.* 1985;41:665-671.

90. Pratt JP, Hamil BM, Moyer EZ, et al. Metabolism of women during the reproductive cycle. XVIII. The effect of multi-vitamin supplements on the secretion of B vitamins in human milk. *J Nutr.* 1951;44:141-157.

91. Bates CJ, Prentice AM, Paul AA, Sutcliffe BA, Watkinson M, Whitehead RG. Riboflavin status in Gambian pregnant and lactating women and its

implications for Recommended Dietary Allowances. *Am J Clin Nutr.* 1981;34:928-935.

92. Kirksey A, Roepke JLB. Vitamin B6 nutriture of mothers of three breast-fed neonates with central nervous system disorders. *Fed Proc.* 1981;40:864.

93. Metz J, Zalusky R, Herbert V. Folic acid binding by serum and milk. *Am J Clin Nutr.* 1968;21:289-297.

94. Sandberg DP, Begley JA, Hall CA. The content, binding, and forms of vitamin B12 in milk. *Am J Clin Nutr.* 1981; 34:1717-1724.

95. Johnson PR, Jr., Roloff JS. Vitamin B12 deficiency in an infant strictly breast-fed by a mother with latent pernicious anemia. *J Pediatr.* 1982;100:917-919.

96. Higginbottom MC, Sweetman L, Nyhan WL. A syndrome of methylmalonic aciduria, homocystinuria, megaloblastic anemia and neurologic abnormalities in a vitamin B12-deficient breast-fed infant of a strict vegetarian. *N Engl J Med.* 1978;299:317-323.

97. Specker BL, Miller D, Norman EJ, Greene H, Hayes KC. Increased urinary methylmalonic acid excretion in breast-fed infants of vegetarian mothers and identification of an acceptable dietary source of vitamin B12. *Am J Clin Nutr.* 1988;47:89-92.

98. Dallman PR. Iron deficiency in the weaning: a nutritional problem on the way to resolution. *Acta Paediatr Scand.* 1986;S323:59-67.

99. Siimes MA, Salmenpera L, Perheentupa J. Exclusive breast-feeding for 9 months: risk of iron deficiency. *J Pediatr.* 1984;104:196-199.

100. Lonnerdal B, Keen CL, Hurley LS. Iron, copper, zinc, and manganese in milk. *Annu Rev Nutr.* 1981;1:149-174.

101. Krebs NF, Reidinger CJ, Hartley S, Robertson AD, Hambidge KM. Zinc supplementation during lactation: effects on maternal status and milk zinc concentrations. *Am J Clin Nutr.* 1995;61:1030-1036.

102. Mannan S, Picciano MF. Influence of maternal selenium status on human milk selenium concentration and glutathione peroxidase activity. *Am J Clin Nutr.* 1987;46:95-100.

103. Gushurst CA, Mueller JA, Green JA, Sedor F. Breast milk iodide: reassessment in the 1980's. *Pediatrics.* 1984; 73:354-357.

104. Hillman LS, Chow W, Salmons SS, Weaver E, Erickson M, Hansen J. Vitamin D metabolism, mineral

homeostasis, and bone mineralization in term infants fed human milk, cow milk-based formula, or soy-based formula. *J Pediatr.* 1988;112:864-874.

105. Venkataraman PS, Luhar H, Neylan MJ. Bone mineral metabolism in full-term infants fed human milk, cow milk-based, and soy-based formulas. *Am J Dis Child.* 1992;146:1302-1305.

106. Greer FR, Searcy JE, Levin RS, Steichen-Asche JJ, Tsang RC. Bone mineral content and serum 25-hydroxyvitamin D concentration in breast-fed infants with and without supplemental vitamin D. *J Pediatr.* 1981;98:696-701.

107. Greer FR, Searcy JE, Levin RS, Steichen JJ, Steichen-Asche PS, Tsang RC. Bone mineral content and serum 25-OHD concentrations in breast-fed infants with and without supplemental vitamin D: One year follow-up. *J Pediatr.* 1982;100:919-922.

108. Popkin BM, Adair L, Akin JS, Black R, Briscoe J, Flieger W. Breast-feeding and diarrheal morbidity. *Pediatrics.* 1990;86:874-882.

109. Glass RI, Stoll BJ. The protective effect of human milk against diarrhea. *Acta Paediatr Scand.* 1989;351:131-136.

110. Cunningham AS. Morbidity in breast-fed and artificially fed infants. *J Pediatr.* 1977;90:726-729.

111. Cunningham AS. Morbidity in breast-fed and artificially fed infants. II. *J Pediatr.* 1979;95:685-689.

112. Cunningham AS, Jelliffe DB, Jelliffe EFP. Breast-feeding and health in the 1980's: a global epidemiologic review. *J Pediatr.* 1991;118:659-666.

113. Dewey KG, Heinig MJ, Nommsen-Rivers LA. Differences in morbidity between breast-fed and formula-fed infants. *J Pediatr.* 1995;126:696-702.

114. Kovar MG, Serdula MD, Marks JS, Fraser DW. Review of the epidemiologic evidence for an association between infant feeding and infant health. *Pediatrics.* 1984;74: S615-S638.

115. Howie PW, Forsyth JS, Ogston SA, Clark A, Florey CV. Protective effect of breast-feeding against infection. *Br Med J.* 1990;300:11-16.

116. Frank AL, Taber LH, Glezen WP, Kasel GL, Wells CR, Paredes A. Breast-feeding and respiratory virus infection. *Pediatrics.* 1982;70:239-245.

117. Wright AL, Holberg CJ, Martinez FD, Morgan WJ, Taussig LM, Group Health Medical Associates. Breast feeding and lower respiratory tract illness in the first year of life. *Br Med J.* 1989;299:945-948.

118. Rubin DH, Leventhal JM, Krasilnikoff PA, et al. Relationship between infant feeding and infectious illness: a prospective study of infants during the first year of life. *Pediatrics.* 1990;85:464-471.

119. Duncan B, Ey J, Holberg CJ, Wright AL, Martinez FD, Taussig LM. Exclusive breast-feeding for at least 4 months protects against otitis media. *Pediatrics.* 1993;91: 867-872.

120. Pisacane A, Graziano L, Mazzarella G, Scarpellino B, Zona G. Breast-feeding and urinary tract infection. *J Pediatr.* 1992;120:87-89.

121. Coppa GV, Gabrielli O, Giorgi P, et al. Preliminary study of breast-feeding and bacterial adhesion to uroepithelial cells. *Lancet.* 1990;335:569-571.

122. Goldblum RM, Schanler RJ, Garza C, Goldman AS. Human milk feeding enhances the urinary excretion of immunologic factors in low birth weight infants. *Pediatr Res.* 1989;25:184-188.

123. Lucas A, Cole TJ. Breast milk and neonatal necrotizing enterocolitis. *Lancet.* 1990;336:1519-1523.

124. Eibl MM, Wolf HM, Furnkranz H, Rosenkranz A. Prevention of necrotizing enterocolitis in low-birth-weight infants by IgA-IgG feeding. *N Engl J Med.* 1988; 319:1-7.

125. Narayanan I, Prakash K, Bala S, Verma RK, Gujral VV. Partial supplementation with expressed breast-milk for prevention of infection in low-birth-weight infants. *Lancet.* 1980;II:561-563.

126. Narayanan I, Prakash K, Gujral VV. The value of human milk in the prevention of infection in the high-risk low-birth-weight infant. *J Pediatr.* 1981;99:496-498.

127. Narayanan I, Prakash K, Verma RK, Gujral VV. Administration of colostrum for the prevention of infection in the low birth weight infant in a developing country. *J Trop Pediatr.* 1983;29:197-200.

128. Davis MK, Savitz DA, Graubard BI. Infant feeding and childhood cancer. *Lancet.* 1988;1:365-368.

129. Koletzko S, Sherman P, Corey M, Griffiths A, Smith C. Role of infant feeding practices in development of Crohn's disease in childhood. *Br Med J.* 1989;298:1617-1618.

130. Gerstein HC. Cow's milk exposure and type I diabetes mellitus. *Diabetes Care.* 1994;17:13-19.

131. Kramer MS. Does breast feeding help protect against atopic disease? Biology, methodology, and a golden jubilee of controversy. *J Pediatr.* 1988;112:181-190.

132. Saarinen UM, Backman A, Kajosaari M, Siimes MA. Prolonged breast-feeding as prophylaxis for atopic disease. *Lancet.* 1979;11:163-166.

133. Karjalainen J, Martin JM, Knip M, et al. A bovine albumin peptide as a possible trigger of insulin-dependent diabetes mellitus. *N Engl J Med.* 1992;327:302-307.

134. Rogan WJ, Gladen BC. Breast-feeding and cognitive development. *Early Hum Dev.* 1993;31:181-193.

135. Lucas A, Morley R, Cole TJ, Gore SM. A randomised multicentre study of human milk versus formula and later development in preterm infants. *Arch Dis Child.* 1994;70:F141-F146.

136. Lucas A, Morley R, Cole TJ, Lister G, Leeson-Payne C. Breast milk and subsequent intelligence quotient in children born preterm. *Lancet.* 1992;339:261-264.

137. Crawford MA. The role of essential fatty acids in neural development: implications for perinatal nutrition. *Am J Clin Nutr.* 1993;57:S703-S710.

138. Anderson GJ, Connor WE, Corliss JD. Docosahexaenoic acid is the preferred dietary n-3 fatty acid for the development of the brain and retina. *Pediatr Res.* 1990;27:89-97.

139. *Growth Curves For Children, Birth-18 Years.* Washington, DC; National Center For Health Statistics (NCHS). U.S. Department of Health, Education, and Welfare: 1977. DHEW Publication No. PHS 78-1650.

140. Ahn CH, MacLean WC. Growth of the exclusively breast-fed infant. *Am J Clin Nutr.* 1980;33:183-192.

141. Dewey KG, Heinig MJ, Nommsen LA, Peerson JM, Lonnerdal B. Growth of breast-fed and formula-fed infants from 0 to 18 months: The DARLING study. *Pediatrics.* 1992;89:1035-1041.

142. Nelson SE, Rogers RR, Ziegler EE, Fomon SJ. Gain in weight and length during early infancy. *Early Hum Dev.* 1989;19:223-239.

143. Salmenpera L, Perheentupa J, Siimes MA. Exclusively breast-fed healthy infants grow slower than reference infants. *Pediatr Res.* 1985;19:307-312.

144. Whitehead RG, Paul AA, Cole TJ. Diet and the growth of healthy infants. *J Hum Nutr Diet.* 1989;2:73-84.

145. *An Evaluation of Infant Growth.* Geneva; Working Group on Infant Growth. World Health Organization. WHO: 1994. Nutrition Unit, WHO.

146. Krebs NF, Reidinger CJ, Robertson AD, Hambidge KM. Growth and intakes of energy and zinc in infants fed human milk. *Pediatrics.* 1994;124:32-39.

147. Persson LA. Infant feeding and growth - a longitudinal study in three Swedish communities. *Ann Hum Biol.* 1985;12:411-452.

148. Yeung DL. Infant nutrition. Ottawa; Canadian Public Health Association: 1983.

149. Heinig MJ, Nommsen LA, Peerson JM, Lonnerdal B, Dewey KG. Intake and growth of breast-fed and formula-fed infants in relation to the timing of introduction of complementary foods: the DARLING study. *Acta Paediatr.* 1993;82:999-1006.

150. Gartner LM. On the question of the relationship between breast-feeding and jaundice in the first 5 days of life. *Semin Perinatol.* 1994;18:502-509.

151. Lascari AD. Early breast-feeding jaundice: Clinical significance. *J Pediatr.* 1986;108:156-158.

152. DeCarvalho M, Klaus MH, Merkatz RB. Frequency of breast-feeding and serum bilirubin concentration. *Am J Dis Child.* 1982;136:737-738.

153. Gartner LM, Arias IM. Studies of prolonged neonatal jaundice in the breast-fed infant. *J Pediatr.* 1966;68:54-66.

154. Riordan J. Anatomy and psychophysiology of lactation. In: Riordan J, Auerbach KG, eds. *Breast-feeding and Human Lactation.* Boston: Jones and Bartlett; 1993: 81-104.

155. Wang IY, Fraser IS. Reproductive function and contraception in the postpartum period. *Obstet Gynecol Survey.* 1994;49:56-63.

156. Campbell OM, Gray RH. Characteristics and determinants of postpartum ovarian function in women in the United States. *Am J Obstet Gynecol.* 1993;169:55-60.

157. Dewey KG, Heinig MJ, Nommsen LA. Maternal weight-loss patterns during prolonged lactation. *Am J Clin Nutr.* 1993;58:162-166.

158. Ohlin A, Rossner S. Maternal body weight development after pregnancy. *Int J Obes.* 1990;15:159-173.

159. Greene GW, Smicklas-Weight H, School TO, Karp RJ. Postpartum weight change: how much of the weight gained in pregnancy will be lost after delivery? *Obstet Gynecol.* 1988;71:701-717.

160. Rookus MA, Rokebrand P, Burema J, Deurenberg P. The effect of pregnancy on the body mass index 9 months postpartum in 49 women. *Int J Obes.* 1987;11: 609-618.

161. Potter S, Hannum S, McFarlin B, Essex-Sorlie D, Campbell E, Trupin S. Does infant feeding method influence maternal weight loss? *J Am Diet Assoc.* 1991;91: 441-446.

162. Dugdale AE, Eaton-Evans J. The effect of lactation and other factors on post-partum changes in body-weight and triceps skinfold thickness. *Br J Nutr.* 1989;61:149-153.

163. Manning-Dalton C, Allen LH. The effects of lactation on energy and protein consumption, postpartum weight change and body composition of well nourished North American women. *Nutr Res.* 1983;3:293-308.

164. Kent GN, Price RI, Gutteridge DH, et al. Human lactation: forearm trabecular bone loss, increased bone turnover, and renal conservation of calcium and inorganic phosphate with recovery of bone mass following weaning. *J Bone Min Res.* 1990;5:361-369.

165. Lamke B, Brundin J, Moberg P. Changes in bone mineral content during pregnancy and lactation. *Acta Obstet Gynecol Scand.* 1977;56:217-219.

166. Specker BL, Tsang RC, Ho ML. Changes in calcium homeostasis over the first year postpartum: effect of lactation and weaning. *Obstet Gynecol.* 1991;78:56-62.

167. Sowers MF, Corton G, Shapiro B, et al. Changes in bone density with lactation. *JAMA.* 1993;269:3130-3135.

168. Aloia JF, Cohn SH, Vaswani A, Yeh JK, Yuen K, Ellis K. Risk factors for postmenopausal osteoporosis. *Am J Med.* 1985;78:95-100.

169. Feldblum PJ, Zhang J, Rich LE, Fortney JA, Talmage RV. Lactation history and bone mineral density among perimenopausal women. *Epidemiol.* 1992;3:527-531.

170. Kreiger N, Kelsey JL, Holford TR, O'Connor T. An epidemiologic study of hip fracture in postmenopausal women. *Epidemiol.* 1982;116:141-148.

171. Cumming RG, Klineberg RJ. Breast-feeding and other reproductive factors and the risk of hip fracture in elderly women. *Int J Epidemiol.* 1993;2:684-691.

172. Bauer DC, Browner WS, Cauley JA, et al. Factors associated with appendicular bone mass in older women. *Ann Intern Med.* 1993;118:657-665.

173. Fox KM, Magaziner J, Sherwin R, et al. Reproductive correlates of bone mass in elderly women. *J Bone Min Res.* 1993;8:901-908.

174. Kritz-Silverstein D, Barett-Connor E, Hollenbach KA. Pregnancy and lactation as determinants of bone mineral density in postmenopausal women. *Am J Epidemiol.* 1992;136:1052-1059.

175. Byers TS, Graham S, Rzepka T, Marshall J. Lactation and breast cancer: evidence for a negative association in premenopausal women. *Am J Epidemiol.* 1985;121:664-674.

176. Layde PM, Webster LA, Baughman AL, Wingo PA, Rugin GL, Ory HW. The independent associations of parity, age at first full term pregnancy, and duration of breast-feeding with the risk of breast cancer. Cancer and Steroid Hormone Study Group. *J Clin Epidemiol.* 1989; 42:963-973.

177. McTiernan A, Thomas DB. Evidence for a protective effect of lactation on risk of breast cancer in young women: results from a case control study. *Am J Epidemiol.* 1986;124:353-358.

178. Yoo K, Tajima K, Kuroishi T, et al. Independent protective effect of lactation against breast cancer: A case control study in Japan. *Am J Epidemiol.* 1992;135:726-733.

179. Newcomb PA, Storer BE, Longnecker MP, et al. Lactation and a reduced risk of premenopausal breast cancer. *N Engl J Med.* 1994;330:81-87.

180. Kvale G, Heuch I. Lactation and cancer risk: is there a relation specific to breast cancer? *J Epidemiol Community Health.* 1987;42:30-37.

181. Wynder EL, MacCornack FA, Stellman SD. The epidemiology of breast cancer in 785 United States Caucasian women. *Cancer.* 1978;41:2341-2354.

182. Brinton LA, Hoover R, Fraumeni JF. Reproductive factors in the aetiology of breast cancer. *Br J Cancer.* 1983; 47:757-762.

183. London SJ, Colditz GA, Stampfer MJ, et al. Lactation and risk of breast cancer in a cohort of US women. *Am J Epidemiol.* 1990;132:17-26.

184. Siskind V, Schofield F, Rice D, Bain C. Breast cancer and breast-feeding: results from an Australian case-control study. *Am J Epidemiol.* 1989;130:229-236.

185. Thomas DB, Noonan EA. Breast cancer and prolonged lactation. The WHO Collaborative Study of Neoplasia and Steroid Contraceptives. *Int J Epidemiol.* 1993;22: 619-626.

186. Ruff AJ. Breastmilk, breast-feeding, and transmission of viruses to the neonate. *Semin Perinatol.* 1994;18:510-516.

187. Dworsky M, Yow M, Stagno S, Pass RF, Alford C. Cytomegalovirus infection of breast milk and transmission in infancy. *Pediatrics.* 1983;72:295-299.

188. Krogh V, Duffy C, Wong D, Rosenband M, Riddlesberger KR, Ogra PL. Postpartum immunization with rubella virus vaccine and antibody response in breast-feeding infants. *J Lab Clin Med.* 1989;113:695-699.

189. Martino MD, Appendino C, Resti M, Rossi ME, Muccioli AT, Vierucci A. Should hepatitis B surface antigen positive mothers breast feed? *Arch Dis Child.* 1985;60:972-974.

190. Dunn DT, Newell ML, Ades AE, Peckham CS. Risk of human immunodeficiency virus type 1 transmission through breast-feeding. *Lancet.* 1992;340:585-588.

191. Palasanthiran P, Ziegler JB, Stewart GJ, et al. Breast-feeding during primary maternal human immunodeficiency virus infection and risk of transmission from mother to infant. *J Infect Dis.* 1993;167:441-444.

192. Oxtoby MJ. Human immunodeficiency virus and other viruses in human milk: placing the issues in broader perspective. *Pediatr Infect Dis J.* 1988;7:825-835.

193. American Academy of Pediatrics, Committee on Drugs. The transfer of drugs and other chemicals into human milk. *Pediatrics.* 1994;93:137-150.

194. DeCarvalho M, Hall M, Harvey D. Effects of water supplementation on physiological jaundice in breast-fed babies. *Arch Dis Child.* 1981;56:568-569.

195. Bachrach S, Fisher J, Parks JS. An outbreak of vitamin D deficiency rickets in a susceptible population. *Pediatrics.* 1979;64:871-877.

196. Roberts CC, Chan GM, Folland D, Rayburn C, Jackson R. Adequate bone mineralization in breast-fed infants. *J Pediatr.* 1981;99:192-196.

197. American Academy of Pediatrics, Committee on Nutrition. Human milk banking. *Pediatrics.* 1980;65:854-857.

198. Arnold LDW. *Guidelines For The Establishment of a Donor Human Milk Bank.* West Hartford, CT; Human Milk Banking Association of North America Inc: 1994.

199. Arnold LDW. *Recommendations For Collection, Storage, and Handling of a Mother's Milk For her Own Infant in the Hospital Setting.* West Hartford, CT; Human Milk Banking Association of North America Inc: 1993.

200. Schanler RJ, Hurst NM. Human milk for the hospitalized preterm infant. *Semin Perinatol* 1994;18:476-484.

201. Schanler RJ. Special methods in feeding the preterm infant. In: Tsang RC, Nichols BL, eds. *Nutrition During Infancy.* Philadelphia: Hanley & Belfus; 1988:314-325.

202. Powers NG, Naylor AJ, Wester RA. Hospital policies: crucial to breast-feeding success. *Semin Perinatol.* 1994;18:517-524.

203. *Protecting, Promoting, and Supporting Breast-feeding: The Special Role of Maternity Services.* Geneva, Switzerland; World Health Organization, UNICEF: 1989. World Health Organization ISBN-92-4-1561-30-0 ed.

204. *Innocenti Declaration on the Protection, Promotion, and Support of Breast-feeding.* New York; UNICEF: 1990. UNICEF, Nutrition Cluster (H-8F).

205. Take the Baby-Friendly Hospital Initiative! A global effort with hospitals, health services, and parents to breast-feed babies for the best start in life. New York; UNICEF: 1991.

206. American Academy of Pediatrics, Committee on Nutrition. Zinc. *Pediatrics.* 1978;62:408-412.

207. Blanc B. Biochemical aspects of human milk - comparison with bovine milk. *World Rev Nutr Diet.* 1981;36:1-89.

208. Dallman PR. Nutritional anemia in infancy: iron, folic acid, and vitamin B12. In: Tsang RC, Nichols BL, eds. *Nutrition During Infancy.* Philadelphia: Hanley & Belfus; 1988:216-235.

209. Schanler RJ. Water soluble vitamins: C, B1, B2, B6, niacin, biotin, and pantothenic acid. In: Tsang RC, Nichols BL, eds. *Nutrition During Infancy.* Philadelphia: Hanley & Belfus; 1988:236-252.

Management of Breast-feeding

Judy Hopkinson Ph.D.,[1] Kay James M.S., C.C.C.,[2]
and J. Paul Zimmer Ph.D.[3]

Children's Nutrition Research Center at Baylor College of Medicine; Houston, Texas,[1]
Pediatric Therapy Center, Houston, Texas,[2]
and University of Alabama at Birmingham, Birmingham, Alabama[3]

Reviewed by Winston W. Koo M.B.B.S., Sandra J. Bartholmey Ph.D. and Margit Hamosh Ph.D.

This work is a publication of the U.S. Department of Agriculture (USDA)/Agricultural Research Service (ARS) Children's Nutrition Research Center (CNRC); Department of Pediatrics, Baylor College of Medicine (BCM); and Texas Children's Hospital (TCH), Houston, Texas, USA. This project has been funded in part with federal funds from the USDA/ARS under Cooperative Agreement number 58-6250-6-001. The contents of this publication do not necessarily reflect the views or policies of the USDA, nor does mention of trade names, commercial product, or organization imply endorsement by the U.S. Government.

Abstract

Assessing and managing of breast-feeding are reviewed in this chapter. Demographics and health benefits of breast-feeding are discussed in the introduction. The hospital period and early breast-feeding assessment are covered in some detail. The period of transition between hospital discharge and the first well-baby visit is a time of high risk for breast-feeding problems; guidelines for telephone triage are provided. Normal changes in maternal milk production and breast comfort, as well as feeding, stool and behavior patterns of breast-fed infants, are examined at subsequent feeding stages. Common problems, maternal and infant illness, vitamin and mineral supplementation, working mothers, and milk storage are discussed in the final sections of the chapter.

Introduction

Although breast-feeding is universally acknowledged as the most beneficial method of infant feeding, it is also the most difficult to prescribe, evaluate, and modify. Effective alteration of breast milk intake requires an understanding of mammary physiology, milk composition, maternal-infant interaction, infant oral-motor development and the process of milk transfer during breast-feeding. Medical education rarely provides sufficient information of practical value regarding breast-feeding management. In a recent survey of pediatricians in the United States, the majority reported that they do not feel they have the skills to effectively intervene when breast-feeding problems arise.[1] This chapter provides practical information in the following areas: 1) increasing the incidence of breast-feeding in a client base; 2) facilitating early lactation through appropriate hospital policies; 3) evaluating breast-feeding effectiveness; 4) anticipating, recognizing and managing common breast-feeding problems and challenges in all stages of lactation.

Incidence of Breast-feeding

In developed countries, the incidence of breast-feeding declined markedly during the early and middle part of this century. Reasons for the decline are complex, but include urbanization, loss of extended families and the emphasis on measurement and technology in infant feeding that accompanied the development of nutrition science. Similar influences are apparent in third-world countries. Breast-feeding is more prevalent among rural women, and declines as populations migrate to urban settings. Rates of breast-feeding have increased significantly in western countries during the last 25 years. With the support of the World Health Organization, many countries have organized initiatives to increase breast-feeding rates. At this time the demography of breast-feeding is qualitatively similar in Australia, Western Europe, and North America, and quite different in most underdeveloped countries. Middle and upper-socioeconomic groups are more likely to breast-feed in developed countries, while the rural poor are more likely to breast-feed in third-world countries.

The United States currently reports one of the lowest breast-feeding rates in the developed world. The percentage of mothers in the United States who initiated breast-feeding rose from a nadir of 22% in 1972 to approximately 60% in 1995.[2-7] Only 22% of U.S. infants received breast milk for six months or longer in 1995. Breast-feeding rates are higher among middle- and upper-income women, women living in the far western United States and women with more formal education.[2, 7, 8] Anglo-Americans are more likely to choose breast-feeding than blacks or Hispanics. Interestingly, acculturation of South American immigrants is associated with a decline in breast-feeding.[9] Although breast-feeding initiation rates are similar among employed and nonemployed mothers, by six months postpartum, full-time maternal employment is associated with a 50% deficit in continuation of lactation.[6]

> *At the Society for Pediatric Research Milk Club presentation in 1990, Dr. Frank Oski was speaking on the importance of feeding human milk to infants and emphasizing studies of cognitive development and IQ improvements.*
>
> *Question from the Audience: Do you really think that a few IQ points would make a difference?*
> *Answer: I do not know about you, but when I struggle in the middle of the night with the discussion section of the paper I am writing, I wish I would be just a few IQ points smarter.*
>
> Margit Hamosh Ph.D.
> Georgetown University
> Children's Medical Center
> Washington D.C.

Impact of Breast-feeding on Infant Health

The World Health Organization, the U.S. surgeon general, the American Academy of Pediatrics, the American College of Obstetricians and Gynecologists and health ministries from around the world support exclusive breast-feeding for term infants.[2, 10] Four to six months of exclusive breast-feeding are recommended before introducing infant foods. Support for this recommendation comes from an ever-growing body of evidence that breast-feeding promotes optimal infant health regardless of the setting in which the infant is raised.

Human milk is the nutritional "gold standard" against which all forms of artificial feeding are compared. The nutrient composition of human milk is covered extensively in Chapter 16, *The Rationale for Breast-feeding,* and will not be further described here. It is important to recognize, however, that the nutrient composition of human milk does not adequately describe its contribution to infant development. Many of the organic components act as growth stimulators, transport molecules, digestive aids or anti-infective agents prior to their digestion and absorption as simple nutrients. These include immuno-globulins, epidermal growth factor, mucopolysaccharides, lipases, fatty acids and many others. Most, but not all, of these components act through species-specific interactions. Thus, duplication in infant formulas is difficult, if not impossible. Many of the reported beneficial effects of human milk, such as promotion of cognitive development[11, 12] and reduction of food allergies,[13] are difficult to explain, but may be related to some of the thousands of human milk components yet to be examined.

Infant formulas were initially designed to mimic the composition of human milk. However, since the impact of human milk is not predicted by its nutrient content alone, adjustments must be made where necessary and possible. For example, transport of iron is aided by human milk proteins such that bioavailability of iron is higher than from any other food source. Iron levels must be substantially elevated in infant formulas to achieve a comparable net iron absorption.

Lactoferrin, lysozyme and several other milk components protect the infant by withholding iron from bacteria, binding or lysing foreign cells. Other factors such as leukocytes, cytokines, nucleotides and hormones have undefined but important roles in the development of the infant's immune system. Such immunological protection may also play a role in reducing the risk of lymphoma, Crohn's disease and Type I diabetes among breast-fed infants.[14-16]

The concentration of specific antibodies in human milk is directly related to the degree of protection the infant receives against a specific pathogen. The immunoglobulins in human milk reflect the pathogens in the mother's environment. Antibody-producing cells in the mother's gut, lungs and other mucosal sites are induced to migrate to the mammary gland by pro-lactin[17]. Once there, they produce IgA-type antibodies for export into the lumen of the secretory lobule where milk is stored prior to feeding. The process of maternal antigen exposure followed by the appearance of anti-body in milk continues as long as the mother is lactat-ing and has been demonstrated even in the second year of lactation.[18] Through this mechanism, each infant receives specific immunoglobulins against infective agents as they arise in the child's environment. Failure to provide the immunological protection of human milk exposes the infant to additional environmental pathogens, which will eventually result in the infant's immunity if he survives these challenges.

In underdeveloped countries, human milk not only ensures the presence of anti-infective agents, but also reduces the exposure to pathogens present in local water supplies. In such areas, breast-feeding is a matter of life and death. In developed countries with clean water supplies and good medical care, differences in mortality between breast-fed and formula-fed infants are not commonly reported. However, differences in morbidity are well established. The list of specific ill-nesses purported to be reduced among breast-fed infants in developed countries is extensive.[19] Because of marked differences between families who choose breast- and formula-feeding, and because of confusion regarding definitions of breast-feeding, definitions of illness and appropriate statistical analyses, many older studies are unreliable.[20] Recent research utilizing rigor-ous study designs substantiates and expands previous observations that breast-feeding is protective against specific illnesses including otitis media, childhood lymphoma, gastrointestinal illness, Sudden Infant Death Syndrome and numerous others.[14, 19, 21-27] In Scotland, infants breast-fed for 13 weeks or longer were one-third as likely to be readmitted to the hospital for

Areas of concern associated with the decision not to breast-feed.	
Lack of confidence	The woman does not believe she will be able to breast-feed.
Embarrassment to breast-feed in public	She believes she will have to expose her breasts in public.
Loss of freedom	The woman believes she will be unable to resume her former activities.
Concerns about dietary and health practices	She believes breastfeeding requires dietary restrictions or that she cannot breast-feed because she smokes cigarettes, etc.
Influence of family and friends	The woman relies heavily on the emotional support of her husband, boyfriend, mother, or others and believes, rightly or wrongly, that they disapprove of breast-feeding.

Table 1: Among lower socioeconomic groups, the desire to establish a special closeness with the infant has been shown to be a powerful motivation for breast-feeding. Conversely, the areas of concern listed above are associated with the decision not to breast-feed.[38]

any reason in the first year of life.[28] It is probable that significant savings in health care costs may be realized by increasing breast-feeding rates. However, consider-able research is needed to identify the duration and pattern of breast-feeding that offers maximum disease protection, and those factors that maximize the immunoprotective properties of human milk.

Feeding Decisions
Common Misconceptions about Breast-feeding

For the individual clinician, increasing the percentage of breast-fed infants in his/her practice is an obvious advantage. However, influencing feeding decisions can be a daunting task. A wide range of demographic, soci-ological, and psychological factors have been shown to influence breast-feeding decisions.[3,29-34] The primary factor influencing women and their husbands to choose breast-feeding is the belief that breast-feeding is healthier for babies. Women who do not breast-feed

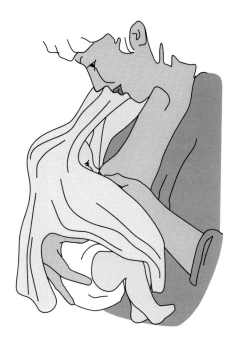

Figure 1: Breast-feeding can be done discreetly anywhere and anytime the baby is hungry.

are less likely to believe that human milk is beneficial to infant health, and are often rejecting breast-feeding rather than making a positive choice for formula. One or more of the following misconceptions frequently underlie rejection of breast-feeding: breast-feeding is painful, breast-feeding causes breasts to sag, breast-feeding is socially confining, breast-feeding precludes sexual activity, breast-feeding requires public breast exposure or breast-feeding requires marked dietary restrictions. None of these is accurate. Perhaps least understood is the relationship between maternal diet and breast-feeding. Maternal diet during breast-feeding has relatively little impact on milk composition. While fluctuations in specific nutrients do occur as a result of dietary choices, they are usually minor and do not override the advantages of human milk.

In addition to the concerns listed above, many women are simply unsure of their ability to breast-feed. Effective behavior-change strategies based on women's reasons for choosing or rejecting breast-feeding have been demonstrated.[35-37]

Pediatricians are uniquely qualified to influence parental beliefs regarding the influence of early nutrition

Three-step strategy for prenatal counseling
1. Elicit the mother's concerns.
2. Acknowledge the mother's feelings.
3. Educate with targeted messages.

Table 2: A three-step strategy for pre-natal counseling which has proven effective in a variety of settings.

on infant health. However, the manner in which breast-feeding information is presented appears to have an overriding influence on the effectiveness of prenatal counseling interactions. When health professionals ask women about their feeding choice before initiating discussions of infant nutrition, the woman may feel forced to make a commitment without considering the information her health provider has to offer. Moreover, once a preference for formula feeding is indicated, most health professionals refrain from providing additional information about breast-feeding. Thus, while as many as three fourths of expectant mothers have identified a feeding choice by the first trimester of pregnancy, these choices are not necessarily well-informed or well-considered.[34]

Techniques to Encourage Breast-feeding

A three-step strategy for prenatal counseling which has proven effective in a variety of settings is outlined below:[38]
1. Elicit the woman's concerns.

Open-ended questions such as "What do you know about breast-feeding?" will initiate discussions which reveal concerns or misconceptions regarding breast-feeding.
2. Acknowledge the woman's feelings.

Acknowledging the woman's feelings establishes trust and facilitates teaching, e.g., "You feel like you won't be able to produce enough milk because your breasts are small." "It does seem logical that women with small breasts would produce less milk."
3. Educate using carefully targeted messages.

Information that specifically addresses the woman's concerns saves time, maintains focus, and empowers the client to make an informed, unencumbered choice.

Another effective prenatal counseling strategy is the physician-led discussion group. Such groups have been reported to increase breast-feeding rates as much as four-fold.[39] The objective in prenatal counseling for infant feeding choice is to ensure that the mother makes a decision based on medically sound, accurate information. It is not to entice every woman to breast-feed. Personal issues and family stress sometimes override medical and nutritional concerns.

Early breast-feeding may be especially challenging, and women should not be enticed into breast-feeding by the false promise that their experience will be problem-free. Rather, the health professional should provide the support to guide the family through the entire course of the breast-feeding experience.

Perinatal Management of Breast-feeding Dyads
Prenatal Examination

When the decision to breast-feed has been made, a breast examination will help to identify women requiring special follow-up. During a prenatal breast exam, the examiner looks for flat, rigid or inverted nipples (see figure 2),; asymmetry; or scar tissue, and asks the mother whether she has experienced breast enlargement during gestation.

The external features of the breast include the breast skin with the darker pigmented nipple and areola, the nipple pores or openings through which the milk will flow, and the Montgomery's glands on and surrounding the areola. The Montgomery's glands secrete an oily substance which lubricates the nipple and small amounts of milk containing secretory immunoglobulin A (SIgA) and other protective components. As a result, the bacterial count of the nipple and areola are an order of magnitude below the remainder of the body. During pregnancy, pigmentation of the areola and nipple darkens, the size of the areola expands and the Montgomery's glands enlarge to resemble inflamed sebaceous glands. In addition, the sensitivity of the nipple increases markedly. The size of the non-pregnant woman's breast depends primarily on the amount of adipose tissue. During pregnancy, proliferation and maturation of mammary-producing tissue results in an increase in breast size. As lactation progresses toward weaning, the Montgomery's glands recede, pigmentation of areola and nipple lightens somewhat, and the size of the breast and areola decrease. While the breasts generally return to their

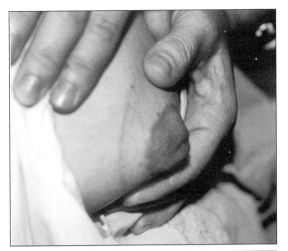

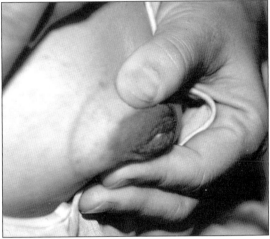

Figure 2: Prenatal breast exam for inverted nipples. Inverted nipples recede on compression and may cause difficulty with latch on. Breast shells used for two months prior to delivery did not correct nipple inversion in this mother.

pre-pregnancy size, nipple and areola may remain somewhat darker and larger.

Flat, rigid or inverted nipples may cause problems when starting lactation because the infant may be unable to achieve or maintain an effective latch-on. Flat nipples do not protrude when stimulated. Rigid nipples are surrounded by a non-protratile areola such that the combined nipple-areolar unit moves together without elongating when pulled gently. Inverted nipples recede on compression. Particular care is needed to distinguish pseudo- from true inversion. The pseudo-inverted nipple is dimpled or creased in the center but does not recede

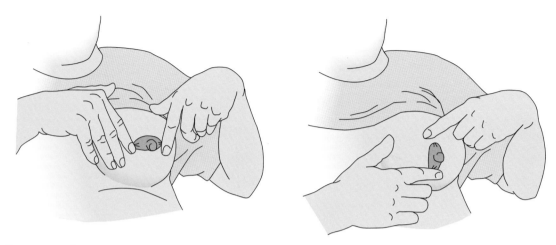

Figure 3: Hoffman's exercises may cause immediate eversion of pseudo-inverted nipples. Exercises are performed by placing a finger on either side of the areola and stretching it while pressing inward toward the chest.

when compressed. Pseudo-inverted nipples are not problematic for nursing. Moreover, for some infants, virtually no nipple is problematic. Two simple exercises ("nipple rolling" and Hoffman's exercises) and breast shells are frequently used to correct flat or inverted nipples before or after delivery. Exercises may be done for a few minutes several times each day, and shells may be worn inside the brassiere for approximately two hours at a time. In theory, forcing the nipple out through the breast shell's central opening stretches or weakens Hoffman's ligaments and facilitates nipple protrusion. However, the shell's efficacy for severely inverted nipples has not been demonstrated. Rubbing the nipples in an attempt to "toughen" them in the hope of preventing nipple soreness does not work and may damage the Montgomery's glands.

Underlying the breast skin and embedded in the adipose tissue are numerous exocrine glands whose secretory ducts terminate at the nipple and areola (see Figure 4). Each exocrine gland, called a mammary lobule, is well supplied with blood from the internal mammary, thoracic and several intercostal arteries, with extensive lymphatic drainage to nodes surrounding the breast tissue. Sensory nerve fibers from several intercostal nerves are found in the nipple, areola, and to a lesser extent, the surrounding skin, with the interior of the gland containing autonomic innervation. Milk constituents are produced and temporarily held in the lobuli, the smallest units of the mammary

lobule. Surrounding each lobulus are myoepithelial cells whose contractions move milk from the lobuli into milk ducts. Myoepithelial cells also line the ducts longitudinally. Milk ducts join and eventually open into several lactiferous sinuses underlying the areola and nipple. When oxytocin is released in response to nipple and areola stimulation, the myoepithelial cells contract, causing milk ejection.

Scars from past surgeries or wounds may indicate interruption of nipple innervation or ducts. If the nipples do not become erect on stimulation, innervation has been interrupted. Such insults may interfere with hormonal response to suckling or milk flow.[2] Suggestive scars and interrupted nipple innervation should be noted, and patients monitored closely for signs of poor infant growth or poor milk production. Significant mammary disproportion and other breast anomalies have been associated with lactation failure.[40-42]

Breast implants may or may not interrupt nipple innervation. At the present time there is not sufficient evidence to determine whether breast-feeding with silicone implants is contraindicated.[43-45]

Breast enlargement is expected during pregnancy. When a woman reports that her breast size has not changed during pregnancy, mammary gland development may be incomplete, and may result in lactation failure.[41] In the authors' experience, however, these reports may be inaccurate and, therefore, nondiagnostic.

When the potential for problems is observed, the woman should be targeted for special follow-up in the early postpartum period. Either the physician or a lactation consultant should observe one or several breast-feedings prior to hospital discharge. In addition, the physician's office should initiate phone contact within three days of hospital discharge to evaluate progress before the first well-baby visit. If any problems with latch-on or early milk production occur, the physician or a lactation specialist should work with the mother to resolve the problem, and the infant should be monitored closely for signs of dehydration or other indicators that formula supplementation is at least temporarily indicated.

Influence of Hospitals and Maternity Services

Numerous studies have demonstrated that hospital policies can have a profound effect on initiation and duration of breast-feeding; however, controversy persists regarding some specific policies and routines. Early initiation of breast-feeding, maternal-infant cohabitation and unlimited, on-demand feeding are clearly established as policies that have a positive influence on breast-feeding success. Conversely, the use of pacifiers or "dummies" in the early postpartum period has received relatively little scientific scrutiny with respect to breast-feeding.

Under ideal circumstances, the newborn human infant is capable of crawling up the mother's abdomen unassisted, locating and attaching to the breast, and initiating effective suckling within the first 30 to 60 minutes after birth.[46-47] When infants were removed for bathing and returned after 20 minutes, alertness, mobility and suckling were adversely affected at the first feeding. (A striking video of this behavior can be obtained from Geddes Productions, 10546 McViney, Sunland, CA, 91040, USA). Thus, the normal course of breast-feeding initiation is facilitated when infants and mothers remain in continuous physical contact for at least one hour after birth. Whether or not the infant effectively suckles during this time period will depend on a number of factors including the duration of labor,[47] and type of maternal anesthesia.[2, 48, 49] Maternal behavior toward the offspring is apparently affected positively if

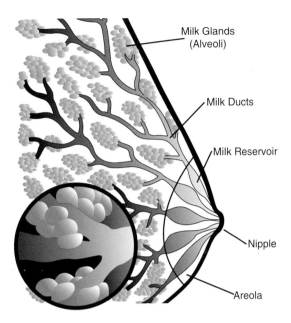

Figure 4: Embedded in the adipose tissue are numerous exocrine glands whose secretory ducts terminate at the nipple and areola.

the infant contacts the nipple and areola in the first one to two hours regardless of suckling effectiveness.[50]

The extent of maternal infant contact throughout hospitalization impacts the duration of breast-feeding.[51-55] When mothers and infants remain in the same room during hospitalization, breast-feeding durations increase. This is consistent with a large body of evidence demonstrating that significant long-term positive effects on maternal behavior result from increased maternal-infant contact during hospitalization.[56]

Although controversy persists, there is no evidence that routine formula or water supplementation is necessary for healthy term breast-fed infants[2]. Routine water supplementation does not affect infant bilirubin levels, contrary to popular misconception, and supplementary formula feedings in the immediate puerperium have been associated with an increased incidence of feeding difficulties and/or lactation failure.[57-61] On the other hand, supplementary water provided *ad libitum* in at least one study did not delay the onset of milk production.[62] Whether supplementary formula feedings during postpartum hospitalization cause difficulties or result from underlying feeding

Ten Steps to Successful Breast-feeding
Every facility providing maternity services and care for newborn infants should:
1. Have a written breast-feeding policy that is routinely communicated to all health-care staff.
2. Train all health-care staff in skills necessary to implement this policy.
3. Inform all pregnant women about the benefits and management of breast-feeding.
4. Help mothers initiate breast-feeding within a half-hour of birth.
5. Show mothers how to breast-feed and how to maintain lactation if they should be separated from their infants.
6. Give newborn infants no food or drink other than human milk, unless medically indicated.
7. Practice rooming in. Allow mothers and infants to remain together 24 hours a day.
8. Encourage breast-feeding on demand.
9. Give no artificial teats or pacifiers (also called dummies or soothers) to breast-feeding infants.
10. Foster the establishment of breast-feeding support groups and refer mothers to them on discharge from the hospital or clinic.

Table 3: The Baby-Friendly Initiative. Protecting, Promoting and Supporting Breast-feeding: The Special Role of Maternity Services, a joint WHO/UNICEF STATEMENT 1989.

problems is not clear. A meta-analysis of the influence of hospital feeding policies on breast-feeding success concluded that in-hospital formula supplementation of 48 ml per day was not associated with reduced breast-feeding durations; however, providing commercial discharge packs was associated with shorter duration.[63] In one study of low-income urban women in the United States, discharge packs containing infant formulas were associated with higher rates of infant rehospitalization (14% vs 1%) than similar packs which did not contain formulas when the latter was combined with breast-feeding counseling.[64]

The psychological effect of the hospital staff's implicit approval of supplementary feedings has been cited as a contributory factor in the premature cessation of breast-feeding.[65] Regardless of the rationale for the use of supplementary feedings, the extent to which they are required in hospital is an indication of existing or potential breast-feeding problems. Breast-feeding infants who receive formula during hospitalization warrant careful monitoring until breast-feeding is well established.

In recognition of the profound influence of breast-feeding on infant health and the impact of maternity services on breast-feeding success, the World Health Organization and UNICEF jointly issued a statement in 1989, describing the "Ten Steps to Successful Breast-feeding" (see Inset). A modification of the 10 steps has been proposed for U.S. hospitals.

Evaluation of and Assistance with Early Breast-feeding

The first nursing episode on the delivery table is generally neither an appropriate nor an effective time to teach the details of latch-on and positioning. Minor assistance may be offered if warranted; however, teaching efforts will be less intrusive and usually more productive later.

Coordination of sucking, swallowing and breathing is essential for safe and efficient feeding. This appears to be relatively effortless in most term infants. However, each of these tasks is physiologically and anatomically complex. In order to work smoothly and effectively, they require highly accurate timing and coordination, and normally developed, well supported, stable oral structures.[66, 67]

Each breast-feeding episode is composed of a series of nonverbal interactions between mother and infant. Chris Mulford has divided these interactions into five sequential steps: signaling, positioning, latch-on, milk transfer and ending.[68] Breakdown of the breast-feeding interaction can occur at any point in the sequence, and each problem deserves attention.

Signaling

The decision to initiate a feeding is, paradoxically, both the most obvious and the most ignored step in a breast-feeding episode. Since the cooperation of the infant is required to draw the nipple and areola into a teat and extract milk, the breast-fed infant must be hungry, alert, and attentive for the feeding to proceed efficiently. Conversely, since the infant exerts control over maternal milk production in large part by varying the frequency of feedings, if the mother fails to observe or rejects his hunger cues, she runs the risk of reducing the supply of milk below his requirements. Arbitrary feeding schedules may, but generally do not, coincide with infant readiness to feed. Maternal attention to infant hunger cues has resulted in more frequent feeding and better weight gain during the first two weeks of life.[69] Infant-initiated feeding has been associated with greater weight gain than scheduled feedings, even when feeding frequency was comparable, in at least one study.[52]

An effective breast-feeding episode begins when the mother correctly identifies infant hunger signals. Hunger signals include increased restlessness, sucking motions of the lips and tongue, hand-to-mouth movements, sucking on fists or fingers and crying. For some infants, the cues may remain extremely subtle and the infant may not wake. In the latter case, mothers are more likely to require assistance in signal detection. Once hunger is identified or suspected, the mother's next task is to assist the infant to achieve a quiet, alert behavioral state appropriate for feeding. This may involve calming a crying infant by swaddling, rocking, etc., or it may involve placing a sleeping infant in skin-to-skin contact on the mother's chest until he arouses sufficiently to proceed. For the sleeping infant, sucking on a pacifier may assist arousal when the infant is hungry. Numerous other techniques are utilized by both mothers and nursing staff. A quiet, alert state is characterized by focused gaze, and relative inactivity. In a few instances, a screaming infant may calm immediately when the nipple is placed in the mouth, but more often he will be unable to respond in his agitated state. Attempting to proceed before the appropriate behavioral state is attained generally results in frustration.

If the mother responds appropriately to infant cues, the infant has the opportunity to adjust both the volume and caloric density of feeds to meet his needs. The amount of suckling stimulation required to maintain a given milk production rate varies from one woman to another, and this sensitivity to stimulation will affect the infant's chosen feeding frequency. Moreover, the fat content of milk extracted from a breast

increases with less time between feedings,[70] as well as with the degree of breast emptying.[71] Given the degree of control exercised by the infant over both the volume and fat content of the milk consumed,[72] it is not surprising that the fat content of milk is a poor predictor of infant growth rates.[73] The wide variability in feeding frequencies of normally growing, breast-fed infants is a physiologic adaptation to maternal lactation performance as well as infant needs.

Signal detection failure can result in insufficient feeding frequency and subsequent poor growth or inadequate milk supply. The latter is the most common reason given by women for weaning their infants prematurely.[29, 74, 75] In practice, breast-fed infants are nursed more frequently in the first few weeks, as mothers fine-tune their signal-detection skills and infants increase their feeding effectiveness. Mothers can safely be reassured that during the first few weeks many of the feedings are simply "practice" and the frequency will decline as the relationship develops.

Interestingly, a mother's recognition of and response to infant hunger signals in early infancy is associated not only with greater breast-feeding success, but also with secure mother-child attachment patterns at one year of age and appropriate childhood behavior and psychological adjustment. It is perhaps not surprising that both successful breast-feeding and the infant's psychological development rely to some extent on the same early mothering skills. Both are improved when infants and mothers remain together during hospitalization.[56]

Positioning

Once both parties are ready, the mother positions the baby for feeding. Her task at this stage is to ensure that the nipple and areola are within easy grasp and to provide the necessary support for her infant to maintain body alignment and flexion so that sucking, swallowing, and breathing may proceed with ease.

Suckling efficiency is enhanced when oral structures are given full range of motion as well as adequate stability and support. Range of motion and stability of oral structures can be influenced by the way the infant is positioned during suckling.[76] If the shoulders are too far forward or back, relaxation and extension of the tongue is inhibited, and the infant experiences difficulty posi-

Ideal Positioning for Breast-feeding
1. The baby faces the breast directly without turning his head to the side. He rests in a side-lying or 3/4 side-lying position.
2. The baby's spine is gently curved and his hips are flexed in an approximation of the fetal position.
3. The baby's head, neck and shoulders are aligned. His neck is straight or slightly tilted forward. His shoulders are relaxed in their natural position at the sides of the body.
4. The baby has easy access to the nipple. It is unnecessary to move the nipple either to the right or the left of its natural position or to stretch the breast to attain latch-on.
5. The baby is well supported and the head and neck are stable.

Table 4: Positioning tips for breast-feeding.

tioning the tongue for effective latch-on, suckling and swallowing a bolus of milk. The extra effort required to latch-on and maintain suckling when the infant must use his body strength to achieve alignment or to stabilize the neck may be too much for a marginal or weak infant. In other cases, the baby may nurse with an altered tongue position, which is both less efficient and traumatic to the mother's nipples. Providing greater stability in the upper body facilitates efficient jaw movement and will positively affect a weaker infant's ability to suck longer before becoming fatigued.

Flexion of the spine and hip and holding the infant in a side-lying or three-quarters side-lying position allows maximum anterior-posterior movement of the thoracic cavity, thus facilitating normal infant respiration.[77]

Infants who require more postural support than others include premature infants, less well-developed infants, infants with less muscle tone, and infants with weaker or malformed oral musculature. Older infants generally require less attention to positioning as muscle tone, strength and oral-motor functioning advance. Swaddling may be helpful in maintaining alignment in young infants; however, care should be taken to ensure that the infant's shoulders remain in midline.

To assist maternal understanding of the principles involved, a few simple exercises are helpful. Mothers may be instructed to attempt to swallow or move the tongue out and down while saying "Ah" (the equivalent of the infant preparing to latch-on to the breast) with their shoulders thrust forward or backward, or their heads tilted forward or backward in order to experience some of the difficulty the infant will face if he is forced to nurse with his head, neck, and shoulders out of alignment. Because of the differences in placement of the infant and adult diaphragm,[78] and the greater stability of structures which support adult oral-pharyngeal function, mothers will be unable to experience the value of hip flexion in enhancing ease of infant feeding. The "football hold" (See Figure 5a) is an excellent position for ensuring alignment, flexion, and easy grasp of the nipple if difficulty is encountered with the standard "cradle hold" (See Figure 5b). Any one of a number of positions may be used to accommodate needs of mother and infant. The mother herself must be comfortable during feedings. If she is strained or in pain, her milk ejection reflex may be impaired. Following cesarean section, mothers may be more comfortable lying down to nurse with a pillow placed between her legs to reduce stress on the incision (see Figure 5c).

Latch-On

In order to empty the breast efficiently, the infant must draw the nipple and enough of the areola into the mouth to form a teat which includes the mother's lactiferous sinuses. The location of the sinuses will differ somewhat from mother to mother, but in general, approximately 1-2 cm of tissue beyond the base of the nipple is drawn into the mouth.

The mother's fingers must be placed far enough behind the areola that they do not interfere with the infant's access (see Figure 5d). Attachment to the breast begins with the infant's rooting reflex. If not displayed spontaneously, the reflex may be elicited by brushing the nipple gently against the lips. Excessive stimulation of the lips and face with the nipple can be counterproductive, causing some infants to "shut down." Reluctant infants may be encouraged to open their mouths by expressing a small amount of milk onto the lips. As the infant's mouth opens wide, with the tongue exhibiting a midline grove and extended down and forward, the mother pulls the infant close

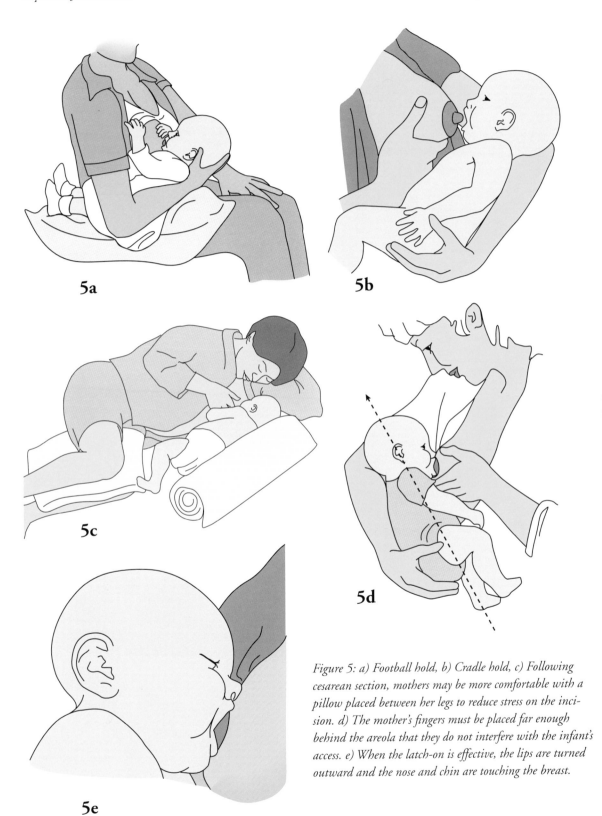

Figure 5: a) Football hold, b) Cradle hold, c) Following cesarean section, mothers may be more comfortable with a pillow placed between her legs to reduce stress on the incision. d) The mother's fingers must be placed far enough behind the areola that they do not interfere with the infant's access. e) When the latch-on is effective, the lips are turned outward and the nose and chin are touching the breast.

Signs of a Good Latch-on
1. Lips turned outward.
2. Nose and chin touch breast.
3. 1-2 cm beyond base of nipple enclosed.
4. Tongue visible if lower lip is pulled down.

Table 5: Signs of good latch-on.

and places the nipple and areola far into the mouth. The infant closes his mouth around the nipple and areola drawing them into a teat which he holds against the palate with his tongue. Ultrasound measurements of suckling by Smith et al indicate that three-month old infants form teats approximately two times the length of the nipple.[79, 80] When the latch-on is effective, the lips are turned outward and pressed against the breast, the nose is usually in close contact with the breast, and the tongue is just visible when the lower lip is pulled down (see Figure 5e). With the onset of non-nutritive suckling, negative pressure is created when the mandible is depressed and the nipple may be drawn further into the mouth sliding over the moist mucosal tissue on the inside of the lower lip. Once a good latch-on is achieved, milk ejection reflex is elicited by the non-nutritive suckling and milk intake can proceed.

Attachment to the breast depends markedly on the successful completion of signaling and positioning. It is not uncommon for this step to fail during a significant percentage of very early breast-feeding attempts.

Suckling and Milk Transfer

Successful milk transfer is indicated by the shift from non-nutritive to nutritive suckling, maternal uterine contractions in the early puerperium, leakage of milk from the contralateral breast and tingling in the breasts (experienced by some but not all women). As milk transfer proceeds, additional signs include passage of gas or stool by the infant, and gradual unfurling of the infant's fists. Gastric motility is stimulated by components in the milk, so that during milk transfer the young infant may become briefly agitated and release his hold on the breast. When stooling is

complete, renewed interest in nursing is apparent. This interlude may cause confusion if mothers misinterpret the agitation and momentary loss of interest as rejection of the breast or completion of the feed.

The oral structures used during sucking are the lips, cheeks, tongue, jaw and palate. The tongue, pharyngeal and laryngeal structures and musculature are used during swallowing. The infant must coordinate the rapid movement/interaction of these oral structures in order to suck, form a bolus, propel the bolus posteriorly and initiate a swallow. The lips receive sensory information, form a loose seal around the breast, and help to stabilize the nipple position. When fully developed, the infant cheek contains a thick padding which provides stability and lateral boundaries and assists with the maintenance of suction and thereby the maintenance of latch-on. If musculature is weak, infants may be unable to produce sufficient suction to achieve or maintain an adequate latch-on. During suckling, the tongue moves in such a way as to create an anterior-posterior peristaltic wave action which helps to form a bolus and propel it posteriorly. Swallowing movements are visible at the level of the hyoid bone.

Suckling patterns of the normal term newborn can be classified into two distinct types – non-nutritive sucking (NNS) and nutritive sucking (NS). Non-nutritive sucking occurs in the absence of milk flow. Once flow is established, the slower NS pattern is evident. NNS is characterized by a sucking rate of two per second with a suck:swallow ratio of 6-8:1. NS occurs at an average rate of one suck per second with a suck:swallow ratio which varies with the rate of flow and the size of the oral cavity.[67, 81-83] The ratio increases when the flow is low and reaches a minimum of 1:1 when the flow is rapid. As the feed progresses and the rate of milk flow changes, the patterns will vary accordingly. If the flow is too rapid, the baby will cough, pull away from the breast or clamp down on the nipple to reduce milk flow.

Ending

When the infant has completed nursing, he is relaxed. In early infancy, the baby will sleep after feedings. Spontaneous release of the breast may occur. Alternatively, the mother may insert a finger into the side of the mouth to break suction before removing the nipple. Stimulation of the oral cavity which occurs as the nipple slides out of the mouth stimulates reflexive sucking movements which may be confused with hunger. If the infant wakens and begins to root for the breast, feeding should resume. For her part, the mother should be able to notice some difference in breast fullness between the beginning and end of the feeding.

In at least one controlled study, when mothers were instructed to feed for a specified number of minutes rather than to terminate feedings in response to infant signals, the total duration of breast-feeding after discharge declined significantly.)[84] Duration of feedings varies markedly between breast-feeding dyads even in later infancy in response to both maternal and infant factors.[85, 86]

Problem Feeding and Oral-Motor Dysfunction

The majority of breast-feeding difficulties encountered shortly after delivery are self-limited. As infants and mothers overcome the rigors of delivery, and physicians, nurses, and lactation consultants provide encouragement, support, advice and assistance, most breast-feeding problems resolve. However, persistent or severe problems may indicate oral-motor dysfunction. When suckling problems do not respond to intervention, infants or mothers may benefit from referral to a physician, speech-language pathologist or other therapist trained in the identification and management of infant feeding problems.

Table 6 lists examples of symptoms and associated breast-feeding problems and/or oral-motor dysfunctions encountered in the authors' practices.

It is also worth noting that infants who exhibit poor weight gain and infants who tire excessively during feedings may be experiencing fatigue and reduced intake secondary to poor oral-motor synchrony.

Discharge Planning
Critical Information

If the mother is aware of the nursing problems that usually arise shortly after release from the hospital and is prepared to manage them, many cases of lactation

Symptom	Possible Causes
Flattened, sore nipples after all feeds.	• Improper latch-on. • Excessive midblade tongue elevation with reduced anterior-posterior peristaltic motion. • Tight frenulum.
Persistent nasal flaring.	• Incoordination of suck/swallow/breathe sequence.
Excessive milk loss during nursing.	• Inadequate seal on the nipple. • Head and trunk out of alignment. • Incoordination of sucking/swallow/breathe sequence. • Overactive milk ejection reflex. *
Clamping on nipple.	• Inability to coordinate oral structures to create negative pressure. • Overactive milk ejection reflex. * • Inadequate positioning.
Gagging, coughing during feeding.	• Uncoordinated or dysfunctional swallowing during feeding. • Sensory involvement. • Gastroesophageal reflux. • Overactive milk ejection reflex. *
Inability to achieve or maintain latch-on.	• Maternal skills deficit. • Inadequate positioning. • Weakness, underdevelopment, or malformation in any or all oral structures. • Difficulty breathing through nose.

* Seen in older infants after mother has achieved full milk production.

Table 6: Examples of symptoms and associated breast-feeding problems and/or oral-motor dysfunctions.

failure may be averted. The decision to terminate breast-feeding early, or to introduce formula prematurely, frequently is made within the first two weeks postpartum.[87] The inappropriate use of formula in managing early problems significantly lessens the probability of long-term breast-feeding.[57].

Women who receive free formula at discharge are more likely to introduce supplementary feedings prematurely when nursing difficulties are encountered.[57, 87]

Prior to discharge, women and their partners should be provided with specific techniques for managing breast engorgement, given clear instructions for identifying infant hunger signals and evaluating infant intake, and provided with a phone number and a list of circumstances under which they should call for assistance. Husbands or family members can be enlisted to aid in monitoring mother and infant status; to shield mother and infant from overintrusive relatives and friends; to provide for the physical needs of the mother, such as meals and clean clothing; and to bathe, change and bond with the infant by holding him in skin-to-skin contact. This will allow the mother to focus her attention on learning her infant's breast-feeding signals and coordinating her milk production with his nutrient requirements. Fathers have a very difficult role in the early period of breast-feeding. However, acknowledgement of and gratitude for his assistance may not be readily forthcoming from an exhausted, preoccupied mother.

Combined Breast- and Bottle-feeding

The choice to combine breast and formula feeding is currently widespread in the U.S. Without careful management, this choice leads rapidly to exclusive formula feeding. Attainment of full milk production requires frequent stimulation and thorough breast emptying for three to four weeks postpartum. If infant hunger is appeased with formula supplements during that time, in the absence of external breast stimulation, attainment of full milk production is compromised. The best course of action is to avoid formula supplementation during the first three weeks. Failing this, breast stimulation with a pump is advisable until maternal supplies meet expectations. Similar considerations apply, albeit with less immediate consequences, in later lactation. If formula supplementation is necessary, careful attention to latch-on and suckling are warranted to circumvent ineffective feeding behaviors sometimes called "nipple confusion."

"Nipple Confusion"

Anecdotal reports of "nipple confusion" abound, as do hypothetical explanations of the phenomenon.[2, 88] Although little scientific scrutiny has been applied to these observations, the widespread nature of the reports and the observation that even slight varia-

> *From a mother of twins: It's great that we have evolved with two breasts, but to nurse two simultaneously you really need four hands!*
>
> Susan Henning Ph.D.
> Department of Pediatrics
> Baylor College of Medicine
> Houston, Texas

tions in nipple size and compressibility are known to affect the characteristics of neonatal suckling[89, 90] suggest caution in switching between breast- and bottle-feeding.

The same oral musculature is used to nurse from either a breast or a bottle. Some authors have suggested differences in tongue movement between breast- and bottle-feeding; however, studies generally have not substantiated significant differences.[67] When an infant nurses from an artificial nipple, his mouth does not have to be wide open. The teat is preformed and may even be inserted between nearly closed lips. For the fully developed term infant, this may be the most significant difference between the two types of feeding. An infant who approaches the breast with a partly open mouth will take in less of the mother's areola and will be less likely to empty the breast effectively. The magnitude of resulting difficulties depends on several factors, e.g., the precise location of the mother's lactiferous sinuses, the infant's oral-motor development and maternal breast-feeding skills. When milk is not removed effectively, the result is milk stasis, decreased milk production and poor infant weight gain. If the infant's tongue and gums compress the mother's nipple rather than the areola, sore or fissured nipples may result.

Bottle-feeding may be introduced after lactation has been established (two to three weeks postpartum is a reasonable estimate). If the infant has difficulty nursing at the breast after receiving a bottle, the mother should ensure that the infant has his mouth positioned well over the lactiferous sinuses and his lower lip turned outward.

Older infants who have never received bottle feedings often refuse to nurse from a bottle. For this reason, women who anticipate a future need to bottle feed their infants should be advised to initiate feedings from a bottle two to three weeks after delivery, and to maintain such feedings on a regular, frequent basis. Use of expressed breast milk for at least initial bottle feedings will often facilitate infant acceptance.

Transition to Office-based Pediatric Care Telephone Triage

After discharge from the hospital, mothers become dependent on the pediatrician, obstetrician and their respective office staffs for help with lactation. It is advisable to train all office staff in basic lactation management. Inaccurate information regarding early breast-feeding can result in serious complications for both mother and infant. Ideally, the first well-baby examination should occur within a week of discharge. Early monitoring is crucial to prevent infant dehydration, which may occur as a consequence of breast-feeding problems. Moreover, timely advice and assistance during the first and second week of breast-feeding can markedly enhance a mother's confidence in health care providers and help ensure maternal compliance if interventions are necessary. A telephone call or home visit within two to three days of delivery is critical for any mother with an identified risk factor (e.g., use of supplements in hospital; poor nursing assessment; flat, rigid or inverted nipples; breast anomalies or scars; premature, small for gestational age or ill infant; poor social support; lack of self-confidence; previous lactation failure; or notable anxiety). All mothers will benefit from a call on the third day postpartum to help in the management of breast engorgement.

During each telephone contact, office staff should record the following basic information for the previous 24-hour period: infant age; infant weight, if known; number of breast-feedings; number, color and estimated volume of infant stools; number of wet diapers; color of infant urine; and average duration of suckling during breast-feeding episodes. Exclusively breast-fed infants should receive an immediate pediatric examination if insufficient intake is suspected in the first few weeks. Possible indications of low milk intake include: fewer than six wet diapers a day after the third day of life; low stool frequency (see table) and/or low stool volume; dark yellow or crystalline urine; and infant not latching onto the breast or falling asleep immediately after latch-on. If a mother reports a feeding frequency below seven per day in the first two weeks, the possibility of inaccurate interpretation or rejection of infant hunger signals should be carefully evaluated and infant growth monitored.

Age (days)	Average	Suggestive Of Low Milk Intake
0-1	3	<2
2-3	3-4	≤2
4-14	4-5	≤3

Table 7: Daily stool frequencies of breast-fed infants.

In addition, if the parents express concern about the baby's intake or health in two separate phone conversations, the infant should be examined.

At the first pediatric visit, the breast-fed infant's hydration status and weight gain are evaluated. Although breast-fed infants lose a greater percentage of their birth weight than formula-fed infants (mean 7.4% vs 4.9%),[91] by two weeks of age they are generally well over birth weight if breast-feeding is progressing satisfactorily.[69]

Breast Engorgement as a Feeding Crisis

On day three postpartum, primiparous women usually experience some breast engorgement resulting from a combination of increased blood and lymph flow and onset of significant milk production (stage III lactogenesis or galactopoiesis). This may occur earlier in multiparous women, but for some, engorgement may not occur for several days. In a certain percentage of women, onset of milk production is so rapid that uncomfortably full breasts are reported within minutes after nursing and the period of engorgement may extend to two or three weeks. Tight-fitting brassieres are often successful inmodulating milk production in the latter case, and analgesics may provide pain relief. If milk expression is necessary to relieve discomfort, frequency of breast stimulation can be minimized by expressing just before or just after nursing. During engorgement breasts become hard and often are painful, the areola may become nonprotractile, and the mother's temperature may increase slightly. In severe cases the infant is unable to latch-on to the distended breast. Without intervention, formula supplementation and discontinuation of breast-feeding are likely to follow. Effective treatment of severe engorgement includes application of moist heat followed by milk expression sufficient to re-establish nipple protractility.

Once the areola is softened, the infant is assisted to achieve an effective latch-on, or milk expression is continued until the breasts are comfortable. Massage concurrent with nursing or pumping aids milk flow. Cold packs may be applied after nursing to reduce swelling and excess milk production. Recently, use of cold cabbage packs has gained considerable attention.[92] Although use of cabbage packs to reduce swelling has an interesting history in veterinary medicine, they were no more effective than cool gel packs in one of the very few published studies.[93]

Feeding Frequency, Duration and Pattern

The mean nursing frequency of exclusively breast-fed infants is approximately eight to 12 times per day during the first two weeks postpartum and eight to nine times per day at four weeks postpartum.[94-96] Feeding frequencies decline with age to approximately seven times per day by four months. However, infants with virtually identical growth patterns may nurse as frequently as 12 times per day or as infrequently as six times per day at almost any age during exclusive breast-feeding. Mothers should be cautioned not to reduce feeding frequency to six per day or less during the first three months without careful attention to milk production and infant growth. Basal serum prolactin concentrations fall and the duration of breast-feeding appears shortened when this low frequency is adopted early in lactation.[97] Above this frequency, no cross-sectional relationships have been observed between frequency and milk volume. For individual mothers, changes in frequency produce changes in milk production over short periods of time.[98, 99]

The usual duration of nursing is four to 20 minutes per breast.[85, 86] Nursings of 25 to 30 minutes or more per breast may be an adaptation to inadequate milk production or ineffective latch-on. The majority of older infants consume 80% of milk within the first four minutes of nursing at each breast.[86] However, because the caloric density of milk increases nonlinearly throughout a feeding, the infant con-

> *Breast-feeding…for two or three years, Then the body will benefit. People today do not use it.*
>
> Tseng Shih-jung,
> Huo-yu K'ou-i, 1294
>
> *Some things never change.*
> Lawrence M. Gartner M.D.
> 1996

sumes disproportionately fewer calories in the early phases of each feeding. The actual number of calories obtained within a given time period at the breast will vary with the mother's milk fat content, the infant's suckling efficiency, the interval between nursings, and the mother's milk production rate. If a feeding is terminated after a set number of minutes rather than in response to infant signals, the infant's caloric intake is disproportionately affected.

Young infants take longer to nurse than older infants on average. Duration of feeding is not predictive of milk volume or of infant growth. Infants usually nurse from both breasts at each feeding, but a significant portion prefer not to do so. This preference has been shown to result from differences in maternal milk fat content and infant requirements;[100] thus, insisting that infants always take both breasts at each feeding may be counterproductive.

For each mother-baby pair, the most effective feeding pattern for achieving appropriate infant growth will depend on several factors, including:

* The infant's age and developmental status
* The mother's 24-hour milk production rate and storage capacity.
* The fat content of the mother's milk.

Jaundice

Elevated concentrations of serum bilirubin in the newborn period occur more often in breast- than formula-fed infants. This is an apparent result of exaggerated physiologic jaundice of the newborn secondary to lower milk intake. Spontaneous feeding frequency during the first three days of life of breast-fed infants is related inversely to the serum concentration of bilirubin at hospital discharge.[94, 101-102] None the less, feeding infants more often did not reduce mean bilirubin levels at three days of life, compared to feeding on demand.[103] Demand-fed infants in this recent study lost less weight in spite of less frequent feedings (mean 6.5 vs 9.0 feedings/24 hours). To date, no studies have examined the relationship between maternal identification of and response to infant hunger signals or early feeding effectiveness on bilirubin levels of breast-fed infants.

In contrast, routine use of water supplements in breast-fed infants had no impact on serum bilirubin concentrations in numerous studies.[104, 105] If the concentration of bilirubin rises sufficiently to be of clinical concern, formula supplements may be used and will serve several purposes. Supplementing the infant's diet with formula prevents increments in bilirubin levels associated with hypocaloric intake, and reduces the enterohepatic circulation of bilirubin.[106, 107]

Discontinuation of breast-feeding for four to 72 hours is of diagnostic value in differentiating breast-milk jaundice from other causes of elevated serum bilirubin concentrations. A rapid drop of serum bilirubin levels following the temporary discontinuation of breast-feeding is pathognomonic of this condition. It is not clear if the discontinuation of breast milk has a direct effect on the liver or if the substitution of formula increases bilirubin excretion. Formula feeding is associated with greater stool volume[108] and net bilirubin elimination. Slight elevations in serum bilirubin are commonly observed when breast-feeding is resumed, and jaundice may persist for several weeks. No detrimental effects of breast-milk jaundice have been reported. Discontinuation of breast-feeding is of no known therapeutic value for this condition. Moreover, even temporary disruption of breast-feeding for diagnostic purposes increases the risk of premature weaning.

If formula feeding is introduced to supplement or replace breast-feeding, the mother's milk production must be maintained by frequent milk expression. Breasts should be nearly emptied approximately eight times per 24 hours. Most mothers will require a high-quality electric breast pump to achieve satisfactory results during this abrupt interruption of normal nursing patterns.

Established Breast-feeding
Vitamin and Mineral Supplements

Healthy, full-term breast-fed infants require little in the way of vitamin or mineral supplementation after hospital discharge. Vitamin K supplements provided immediately after birth are sufficient to restore pro-

Ten Most Common Concerns of Breastfeeding Mothers in the First Month After Delivery	
Breast-feeding Concern	**n=613 % of calls**
Frequency of feeding	14.2
Supplementation (formula or solids)	13.8
Colic/fussy period/spitting up	10.6
Pumping/storing milk	9.0
Maternal diet	8.6
Latch on/positioning	8.2
Vitamins or water supplements	5.1
Weaning	4.7
Working and breastfeeding	3.8
Sore nipples	3.8

Table 8: Maternal concerns expressed during routine screening phone calls to identify eligible participants for nutrition studies. All calls were made between two to four weeks postpartum. Names were selected sequentially from delivery lists from a private hospital in Houston, TX, between 1986 and 1989.

longed prothrombin time to normal values. Vitamin D, although present in low concentrations in human milk, is produced readily in response to minimal exposure to sunlight. Iron absorbed from human milk is sufficient to meet infant needs for at least four to six months, after which addition of iron-fortified cereals to the diet is recommended.

Progressive Changes in Behavior of Breast-fed Infants
Stools

During the first six weeks of life, breast-fed infants exhibit more rapid gastrointestinal transit. The softer stool of the breast-fed infant is attributed primarily to their markedly lower content of calcium soaps of palmitic and stearic acid. The harder stool of the formula-fed infant has been suggested as a possible cause for bowel obstruction in premature infants.[109]

The following behaviors are significant in managing term infants. The normal breast-fed infant may have a bowel evacuation at each nursing during the first four to six weeks of life. Therefore, ten or more stools per day are common in this population, although the mean frequency is close to four.[110] The frequency of evacuations may decrease suddenly to two per day, one per week or even fewer in later lactation. A low stool frequency and volume in the first month of lactation (<4 per day and <1 to 2 T.) is suggestive of inadequate milk intake. Stools of breast-fed infants are usually unformed, yellow-brown or green, seedy and inoffensive in odor until supplements are introduced.

Changing Patterns of Nursing

As the infant matures, nursing behaviors change. At approximately three months of age, infants gain the ability to independently rotate the head and shoulders, which may move in and out of alignment several times while nursing. The infant may frequently loosen and reestablish the seal between the lips and the breast. In addition, the infant takes on more responsibility for maintaining his stability; the mother's role in positioning the infant becomes less critical. When distracted during nursing, the baby will now turn his head. The increased strength of the lips, cheeks and tongue facilitate maintenance of suction as the head rotates. The tongue assumes more of the responsibility for suction and is more often visible during nursing as the lips now form a looser seal. With increasing age, feeding frequency and duration decline. Thus, breast-feeding behavior of the older infant is noticeably different from that of the newborn.

Nursing Strikes

The older infant may refuse to nurse during teething, when congested, if he develops thrush, or in other circumstances. These "nursing strikes" are temporary, usually lasting no more than a day or two. The cause may be difficult to determine in some cases; however, illness, oral pain or obstructed breathing are common.[2]

Sleep Patterns

At four weeks, feedings usually are distributed erratically through a 24-hour period; the mean interval is approximately three hours.[38] Night feedings are less common after three months of age; however, many breast-fed infants do not sleep through the night until they are weaned. For the older breast-fed infant, the usual period of continuous sleep each night is approximately five to seven hours. According to a study by Elias et al, when breast-feeding is discontinued, the sleep period increases to approximately eight hours.[111] A successful technique for training breast-fed infants to sleep through the night during early infancy has been reported.[112] In this study, no reduction in milk production was observed. Contrary to popular misconception, introduction of solid foods to breast-fed infants does not increase the duration of night sleep.[113]

Growth and Intake

Exclusively breast-fed infants initially grow faster than formula-fed infants, but not as fast after three to six months. By two years of age, weights are comparable.[95, 113, 114] Breast-milk consumption averages 750 ml per day throughout exclusive breast-feeding. By four months, this represents slightly over three fourths of the intake of formula-fed infants. The explanation for the difference in intake is not entirely clear. Growth differences explain only a part of the differences in energy intake. It is important to recognize that growth differences between breast- and formula-fed infants are relatively minor, and growth faltering in a breast-fed infant should not be ignored. If a significant growth deficit is noted, efforts to increase maternal milk production are an appropriate first intervention. A minimum of two weeks of intensive effort should be allowed to effect an increase in milk volume. This can be accomplished by increasing the frequency and degree of breast emptying.[2, 98, 99] If the infant is vigorous, increasing nursing frequency should suffice. If the infant is nursing ineffectively, use of a breast pump is indicated. A lactation consultant should work closely with the mother to assess nursing effectiveness, recommend a viable regimen for increasing milk production and provide emotional support.

Supplementary Bottle-feeding

The introduction of bottle-feeding after the second week postpartum and at weekly intervals thereafter aids the infant in retaining the skill and disposition to nurse from a rubber nipple. Use of expressed breast milk is appropriate. Breast- and bottle-feeding can be integrated successfully if milk volumes are maintained. Periodic increases in nursing frequency (e.g., on weekends for the woman working outside the home) may be sufficient to maintain milk volume. The range of feeding frequency when both modes of feeding are integrated is broad; some women maintain desired milk volumes with only a few feedings per day. While others require more frequent stimulation to prevent decreased milk production. When formula supplementation is desired, any standard formula is appropriate in the absence of demonstrated sensitivity to cow-milk protein.

Management of Common Complications
Sore Nipples

The majority of mothers experience some nipple tenderness during the first two weeks postpartum. Discomfort is usually most pronounced for the first 30 seconds to a minute after latch-on and subsides during the remainder of the nursing. Prenatal preparation of the breast does not affect the incidence or severity of sore nipples. In the absence of complications, nipple discomfort is mild and transient. Poor latch-on or abnormal suckling techniques, with subsequent trauma to the nipple/areola, and bacterial or fungal infections are the most common etiologies of severe nipple pain.

Cracks, bruises, fissures and abrasions may result from inappropriate breast-feeding techniques. When these occur, prevention of secondary infection is of paramount importance. This is best accomplished by rinsing the affected nipple after nursing and thoroughly drying the nipple and areola. Explicit instructions to allow a minimum of 10 minutes of air exposure after rinsing and drying with a clean towel may be required to obtain adequate compliance. Similar instructions are needed to successfully combat Candida albicans infections of the nipple. Pain may become exquisite, the risk of mastitis is increased, and nipple ulceration can occur when sore nipples are left untreated. When extremely sore nipples are reported, an examination should be scheduled at the earliest opportunity.

Examination of painful nipples includes a dermatologic inspection and observation of a nursing episode. The nipple, like any other portion of the body surface, is subject to rashes, irritations and infections, many of which may be exacerbated by the high moisture level associated with nursing. We have observed a variety of skin conditions including chemical irritation, rashes, ringworm, and herpes lesions on the nipples and areolas of nursing mothers. Referral to a dermatologist may be appropriate in some cases. When infected cracks or fissures are identified, a topical antibiotic may prove helpful; treatment with an antifungal agent such as nystatin is indicated in the case of yeast infection. In the latter circumstance, concurrent treatment of the infant is necessary to prevent reinfection, and careful attention to hygiene and moisture reduction is critical. An active herpes lesion on the nipple is an indication to temporarily suspend breast-feeding on the affected breast and to pump and discard milk from that breast.

Appropriate latch-on and positioning help prevent sore nipples, and are essential in treatment. Observation of an entire nursing episode together with an adequate history are necessary to identify poor latch-on, inappropriate suckling technique, and periodic clamping, biting, or stretching, which may be responsible for initial and/or repeated trauma. Although infection and pain can be treated with medication, nursing problems must be corrected to prevent recurrence. Mothers experiencing persistently sore nipples should work with a lactation consultant.

Milk Stasis and Localized Tenderness

In later lactation, if an individual duct is obstructed or the breast is drained unevenly, milk may be retained in the contiguous lobule, producing a palpable, tender lump. Generalized milk stasis similar to initial engorgement occurs following extended feed intervals. When milk stasis is localized, nursing with the infant's chin next to the painful area facilitates drainage of that part of the breast by focusing the pressure exerted by the tongue on the ampullae contiguous with the blocked duct. Tenderness and inflammation are common sequelae when drainage is uneven or incomplete. If the condition remains untreated, mastitis may follow. The mother's temperature and general condi-

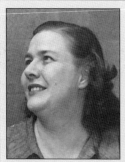

Niles A. Newton Ph.D. (1922-1994) received her doctorate from Columbia University after her first two children were born. She was mentored by Margaret Mead. Newton was Professor of Behavioral Sciences at Northwestern University Medical School where she became a leading authority on physiology and psychophysiology of lactation. She taught that it is possible to enjoy femininism both at the professional and personal levels. Newton wrote, "We can usually arrange to be full-time mothers to our babies," *Newton on Birth and Women*, Selected works Birth and Life Bookstore, Seattle, 1990.

tion should be monitored for a few days to identify any early signs of mastitis when marked breast engorgement or tenderness is reported.

Mastitis

Symptoms of mastitis include fever and body aches similar to flu. A red, tender area of the breast which is warm to the touch, fever of 38.5°C or greater plus flu-like symptoms are diagnostic. The condition is generally unilateral. Treatment of mastitis includes frequent and complete emptying of the breast together with antibiotic therapy. Less virulent strains of Staphylococcus aureus and Escherichia coli are the predominant etiologic agents in spontaneous mastitis. Streptococcus is less common. Tuberculous mastitis is reportedly rarely in endemic areas.[2] In the rare event of epidemic puerperal mastitis, a highly virulent Staphylococcus aureus strain or other pathogen may be involved. Continued nursing from a mastitic breast is recommended.[2, 115] In most cases, penicillin, ampicillin or erythromycin is the initial treatment. After the agent is identified, amoxicillin, dicloxacillin, or nafcillin may be required for severe staphylococcal infections. Because the drug will pass into the milk, the infant should be considered when choosing treatment. Sulfa drugs should be avoided when the infant is less than one month old. Bed rest and ample fluids are mandatory. Appropriate analgesics may be used together with heat packs before nursing and heat or ice packs to

relieve discomfort between feedings. Women should be advised to complete the course of antibiotics even though symptoms may disappear within a few days of treatment. Recurrent mastitis may result from incomplete treatment. Multiple recurrences of mastitis in the same location which respond abnormally or fail to respond to antibiotic treatment may indicate blockage by some obstruction, such as cancerous nodules.

Untreated mastitis may progress to a breast abscess. If an abscess is diagnosed, incision and drainage are indicated. With care, breast-feeding may continue in most cases.[2]

Low Milk Production

The most common reason a woman stops breast-feeding prematurely is that she believes she isn't producing enough milk. If a mother expresses concern about her milk supply in spite of adequate infant growth, it is appropriate to analyze the infant behavior that prompted her concern. The definitive determination of milk insufficiency is inadequate growth in an otherwise healthy infant. Thus, the first step in evaluating growth faltering in a breast-fed infant is a thorough medical examination. While early failure to thrive is usually associated with insufficient nursing frequency or inadequate breast emptying, late-onset failure to thrive is more often caused by underlying illness. If low milk production or lactation failure is confirmed, management depends on the underlying cause, and requires an understanding of lactation physiology.

Development of the mammary gland during pregnancy requires the orchestrated interaction of pituitary, pancreatic, adrenal and placental hormones. By the sixteenth week of pregnancy, mammogenesis is complete and the breast is prepared for milk production. While it is not uncommon for women to experience leakage of a small quantity of milk in the latter stages of pregnancy, complete milk production is precluded by high levels of placental progesterone and estrogen that inhibit the lactogenic functions of prolactin on secretory cells in the lobuli. After the placenta is delivered, the circulating levels of these hormones begin to fall over the next one to three days. During this time, the mother produces colostrum, a high-protein milk precursor enriched in immunologically protective factors. Copious milk production begins when progesterone and estrogen have fallen to baseline levels within the first week. Early lactation failure may result from retained placental fragments which continue to release progesterone and estrogens into the maternal circulation. Other causes of low-milk production in early lactation include pharmacologic agents and interrupted nipple innervation, which prevent suckling-induced release of oxytocin and prolactin. In addition, copious blood loss during delivery has been associated with early lactation failure.[116] Possible explanations for the latter phenomenon include damage to the pituitary gland analogous to but less severe than Sheenan's syndrome.

Normal development of full milk production rates and later maintenance of milk production are governed primarily by circulating prolactin and oxytocin levels and cyclic decreases in intramammary pressure.

Prolactin is regulated by tactile stimulation to the nipple, which causes inhibition of hypothlamic dopamine release, facilitating release of prolactin from the anterior pituitary gland. Circulating prolactin acts on the secretory cells in each lobulus to promote casein synthesis and regulate milk osmolality and volume. "Non-nutritive" suckling prior to and after milk delivery increases prolactin levels and milk production for subsequent feedings. Prolactin is also elevated during sleep. Thus, frequency and duration of feeding and maternal sleep periods are factors to be considered in identifying a cause for low milk production. The number of daily feedings required to maintain adequate milk production will vary from one mother-child dyad to another.

Oxytocin is also released from the pituitary gland in response to suckling. It causes milk ejection by inducing contraction of myoepithelial cells surrounding lobuli and ducts. Oxytocin is also released in response to conditioned reflexes. For example, a mother may experience milk ejection in response to a child's cry. Release of the hormone is blocked by maternal stress response. In one study, the influence of the hospital setting alone was sufficiently stressful to block the milk ejection reflex and temporarily reduce milk output.[117] When maternal stress inhibits milk ejection, nursing during the night while the mother is only partially awake, is usually more successful. Relaxation techniques may be helpful in modulating stress response and increasing milk ejection. Relaxation audio tapes have

Causes of Early Lactation Failure
1. Inadequate nursing frequency.
2. Elevated intramammary pressure (secondary to insufficient milk removal.)
3. Retained placenta.
4. Interrupted nipple innervation.
5. Insufficient glandular development.
6. Postpartum hemorrhage.
7. Pharmacologic agents.

Table 9: Causes of early lactation failure or low milk production in the first two weeks are most often caused by inadequate nursing frequency and/or inefficient milk extraction. Less often, underlying hormonal, anatomical or pharmacologic factors may be responsible.

been used successfully to increase release of milk from the mammary gland in mothers of premature infants.[118]

Intramammary pressure is regulated by nursing frequency and efficiency of breast emptying. Failure to frequently and effectively remove milk from the breast causes the mammary lobules to become engorged with milk. Blood vessels surrounding the lobuli are constricted, reducing availability of glucose and other nutrients, fluid, oxytocin, prolactin, and other factors necessary for milk production. When engorgement is severe and prolonged, contact with the basal membrane surrounding the alveoli is disrupted and mammary involution is initiated. Efficiency of breast emptying may be evaluated by milk expression after nursing. When significant volumes of milk are consistently extracted from each breast after nursing, inadequate emptying may be contributing to low milk production. If the infant is unable to empty the breast an alternative mechanism (a breast pump or hand expression) must be employed to assure regular, cyclic decreases in intramammary pressure and to prevent feed-back inhibition.

A number of circumstances may precipitate less frequent nursing and ineffective milk removal. These include the mother's employment, imposed feeding schedules, infant or maternal illness, thrush, teething,

Common Causes of Late-Onset Lactation Failure
1. Infant illness.
2. Reduced nursing frequency.
3. Pharmacologic agents.
4. Maternal illness, fatigue or stress.

Table 10: Late onset lactation failure most frequently results from underlying infant illness, and less often from maternal factors.

excessive use of pacifiers and prolongation of night-time sleep periods, to name a few.

When infant growth faltering is marked and maternal milk supply does not respond adequately to increased frequency and effectiveness of breast empty-ing or other interventions, formula supplementation may be required to achieve catch-up growth. If the mother is committed to exclusive breast-feeding, maternal compliance with supplementation is best obtained by continuing to emphasize efforts to increase her milk supply. Giving formula *ad libitum* is the fastest way to complete catch-up growth and reestablish exclusive breast-feeding. Once infant requirements decrease to a level consistent with normal growth rates, maternal milk production is more likely to meet infant needs.

Maternal or Infant Illness

In most cases, the risk of an infant acquiring an infectious disease from the mother's milk is minimal. Transplacentally acquired IgG antibodies and maternal immune factors in human milk provide the infant with immunological defenses against the range of pathogens in the mother's environment. While pathogens like shigella, salmonella, cytomegalovirus, rubella, and hepatitis B virus have been found in human milk in areas where these are prevalent, it is unusual for an infant to develop symptomatic infection by these agents. Breast-feeding, when supplemented by standard immunization protocols for diseases like hepatitis B and rubella, is effective in promoting infant health and is preferable to artificial feedings, which provide no immunological benefit to the infant. As a general rule, nursing should be continued throughout maternal or infant illness.

In developed countries, the following maternal illnesses are considered contraindications to breast-feeding: maternal AIDS (acquired immune deficiency syndrome); active untreated tuberculosis; untreated gonorrhea; herpes lesions on the nipple, areola or other regions of the breast, primary disseminated herpes, and positive human immunodeficiency virus (HIV) or human lymphocytotropic virus type 1. While HTLV-1+ is still rare in the United States, the risk of transmitting the virus to the infant through human milk is apparently significant,[119] and until more information is available, it is sound medical practice to discourage HTLV-1+ women from breast-feeding. The data on HIV transmission in human milk is more controversial, and has led to conflicting recommendations. Given the lack of conclusive information, the U.S. Centers for Disease Control[120] recommends that HIV+ women in the U.S. not breast-feed.

Hepatitis C (non-A, non-B) also falls into the category of untreatable diseases for which breast-feeding is considered contraindicated; however, transmission via breast milk was not reported on any subjects in a recent study of 11 infants breast-fed by HCV-positive mothers.[121] While it has also been suggested that nursing should be discontinued during maternal hepatitis, from a practical standpoint, infant exposure preceding clinical illness in the mother is very likely. Moreover, there is no current evidence that breast-feeding poses any additional risks to infants of HBV carrier mothers (Table 11). In the case of maternal tuberculosis, breast-feeding may be reinstated following the initiation of treatment.

In countries where medical services are less readily available and conditions are less hygienic, a different standard applies. In these countries, the risk of death associated with not breast-feeding far outweighs the theoretical risk of disease transmission via breast milk. The World Health Organization[122] recommends that HIV+ women in developing countries continue to breast-feed to protect the infant against other pathogens.

Infants with galactosemia cannot receive breast milk. Infants with maple syrup urine disease or phenylketonuria can be partially breast-fed with careful monitoring.[123]

Drugs and Contaminants

Medication should not be prescribed for nursing mothers unless absolutely necessary. When it is required, the safest alternative should be chosen. A number of considerations are important in selecting an appropriate drug. These include oral availability, milk/plasma ratios and half-life, as well as the potential impact on infant health and maternal milk production. Premature infants may be particularly sensitive to certain drugs because of their reduced ability to systematically clear them or convert them to inactive metabolites. In addition, the possibility of interaction between the infant's medications and those in the mother's milk must be carefully evaluated.

The American Academy of Pediatrics (AAP) divides drugs into seven categories based on their transfer into mother's milk and their potential consequences for nursing infants. In its 1994 publication, the AAP includes in Category 6, "Maternal medication usually compatible with breast-feeding," such commonly prescribed drugs as acetaminophen, amoxicillin, codeine, digoxin, erythromycin, ibuprofen, prednisone, streptomycin, tetracycline, and warfarin[128] along with many others. Interestingly, aspirin is classified as a Category 5 drug which should be given to nursing mothers with caution because one case of metabolic acidosis in a breast-fed infant was reported following maternal ingestion. Although most maternal medications are compatible with breast-feeding, antineoplastic agents, some radiopharmaceuticals,[129] antiprotozoan agents, some antithyroid agents and certain other drugs are contraindicated. When temporary treatment with contraindicated drugs is required, the mother should be advised to pump and discard milk for a specified period of time until the agent has cleared her system. The physician is encouraged to consult the text *Drugs in Pregnancy and Lactation*[130] and *Breast-feeding: A Guide for the Medical Professions*[2] to determine if the agent is transmitted in mother's milk and if it poses any risk to the infant. In addition, the Lactation Study Center in Rochester, NY, (716-275-0088) maintains a computer data base of pharmacologic research on lactating women. In many cases, acceptable agents can be substituted for contraindicated drugs.

The amount of drug transferred to the infant can often be minimized by timing the mother's intake to ensure the lowest possible concentration in milk at the beginning of each feeding. For example, she may take the medication right after nursing or before bedtime. In some cases it is advisable to monitor the infant's blood levels.[128]

Massive exposure to some nonpharmaceutical chemical agents poses a special concern for lactating women. Heavy metals, pesticides, polychlorinated biphenyls (PCBs) and dioxins are readily transferred to human milk. Nonetheless, levels of exposure characteristic of urban living present no apparent problem for infant health.[131] Some level of contamination is virtually ubiquitous. Breast-feeding is contraindicated only after massive exposure to hazardous contaminants has been confirmed by testing. Illegal drugs such as heroin, cocaine and marijuana place the infant at significant risk. Mothers who abuse drugs should be discouraged from breast-feeding. Particular care should be taken to screen mothers of premature infants who supply milk to feed their hospitalized neonates. Low doses of caffeine (one to two beverages/day) or alcohol (one to two drinks/week) have not yet been associated with infant health problems.[128, 132] Although alcohol has been promoted as a relaxant, it has been shown to inhibit oxytocin release and reduce infant breast milk intake.[133, 134] Maternal cigarette smoking endangers infant health primarily through passive smoke exposure, although other concerns exist.[135] Nicotine and cotinine are found in milk, and both volume and milk fat content have been reported to be reduced in early lactation in women who smoke cigarettes.[136, 137] Mothers who smoke are less likely to breast-feed their infants.[138] Paradoxically, infants of smokers who continue to breast-feed grew more rapidly than controls in one study.[139] Any smoking in the presence of infants and children dramatically increases the risk of respiratory disease and should be avoided whether or not breast-feeding is involved.

Breast-feeding During Mother-Infant Separation

Working Mothers

Breast-feeding is compatible with work outside the home, however, the combination requires planning and preparation. Several options are available. Mothers may continue

Illness	Continue Breastfeeding	Comment/Reference
Infant Illness		
Galactosemia	No	(123)
PKU	Partial Breastfeeding	Monitor infant & adjust volume of breastmilk intake. (124)
Maple Syrup	Partial Breastfeeding	Monitor infant & adjust volume of breastmilk intake. (123)
HIV/AIDS	Controversial	(122,126,125,120,2)
Herpes Simplex (oral lesion)		Give expressed breastmilk until infant's oral lesions heal. (127)
Maternal Illness		
Minor bacterial infections	Yes	
Salmonella	Yes	If culture negative. (2)
Shigella	Yes	If culture negative. (2)
Group B-Staphylococcus	Yes	See Lawrence (2) for special precautions for premature or compromised newborns when mother has possible cervical culture and obstetric history.
Group A-Streptococcus	Yes	Give expressed breast milk until the mother has 24 hr of treatment. (2)
Gonorrhea	Yes	Give expressed breast milk until mother receives 24 hr of treatment and passes acute stage. (125,2)
Syphilis mother treated	No	(2)
Syphilis stage 2 or skin lesions mother untreated		Give expressed breast milk, if mother is isolated from infant, or if active lesions on breast. (2)
Herpes simplex without breast lesion	Yes	
Herpes simplex with breast lesion		Give expressed breast milk until breast lesion heals. (125,2,123)
Chicken Pox	Yes	See (2,125) for isolation protocols for newborn hospitalized infants.
Tuberculosis	Yes	After 24 hrs of treatment or if inactive disease, give expressed breast milk if mother is isolated from infant. (2,125,123)
Hepatitis A	Yes	(125)
Hepatitis B	Yes	If infant receives HBIG and Heptavax. (125)
Hepatitis C	Controversial	(125,2,121)

Illness	Continue Breastfeeding	Comment/Reference
Maternal Illness		
Leprosy	Yes	(2)
Toxoplasmosis	Yes	(2)
Mastitis	Yes	(123,2)
Breast abscess	Partial	Feed from unaffected breast. (123,2)
Breast cancer	Yes	Unless drug therapy contraindicates. (2)
HIV/AIDS	Controversial	No in U.S. (1995) Consult recent references. (125,122,126)
CMV	Yes	(2)
HTLV-1	Controversial	(119)

Table 11: Recommendations regarding breast-feeding during illness based on information available in 1995-96. (adapted from Lactation Management Curriculum: A Faculty Guide for Schools of Medicine, Nursing and Nutrition. *Woodward-Lopez, Gail, Greer, A Elizabeth, ed. San Diego, CA: Wellstart International; 1994.)*

exclusive breast-feeding by bringing their infants to work, placing them in work-site day-care centers, or expressing milk during breaks in the workday. They may combine breast and formula feeding for extended periods by monitoring their milk production and stimulating their supply when milk volumes decline. They may introduce formula when they return to work and gradually switch to exclusive formula feeding as their milk production decreases. While maternity leave policies in many countries allow ample time for extended breast-feeding, most working women in the United States are required to return to work within four to eight weeks after delivery. The transition can be eased if the mother arranges to return to work on a Wednesday or Thursday and take a day off in the middle of week for the first few weeks. This allows her to monitor and correct milk production deficits. In addition, mothers should begin milk expression and storage at least two weeks before returning to work to facilitate exclusive breast-feeding while separated from their infants. The stored milk and the increased milk production rates which result will carry them through the first week or two.

Initiating milk collection at the early morning feeding usually is best. Mothers may begin by nursing the infant on one breast and pumping the other either simultaneously or as soon as possible after the infant has finished one side. The infant's stimulation of milk-ejection reflex increases the effectiveness of the milk expression and assists in conditioning the reflex to pump use. After expressing milk, the infant should be allowed to nurse at the breast from which milk has been expressed to stimulate additional production. Expressed milk can be frozen and the date of collection recorded on the container.

Meanwhile, the mother can negotiate with her employer to identify locations and times for milk expression at work. Intervals between milk expressions should be short (three to five hours) and regular, especially in the first few days, to avoid plugged ducts and mastitis. The mother may nurse her baby before she leaves home or at the child care facility. She may then (ideally) express milk two or three times during the day and nurse as soon after work as possible.

Premature Delivery
Maintaining Milk Production After Premature Delivery
Premature delivery presents unique breast-feeding problems. Lactation must be initiated and maintained in the absence of suckling while the mother is under significant stress. Prolonged delays in the initiation of milk expression (more than four days) result in temporarily low milk production or potential involution of the mammary

gland.[98] It is not necessary to initiate milk expression during the first 24 hours after delivery. These guidelines are recommended for mothers of premature infants:

1) Begin milk expression within two to three days after delivery.

2) Express milk six or more times per day, approximately every three hours.

3) Empty both breasts thoroughly at each expression (100 minutes/day total pumping minimum for single pumping, with adjustment downward for double pumping).

4) Pump during the night if breasts become uncomfortably full; otherwise, allow a prolonged nighttime sleep period.

If milk volumes are low or begin to decline, mother may be advised to increase expression frequency to eight times per 24 hours. Metoclopramide has been used with some success to increase milk production in mothers of premature infants.[2] Skin-to-skin contact between mother and infant has been associated with greater maternal milk production.[140]

Initiation of Suckling After Premature Delivery

Use of extended skin-to-skin contact has been shown to increase nursing effectiveness and breast-feeding duration of premature infants.[140-142] During skin-to-skin contact, alert inactivity increased nearly fourfold.[143] Each stage of a feeding episode is more complex when the infant is premature. Hunger signals are more subtle, the infant's behavior state is more tenuous and the quiet alert state is generally shorter. Latch-on is more difficult because buccal pads are less developed and oral musculature is weaker, making sustained suction difficult. Finally, sucking, swallowing, and breathing are less well coordinated. Development of mature suckling patterns in premature infants has been examined and differences between suckling patterns of premature and term infants have been described.[79, 80] Although premature infants have been reported to suckle successfully at body weights as low as 1300 gm,[144, 145] most are unable to coordinate suckling and swallowing until they are at least 1,500 to 1,800 gm. The ability to nurse adequately depends on a variety of factors: coordination of sucking/swallowing/breathing, strength and stability of oral musculature, freedom from ventilatory support, wakefulness of the infant, maternal milk volume and nipple anatomy, and

the mother's breast-feeding skills. Assessment and/or therapeutic intervention by a speech pathologist or physical therapist who specializes in breast-feeding may be useful when significant difficulties are encountered. In premature infants, coordination of suckling and breathing differs during breast-feeding and feeding from artificial nipples. Inability to feed from a bottle does not necessarily correlate with inability to feed from the breast. The decision to initiate suckling should be made after carefully evaluating both infant's and mother's readiness. Once sucking is initiated, nursery staff should set aside certain feedings for the mother to breast-feed her infant. When promises have been made to reserve feedings, they should be kept. These interludes are considerably more meaningful to parents than to staff.

Elements of Lactation Support for Mothers of Preterm Infants

Practical support for the lactating mother of a preterm infant includes clear instructions for collecting, labeling, storing, transporting, and delivering expressed milk and providing (or identification of sources for) breast pumps and collection and storage containers. It also includes space dedicated for milk expression during hospital visits. Appropriate use and cleaning of milk collection equipment are best reviewed with each mother, since equipment rental agencies frequently provide little or inadequate information in these important areas. Finally, records of milk delivered by mothers for their infants should be maintained by the support service which helps the mother initiate and maintain lactation.

Psychological support for the preterm mother is more difficult to define. Providing practical support for milk expression as described above will validate and encourage the mother's efforts. Skin-to-skin contact is also a source of psychological comfort to parents. Greater maternal and paternal comfort with infant care and longer letters of thanks to hospital staff have been reported in studies of parents who were given the opportunity for skin-to-skin contact with their hospitalized premature infants.[140, 141, 146-148]

Discharge Planning for the Nursing Preterm Infant

The mother of a premature infant may gain confidence in her breast-feeding and parenting skills by caring for her infant in the hospital for one or two days prior to discharge. In addition, a period of rooming-in allows the physician to evaluate the need for supplementary feedings and home visits by the lactation support staff.

Exclusive breast-feeding after discharge is possible for some, but not all, premature infants. If the mother is either not producing sufficient milk or expresses significant doubt that the infant is receiving enough milk, a supplemental nursing device may be a viable alternative to supplemental bottle-feeding. Such a device (See Figure 6) delivers milk through a small tube leading from a milk reservoir to infants mouth as he suckles the mother's nipple. It provides a mechanism for the infant to stimulate increased milk production through suckling, while receiving supplementary feeds at the breast. Moreover, the visual confirmation of milk intake reduces maternal anxiety. Supplementary feedings, whether from bottles, cups, or nursing devices, may be discontinued gradually as the mother's milk supply and the infant's nursing skills improve.

Expressing and Storing Human Milk For Home Use

Recommendations for storing and handling human milk vary depending on infant status, the length of time the milk is to be stored, and the relationship between the recipient and the donor. Milk for hospitalized infants should be collected and stored under the guidance of the hospital staff. The Human Milk Banking Association of North America has published guidelines for hospital milk banks which cover all details of milk handling and preparation for compromised infants.[149, 150]

Expressing and storing milk for home use requires less rigorous attention to detail. Fortunately, human milk is inherently resistant to bacterial growth. Breast milk may be expressed by hand or by using any of a number of breast pumps. Pumps and attachments must be cleaned thoroughly to prevent contamination. Milk may be stored in glass containers, hard plastic containers, or baggie bottles. When baggie bottles are used, care should be taken to prevent puncture. Some loss of specific secretory IgA has been reported when breast milk is stored in polyethylene baggies.[151] This may be a significant consideration when expressed milk is fed to premature or compromised infants in hospital, but is of little consequence for occasional

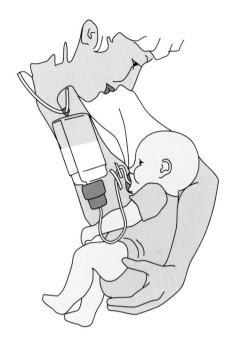

Figure 6: Supplemental nursing device. These devices deliver supplemental milk to the baby while the baby stimulates maternal hormone release and milk production.

feeding of healthy infants in a home setting. No studies have been reported to date regarding adhesion of cells or immunologic components to baggie bottles made of substances other than polyethylene.

Pardou et al have reported that freshly expressed milk stored at 4°C exhibits no bacterial growth for up to eight days under laboratory conditions.[152] This remarkable resistance to bacterial growth is due to anti-infective agents in human milk. As a pragmatic measure, however, it may be advisable for mothers to freeze milk when feeding within the next four to five days is not anticipated. This will eliminate the possibility of inadvertently prolonged storage and also reduce lipid peroxidation which becomes significant after four days of refrigeration.[153] Frozen milk may be thawed by gently shaking under warm running water. With this method it requires approximately four minutes to thaw three ounces of breast milk frozen in a glass bottle. Alternatively, frozen milk may be placed in the refrigerator to thaw. Leaving frozen breast milk to thaw at room temperature is not recommended because of the possibility that it will be inadvertently left for long time periods. Microwaving is

Directions for Hand Expression
1. Gently massage or stroke the breast or apply warm, moist compresses.
2. Place the fingers below and thumb above the nipple, 1-2 cm from the base.
3. Press back toward the chest wall.
4. Compress.
5. Roll fingers and thumb slightly forward.
6. Repeat rhythmically.
7. Adjust position of fingers and thumb as needed to access milk sinuses and empty all areas of the breast.

Table 12: Directions for hand expression. With practice, this can be an economical and effective technique for expressing milk.

not recommended for human milk feeding or formula feeding. Severe burns with destruction of oral tissues have been reported for infants fed bottles of milk heated in microwave ovens. Microwaving human milk is further contraindicated because some of the anti-infective components of human milk can be damaged. Even at low temperatures (20 to 53ºC), microwaving reportedly reduced specific IgA to some E coli serotypes. It also decreased lysozyme and increased growth of E coli to five times that of controls. Microwaving at high temperature (72 to 98ºC) was even more destructive.[154] Once frozen and thawed, breast milk is markedly less resistant to bacterial growth, and should be kept in the refrigerator until used within a day or two, at most.

Case Studies

Case Study #1

Complaint: *An otherwise healthy female infant presented with a net 65 gm weight loss at two weeks postpartum. Mother reported that the baby had difficulty with latch-on, sometimes became agitated and sometimes fell asleep during nursing.*

History: *Birth weight: 3145 gm. Apgar 8 at one minute, 9 at five minutes. Infant was born at term of a 31-year-old primigravida by an uncomplicated vaginal delivery. Breast-feeding was initiated six hours postpartum and*

continued on demand at a frequency of seven to eight times per 24 hours. Nursing episodes varied in length between 20 minutes and one and a half hours and were problematic. Mother experienced severe engorgement on day three and began milk expression to relieve discomfort. Expression continued on a daily basis. At the time of presentation, the mother was expressing and storing seven ounces of breastmilk per day.

Examination: *Infant: Infant was well hydrated and in good health.*

Breasts: *Breasts and nipples were average in shape and protractility. A small fissure was visible on the left nipple. Milk was readily expressed. Hand expression indicated that milk sinuses were located approximately 1 cm from the base of the nipple.*

Nursing: *The mother offered the breast with her fingers blocking access to the areola (Figure 7a). Latch-on was poor, encompassing little more than the nipple. The infant's lower lip was sucked into the mouth during nursing (Figure 7b). The baby took a few sucks and fussed/ cried, and repeated this pattern several times. Finally the baby settled and nursed with barely audible swallowing for several minutes. The nursing episode (left breast only) lasted 15 minutes. Total milk intake was 17 grams.*

Diagnosis: *Inappropriate latch-on.*

Management: *The mother was shown how to offer the breast without interfering with the infant's access. Latch-on was improved, but the lower lip was again tucked inside the mouth. This was corrected by pulling down the infant's chin and wedging more of the areola into the mouth (Figure 7c). The baby hesitated and did not initiate suckling until breast massage was used to express milk into the mouth while the infant remained in a correct latch-on (Figure 7d). At that point the infant swallowed and began to nurse with rhythmic, audible swallows. When asked to describe the difference, the mother replied, "It doesn't hurt this way," and "It feels like a deeper pull." After demonstration, the mother was able to attain a correct latch-on unassisted.*

Outcome: *The infant gained 300 g during the next week with no supplementation, and 350 g the following week to return to 50% weight for height. Nursing frequency initially increased and then returned to seven to eight nursings per 24 hours. Nursing durations decreased to eight to 10 minutes per breast.*

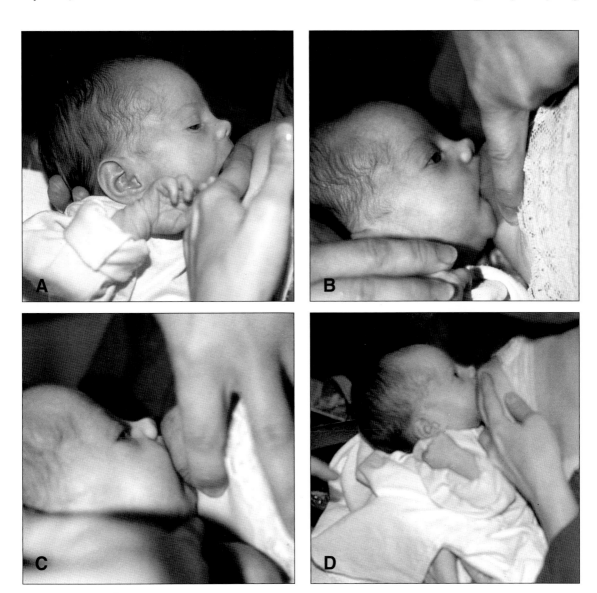

Figure 7: Case study #1.

Case Study #2:

Complaint: *A 26-year-old primigravida presented with redness and localized tenderness in her left breast.*

   History: *Patient reported two prior episodes of mastitis in the left breast and mild, bilateral nipple soreness during the two months since delivery of a 3.14 kg baby boy. No prior breast surgery or breast injury reported. Milk production was adequate to support infant gain greater than 4.5 kg/month. Previous consultation for poor latch-on provided some relief of early nipple discomfort.*

Examination:

Temperature: *98.9°F*

   Breasts: *Left breast was red and warm to touch. A large (3cm), palpable lump consistent with milk stasis in lower medial quadrant was tender to touch. The left nipple was slightly abraded. No signs of thrush were noted. There was a scar at the base of breast in the lower medial quadrant. Right breast and nipple were normal. On questioning, the patient reported that her scar was caused by a clip on her brassiere which had caused an abrasion followed by an infection and considerable discomfort during pregnancy.*

Infant: *The infant was a healthy, 6.8 kg, two-month-old male. Finger feeding examination revealed exaggerated midblade tongue elevation and compression during suckling.*

Nursing: *The mother placed the infant in a standard cradle hold, with the infant positioned horizontally. Latch-on was marginal with only 1/2 cm of areola beyond base of nipple encompassed. The infant did not cup and extend the tongue during latch-on. Extension of the tongue past the lower gums was not observed. Milk flow was rapid, and the infant swallowed loudly and occasionally struggled at the breast. The mother maintained positioning and latch-on during the infant's agitation but flinched and clinched her teeth. On questioning, she reported that the infant had "clamped down" on her nipple which he did regularly while nursing. The infant consumed four ounces of breast milk from the left breast within seven minutes and refused the second breast. Mother reported that the infant usually nursed from only one side. Immediately following nursing, the nipple was flattened and blanched. It gradually changed from blanched white to bright red and back over the course of a minute. This spasmodic vasoconstriction continued for several minutes after feeding.*

Diagnosis: *Plugged duct with incipient unilateral mastitis secondary to milk stasis and nipple trauma.*

Possible causes of milk stasis:

1. Uneven breast emptying combined with long internursing episodes resulting from alternate breast nursing pattern.

2. Inflammation or scar tissue blocking free flow of milk through duct.

Possible causes of nipple trauma:

1. Clamping of infant jaw during nursing to reduce rapid milk flow caused by overactive milk ejection reflex.

2. Poor latch-on, promoting consistent midblade tongue elevation and abnormal tongue movement.

Management: *The patient was shown how to achieve a better latch-on and how to hold the infant upright in order to give him greater control over the direction of milk flow. Moist heat and massage were utilized in conjunction with an electric breast pump to remove the palpable knot of residual milk in the left breast. The patient was instructed to massage breasts at the end of each nursing to assure even drainage; repeat treatment of moist heat and massage at the first sign of subsequent plugged ducts; break suction immediately when the infant became agitated to prevent clamping on the nipple; and to rinse and air-dry the nipples for a minimum of 10 minutes postfeeding to prevent secondary infection of abraded nipple.*

Outcome: *Body aches and breast tenderness disappeared before bedtime (eight hours post treatment.) Over the following two months, the mother reported two episodes of plugged ducts, which resolved promptly on management. Nipple blanching and creasing post-nursing occurred sporadically, but with decreasing frequency over the next month and did not recur thereafter.*

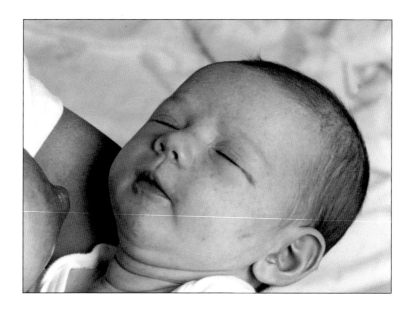

References

1. Freed GL, Clark SJ, Curtis PJ, Sorenson JR. Breast-feeding education and practice in family medicine. *J Fam Pract.* 1995;40(3):263-269.

2. Lawrence RA. *Breast-feeding: A guide for the medical profession.* Fourth Edition. St. Louis: Mosby; 1994:878.

3. Martinez GA, Kreiger FW. Milk-feeding patterns in the United States. *Pediatr.* 1984;76:1004-1008.

4. Hendershot GE. Trends in breast-feeding. *Pediatr.* 1984; 74(Suppl):591-602.

5. Ryan AS, Pratt WF, Wysong JL, Lewandowski G, McNally JW, Krieger FW. A Comparison of Breast-Feeding Data from the National Surveys of Family Growth and the Ross Laboratories Mothers Surveys. *Am J Public Health.* 1991;81(8):1049-1052.

6. Ryan AS, Martinez GA. Breast-Feeding and the Working Mother: A Profile. *Pediatr.* 1989;(83):524-531.

7. Ryan AS. The Resurgence of Breast-feeding in the United States. *Pediatr.* 1997;99(4) e12.

8. Wright AL, Holberg C, Taussig LM, et al. Infant-Feeding Practices Among Middle-Class Anglos and Hispanics. *Pediatr.* 1988;82(3):496-503.

9. Rassin DK, Markides KS, Baranowski T, Bee DE, Richardson CJ, Mikrut WD, Winkler BA. Acculturation and breast-feeding on the United States-Mexico border. *Am J Med Sci.* 1993;306(1):28-34.

10. Institute of Medicine. *Nutrition during lactation.* Washington, DC: National Academy Press; 1991.

11. Morrow-Tlucak M, Haude RH, Ernhart CB. Breast-feeding and cognitive development in the first two years of life. *Soc Sci Med.* 1988;26:635-639.

12. Rogan WJ, Galden BC. Breast-feeding and cognitive development. *Early Hum Dev.* 1993;(31):181-193.

13. Kramer MS. Does breast-feeding help protect against atopic disease? Biology methodology, and a golden jubilee of controversy. *J Pediatr.* 1988;112:181-190.

14. Davis MK, Savitz DA, Graubard BI. Infant feeding and childhood cancer. *Lancet.* 1988;2:365-368.

15. Mayer EJ, Hammon RF, Gay EC, Lezotte DC, Savitz DA, Klingensmith GK. Reduced risk of IDDM among breast-fed children: The Colorado IDDM Registry. *Diabetes.* 1988;37:1625-1632.

16. Koletzko S, Sherman P, Corey M, Griffiths A, Smith C. Role of infant feeding practices in development of Crohn's disease in childhood. *Br Med J.* 1989;298: 1617-1618.

17. Weiss-Carrington P, Roux ME, McWilliams M, Phillips-Qugliata JM, Lamm ME. Hormonal induction of the secretory immune system in the mammary gland. *Proc Natl Acad Sci USA.* 1978;75:2928-2932.

18. Goldman AS, Goldblum RM, Garza C. Immunologic components of human milk during the second year of lactation. *Acta Paediatr Scand.* 1983;72:461-462.

19. Cunningham AS, Jelliffe D, Jelliffe E. Breast-feeding and health in the 1980's: A global epidemiologic review. *J Pediatr.* 1991;118(5):659-666.

20. Bauchner H, Leventhal JM, Shapiro ED. Studies of breast-feeding and infections: how good is the evidence? *JAMA.* 1986;256(7):887-892.

21. Paradise J, Elster BA, Tan L. Evidence in Infants with cleft palate that breast milk protects against otitis media. *Pediatr.* 1994;94:853-860.

22. Owen MJ, Baldwin CD, Swank PR, Pannu AK, Johnson DL, Howie VM. Relation of infant feeding practices, cigarette smoke exposure, and group child care to the onset and duration of otitis media with effusion in the first two years of life. *J Pediatr.* 1993;123:702-711.

23. Duncan B, Ey J, Holberg CJ, Wright AL, Martinez FD, Taussig LM. Exclusive breast-feeding for at least 4 months protects against otitis media. *Pediatr.* 1993;91: 867-872.

24. Ford RPK, Taylor BJ, Mitchell EA, Enright SA, Stewart AW, Becroft DMO, Scragg R, Hassall IB, Barry DMJ, Allen EM, Roberts AP. Breast-feeding and the risk of sudden infant death syndrome. *Int J Epidemiology.* 1993; 22(5):885-890.

25. Beaudry M, Dufour R, Marcoux S. Relation between infant feeding and infections during the first six months of life. *J Pediatr.* 1995;126:191-197.

26. Habicht J-P, DaVanzo J, Butz WP. Mother's milk and sewage: their interactive effects on infant mortality. *Pediatr.* 1988;81:456-461.

27. Forsyth JS. Is it worthwhile breast-feeding? *Eur J Clin Nutr.* 1992;46(suppl.1):S19-S25.

28. Howie PW, Forsyth JS, Ogston SA, Clark A, Florey C. Protective effect of breast feeding against infection. *Br Med J.* 1990;300:11-16.

29. Simopoulos AP, Grave GD. Factors associated with the

choice and duration of infant-feeding practice. *Pediatr.* 1984;74(Suppl):603-614.

30. Losch M, Dungy CI, Russell D, Dusdieker LB. Impact of attitudes on maternal decisions regarding infant feeding. *J Pediatr.* 1995;126(4):507-514.

31. Jones DA. The choice to breast feed or bottle feed and influences upon that choice: a survey of 1525 mothers. *Child Care, Health and Development.* 1987;13:75-85.

32. Radius SM, Joffe A. Understanding adolescent mothers' feelings about breast-feeding. *J Adolescent Health Care.* 1988;9:1256-1260.

33. Freed GL, Jones TM, Schanler RJ. Prenatal determination of demographic and attitudinal factors regarding feeding practice in an indigent population. *Am J Perinatol.* 1992; 9(5/6):420-424.

34. Bryant C, Lazarov M, Light R, Bailey D, Coreil J, D'Angelo SL. Best start: breast-feeding for healthy mothers, healthy babies - a new model for breast-feeding promotion. *J Tenn Med Assoc.* 1989;82(12):6423.

35. Sciacca JP, Phipps BL, Dube DA, Ratliff MI. Influences on breast-feeding by lower-income women: An incentive-based, partner-supported educational program. *J Am Diet Assoc.* 1995;95:323-328.

36. *WIC Breast-feeding Promotion Study and Demonstration. Phase IV Report.* Volume 1. USDA/FNS; 1990:166.

37. *Promoting Breast-feeding in WIC: A Compendium of Practical Approaches.* USDA FNS, FNS-256. June, 1988:166.

38. Bryant C, Roy M. *Breast-feeding for Healthy Mothers Healthy Babies: Training Manual.* Tampa, Fl: Best Start Inc; 1990.

39. Haider SA. Encouragement of breast-feeding (letter). *BMJ.* 1976;1:650.

40. Neville NC, Neifert MR, eds. *Lactation: Physiology, Nutrition and Breast-feeding.* New York: Plenum Press; 1983.

41. Neifert MR, Seacat JM, Jobe WE. Lactation failure due to insufficient glandular development of the breast. *Pediatr.* 1985;76:823-301.

42. Neifert MR, Seacat JM. A guide to successful breast-feeding. *Contemp Pediatr.* 1986;3:26-45.

43. Levine JJ, Ilowite NT. Sclerodermalike esophageal disease in children breast-fed by mothers with silicone breast implants. *JAMA.* 1994;271(3):213-216.

44. Flick JA. Silicone implants and esophageal dysmotility: Are breast-fed infants at risk? *JAMA.* 1994;271(3):240-241.

45. FDA Talk Paper (t94-6): 1/21/1994.

46. Righard L, Alade MO. Effect of delivery room routines on success of first breast-feed. *Lancet.* 1990;336:1105-1107.

47. Widstrom AM, Ransjo-Arvidson AB, Christensson K, Mattiesen AS, Winberg J, Uvnas-Moberg K. Gastric suction in healthy newborn infants: Effects on circulation and developing feeding behavior. *Acta Paediatr Scand.* 1987;76:566-572.

48. Nissen E, Lilja G, Matthiesen A-S, Ransjo-Arvidsson A-B, Uvnas-Moberg K, Widstrom A-M. Effects of maternal Pithidine on infants' developing breast feeding behavior. *Acta Paediatr.* 1995;84:140-145.

49. Dubignon J, Campbell D, Curtis M, Partington MW. The relation between laboratory measures of suckling, food intake and perinatal factors during the newborn period. *Child Dev.* 1969;40:1107-1120.

50. Widstrom AM, Wahlberg V, Matthiesen AS, Eneroth P, Uvnas-Moberg V, Werner S, Winberg J. Short-term effects of early suckling and touch of the nipple on maternal behavior. *Early Hum Dev.* 1990;21:153-163.

51. de Chateau P, Wiberg B. Long term effect on mother-infant behavior of extra contact during the first hour postpartum. II. A follow-up at 3 months. *Acta Paediatr Scand.* 1977;66:145-151.

52. Illingsworth RS, Stone DGH, Jowett GH, Scott JF. Self-demand feeding in a maternity unit. *Lancet.* 1952;1: 683-687.

53. Johnson NW. Breast-feeding at one hour of age. *Am J Matern Child Nurs.* 1976;1:12-16.

54. Salariya EM, Easton PM, Cater JI. Duration of breast-feeding after early initiation and frequent feeding. *Lancet.* 1978;2:1141-1143.

55. Sosa R, Kennell JH, Klaus M, Urrutia JJ. The effect of early mother-infant contact on breast-feeding, infection and growth. In: *Breast-feeding and the Mother. Ciba Foundation Symposium 45.* Elsevier, North Holland: Excerpta Medica; 1976:79-187.

56. Thomson M, Westreich R. Restriction of mother-infant contact in the immediate postnatal period. In: Chalmers I, Enkin M, Keirse MJNC, eds. *Effective Care in Pregnancy and Childbirth.* New York: Oxford U Press; 1989.

57. Bergevin Y, Dougherty C, Kramer MS. Do infant formula samples shorten the duration of breast-feeding? *Lancet.* 1983;2(8334):1148-1151.

58. Feinstein JM, Berkehamer JE, Gruszaka ME, et al. Factors related to early termination of breast-feeding in an urban population. *Pediatr.* 1986;78:210-2151.

59. Loughlin HH, Clapp-Channing NE, Gehlback SH, et al. Early termination of breast-feeding: identifying those at risk. *Pediatr.* 1985;75:508-513.

60. Gray-Donald K, Kramer MS, Munday S, Leduc DG. Effect of formula supplementation in the hospital on the duration of breast-feeding: a controlled clinical trial. *Pediatr.* 1985;75:514-518.

61. Herrera AJ. Supplemented versus unsupplemented breast-feeding. *Perinatol Neonatol.* 1984;8:70-74.

62. Schutzman DL, Hervada AR, Branca PA. Effect of water supplementation of full-term newborns on arrival of milk in the nursing mother. *Clin Pediatr.* 1986;25(2): 78-80.

63. Perez-Escamilla R, Pollitt E, Lonnerdal B, Dewey K. Infant feeding policies in maternity wards and their effect on breast-feeding success: an analytical overview. *Am J Public Health.* 1994;84(1):89-97.

64. Frank DA, Wirtx SJ, Sorenson JR, Heeren T. Commercial discharge packs and breast-feeding counseling: effects on infant-feeding practices in a randomized trial. *Pediatr.* 1987;80(6):845-854.

65. Reiff MI, Essock-Vitale SM. Hospital influences on early infant-feeding practices. *Pediatr.* 1985;76: 872-879.

66. Arvedson J, Brodsky L. *Pediatric Swallowing and Feeding.* San Diego, CA: Singular Pub Group Inc; 1993.

67. Wolf LS, Glass RP. *Feeding and Swallowing Disorders in Infancy: Assessment and Management.* Therapy Skill Builders; 1992.

68. Mulford C. The mother-baby assessment (MBA): an "Apgar score" for breast-feeding." *J Human Lact.* 1992;8: 79-82.

69. De Carvalho M, Robertson S, Friedman A, Klaus M. Effect of frequent breast-feeding on early milk production and infant weight gain. *Pediatr.* 1983;72:307-331.

70. Michaelsen KF, Larsen PS, Thomsen BL, Samuelson G. The Copenhagen cohort study on infant nutrition and growth: duration of breast feeding and influencing factors. *Acta Paediatr.* 1994;83:565-571.

71. Daly SJ, DiRosso A, Owens RA, Hatmann PE. Degree of breast emptying explains changes in the fat content, but not fatty acid composition, of human milk. *Exper Physiol.* 1993;78:741-755.

72. Dewey KG, Heinig MJ, Nommsen LA, Lonnerdal B. Maternal versus infant factors related to breast milk intake and residual milk volume: the DARLING study. *Peadiatr.* 1991;87(6):829-837.

73. Dewey KG, Heinig MJ, Nommsen LA, Peerson JM, Lonnerdal B. Breast-fed infants are leaner than formula-fed infants at 1 yr of age: the DARLING study. *Am J Clin Nutr.* 1993;57(2):140-145.

74. Newman J. Breast-feeding: The problem of "not enough milk." *Can Fam Phys.* 1986;32:571-574.

75. Martin J. *Infant Feeding 1975: Attitudes and Practice in England and Wales.* London: Office of Population Censuses and Surveys, Social Survey Division, Her Majesty's Stationery Office; 1978.

76. Alexander R. Developing pre-speech and feeding abilities in children. In: Shanks S, ed. *Nursing and the Management of Pediatric Communication Disorders.* Waltham, MA: College-Hill Press/Little Brown & Co; 1983.

77. Davis LF. Respiration and phonation in cerebral palsy: a developmental model. *Seminars in Speech and Language.* 1987;8(1):101-106.

78. Devlieger H, Daniels H, Marchal G, Moerman P, Casaer P, Eggermont E. The diaphragm of the newborn infant: anatomical and ultrasonographic studies. *J Dev Physiol.* 1991;16(6):321-329.

79. Smith WL, Erenberg A, Nowak A. Imaging evaluation of the human nipple during breast-feeding. *Am J Dis Child.* 1988;142:76-84.

80. Smith WL, Erenberg A, Nowak A. Physiology of sucking in the normal term infant using real-time U.S. *Radiol.* 1985;156:379.

81. Bowen-Jones A, Thompson C, Drewett RF. Milk flow and sucking rates during breast-feeding. *Dev Med Child Neurol.* 1982;24:626-633.

82. Woolridge MW, How TV, Drewett RF, Rolfe P, Baum JD. The continuous measurement of milk intake at a feed in breast-fed babies. *Early Hum Dev.* 1982;6: 365-373.

83. Drewett RF, Woolridge M. Sucking patterns of human babies on the breast. *Early Hum Dev.* 1979;3/4:315-320.

84. Slaven S, Harvey D. Unlimited suckling time improves breast feeding. *Lancet.* 1981;1(8216):392-393.

85. Woolridge MW, Baum JD, Drewett RF. Individual patterns of milk intake during breast-feeding. *Early Hum Dev.* 1982;7:265-272.

86. Lucas A, Lucas PJ, Baum JD. Pattern of milk flow in breast-fed infants. *Lancet.* 1979;298(133):57-58.

87. Samuels SE, Margen S, Schoen EJ. Incidence and duration of breast-feeding in a health maintenance organization population. *Am J Clin Nutr.* 1985;42:504-510.

88. Frantz KB. An easy solution to an early problem. In: Freier S, Eidelman AI, eds. *Human Milk, Its Biological and Social Value.* Amsterdam: Excerpta Medica; 1980.

89. Christensen S, Dubignon J, Campbell D. Variations in intraoral stimulation and nutritive sucking. *Child Dev.* 1976;47:539-542.

90. Dubignon J, Campbell D. Intraoral stimulation and sucking in the newborn. *J Exp Child Psychol.* 1968;6:154-166.

91. Podratz RO, Broughton DD, Gustafson DH, Bergstralh EJ, Melton LJ. Weight loss and body temperature changes in breast-fed and bottle-fed neonates. *Clin Pediatr.* 1986;25(2):73-77.

92. Nikodem VC, Danziger D, Gebka N, Gulmezoglu AM, Hofmeyr GJ. Do cabbage leaves prevent breast engorgement? a randomized, controlled study. *Birth.* 1993;20(2);61-64.

93. Roberts KL. A comparison of chilled cabbage leaves and chilled gelpaks in reducing breast engorgement. *J Hum Lact.* 1995;11(1):17-20.

94. Yamouchi Y, Yamanouchi I. Breast-feeding frequency during the first 24 hours after birth in full-term neonates. *Pediatr.* 1990;86(2):171-175.

95. Butte NF, Garza C, Smith EO, Nichols BL. Human milk intake and growth in exclusively breast-fed infants. *J Pediatr.* 1984;104:187-195.

96. Butte NF, Wills C, Jean CA, et al. Feeding patterns of exclusively breast-fed infants during the first four months of life. *Early Hum Dev.* 1985;12:291-300.

97. Delvoye P, Demaegd M, Delogne-Desnoeck J, Robyn C. The influence of the frequency of nursing and of previous lactation experience on serum prolactin in lactating mothers. *J Biosoc Sci.* 1977;9:447-451.

98. Hopkinson JM, Schanler RJ, Garza C. Milk production by mothers of premature infants. *Pediatr.* 1988;81(6):815-820.

99. De Carvalho M, Anderson DM, Giangreco A, Pittard WB. Frequency of milk expression and milk production by mothers of nonnursing premature neonates. *Am J Dis Child.* 1985;139:483-485.

100. Woolridge MW, Ingram JC, Baum JD. Do changes in pattern of breast usage alter the baby's nutrient intake? *Lancet.* 1990;336:395-397.

101. De Carvalho M, Klaus MH, Merkatz RB. Frequency of breast-feeding and serum bilirubin concentration. *Am J Dis Child.* 1982;136:737-738.

102. Varimo P, Simila S, Wendt L, Kolvisto M. Frequency of breast-feeding and hyperbilirubinemia. *Clin Pediatr.* 1986; 25:112.

103. Maisels MJ, Vain N, Acquavita AM, deBlanco NV, Cohen A, DiGregorio J. The effect of breast-feeding frequency on serum bilirubin levels. *Am J Obstet Gynecol.* 1994;170:880-883.

104. De Carvalho M, Hall M, Harvey D. Effects of water supplementation on physiological jaundice in breast-fed babies. *Arch Dis Child.* 1981;56:568-569.

105. Nicoll A, Ginsburg R, Tripp JH. Supplementary feeding and jaundice in the newborn. *Acta Paediatr Scand.* 1982; 71:759-761.

106. Gartner LM, Lee K, Moscioni AD. Effect of milk feeding on intestinal bilirubin absorption in the rat. *J Pediatr.* 1983;103:464-471.

107. Lascari AD. "Early" breast-feeding jaundice: clinical significance. *J Pediatr.* 1986;108:156-158.

108. Sievers E, Oldigs H-D, Schulz-Lell G, Schaub J. Faecal excretion in infants. *Eur J Pediatr.* 1993;152:452-454.

109. Quinlan PT, Locton S, Irwin J, Lucas AL. The relationship between stool hardness and stool composition in breast and formula-fed infants. *J Pediatr Gastro Nutr.* 1995;20:81-90.

110. Weaver LT, Ewing G, Taylor LC. The bowel habit of milk-fed infants. *J Pediatr Gastro Nutr.* 1988;7:568-571.

111. Elias MF, Nicolson NA, Bora C, Johnston J. Sleep/wake patterns of breast-fed infants in the first two years of life. *Pediatr.* 1986;77:322-329.

112. Pinilla T, Birch LL. Help me make it through the night: Behavioral entrainment of breast-fed infants' sleep patterns. *Pediatr.* 1993;91:436-444.

113. Heinig MJ, Nommsen LA, Peerson JM, Lonnerdal B, Dewey KG. Intake and growth of breast-fed and

formula-fed infants in relation to the timing of introduction of complementary foods: the DARLING study. *Acta Paediatr.* 1993;82:999-1006.

114. Stuff JE, Nichols BL. Nutrient intake and growth performance of older infants fed human milk. *J Pediatr.* 1989;115(6):959-968.

115. Marshall BR, Heppler JK, Zirbel CC. Sporadic puerperal mastitis, an infection that need not interrupt lactation. *JAMA.* 1975;233:1377-1379.

116. Willis C, Livingstone VH. Infant insufficient milk syndrome associated with maternal postpartum hemorrhage. *J Hum Lact.* 1995;11:123-126.

117. Lindbland BS, Ljungquist A, Gebre-Medhin M, Rahimtoola RJ. The composition and yield of human milk in developing countries. In: Hambraeus L, Hanson LA, McFarlane H, eds. *Food and Immunology: Symposium of the Swedish Nutrition Foundation XIII.* Uppsala, Sweden: Almquist & Wiksell; 1877:125.

118. Feher SD, Berger LR, Johnson JD, Wilde JB. Increasing breast milk production for premature infants with a relaxation/imagery audiotape. *Pediatr.* 1989;83:57-60.

119. Hino S. Milk-borne transmission of HTLV-1 as a major route in the endemic cycle. *Acta Paediatr Jpn.* 1989;31:428-435.

120. CDC (Centers for Disease Control). Recommendations for assisting in the prevention of perinatal transmission of human T-lymphotropic virus type III/lympha-denopathy-associated virus and acquired immunodeficiency syndrome. *Morib Mortal Wkly Rep.* 1985;34:721-732.

121. Ho-Hsiung L, Kao J-H, Hsu H-Y, Ni Y-H, Chang M-H, Huang S-C, Hwang L-H, Chen P-J, Chen D-S. Absence of infection in breast-fed infants born to hepatitis C virus-infected mothers. *J Pediatr.* 1955;126(4):589-591.

122. WHO (World Health Organization). Breast-feeding/breast milk and human immunodeficiency virus (HIV). *Weekly Epidemiol Rec.* 1987;62:245-246.

123. World Health Organization/UNICEF. Guidelines concerning the main health and socioeconomic circumstances in which infants have to be fed on breastmilk substitutes. WHO: April 10, 1986. A39/8 ADD. 1.

124. Ernest AE, McCabe ERB, Neifert MR, et al. *Guide to breast feeding the infant with PKU.* Washington, DC: US Government Printing Office; 1980.

125. American Academy of Pediatrics, Committee on Infectious Disease. *Report of the Committee*, 22nd ed. Elk Grove Village, IL: 1991.

126. World Health Organization/UNICEF Consensus statement from the WHO/UNICEF consultation on HIV transmission and breast-feeding. Geneva: April 30-May 1, 1992.

127. Quinn PT, Lofberg JV. Maternal herpetic breast infection: another hazard of neonatal herpes simplex. *Med J Aust.* 1978;2:411.

128. American Academy of Pediatrics Committee on Drugs: The transfer of drugs and other chemicals into human milk. *Pediatr.* 1994;93:137-150.

129. Harding LK, Bossuyt A, Pellet S, Reiners C, Talbot JN. Recommendations for nuclear medicine physicians regarding breast-feeding mothers. *Eur J Nucl Med.* 1995;22(5):BP17.

130. Briggs GG, Freeman RK, Yaffe SJ. *Drugs in Pregnancy and Lactation: A Reference Guide to Fetal and Neonatal Risk.* Fourth Edition. Baltimore, MD: Williams and Wilkins; 1994:975.

131. Rogan WJ, Gladen BC, McKinney JD, Carreras N, Hardy P, Thullen J, Tingelstad J, Tully M. Polychlorinated biphenyls (PCBs) and dichorodiphenyl dichloroethene (DDE) in human milk: effects on growth, morbidity, and duration of lactation. *AJPH.* 1987;77(10):1294-1297.

132. Nehlig A, Debry G. Consequences on the Newborn of Chronic Maternal Consumption of Coffee during Gestation and Lactation: A Review. *J Am Col Nutr.* 1994;13(1):6-21.

133. Cobo E. Effect of different doses of ethanol on the milk ejecting reflex in lactating women. *Am J Obstet Gynecol.* 1973;115:817-819.

134. Mennella JA, Beauchamp GK. Beer, Breast Feeding, and Folklore. *Dev Phsychobiology.* 1993;26(8):459-466.

135. Luck W, Nau H. Nicotine and cotine concentrations in the milk of smoking mothers: influence of cigarette consumption and diurnal variation. *Eur J Pediatr.* 1987;146:21-26.

136. Hopkinson JM, Schanler R, Fraley K, Garza C. Milk production by mothers of premature infants: influence of cigarette smoking. *Pediatr.* 1992;90:934-938.

137. Vio F, Salazar G, Infante C. Smoking during pregnancy

and lactation and its effects on breast-milk volume. *Am J Clin Nutr.* 1991;54:1011-1016.

138. Counsilman JJ, Mackay EV. Cigarette smoking by pregnant women with particular reference to their past and subsequent breast feeding behavior. *Aust NZ J Obstet Gynaecol.* 1985;25:101-107.

139. Little RE, Lambert MD, Worthington-Roberts B, Ervin CH. Maternal smoking during lactation: relation to infant size at one year of age. *Am J Epidemiol.* 1994;140: 544-554.

140. Schmidt E, Wittreich G. *Care of the abnormal newborn.* A random controlled trial study of the "Kangaroo method of care for low-birth-weight newborns." Paper presented at the Euro-Amer Symposium on Appropriate Technology Following Birth. Trieste; October 7-11, 1986.

141. Whitelaw A, Heisterkamp G, Sleath K, Acolet D, Richards M. Skin-to-skin contact for very low birth weight infants and their mothers: A randomized trial of "kangaroo care." *Arch Dis Child.* 1988;63:1377-1381.

142. Whitelaw A. Kangaroo baby care: just a nice experience or an important advance for preterm infants? *Pediatr.* 1990;85(4):604-605.

143. Ludington-Hoe SM, Hadeed AJ, Anderson GC. Physiologic responses to skin-to-skin contact in hospitalized premature infants. *J Perinatol.* 1990;11(1):19-24.

144. Bowen-Jones A, Thomas C, Drewett RF. Milk flow and sucking rates during breast-feeding. *Dev Med Child Neurol.* 1982;24:626-633.

145. Pearce JL, Buchanan LF. Breast milk and breast feeding in very low birthweight infants. *Arch Dis Child.* 1979;54: 897-899.

146. Rey ES, Martinez HG. *Rational management of the premature infant.* Paper presented at the First Course of Fetal and Meonatal Medicine. Bogota, Colombia: March 17-19, 1983.

147. Bosque EM, Brady JP, Affonso DD, Wahlberg V. Continuous physiologic measures of Kangaroo versus incubator care in a tertiary level nursery. *Pediatr Res.* 1988;23(4, part 2):402A(Abstract 1204).

148. Anderson GC. Current knowledge about skin-to-skin (kangaroo) care for preterm infants. *J Perinatol.* 1991; 11(3):216-226.

149. Arnold LD, Tully MR. *Guidelines for the establishment and operation of a human milk bank.* West Hartford, CT: Human Milk Banking Association of North America Inc; 1994.

150. Arnold LD, Tully MR. *Recommendations for collection, storage, and handling of a mother's milk for her own infant in the hospital setting.* West Hartford, CT: Human Milk Banking Association of North America Inc; 1993.

151. Goldblum, RM, Garza C, Johnson CA, Nichols BL, Goldman AS. Human Milk Banking II. Relative stability of immunologic factors in stored colostrum. *Acta Paediatr Scand.* 1982;71:143-152.

152. Pardou A, Serruys E, Mascartlemone F, Dramaix M, Vis HL. Human milk banking: Influence of storage processes and of bacterial contamination an some milk constituents. *Biol Neonate.* 1994;65(5):302-309.

153. Van Zoeren-Grobben D, Moison RMW, Ester WM, Berger HM. Lipid peroxidation in human milk and infant formula-effect of storage, tube feeding and exposure to phototherapy. *Acta Paediatr.* 1993;82(8): 645-649.

154. Quan R, Yang C, Rubinstein S, Lewiston NJ, Sunshine P, Stevenson D, Kerner JA. Effects of microwave radiation on anti-infective factors in human milk. *Pediatr.* 1992; 89:667-669.

Weaning - Transition to the Table

Sandra J. Bartholmey Ph.D.

Manager of Nutrition Science, Research and Development,
Gerber Products Company,
Fremont, Michigan

Reviewed by Judy Hopkinson Ph.D., Nancy F. Butte Ph.D. and Janice E. Stuff M.S.R.D.

Weaning

What is weaning? the transition from exclusive milk feeding to the foods of one's culture

Why to wean? to maintain normal infant growth and development, to introduce the infant to family society and to the foods of the family's culture

When to wean? when the infant is developmentally ready and when it is safe to do so

How to wean? with safe, hygienic foods of appropriate nutrient density and variety, with texture and consistency appropriate to the infant's feeding skills

Introduction

"The definition of weaning is cloudy, optimal measurements for success are unknown, and outcome...occurs in the distant future."

"Empirically, {in an ideal world} it is anticipated that wide variations would be noted, and almost any regimen would be found to be appropriate."

Lewis A. Barness, 1990

The human race survives and thrives on widely diverse foods and varied times of introduction during the weaning period (Table 1).[2, 3] The human infant, a marvel of adaptation, thrives best on exclusive breast-feeding in the first months of life. But necessity and experience show us that infants survive and even thrive amidst a wide range of circumstances during the crucial first year of life. For example, we tolerate and grow on the milk of other mammals. Foods can be introduced early or late during the first year with enormous impact on health, growth and development, depending on the quality of the foods[4] and the level of sanitation and hygiene in the environment.[5, 6]

According to cultural practice and the availability of caregivers, infants may be fed "on demand," every four hours, or only two or three times a day. Infants are weaned in a social context, too. Initially, they are totally influenced by intimate contact with the mother during suckling. Later on, other family members and caregivers serve as models for eating behavior, food acceptance and preferences. Infants slowly assume the culture's "rules of cuisine." The dynamic of the infant's environment affects the weaning process.[7]

The cultural setting of infant feeding practices has a direct effect on the health status of the growing child[8] and, therefore, great relevance to the timing of weaning. Accessibility to safe, wholesome, nutritious weaning foods prepared in an hygienic environment enhances the benefits of weaning.[9, 10] The risks of an adverse effect of weaning are increased[11] in situations where appropriate weaning foods are not available, or where basic hygiene and sanitary food preparation are not practiced. Within increasingly heterogeneous societies, as in the U.S., England, Germany and Australia, more than one cultural setting is the norm, as recent arrivals continue their traditional weaning practices within a new homeland. Health care professionals must meet the challenge of understanding and accommodating these differing cultural practices and beliefs to provide the best care for their patients.

Considering the wide variations in weaning practices around the world and within each country, we can ask the following questions: How do we define weaning? Is there one "best" weaning recommendation for all infants? What criteria can we use to assess when an infant is ready for weaning? Which criteria take precedence when evalu-

Trends in Complementary Infant Feeding Practices		
Country	Age of Introduction of Complementary Foods	First Complementary Foods Offered
Austria	3 months	fruits, vegetables
Belgium	4 months	cereals, fruits
Caribbean	before 3 months	malted milk drink, fruit juices, commercial cereal
Finland	3 months	vegetables
France	2-3 months	cereals, fruit
Germany	3-4 months	meats, vegetables
Greece	2-3 months	fruits
Hungary	2-3 months	fruits
India	3 months	commercial cereal
Ireland	3-4 months	cereals, fruits
Italy	3 months	cereals, fruits
Kenya	1-3 months	sorghum, millet or maize gruel, commercial cereal
Malaysia	before 3 months	commercial cereal
Mexico	2-3 months	cereal, soup-soaked tortilla
Netherlands	4-5 months	fruits
Nigeria	by 6 months	maize or sorghum pap
Norway	5 months	vegetables
Poland	3 months	fruits, cereals
Spain	3-4 months	cereals, fruits
Sweden	3 months	vegetables
Switzerland	3-4 months	fruits, vegetables
Turkey	6 months	cereals, fruits
United Kingdom	4 months	cereals
Zaire	before 3 months up to 6 months	starchy gruel

Adapted from Ballabriga A, Schmidt E. Actual trends of the diversification of infant feeding in industrialized countries in Europe. In Weaning: Why, What, and When? (Ballabriga A, Rey J, eds.). Nestlé Nutrition Workshop Series, Volume 10. Nestlé Nutrition, Vevey. Raven Press, New York. 1987. pp.129-153 and King J, Ashworth A. Contemporary feeding practices in infancy and early childhood in developing countries. In Infant and Child Nutrition Worldwide: Issues and Perspectives. (Falkner F. ed.). CRC Press, Boca Raton, Fl. 1991. pp.141-174.

Table 1: Trends in complementary infant feeding practices.

ating when an infant in a particular environment should be weaned? This chapter will look at the interplay of factors that affect weaning: the nutritional, developmental, and social environments of the infant; health and safety issues; and cultural practices. The weight placed on each of these factors will vary depending on the environment.

Infants are born and survive in every environment known to man – from Tierra del Fuego, Argentina, to Hammerfest, Norway. This perspective may help explain why weaning practices and recommendations often differ; it may also guide our thinking on how to evaluate and accommodate the differences.

Definitions of Weaning

Wean - "1. to accustom (a child or young animal) to the loss of its mother's milk…"

Oxford English Dictionary, 1971[12]

Every child must make the transition from suckling to eating a varied diet of semi-solid and solid foods. How and when this transition occurs is controlled by cultural beliefs and practices, including those of the medical community, mothers' perceptions of their babies' needs, and mothers' ability and willingness to respond to those perceived needs. In the U.S. and other industrialized countries, the total transition to family foods usually occurs at the end of the first year and continues during the second year of life.

Although the weaning period is strictly defined as the time when any food other than human milk is introduced in the infant diet, in practice, weaning can describe three patterns. The first is the transition from human milk to other forms of milk, such as infant formulas or other milks. Formula or other milk feeds may replace breast-feedings partially or entirely. In the latter case, the infant is considered weaned from the breast.

A second definition of weaning is the transition from a liquid, total milk diet, whether human milk or formula, to a diet that includes complementary semi-solid or solid foods. Human milk or formula continues to supply the major source of nutrients to the infant. The added foods complement (add to) and supplement (begin to replace) the liquid diet in three major ways: 1) to provide additional energy and nutrients to meet the growing needs of the infant, 2) as a means of

teaching the infant to chew and swallow foods of varied consistency and texture, and 3) to introduce the tastes and flavors enjoyed by family members, or, in other words, the "rules of cuisine."

The third definition of weaning is that of weaning from the milk used in infancy, be it human milk or infant formula. Complementary foods or family foods are already part of the infant diet when this form of weaning occurs. Weaning from human milk or formula may occur as early as six to eight months of age, if cow milk is introduced and totally replaces human milk or formula.[13, 14, 15] This practice has led to a resurgence in iron deficiency anemia, however, and is not recommended.[16] Weaning from human milk may not occur until the second or third year, as is common in some non-industrialized countries.[17, 18]

Weaning usually occurs during a period of rapid growth. Negotiating this transition during the rapid growth of infancy would seem risky, but the vast majority of children, at least in industrialized countries, successfully negotiate the transition despite enormous dietary change.[7] Even under less than optimal conditions, infants can continue to grow and develop, albeit at a sub optimal rate, unless the conditions are very severe.[19]

It is the pattern of gradual weaning from milk as the sole source of nourishment to foods of the culture that most commonly defines the weaning period[20] and it is this definition that will be considered in this chapter.

Role of Complementary Foods

There is evidence that a diet high in variety from infancy will result in the development of food preferences favoring a more diverse and nutrient-rich diet in adulthood.

Paul Rozin, 1990[21]

Complementary or weaning foods have several roles – from meeting nutritional needs to challenging developmental abilities and educating infants' tastes for the gastronomic delights and cultural eating patterns of their families. Introducing complementary foods should not, however, be an early vector for introducing disease; safe, hygienic preparation of suitable foods for all infants is a primary concern.

Human milk defines the standards for infant feeding. Its dynamic and complex nature make human milk the best sole source of nutrition for infants during the first

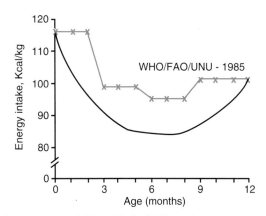

Adapted from *Journal of Human Nutrition* (1981) 35, 339-348.

Figure 1: A comparison of smoothed actual intake data (quadratic regression) and theoretical energy requirements developed by WHO/FAO/UNU in 1985.

months of life and longer, in areas where problems with sanitation and hygiene present health hazards in the preparation of alternative milks and complementary foods.[11, 22] Human milk continues as the best milk source throughout the weaning period and as long as breast-feeding suits the mother and baby.

Nutritional Benefits

Ideally, complementary foods supply nutrients that may be low in human milk but needed in increasing amounts by the rapidly growing infant. These foods should be of appropriate texture and consistency so as to help the infant safely master new feeding skills and to learn to accept the tastes of a variety of foods.

Weaning to complementary foods is a process that does not mean the end of breast-feeding. As the weaning process begins, foods introduced to the infant can assure that nutritional needs are met while the infant continues to enjoy the benefits of breast-feeding or, if breast-feeding is not possible, of infant formula.

Provide Nutrients Limiting in Liquid Diet

The nutrients that have been proposed as eventually limiting to infant growth in the exclusive milk diet are energy, protein, iron, and zinc. When these additional nutrients are needed is the focal point of long-standing and lively debate.

The Energy Issue

Assuring adequate energy intake is of primary concern because we assume that if infants satisfy their energy needs from nutrient-replete foods, nutrient intake, in general, will likely be adequate. In non-industrialized countries where food availability is marginal and mothers may be under-nourished, the risk of malnutrition and growth faltering during the first year is far greater than in developed countries.[23] In industrialized countries, infants are more likely to have access to milk of well-nourished mothers or to hygienically-prepared infant formulas. In both circumstances, energy requirements of infants have been re-examined primarily because of two observations: 1) breast-fed infants consistently consume less energy than formula-fed infants in the first six months and generally do not meet recommended theoretic energy intakes after the first month;[24, 25, 26, 27] and 2) infants regulate their food intakes in an attempt to meet their energy needs.[28] Consequently, a decrease in milk consumption often occurs when complementary foods are introduced.[9, 25, 26] Each of these observations will be examined separately.

Energy Intake of Breast-fed Babies

When measured on a body weight basis, daily milk intake of breast-fed infants declines from just more than 100 kilocalories per kilogram body weight at one month of age to less than 90 kcal/kg/d at four months.[26] These intakes are less than the recommended energy intake of 116 kcal/kg/d for infants zero to three months of age and the 99 kcal/kg/d recommended for infants three to six months of age.[26, 29] Formula-fed infants have a greater growth velocity in the third to fourth month than breast-fed infants.[30, 31] The question is: are formula-fed infants overweight, or are breast-fed infants faltering?

The energy issue generated an explosion of research on the question of what constitutes normal infant growth and the differences between breast-fed and formula-fed infants in energy utilization and growth. This issue is summarized in Whitehead's review[32] and is briefly summarized here.

Partial clarification of the discrepancies observed between recommended energy intake and actual intakes of young infants came from an analysis of energy intake data compiled by Whitehead, Paul and

Cole;[33] this was validated by analysis of energy expenditure data obtained by direct measurement.[34] When the energy expenditure data were adjusted to include a factor for energy content of new tissue, the new data formed the basis for revising estimates of daily energy requirements downward and closer to actual intakes (Figure 1), from a high of 115 kcal/kg/d at one month to approximately 95 kcal/kg/d at four months and 85 kcal/kg/d at six months.[32] Although these requirements are more realistic, actual measurements of the energy intake of exclusively breast-fed infants vary considerably around these estimates, depending on methods used to assess milk intake and energy content of human milk.[35] These estimates are still higher than reported energy intakes of breast-fed infants.[36] Formula-fed infants also may not attain recommended energy intakes and reference growth rates,[37] which supports the idea that reference standards for energy intake may be exaggerated.

A 1996 review of energy requirements[38] suggests that estimated energy requirements of infants based on total energy expenditure and growth are 9 to 39% lower than the 1985 FAO/WHO/UNU recommendations, and that energy requirements of breast-fed infants may be lower than those of formula-fed infants.

Revised estimates of energy requirements have not been adopted as recommendations, however, because recommendations are often used prescriptively and as a guide to how much food children should be given at different stages during infancy.[32] As such, the recommendations do not address the variability of energy intake of exclusively breast-fed infants in the first six months of life.[39] Research continues on why and how energy intakes and expenditure differ between human milk-fed and formula-fed infants,[40] how growth rates vary among infants,[41] for how long human milk alone can support "normal" growth, and when complementary or supplementary feeding should begin.[9, 42]

Regulation of Energy Intake and Introduction of Complementary Foods

In considering when complementary feeding should begin, it is worth noting that after about six weeks of age, young infants are able to regulate food intake to meet their energy needs.[43] When weaning foods are

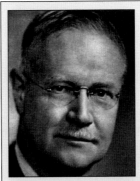

Frederick F. Tisdall M.D. (1893-1949) trained in pediatric research under Howland. He returned to the Hospital for Sick Children (HSC), Toronto, where he continued to study rickets and "metabolism studies to determine the utilization of various food components in chronic intestinal indigestion." Tisdall reported that an acidosis due in part to decrease in total fixed base through loss of alkaline secretions may occur in severe diarrhea. He became convinced of the importance of prevention of nutrient deficiencies and developed a fortified cereal, Pablum, for weaning infants. He wrote, "the normal infant should be weaned some time between the eighth and ninth month." He lead the program to rebuild the HSC and the hospital research laboratories are named in his memory. Pediatric Profiles editor B. S. Veeder, Mosby St. Louis, 1957, 244-246 (Photo courtesy of HSC)

added to the infant diet before six months, infants tend to consume less human milk or formula to compensate for the additional energy intake rather than increase their caloric intake.[9, 25, 26] Although average milk intake tends to increase during the first four months, decreases in total milk intake/24 hours between two and four months of age were also observed in healthy, full-term breast-fed infants receiving no complementary foods.[39] For an individual infant, energy needs are almost totally unpredictable.[44] Infant growth rate remains the best indicator of adequate nutrient intake. Deviations from a characteristic trajectory should signal counseling of the mother on intervention strategies.

Nutrients Other Than Energy

If infants do not need extra energy, why add additional foods? The answer lies in the complex nature of the weaning process itself and in the multitude of factors that determine when an individual infant will start the weaning process. Is energy the only reason to give additional foods? Nutrients other than energy, factors other than nutritional need, and what the mother can and will provide are part of the total weaning picture and need to be considered in answering this question.

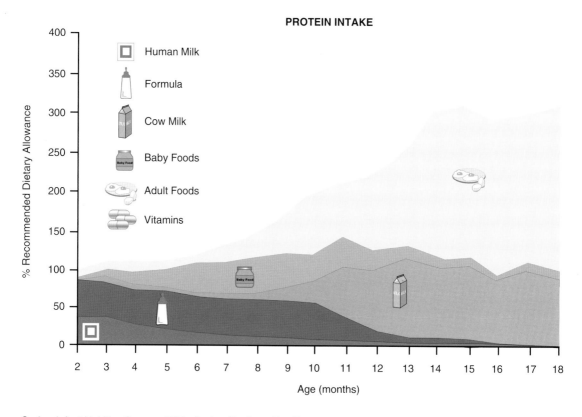

Gerber Infant Nutrition Survey, 1994. Gerber Products Co., Fremont, MI
National Research Council 1989 RDA for Protein: 0-5 mos., 2.2 g/kg body weight; 6-11 mos., 1.6 g/kg body weight;
1-3 yrs., 1.2 g/kg body weight

Figure 2: Protein intake of U.S. infants 2 to 18 months of age by food source.

As lactation progresses, nutrient content of human milk tends to decline.[45, 46] Even though the infant's total intake of human milk increases, he may not be able to consume a large enough volume of milk to maintain robust growth. The nutrients that first become limiting and of concern, particularly for the breast-fed infant and eventually for the formula-fed infant, are protein, iron and zinc.

Protein

In the U.S., the milks of infancy meet the infant's requirements for protein in the first six months and continue to meet most of the protein requirements in the second six months, even as protein-rich foods are slowly added to the infant diet (Figure 2).[47, 48] The average breast-fed infant receives approximately 1.0[39] to 1.5 grams of protein per kilogram of body weight

per day, and the formula-fed infant receives a generous 2.2 grams of protein/kg/d.[1] Within this range of protein intake, growth is equally satisfactory for both human milk-fed and formula-fed infants, and other protein-rich foods are seldom needed in the first six months. Weaning foods are traditionally carbohydrate-rich foods – grains, fruits and vegetables – which provide small amounts of protein. Protein intake becomes limiting in the second six months for the breast-fed infant[49] and for any infant for whom milk intake is limited; therefore, protein-rich weaning foods assume more importance in the infant diet after the first six months.[50]

A recent review of protein requirements of infants and children[42] suggests that protein requirements for infants may be 27 to 35% lower than the 1985 FAO/WHO/UNU recommendations. Estimates of protein

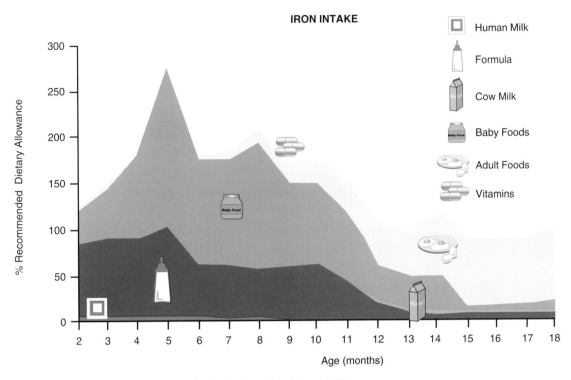

Gerber Infant Nutrition Survey, 1994. Gerber Products Co., Fremont, MI
National Research Council 1989 RDA for Iron: 0-5 mos., 6 mg; 6-11 mos., 10 mg; 1-3 yrs., 10 mg

Figure 3: Iron intake (% RDA) of U.S. infants 2 to 18 months of age by food source.

intake for the first six months of life for exclusively breast-fed infants were also reported to be 10 to 26% lower than intake data presented in the 1985 report. The reviewers recommended that the 1985 requirements be reconsidered.

Iron

Human milk contains low levels of highly bioavailable iron[51] and supplies adequate iron during the early months when neonatal iron stores are being mobilized. Some infants exclusively breast-fed after six months appear to adapt to low iron intakes,[52] but iron supplementation is recommended for the breast-fed infant between four and six months of age.[53]

For all infants, the concern about sufficient iron intake in the first year is to prevent iron deficiency anemia, the most prevalent nutrient deficiency in children throughout the world.[54] Iron deficiency anemia is less common in infants and young children in the U.S., its prevalence having decreased in the last two decades

from 9 to 3%.[55, 56] Infants in the lower socioeconomic groups have benefited most from the iron-fortified infant formulas and infant cereals provided as part of the U.S.D.A. Supplemental Food Program for Women, Infants and Children (WIC).[57] Dietary iron is needed to replace normal losses, support the rapid metabolism and growth typical of the first year, and maintain adequate iron stores through the second year. The risk of not receiving adequate iron throughout the first year is documented in slowed growth[58] and the long-term cognitive and psychomotor deficits that are associated with iron deficiency anemia during infancy.[59, 60]

To prevent depleted iron stores and iron deficiency anemia from occurring in the second six months, most U.S. pediatricians recommend iron supplementation of 1.0 mg/kg/day or dietary iron from iron-fortified infant cereal[61] or meat[55] for all term infants from four months of age. In the U.S., human milk and iron-fortified infant formula are the only acceptable milks during the first year; and infant cereals are recom-

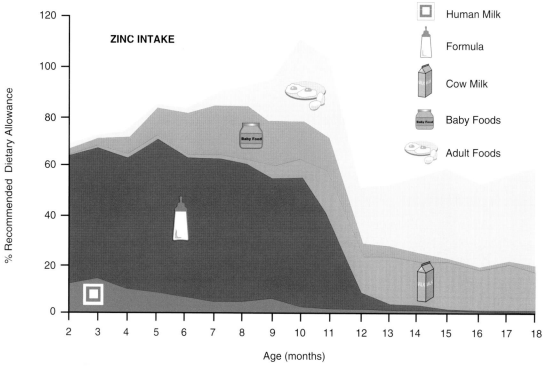

Gerber Infant Nutrition Survey, 1994. Gerber Products Co., Fremont, MI
National Research Council 1989 RDA for Zinc: 0-11 mos., 5 mg; 1-3 yrs., 10 mg

Figure 4: Zinc intake (% RDA) of U.S. infants 2 to 18 months of age by food source. The drop in % RDA for zinc intake at 12 months occurs because the RDA for zinc doubles at one year of age but zinc intake does not double.

mended for the first two years[62] as a useful source of bioavailable iron to prevent anemia[63] (Figure 3).[41]

Zinc

Similar to iron, zinc in human milk is highly bioavailable, but the low zinc content of milk in later lactation[45, 46] and in weaning foods[64] has generated concern for when zinc may be a limiting nutrient for infants.[64, 65, 66] Zinc supplementation trials suggest that the decreased growth velocity of breast-fed infants in early infancy may be due to inadequate zinc intake or to poor bioavailability of zinc from unfortified weaning foods.[64, 67, 68]

According to a U.S. survey of infant dietary intake, about 22% of infants six to 12 months of age receive less than two-thirds the RDA for zinc. Approximately 74% of children one to two years of age fail to receive adequate zinc (Figures 4 and 5).[47] In countries where

food availability is not an issue, meats are an excellent source of bioavailable zinc, and some infant cereals in the U.S. are now fortified with bioavailable zinc. In areas of the world where unfortified grains and legumes make up the majority of the weaning diet, human milk continues to be the best source of bioavailable zinc for the infant.

Accommodate Patterns of Growth

"Human growth may reflect an example of mathematical chaos."
"Growth...occurs in a pattern of bursts punctuated by periods of stasis that is unique for each child."

Michelle Lampl, 1995[41]

New research into infant growth patterns sheds some light on possible reasons for the well-documented variability in patterns of growth and development of chil-

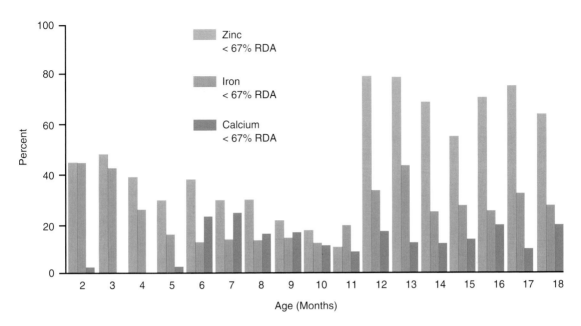

Gerber Infant Nutrition Survey, 1994. Gerber Products Co., Fremont, MI

Figure 5: Percent of infants not meeting ⅔ of the National Research Council 1989 Recommended Dietary Allowances (RDA) for zinc, iron and calcium by age.

dren in different parts of the world. "Saltatory" growth, described by measurements of infants and children taken at daily and weekly intervals, documents that the periods of rapid growth are characterized by rapid bursts of incremental growth in length interspersed with intervals of stasis or no growth (Figure 6).[69] Examples of the individualized nature of growth are shown in Figure 7 in the patterns of growth spurts of three infants.[41, 69] This explains growth as a unique series of episodes distinctive in both amplitude and timing that accord with each child's genetic potential and environmental circumstance. The timing of these events and the amount of growth at each event determine each child's growth velocity. Such an individualized basis of growth velocity favors an individualized approach to infant feeding.

Based on Lampl's observations, the growth spurts are preceded by changes in behaviors that mothers interpret as signals to begin complementary or supplementary feeding[70] – "frenzy eating" (the infant demands to eat more frequently and vigorously), crankiness, fussiness and decreased time sleeping. Following the growth spurts, feeding patterns return to

normal and sleeping time increases. Parents in Lampl's studies also observed that their infants achieved new developmental milestones at the conclusion of each growth spurt. New plateaus of neuromuscular coordination, cognitive abilities and social skills were reported to occur after a growth spurt. That the pattern of growth spurts of an individual infant may be the organizing principle that directs the timing of an infant's development, and thus the timing of weaning, is an intriguing hypothesis that is consistent with observations in developmental biology.[71]

Developmental Biology - the Chicken or the Egg

The physiological, neurological and morphological adaptations exhibited by the weanling human infant can be viewed as characteristics that can be stimulated or induced by nutritive substrates. For example, exposure to oral feedings changes the hormones and enzymes of the neonatal gut as the presence of milk in the newborn's GI tract stimulates shifts in physiology.[72, 73] In this case, a change in nutrient supply from trans-placental glucose feeding in utero to high-fat

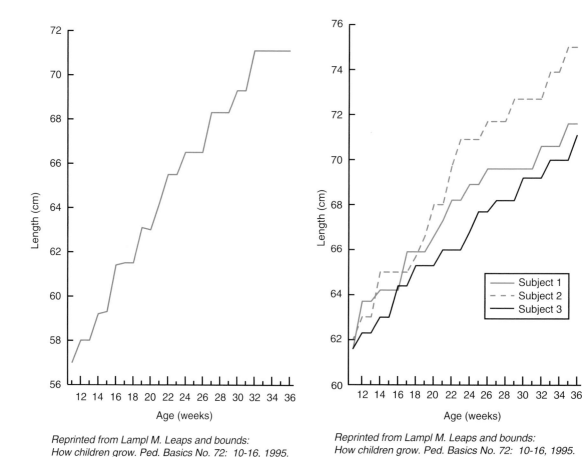

Reprinted from Lampl M. Leaps and bounds:
How children grow. Ped. Basics No. 72: 10-16, 1995.

Figure 6: Postnatal infant growth assessment.

Reprinted from Lampl M. Leaps and bounds:
How children grow. Ped. Basics No. 72: 10-16, 1995.

Figure 7. Individual variability in growth patterns.

milk feeding during suckling drives changes in gut physiology and development. A second example of induced adaptation is the observation that preterm infants receiving enteral feedings at three to five days of age had more mature intestinal motor patterns and higher plasma concentrations of gut hormones at 10 days than infants not receiving enteral feeds.[74] Likewise, the shift at weaning from human milk or formula as a sole source of nourishment to a diet that includes other foods is a dramatic transition through a series of enzymatic, hormonal, morphological and behavioral changes that induces the infant's physiological adaptation to use foods other than milk.

As the infant's environment and experiences offered by the caregiver change during early development, these changes require adaptive modifications. An example of physiologic adaptation is when infant cereal, a source of complex carbohydrate, is fed to infants as early as four weeks of age.[75] Even with low levels of pancreatic amylase present at this age, consumption of complex carbohydrate induces an increased activity of glucoamylase[76] and colonic fermentation, thereby increasing net absorption of the carbohydrate.[75]

An example of behavioral adaptation is taken from a U.S. survey of infant feeding practices[77] in which wide variations were noted in the appearance of developmental markers for complementary feeding, i.e., takes pureed foods from a spoon or closes lips around spoon. The wide differences noted between infants were due to the fact that some mothers challenged their babies with spoon feeding earlier than did others. Thus, some behaviors are learned only when the caregiver provides the opportunity for these behaviors to occur.[77]

Knowing that the human infant is highly adaptable reassures us that the human race will continue to survive, but it does not address the optimum timing for weaning. Knowing which developmental markers are easily identified by caregivers and health care professionals, and that they correlate with adequate maturity of the immunological, digestive, absorptive and renal systems, would be enormously useful.

Specific ontogenetic changes in muscular development and coordination can be used as markers of an infant's developmental maturity for complementary and supplemental feeding (Table 2).[78] These behavioral changes can be seen in some infants as early as three months, but are generally observed in most infants by four months of age when adequate intestinal and renal maturity are established.[79, 80]

Many behavioral changes observed in infants during their first year have been evaluated by mothers as cues of infant development. Some appear to be useful as markers of the infant's ability to begin complementary feeding.[77] Three such developmental markers, long recognized by pediatricians, reflect the early trunk control and postural stability associated with oral-motor control and the physical skill required for eating complementary foods. These markers are the baby's ability to sit with support; to hold up the head and support weight on straight elbows when placed on the stomach; and to control head and neck movements to express satiety by turning away from food, or to express hunger by leaning toward the food.[78, 81] These and other developmental markers are shown in Table 2.

The idea of an infant-driven optimum time to introduce complementary foods resonates with the concept of a "critical period of development" defined as the period during which infants can and must learn to accept and tolerate foods orally. Evidence for a "critical period" is based on observations of infants who, for medical or surgical reasons, cannot have solid foods introduced during the early months. When solids are eventually tried after one year or later, the infants have difficulty accepting them.[82]

Infant-driven developmental markers have been correlated with appropriate timing of complementary feeding[77] overlapping with the appearance of opportunistic markers resulting from feeding challenges initiated by the caregiver. The optimum timing to initiate complementary feeding would ideally rely on the mother's observation and understanding of her infant's behavioral cues, which arise from the baby's individual pattern of growth and development.

Exposure to Foods of One's Culture

"Food is at the center of infant life...and retains a central role in daily life."

Paul Rozin, 1990[21]

Whether omnivores or vegans, we have a multitude of foods available to us to satisfy our nutrient needs, yet we are born with no genetic programming for or recognition of specific foods to assure our survival. In learning about the foods of our culture, we must rely on our elders who have safely negotiated the natural hazards and toxins in our food supply to guide us in selecting foods that will nourish us throughout life.[21]

Learning the "rules of cuisine" of our culture, what is edible and in what contexts, is one of the most important and complex challenges that face a young child.[21] We acquire our food preferences through early and repeated experiences of eating foods and by following the examples of our family and group members to learn the appropriate context and combinations for foods,[83] i.e., what foods are eaten for breakfast, that mustard goes with ham, and beans with rice. The social context in which foods are offered and experienced is, therefore, extremely important in acquiring our patterns of food acceptance or rejection.[83, 84] These patterns can be modified as we are exposed to new cultures and environments.

> *As soon as the Children have any teeth, at six or eight months, they may by degrees be used to a little flesh-meat; which they are always very fond of, much more so at first, than of any confectionary or pastry wares, with which they should never debauch their taste.*
>
> *Pediatrics of the Past*
> An anthology compiled and edited by John Ruhrah M.D., 1925
> Paul B. Hoeber, Inc., Publishers, New York, NY

Periods of Infant Feeding	Physical Development	Feeding Skills	Communication Skills	Food Choices
Nursing *Newborn*	• Poor control of head, neck and trunk. • Most movements are random and reflexive. Randomly moves arms and legs. Reflexively "mouths"hands and toys.	• Roots in search of nipple. • Can suck and swallow only liquids. • Holds liquids in mouth with help of fat pads in cheeks.	• Cries and sucks intensely when hungry. • Releases nipple or falls asleep during feeding when satisfied. • Can regulate food intake to meet caloric needs by six weeks.	• Breast milk.
Transitional *Head Up*	• *Doubles birth weight and weighs at least 13 pounds.* • Emerging postural stability and trunk control. Sits with help. When placed on stomach, lifts head and supports weight with straight elbows. • Newborn reflexes diminish. Purposely bats objects with fisted hands. Deliberately "mouths" hands and toys.	• Opens mouth as spoon approaches. • Quickly learns to suck thin purees from spoon. • Uses tongue to move food to the back of the mouth to swallow without gagging.	• Changes established feeding patterns. Seems hungry after actively breast-feeding 8-10 times a day, or drinking 32 oz. of formula. • Moves forward as spoon approaches to signal hunger. Pushes feeder's hand away when satisfied.	• Breast milk or instant formula. • Single-ingredient cereals and fine purees. • Avoid foods containing egg, soy and wheat. • Easily eats a variety of thin purees.
Sitter	• Good postural stability. Sits alone. • Developing independent mobility. Rolls from back to front and "creeps" on stomach. • Emerging hand skills. Rakes small objects towards self into a fisted hand. Transfers objects from one hand to the other.	• Easily eats a variety of thin purees. • Learns to keep thick purees in mouth and swallow without gagging. • Begins drinking from a lidded cup with assistance.	• Grasps spoon as if to say, "I want that!" • Looks for food when parents remove feeding dish.	• Breast milk or instant formula. • Thick purees. • Mixed-ingredient foods, including, egg, soy and wheat. • Mild flavors.
Crawler	• Strong postural stability. Can reach out for a toy without losing balance. • Improving mobility. Crawls well. Pulls self up to stand. • Practicing hand skills. Uses thumb and finger to hold small objects.	• Uses tongue to move food to side of mouth for mashing. • Holds lidded cup while drinking with no help. • Shows interest in self-feeding by reaching out for utensils to mouth or play with them.	• Vocalizes, points or touches parent's hand during mealtimes to control what and how much is being fed.	• Breast milk or instant formula. • Textures that encourage chewing. • More complex seasonings and flavors.
Modified Adult *Toddler*	• *Triples birth weight.* • Good mobility. Walks with assistance. Stands alone. • Efficient hand skills. Uses finger tips to delicately pick up small objects. Reaches out with palms up to receive an object from someone else.	• Keeps lids closed and most of food in mouth when chewing. • Has some upper and lower teeth. Bites through a variety of textured foods. • Can easily feed self using fingers. Learns to spear food with a fork and scoops with a spoon. • Drinks from a cup. Stops bottle feeding.	• Will mimic parents' mealtime behaviors. • Uses words or sounds to express the desire for specific foods.	• Introduce whole cow's milk when a sufficient variety of solid foods is being consumed. • Foods with mature flavors and varied textures for continued chewing practice.
Walker	• Masters gross motor skills. Walks with confidence. • Masters fine motor skills. Hand skills include a variety of grasp patterns. Can manipulate objects within a hand. Shows clear preference for one hand.	• Uses lips, tongue and teeth to draw food and liquid into mouth for efficient eating. • Uses one hand to adjust spoon into more efficient position when scooping a variety of consistencies. • Can bring spoon to the mouth with minimal spilling.	• Expresses mealtime wants with simple phrases, "want that," "more juice," "all done." • Can lead parent to cupboard or refrigerator and point to a desired food or drink. • Develops definite food preferences. May develop erratic eating behaviors.	• Whole cow's milk. • A wide variety of foods with challenging textures and flavors, as well as familiar favorites.

* Ages are not assigned to the periods of infant feeding. Infants will develop skills and reach milestones according to their individual patterns of development.

Adapted from Dietary Guidelines for Infants 1994. Gerber Products Company, Freemont, MI
©1996 Gerber Products Company

Table 2: Developmental feeding plan.

It is postulated that the breast-fed infant experiences dietary variety through the mother's milk which carries the flavors of the foods from the mother's diet.[85] This early introduction to dietary variety via mother's milk may explain why breast-fed infants accept new foods more readily than formula-fed infants.[86]

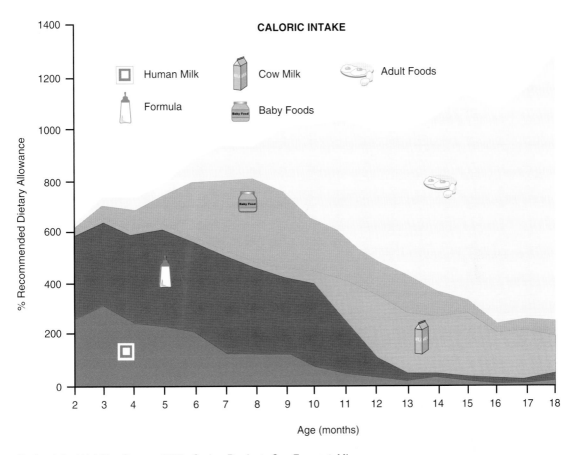

Gerber Infant Nutrition Survey, 1994. Gerber Products Co., Fremont, MI

Figure 8. Caloric intake (% RDA) of U.S. infants 2 to 18 months of age by food source.

By the end of the first year, most infants in the U.S. will be eating from a variety of fruits, vegetables and grain products and small amounts of meats, primarily in casseroles or mixed dishes (Figure 8).[47] Most of the cereals will be consumed at breakfast or early in the day; fruit will be eaten throughout the day; vegetables, breads and meat dishes will be consumed at later meals.[47] Such patterns reflect the rules of cuisine and food preferences and practices of our culture.

Balancing the Risks and Benefits of Adding Complementary Foods to the Infant Diet

Problems during the weaning process fall into two broad categories: poor diets and poor feeding practices.[87] The quality of foods and the level of sanitation available for preparing weaning foods are two of the most important criteria to consider in deciding when complementary feeding is to begin. In more industrialized, affluent regions where modern food processing techniques ensure hygienic preparation of a wide variety of nutrient-replete infant foods, the risks of weaning are reduced to a minimum and the benefits of weaning are maximized. With a variety of safe foods for infants readily available, determinants other than safety can take precedence, for example, infant growth rate, stage of development, and mother's perceptions and needs. The role of exclusive and extended breast-feeding is less critical in such environments, and breast-feeding can be complemented with little risk to the infant.

Conversely, in less industrialized regions, complementary feeding may mean weaning foods of low nutrient density and bioavailability[88] prepared and fed in unhygienic conditions. Such practices introduce the downward spiral of gastrointestinal disease, diarrhea, malnutrition, growth faltering and increased morbidity and mortality,[89] thereby maximizing the risks of weaning and minimizing the benefits. Under these conditions, the protective and nutritional benefits of prolonged breast-feeding offer the safest course.[89, 90] Yet complementary and supplemental feedings are essential to avoid malnutrition and continue growth.

The dilemma for weanlings and their caretakers is in balancing the risk of continuing inadequate energy and nutrient intakes with breast milk alone with the risks of infection and nutritional hazards associated with contaminated, low-nutrient weaning foods.[44] Preventing infectious disease, ensuring sanitation and hygiene and preparing and making available safe, nutritious foods is optimal. Committing the will and the skill to achieve these solutions is the challenge facing us in the next decades if we are to reverse the "silent emergencies" of malnutrition, disease, and illiteracy[23] that exist in many regions and communities; these have tremendous impact on a caregiver's decisions about feeding her baby as well as the baby's health, growth and development.

The Caregiver's Perspective

Cross-cultural studies of infant feeding document wide variation in the timing, type and amounts of supplemental feeds and in beliefs about the appropriate styles of feeding.[20] Factors that influence when a mother chooses to wean are cultural attitudes to child care and maternal factors of age, education and social class.[70] For example, older, more educated, higher income women tend to breast-feed their infants longer than young, less educated, working women.[70, 81, 89, 92]

The quality of interaction between the mother or caregiver and the infant[20, 93] affects how the feeding situation will go because the quality of interaction is a measure of a mother's confidence in her ability to observe, interpret and respond to changes in her baby's behavior and needs.

Reasons Mothers Begin Complementary Feeding

The reasons mothers give most often for introducing complementary foods to their infants fall into four cat-

egories: mother's response to changes in her baby's behavior; her own beliefs about what is best for her baby; mother's confidence in her ability to meet the baby's needs; and the advice and support available to her from her family and community, her employer, the health care advisor or government programs.

Changes in Baby's Behavior

Harris[70] reported that 75% of middle-class mothers taking part in her study in urban Birmingham introduced solid foods to their babies in response to changes in their behavior. The most frequent changes cited were more frequent demand for feeding and return to waking at night. The median age of introduction of solids in this study was 14 weeks. Both behaviors are those described by mothers to Lampl[69] as preceding their infants' growth spurts. Young mothers of lower socio-economic class, in an urban setting, were more likely to respond earlier to these same behavioral changes by giving solid foods than middle-class mothers, at the median age of ten weeks vs 14 weeks, respectively.

Belief About What is Best for Baby

Why the timing of the mothers' responses differed may be explained by differences in mothers' beliefs about what was best for their babies; that is, when to introduce complementary foods.[70] The middle-class women in this study were aware of health care advice not to introduce solid foods too early, and most complied with these recommendations as they responded to their babies' behaviors. Presumably, introducing complementary foods before a given age was not considered an appropriate response to behavioral signals that could have been hunger signs. The lower social class mothers were presumed to be more influenced by family pressure regarding time to introduce complementary foods because they introduced foods earlier as they responded to changes in their baby's behaviors.

Mothers' Confidence in Their Ability to Meet Babies' Needs

Mothers' confidence in their abilities to meet their infants' needs relates initially to lactation success. The reason most nursing women introduce complementary foods is the perceived lack of milk or the perception that their milk is not satisfying the baby.[9, 37, 94] These perceptions are usually based on observed signs of the baby's dissatisfaction during or after nursing. Yet mothers who feed infant formula are more likely to introduce all baby foods earlier than nursing mothers.[95]

Health Care Advice

Health care advisors can affect the mother's decision to continue exclusive breast-feeding or to delay feeding complementary foods. Furthermore, more education, higher income and unemployment correlate with mothers following the infant feeding recommendations of health care advisors.[70]

Support for Breast-feeding

In Scandinavia, with liberal work arrangements that encourage mothers to stay home with their babies and breast-feed, the majority of infants are breast-fed for more than six months and many throughout the second half of infancy.[39] Having to return to the workplace can interrupt the milk flow of the most determined nursing mothers. A combination of education about breast-feeding in the last trimester of pregnancy, a time when mothers are deciding how they will feed their babies, and encouragement from several sources – the family, health care advisor, friends – can help increase breast-feeding rates. If work policies are generous and encourage mothers to stay home for longer periods of time, as in Scandinavia, more babies would benefit from the advantages of longer breast-feeding.

> *We tend to forget that weaning is as innate to a mammal as suckling.*
> Susan Henning Ph.D.
> Department of Pediatrics
> Baylor College of Medicine
> Houston, TX

Recommendations
When to Wean

In the U.S. in the 1950s and 60s, early introduction of complementary foods reached its peak, when infants were fed foods within days of being born! Cereals were begun at two to three days of age and strained vegetables at ten days.[96] Although no demonstrable harm was apparent with this feeding schedule, neither were benefits observed. At the other extreme, infants in some cultures may not routinely receive complementary foods until after the first year.[97]

Range of Recommendations

Traditional pediatric advice seems to be supported by rational science – human milk can reasonably support growth of infants for the first three to four months,[32] even in marginally undernourished populations,[98] to six months,[9] and in some cases longer.[99] Such a wide range of recommendations should not be surprising, given the range of environmental conditions in which infants are born, in their size, growth rate, and nutrient need. Mothers differ in lactational capacity and confidence. The time when additional foods are needed to complement the energy and nutrient intake of human milk will vary with the individual infant and mother. The European community recommends supplementing within the first three to six months.[100] The U.S. Academy of Pediatrics Committee on Nutrition prefers supplementation to begin no earlier than four but not later than six months of age,[61] a recommendation in accord with the World Health Organization recommendation of exclusive breast-feeding for the first four to six months.[101] The needs of the majority of infants are likely to be met within this broad range of recommendations.

In the U.S., bottle feeding is not recommended beyond one year of age, particularly as an aid to sleep, to avoid "nursing bottle caries" that can develop from dependence on bottle feeding.[102] Any beverage with naturally occurring or added sugars, including any type of milk or juice, can contribute to "nursing bottle caries" if fed inappropriately from a bottle. The transition from bottle to cup can begin about six months of age and be completed at the beginning of the second year, depending on the baby's feeding skills.

Use of Cow Milk

Current recommendations in the U.S. encourage breast-feeding or the use of iron-fortified infant formula for the first year of life.[16] The American Academy of Family Physicians also endorses the promotion of breast-feeding and practices that encourage breast-feeding as the standard of infant feeding.[103]

Whole cow milk and low-iron formulas are not recommended during the first year,[16] although small amounts of dairy products such as yogurt are accept-

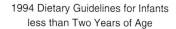

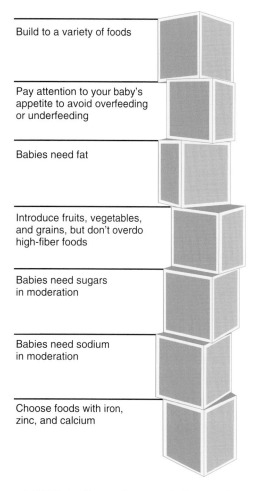

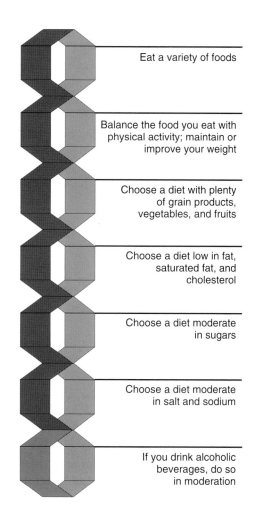

© 1996 Gerber Products Company. Used with permission

Table 3: Dietary guidelines comparison.

able for the older infant when fed as part of a varied diet. Cow milk protein allergy is a concern for some infants, whether it be from whole cow milk or cow milk-based formulas. For infants who are not allergic, the use of whole cow milk can be based on the infant's dietary adequacy and tolerance to lactose.[16]

How to Wean

Parents are responsible for the foods that are presented to children and the context in which they are presented...

Children are responsible for determining the quantity of food eaten.

Ellyn M. Satter, 1988[104]

"...mothers with well-nourished children have more self-confidence; that is, they introduce foods when they believe it is right rather than when the child 'accepts' the foods. They are more likely to persist in feeding their child when the child refuses; and, they are more willing to try new foods and practices."

Marcia Griffiths, 1993[105]

Infant feeding takes place in three overlapping stages: the nursing period, the transitional period and the modified adult period.[61] The rate at which an infant progresses through these three stages will be dictated first by beliefs and practices of the culture in which he is born. Ideally, within the cultural context, the infant's nutritional need, expressed as hunger and developmental progress with feeding skills, will guide the infant's dietary experience and progression to the family table.

In the affluent U.S., the overriding preoccupation is to improve health and prevent chronic disease, particularly obesity, a concern that dominates our public health goals. Therefore, concern for controlling an exuberant appetite is a high priority and finds its way into our dietary guidelines. This concern filters through to recommendations on feeding practices during infancy. We prefer to see an infant self-regulate food intake rather than have a caregiver encourage greater consumption than the infant may demand or require.[106]

At the same time, adult dietary guidelines with recommendations for low fat intake and high-fiber foods have been inappropriately applied to infants, resulting in failure to thrive.[107] The guidelines for infants during weaning, then, differ from those for adults (Table 3).

In contrast to adult dietary guidelines, guidelines for infants in the U.S.[108, 109] follow current U.S. pediatric recommendations that emphasize building slowly to dietary variety; following a baby's cues for hunger and satiety to support the baby's individual growth rate; and not restricting fat in order to meet caloric needs for maintenance and rapid growth. Teaching desirable long-term food selections and preferences are pointed out in the final four guidelines that include introducing a variety of grains, fruits and vegetables; understanding the appropriateness of sugars; using sodium and salt in moderation; and choosing foods that are good sources of minerals that are often limiting in the weaning diet. In the U.S., infants generally are fed iron-fortified infant cereal as the first complementary food, followed by fruits and vegetables before six months of age. This feeding pattern is in line with U.S. pediatric recommendations. These foods complement and supplement the nutrient intake from human milk or infant formula.

In learning how to feed their infants, parents need to understand changes in their babies' behavior that relate to feeding regulation. These behaviors were referred to earlier as developmental markers (Table 2). The practice of introducing one new food at a time and watching for signs of food sensitivity is practical in industrialized countries where a wide range of prepared, single-ingredient infant foods is available. Where infants are introduced to foods from the "family pot," getting enough to eat may be a higher priority than identifying food sensitivities. The quality and safety of available weaning foods must be evaluated for the contribution the foods make to the infant's needs.

The order of food introduction throughout the world (Table 1) seems to depend on food availability and rules of cuisine. Even within cultures, the order of food introduction varies widely.[20] In the U.S., juices and iron-fortified infant cereals are traditionally favored as first infant foods to provide bioavailable iron and additional calories, but fruits and vegetables are also favored.

With continued exposure to complementary foods and continued developmental maturation, the infant learns to accept and manage foods of varied textures, consistencies, and flavors in the move to the family table.[107] The caregiver's interactions with the child during these transitional steps are important influences on a child's acceptance of a food and food intake. Parents' attitudes towards the food and interest in the child's food intake affect a child's food preference and appetite.[7, 83, 93]

The parent/child interaction has a most pervasive influence on a child's feeding behavior, but it is only relatively recently that physiologists and nutritionists have joined forces with psychologists, sociologists and human behaviorists[20, 21] to explore the complex social context of feeding.

The statements by Ellyn Satter and Marcia Griffiths at the beginning of this section appear to represent two opposing schools of thought on the social context of feeding infants and young children. Satter divides the responsibilities into two areas: the parents provide suitable foods, and the child eats as much or as little as she wants. Griffiths' setting seems to describe a type of force feeding that some may frown upon because it appears to deny the child the right of refusal. The paradox is that both modes of feeding are correct and effective, depending once again on context and the environment in which they are practiced.[83, 84]

Where foods are readily available on a daily basis, easy for the infant or child to consume, the feeding environment is relaxed and unhurried, the infant is hungry and the mother correctly interprets her baby's cues for hunger and satiety, or the infant has learned the skills to feed herself, then she can, indeed, determine for herself how much food is enough at a given meal and thrive on following her own internal cues of hunger and satiety.

However, if the child is weakened and undernourished, ill and anorectic, if the food is unvaried in flavor and texture, the mother's success in feeding her child may be determined by the degree of assertiveness she uses in encouraging her child to eat. It is not a democratic process, but it works. Different circumstances demand different remedies. There is no one right way to feed a child; there are many. And each may be best in a given circumstance.

Summary

The time to introduce complementary foods is not fixed to a specific age. Infants are individual in their patterns of growth and development. Caregivers interpret these patterns of growth and behaviors and make changes in feeding practices to help the infant transition to the family table. Infants are highly adaptive and will respond to and thrive on the feeding mode available to them at birth and the variety of foods and feeding challenges they experience throughout weaning. That is, they will thrive as long as the foods provide safe access to adequate and bioavailable nutrients, and the environment and feeding practices do not burden the immature immune system with pathogens. The safety and nutrient content of weaning foods are, therefore, key factors in determining when an infant can move from exclusive breast or formula-feeding to other forms of nourishment. Each mother's beliefs in her capabilities, based partly on cultural and partly on individual experiences, are equally dominant factors in determining the time of infant weaning or complementary feeding.

If our goal is to have actual practices follow infant feeding recommendations and guidelines, then recommendations and guidelines must take into account the experience and knowledge of the mother, the factors that affect the mother's decision-making process, and her motivation and ability to apply recommendations to her individual infant – the only baby ever born, as far as any mother is concerned.

Practical Application

The time to begin weaning with the introduction of complementary foods is a moving target. The European Society for Pediatric Gastroenterology and Nutrition, the Committee on Nutrition of the American Academy of Pediatrics and the World Health Organization give general guidelines of about four to six months of age, but these guidelines are applied to individual babies in your practice. The criteria for introducing complementary feeding to a particular infant in a particular environment can be prioritized based on what you know about the infant's current environment, nutritional status, growth and development characteristics and the mother's beliefs, cultural practices and level of confidence and capabilities. The "decision tree" on the following page is a guide to help evaluate the risks and benefits of introducing complementary foods in a variety of circumstances.

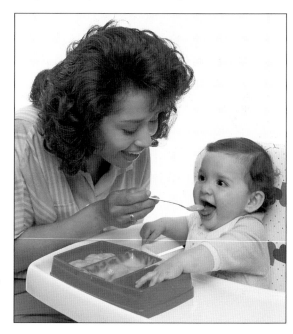

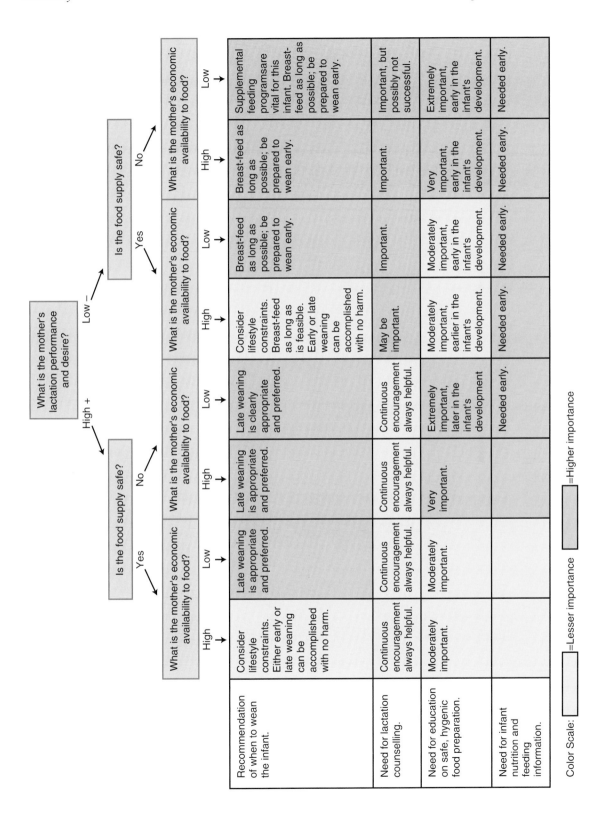

Color Scale: ☐ =Lesser importance ▨ =Higher importance

References

1. Barness LA. Bases of weaning recommendations. *J Pediatr.* 1990;117(2, Part 2):S84-S86.

2. Ballabriga A, Schmidt E. Actual trends of the diversification of infant feeding in industrialized countries in Europe. In: Ballabriga A, Rey J, eds. *Weaning: Why, What, and When?* Nestlé Nutrition Workshop Series, Volume 10. New York: Raven Press; 1987:129-153.

3. King J, Ashworth A. Contemporary feeding practices in infancy and early childhood in developing countries. In: Falkner F, ed. *Infant and Child Nutrition Worldwide: Issues and Perspectives.* Boca Raton, FL: CRC Press; 1991: 141-174.

4. Husaini MA, Karyadi L, Husaini YK, Sandjaja, Karyadi D, Pollitt E. Developmental effects of short-term supplementary feeding in nutritionally-at-risk Indonesian infants. *Am J Clin Nutr.* 1991;54:799-804.

5. Rowland MGM. Epidemiology of childhood diarrhoea in the Gambia. In: Chen LC, Scrimshaw LS, eds. *Diarrhoea and Malnutrition.* New York: Plenum Press; 1982:87-98.

6. Motarjemi Y, Käferstein F, Moy G, Quevedo F. Contaminated food, a hazard for the very young. *World Health Forum.* 1994;15(1):69-71.

7. Birch LL. Development of food acceptance patterns. *Develop Psych.* 1990;26(4):515-519.

8. Ahmad A. Supplementary infant feeding in developing countries. In: Ballabriga A, Rey J, eds. *Weaning: Why, What, and When?* Nestlé Nutrition Workshop Series, Volume 10. New York: Raven Press; 1987:197-204.

9. Cohen RJ, Brown KH, Canahuati J, Rivera LL, Dewey KG. Effects of age of introduction of complementary foods on infant breast milk intake, total energy intake, and growth: a randomised intervention study in Honduras. *Lancet.* 1994;344:288-293.

10. Bartholmey SJ. Breast-feeding and complementary commercially prepared weaning foods. *Lancet.* 1994; 344:1305(Letter).

11. Motarjemi Y, Käferstein F, Moy G, Quevedo F. Contaminated weaning food: a major risk factor for diarrhoea and associated malnutrition. *Bull Wrld Hlth Org.* 1993;71(1):79-92.

12. *The Compact Edition of the Oxford English Dictionary.* Walton Street, Oxford; 1971. Oxford University Press,

OX2 6DP. 3718.

13. Martinez GA, Krieger FW. 1984 milk feeding patterns in the United States. *Pediatrics.* 1985;76:1004-1008.

14. Montalto MB, Benson JD, Martinez GA. Nutrient intakes of formula-fed infants and infants fed cow's milk. *Pediatrics.* 1985;75:343-351.

15. Purvis GA, Bartholmey SJ. Infant feeding practices: commercially prepared baby foods. In: Tsang R, Nichols BL, eds. *Nutrition During Infancy.* Philadelphia: Hanley & Belfus; 1988:399-417.

16. American Academy of Pediatrics, Committee on Nutrition. The Use of Whole Cow's Milk in Infancy. *Pediatrics.* 1992;89(6):1105-1109.

17. United Nations Children's Fund. *The State of the World's Children 1994.* New York: Oxford University Press; 1994: 66-67.

18. Calloway DH, Murphy S, Balderston J, Receveur O, Lein D, Hudes M. *Findings: Children's Intake. Village Nutrition in Egypt, Kenya and Mexico: Looking Across the CRSP Projects.* Final Report to the U.S. Agency for International Development Cooperative Agreement: April, 1992. #DAN 1309-A-00-9090-00;54.

19. Calloway DH, Murphy SP, Beaton GH. *Pregnancy, Lactation and Infancy. Food Intake and Human Function: A Cross-Project Perspective of the Collaborative Research Support Program in Egypt, Kenya and Mexico.* University of California, Berkeley: 1988. Prepared under U.S. Agency for International Development grant # DAN-0262-G-SS-7079-00;59-70.

20. Bentley ME, Black MM. *Children's Appetite and Growth: Individual, Maternal, and Cultural Influences.* (submitted for publication) permission to cite granted.

21. Rozin P. Development in the food domain. *Develop Psych.* 1990;26(4):555-562.

22. VanDerslice J, Popkin B, Briscoe J. Drinking-water quality, sanitation, and breast-feeding: their interactive effects on infant health. *Bull Wrld Hlth Org.* 1994;72(4): 589-601.

23. *The State of the World's Children 1994. Malnutrition: the invisible compromise.* United Nations Children's Fund: 1994. 16-19.

24. Lönnerdal B, Forsum E, Hambraeus L. A longitudinal study of the protein, nitrogen and lactose content of human milk from well-nourished mothers. *Am J Clin*

Nutr. 1976;29:1127-1133.

25. Stuff J, Nichols BL. Nutrient intake and growth performance of older infants fed human milk. *J Pediatr.* 1989;115:959-968.

26. Butte NF, Wong WW, Garza C, Klein PD. Adequacy of human milk for meeting energy requirements during early infancy. In: Atkinson SA, Hanson LA, Chandra RK, eds. *Breast-feeding, Nutrition, Infection and Infant Growth in Developed and Emerging Countries.* ©ARTS. St. John's, Newfoundland, Canada: Biomedical Publishers and Distributors; 1990:103-116.

27. Whitehead RG, Paul AA. Dietary energy needs from 6 to 12 months of age. In: Heird WC, ed. *Nutritional Needs of the Six to Twelve Month Old Infant.* Carnation Nutrition Education Series, Vol. 2. New York: Raven Press Ltd; 1991:135-148.

28. Hofvandeer Y, Hagman U, Hillervik C, Sjölin S. The amount of milk consumed by 1-3 months old breast-or bottle-fed infants. *Acta Paediatr Scand.* 1982;71:953-958.

29. FAO/WHO/UNU Expert Consultation. *Energy and protein requirements.* Geneva; World Health Organization Technical Report Series 724:1985.

30. Chandra RK. Physical growth of exclusively breast-fed infants. *Nutr Res.* 1982;2:275-276.

31. Duncan B, Schaefer C, Sibley B, Fonseca NM. Reduced growth velocity in exclusively breast-fed infants. *Am J Dis Child.* 1984;138:309-313.

32. Whitehead RG. For how long is exclusive breast-feeding adequate to satisfy the dietary energy needs of the average young baby? *Pediatr Res.* 1995;36(2):239-243.

33. Whitehead RG, Paul AA, Cole TJ. A critical analysis of measured food energy intakes during infancy and early childhood in comparison with current international recommendations. *J Hum Nutr.* 1981;35:339-348.

34. Prentice AM, Lucas A, Vasquez-Velasquez L, Davies PSW, Whitehead RG. Are current guidelines for young children a prescription for overfeeding? *Lancet.* 1988;2:1066-1069.

35. Lucas A. Energy requirements in normal infants and children. In: Schürch B, Scrimshaw NS, eds. *Activity, Energy Expenditure and Energy Requirements of Infants and Children.* Lausanne, Switzerland: United Nations University and Nestlé Foundation; 1990:9-34.

36. Stuff J, Garza C, Boutte C, Fraley JK, O'Brian, Smith E, Klein ER, Nichols BL. Sources of variance in milk and

caloric intakes in breast-fed infants: implications for lactation study design and interpretation. *Am J Clin Nutr.* 1986;43:361-366.

37. Leung S, Davies DP. Infant feeding and growth of Chinese infants: birth to 2 years. *Paediatr Perinat Epidem.* 1994;8:301-313.

38. Butte NF. Energy requirements of infants. *Eur J Clin Nutr.* 1996;50,Suppl.1:S24-S36.

39. Michaelsen KF, Larsen PS, Thomsen BL, Samuelson G. The Copenhagen Cohort study on Infant Nutrition and Growth: breast-milk intake, human milk macronutrient content, and influencing factors. *Am J Clin Nutr.* 1994; 59:600-611.

40. Davies PSW. Energy requirements and energy expenditure in infancy. *Eur J Clin Nutr.* 1992;46(Suppl 4):S29-S35.

41. Lampl M. *Leaps and bounds: how children grow.* 1995; Ped Basics No.72:10-16.

42. Dewey KG, Beaton G, Fjeld C, Lönnerdal B, Reeds P. Protein requirements of infants and children. *Eur J Clin Nutr.* 1996;50,Suppl.1:S119-S150.

43. Fomon SJ, Filer LJ Jr, Thomas LN, et al. Influence of formula concentration of caloric intake and growth of normal infants. *Acta Paediatr Scand.* 1975;64:172-181.

44. Poskitt EME. Energy needs in the weaning period. In: Ballabriga A, Rey J, eds. *Weaning: Why, What, and When?* Nestlé Nutrition Workshop Series, Volume 10. New York: Raven Press; 1987:45-61.

45. Karra MV, Udipi SA, Kirksey A, Roepke JLB. Changes in specific nutrients in breast milk during extended lactation. *Am J Clin Nutr.* 1986;43:495-503.

46. Dewey KG, Lönnerdal B. Milk and nutrient intake of breast-fed infants from 1 to 6 months: relation to growth and fatness. *J Pediatr Gastroenterol Nutr.* 1983;2:497-506.

47. *Patterns of food and nutrient intake of infants and toddlers 2 months to 3 years of age.* Fremont, MI; Gerber Infant Nutrition Survey: 1994. Gerber Products Company; unpublished data.

48. Ernst JA, Brady MS, Rickard KA. Food and nutrient intake of 6- to 12- month-old infants fed formula or cow milk: A summary of four national surveys. *J Pediatr.* 1990;117(2),Part 2:S86-S100.

49. Fomon SJ. Human milk and breast-feeding. In: Fomon SJ, ed. *Nutrition of Normal Infants.* St. Louis: Mosby; 1993:409-423.

50. Young VR, Cortiella J. Protein and amino acid requirements of healthy 6- to 12- month-old infants. In: Heird WC, ed. *Nutritional Needs of the Six to Twelve Month Old Infant.* Carnation Nutrition Education Series, Vol. 2. New York: Raven Press Ltd; 1991:149-173.

51. Saarinen UM, Siimes MA, Dallman PR. Iron absorption in infants: high bioavailability of breast milk iron as indicated by the extrinsic tag method of iron absorption and by the concentration of serum ferritin. *J Pediatr.* 1977;91:36-39.

52. Lönnerdal B. Iron intake and requirements: Interactions with other trace elements. In: Heird WC, ed. *Nutritional Needs of the Six to Twelve Month Old Infant.* Carnation Nutrition Education Series, Vol. 2. New York: Raven Press Ltd; 1991:199-211.

53. American Academy of Pediatrics, Committee on Nutrition. Vitamin and mineral supplement needs. In: Barness LA, ed. *Pediatric Nutrition Handbook,* 3rd edition. Elk Grove Village, IL: 1993:34-42.

54. DeMaeyer E, Adiels-Tegman M. Prevalence of anemia in the world. *Child Hlth Stat Qrtly.* 1985;35:302-316.

55. Committee on the Prevention, Detection, and Management of Iron Deficiency Anemia Among U.S. Children and Women of Childbearing Age. *Iron Deficiency Anemia.* Washington, DC; Food and Nutrition Board, Institute of Medicine, National Academy of Sciences: 1993. National Academy Press.

56. Looker AC, Dallman PR, Carroll MD, Gunter EW, Johnson CL. Prevalence of iron deficiency in the United States. *JAMA.* 1997;277:973-976.

57. Yip R, Binkin NH, Fleshood L, Trowbridge FL. Declining prevalence of anemia among low-income children in the United States. *JAMA.* 1987;258:1619-1623.

58. Tulchinsky TH, El Ebweini S, Ginsberg GM, Abed Y, Montano-Cuellar D, Schoenbaum M, Zansky SM, Jacob S, El Tibbi AJ, Abu Sah'aban D, Koch J, Melnick Y. Growth and nutrition patterns of infants associated with a nutrition education and supplementation programme in Gaza, 1987-92. *Bull Wrld Hlth Org.* 1994; 72(6):869-875.

59. Lozoff B, Jimenez E, Wolf A. Long term developmental outcome of infants with iron deficiency. *N Eng J Med.* 1991;325:687-694.

60. Walter T. Early and long-term effect of iron deficiency anemia on child development. In: Fomon SJ, Zlotkin S, eds. *Nutritional Anemias.* Nestlé Nutrition Workshop Series, Volume 30. New York: Raven Press Ltd; 1992: 81-92.

61. American Academy of Pediatrics, Committee on Nutrition. Supplemental foods for infants. In: Barness LA, ed. *Pediatric Nutrition Handbook.* 3rd edition. Elk Grove Village, IL: 1993:34-42.

62. American Academy of Pediatrics, Committee on Nutrition. Iron-fortified infant formulas. *Pediatrics.* 1989; 84:1114-1116.

63. Walter T, Dallman PR, Pizarro F, Leloza L, Peña G, Bartholmey SJ, Hertrampf E, Olivares M, Letelier A, Arredondo M. Effectiveness of iron-fortified infant cereal in prevention of iron deficiency anemia. *Pediatrics.* 1993;91(5):976-982.

64. Michaelsen KF, Samuelson G, Graham TW, Lönnerdal B. Zinc intake, zinc status and growth in a longitudinal study of healthy Danish infants. *Acta Paediatr.* 1994;83: 1115-1121.

65. Krebs NF, Reidinger CJ, et al. Growth and intake of energy and zinc in infants fed human milk. *J Pediatr.* 1994;124:32-39.

66. Dorea JG. Is zinc a first limiting nutrient in human milk? *Nutr Res.* 1993;13:656-659.

67. Walravens PA, Hambidge KM, Koepfer DM. Zinc supplementation in infants with a nutritional pattern of failure to thrive: a double-blind, controlled study. *Pediatrics.* 1989;83(4):532-538.

68. Walravens PA, Chakar A, Mokni R, Denise J, Lemonnier D. Zinc supplements in breast-fed infants. *Lancet.* 1992; 340:683-685.

69. Lampl M. Evidence of saltatory growth in infancy. *Am J Hum Biol.* 1993;5:641-652.

70. Harris G. Determinants of the introduction of solid food. *J Reprod Infant Psychol.* 1988;66:241-249.

71. Alberts JR. Learning as adaptation of the infant. *Acta Paediatr Suppl.* 1994;397:77-85.

72. Lucas A. Breast-feeding and gut hormones. In: Filer LJ Jr, Domon AJ, eds. *The Breast-fed Infant: A Model for Performance. Report of the 91st Ross Conference on Pediatric Research.* Columbus, OH: Ross Laboratories; 1987:73-83.

73. Lin C-H, Tolia K, Correia L, Tolia V, Lee PC, Luk GD.

Induction of small intestinal ornithine decarboxylase (ODC) in early weaning neonatal rats. *Pediatr Res.* 1991; 29:106A.

74. Berseth CL. Effect of early feeding on maturation of the preterm infant's small intestine. *J Pediatr.* 1992;120: 947-953.

75. Shulman RJ, Wong WW, Irving CS, Nichols BL, Klein PD. Utilization of dietary cereal by young infants. *J Pediatr.* 1982;103:23-28.

76. Lebenthal E, Lee PC, Heitlinger LA. Impact of development of the gastrointestinal tract on infant feeding. *J Pediatr.* 1983;102:1-9.

77. Carruth BR, Skinner J, Morris SE, Houck K, Coletta FA, McLeod M, Cotter R. *Infant development and eating readiness: A current view.* Seoul, Korea; Proceedings of the 2nd International Symposium on Infant Nutrition: March 11, 1995. Yonsei University, Res. Inst. of Foods and Nutritional Sciences.

78. Morris SE. Eating readiness cues: Introducing supplemental foods. *Ped Basics.* 1992;61:2-7.

79. Kleinman RE. Immune consequences of dietary protein. In: Heird WC, ed. *Nutritional Needs of the Six to Twelve Month Old Infant.* Carnation Nutrition Education Series, Vol. 2. New York: Raven Press Ltd; 1991:109-120.

80. Rodriguez-Soriano J. Adaptation of renal function from birth to one year. In: Ballabriga A, Rey J, eds. *Weaning: Why, What, and When?* Nestlé Nutrition Workshop Series, Volume 10. New York: Raven Press; 1987:45-62.

81. Kleinman RE. Learning about dietary variety: the first steps. *Ped Basics.* 1994;68:2-11.

82. Illingworth RS, Lister J. The critical or sensitive period, with special reference to certain feeding problems in infants and children. *J Pediatr.* 1964;65:839-848.

83. Birch LL. Children's food preferences: Developmental patterns and environmental influences. In: Vasta R, ed. *Annals of Child Development,* Vol. 4. Greenwich, CT: JAI Press; 1987:131-170.

84. Johnson SL, Birch LL. Parents' and children's adiposity and feeding style. *Pediatrics.* 1994;94(5):653-661.

85. Mennella JA, Beauchamp GK. Maternal diet alters the sensory qualities of human milk and the nursling's behavior. *Pediatrics.* 1991;88:737-744.

86. Sullivan SA, Birch LL. Infant dietary experience and acceptance of solid foods. *Pediatrics.* 1994;93(2):271-277.

87. Huffman SL, Martin LH. First feedings: optimal feeding of infants and toddlers. *Nutr Res.* 1994;14:127-159.

88. Golden BE, Golden MHN. Relationships among dietary quality, children's appetites, growth stunting, and efficiency of growth in poor populations. *Food Nutr Bull.* 1991;13(2):105-109.

89. Mata L. Breast-feeding, infections and infant outcomes: An international perspective. In: Atkinson SA, Hanson LA, Chandra RK, eds. *Breast-feeding, Nutrition, Infection and Infant Growth in Developed and Emerging Countries.* ©ARTS. St. John's, Newfoundland, Canada: Biomedical Publishers and Distributors; 1990:1-23.

90. Molbak K, Gottschau A, Aaby P, Hojlyng N, Ingholt L, José da Silva AP. Prolonged breast feeding, diarrhoeal disease, and survival of children in Guinea-Bissau. *Br Med J.* 1994;308:403-406.

91. Hussain AMZ, Rafiquzzaman M. Determinants of weaning age in rural Bangladesh. *Social Biology.* 1994; 41(1-2):788-782.

92. Lawrence RA, Friedman LR. Breast-feeding practices in industrialized countries. In: Atkinson SA, Hanson LA, Chandra RK, eds. *Breast-feeding, Nutrition, Infection and Infant Growth in Developed and Emerging Countries.* ©ARTS. St. John's, Newfoundland, Canada: Biomedical Publishers and Distributors; 1990:447-455.

93. Birch LL, McPhee L, Shoba BC, Steinberg L, Krehbiel R. "Clean up you plate": Effects of child feeding practices on the development of intake regulation. *Learning and Motivation.* 1987;18:301-317.

94. Piwoz EG, Black RE, Lopez de Romaña G, Creed de Kanashiro H, Brown KH. The relationship between infants' preceding appetite, illness, and growth performance and mothers' subsequent feeding practice decisions. *Soc Sci Med.* 1994;39(6):851-860.

95. Bartholmey SJ, Cotter R. Dietary patterns of infants 2-12 months of age fed human milk vs. those not fed human milk. *FASEB J.* 1991;5(6):A1666, Part III. (abstract 7522).

96. Sackett WW Jr. Results of three years experience with a new concept of baby feeding. *South Med J.* 1953;46:358-363.

97. Ajenifuja B. Weaning practices in developing countries. In: Ballabriga A, Rey J, eds. *Weaning: Why, What, and When?* Nestlé Nutrition Workshop Series, Volume 10. New York: Raven Press; 1987:205-210.

98. Brown KH, Robertson AD, Akhtar NA. Lactational capacity of marginally nourished mothers: Infants' milk nutrient consumption and patterns of growth. *Pediatrics.* 1986;78(5):920-927.

99. Siimes MA, Salmenperä L, Perheentupa J. Exclusive breast-feeding for 9 months: risk of iron deficiency. *J Pediatr.* 1984;104:196-199.

100. Lindquist B. ESPGAN Committee on Nutrition. Guidelines on infant nutrition. III. Recommendations for infant feeding. *Acta Paediatr Scand.* 1981;(Suppl) 284:1-85.

101. Akre J. WHO report on infant and young child nutrition: Global problems and promising developments. *Soz Präventivmed.* 1994;39:397-398.

102. American Academy of Pediatrics, Committee on Nutrition. *Juice in ready-to-use bottles and nursing bottle caries.* Policy Reference Guide, AAP. A joint statement of the AAP and the American Academy of Pedodontics. Elk Grove Village, IL: 1994. 378.

103. Commission on Public Health and Scientific Affairs/ American Academy of Family Physicians. Special Medical Report: Academy Endorses the 10 Steps and Criteria of the Breast-feeding Health Initiative. *Amer Family Phys.* 1994;50(2):457-458.

104. Satter EM. The feeding relationship. *Perspectives in Practice.* 1986;86:352-356.

105. Griffiths M. *Comprehensive strategy framework for improving young child feeding.* Washington, DC; The Manoff Group: 1993. unpublished.

106. Fomon SJ. Recommendations for feeding normal infants. In: Fomon SJ, ed. *Nutrition of Normal Infants.* St. Louis: Mosby; 1993:455-458.

107. Pugliese MT, Weyman-Daum M, Moses N, Lifshitz F. Parental health beliefs as a cause of nonorganic failure to thrive. *Pediatrics.* 1987;80:175-182.

108. Kleinman RE, Fomon SJ, Greenspan SJ, Lauer RM, Baker SS, Glinsmann WH, Beauchamp GK, Finberg L, Lönnerdal B. Dietary Guidelines for Infants. *Ped Basics.* 1994;69:1-29.

109. Glinsmann WH, Bartholmey SJ, Dietary Guidelines for Infants: a timely reminder. *Nutr Rev.* 1996;54(2):50-57.

Human Milk Substitutes

James W. Hansen M.D., Ph.D.[1]
Julia A. Boettcher M.Ed., R.D.[2]

Director, Nutrition & Metabolism[1] and
Principal Product Information Specialist,[2]
Mead Johnson Nutritionals, Evansville, Indiana

Reviewed by Judy Hopkinson Ph.D., William Mclean M.D. and Roger Coleman M.D.

Introduction
History

The importance of breast-feeding has long been recognized. In 1812, Buchannan declared, "Nothing can shew the disposition which mankind have to depart from nature more than their endeavoring to bring up children without the breast. The mother's milk or that of a healthy nurse is unquestionably the best food for an infant. Neither art nor nature can afford a proper substitute for it. Children may seem to thrive for a few months without the breast; but when teething, the small-pox and other diseases incident to childhood come on they generally perish."[1]

Despite the advantages of breast-feeding, some infants are not breast-fed and do not receive human milk. These babies need nutritionally sound and safe alternatives. Humans have always been challenged to find suitable alternatives to breast-feeding and human milk. The earliest known feeding vessel was found in Phoenikas, Cyprus, and is dated circa 2000 BC.[2] Its shape is similar to the Greek vessel circa 500 BC shown in Figure 2. In the 18th century, "pap"- usually a mixture of bread, toast or baked flour and water - was used as an early weaning food. When milk, butter and/or broth were added, the mixture was called "panada." Other ingredients that might have been included were sugar, raw meat juices, beer, wine, Castile soap and drugs "to soothe the baby."[2] In 1784, Underwood criticized this human milk substitute saying, "It was indeed been a wonder to me how the custom of stuffing newborn babies with and such like could become so universal or the idea first enter the mind of a parent that such heavy food could be fit for the babies' nourishment at the age of six or seven months.

This food may be justly considered a poison, which, if not puked up, or very soon voided by stool, may occasion sickness, gripes (inward fits) and all the train of bowel complaints, which may terminate in Worms, Convulsions, Rickets, Scrofula, Slow Fevers, Purging and a fatal Marasmus."[1] In contrast, Underwood recommended cow milk diluted with barley water for the healthy baby. Nutrition knowledge has grown since the days of pap and panada, and infant nutrition is now a science unto itself. Although the science of infant nutrition is much more sophisticated today, the basic challenge remains: develop the best possible human milk substitute for infants who are not breast-fed.

Nutrient Levels in Human Milk Substitutes

Human milk is the standard with which all infant formulas are compared. Consequently, the goal in preparing human milk substitutes is to formulate an acceptable product that is nutritionally as close to human milk as possible (Figure 3). However, many nutrients are absorbed and used more efficiently from human milk than they are from infant formula. Consequently the protein, vitamin and mineral contents in infant formulas are usually somewhat higher than the levels in human milk. This helps assure adequate nutrient intake.

Over the past few decades, the nutrient profile of human milk and the needs of term infants have been relatively well defined. The importance of providing appropriate nutrient levels in infant formulas was dramatically illustrated by two separate occurrences. First, in the early 1950s, the vitamin B_6 content of a popular brand of infant formula was reduced by a

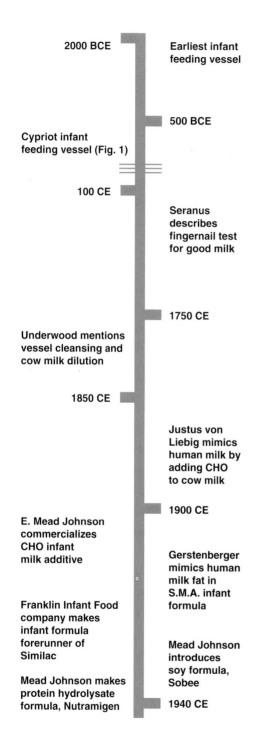

2000 BCE	**Earliest infant feeding vessel**
Cypriot infant feeding vessel (Fig. 1)	**500 BCE**
	100 CE
	Seranus describes fingernail test for good milk
	1750 CE
Underwood mentions vessel cleansing and cow milk dilution	
	1850 CE
	Justus von Liebig mimics human milk by adding CHO to cow milk
	1900 CE
E. Mead Johnson commercializes CHO infant milk additive	
	Gerstenberger mimics human milk fat in S.M.A. infant formula
Franklin Infant Food company makes infant formula forerunner of Similac	
	Mead Johnson introduces soy formula, Sobee
Mead Johnson makes protein hydrolysate formula, Nutramigen	**1940 CE**

Figure 1: Time line for highlighting use of human milk substitutes for feeding infants.

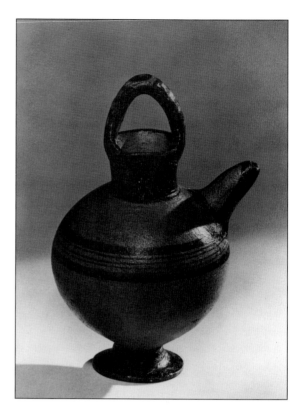

Figure 2: Infant feeding bottle from Cyprus, circa 500 B.C.

new heat processing technique employed by the manufacturer. Infants consuming the formula experienced irritability, gastrointestinal distress and convulsions. The cause of the convulsions was confirmed when they were corrected within minutes by injections of pyridoxine.[3] Second, in 1979, a soy formula was manufactured without adequate chloride. Infants consuming the formula experienced alkalosis, growth retardation, weakness and poor appetite. Most of the infants responded to supplementation with chloride and feedings of an infant formula with adequate chloride content.[4] Prompted by these occurrences, the United States Congress passed the Infant Formula Act in 1980 with revisions in 1985.[5] This law requires that all infant formulas distributed for general use contain levels of nutrients in specific ranges. The nutrient levels specified in the Infant Formula Act were based on the best available estimates of requirements from scientific

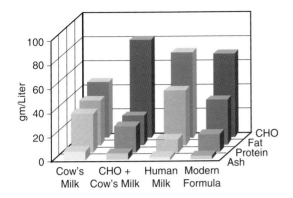

Figure 3: Comparison of the macro nutrient content of cow's milk.

literature or on recommendations of the American Academy of Pediatrics (AAP), Committee on Nutrition (CON). The Infant Formula Act nutrient requirements are listed in Table I. The Infant Formula Act also gives the United States Food and Drug Administration (FDA) authority to establish quality control and recall procedures related to infant formulas.

Some nutrient contents vary in infant formulas and others may decrease during processing or storage through shelf-life. Extra amounts (overages) of such nutrients above levels specified on the label are included in infant formulas to ensure that the nutrient levels are appropriate at the end of shelf-life. The addition of nutrients is carefully controlled during manufacture to assure that none are present at undesirable levels.

Composition of formulas designed to meet unique nutritional needs may differ substantially from the composition of human milk, since infants requiring these formulas may not be able to tolerate one or more of the components. In the United States, these special formulas are exempt from meeting the Infant Formula Act guidelines when the unique need requires nutrient levels deviating from the Act. (Figure 4)

Formulas for Toddlers

During the past decade, formulas have been introduced around the world for the older infant and young child. Such products often contain additional protein and minerals along with flavoring, and some sucrose

Nutrients	Minimum Level*	Maximum Level*
Protein, g	1.8	4.5
Fat, g	3.3	6.0
% of calories	30	54
Linoleic acid, mg	300	-
% of calories	2.7	-
Vitamins		
Vitamin A, IU	250	750
Vitamin D, IU	40	100
Vitamin E, IU	0.7	-
Vitamin K, µg	4	-
Thiamine (vitamin B_1), µg	40	-
Riboflavin (vitamin B_2), µg	60	-
Vitamin B_6, µg	35	-
Vitamin B_{12}, µg	0.15	-
Niacin[1], µg	250	-
Folic acid (folacin), µg	4	-
Pantothenic acid, µg	300	-
Biotin[2], µg	1.5	-
Vitamin C (ascorbic acid), mg	8	-
Choline[2], mg	7	-
Inositol[2], mg	4	-
Minerals		
Calcium, mg	60	-
Phosphorus, mg	30	-
Magnesium, mg	6	-
Iron, mg	0.15	3.0
Zinc, mg	0.5	-
Manganese, µg	5	-
Copper, µg	60	-
Iodine, µg	5	75
Sodium, mg	20	60
Potassium, mg	80	200
Chloride, mg	55	150

* Per 100 Calories
[1] The generic term "niacin" includes niacin (nicotinic acid) and niacinamide (nicotinamide).
[2] Required only for non-milk-based infant formulas.

Table 1: Nutrient levels per 100 calories specified by the Infant Formula Act.

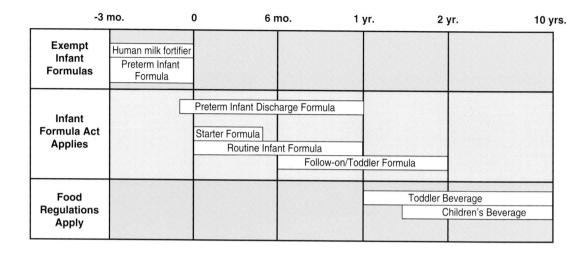

Figure 4: Cow milk-based formulas and beverages provide for the basic nutritional needs of most infants and young children.

and fiber. In the United States, some of these products comply with the Infant Formula Act and thus can be used in the latter part of the first year of life and the second year. Contrary to the recommendations of the AAP,[6] many parents begin feeding cow milk prior to 12 months of life. By encouraging parents to use a toddler beverage that meets Infant Formula Act recommendations, health care professionals can help prevent the negative consequences (such as iron deficiency) associated with early introduction of unmodified cow milk. Other nutritional beverages made for toddlers are food supplements not intended for use as a sole item of diet. Because they contain heat-treated protein and iron, they reduce potential concerns about protein-induced enteropathy and anemia associated with heavy use of whole cow milk. They also help assure appropriate intakes of vitamins that are not abundant in whole cow milk and in some cases, iron.

Complete Tube Feedings and Supplements for Children Ages One to Ten

There are no comprehensive guidelines (such as the Infant Formula Act) to determine the nutrient levels in complete tube feedings and supplements for children over the age of one year. Many nutrition scientists use the Recommended Dietary Allowances set forth by the National Research Council of the National Academy of Sciences[7] as well as patterns of dietary intake when

they determine the nutrient composition of these formulas. They also consider results of nutrition research conducted in the populations most likely to be using the product.

Protein

About 6% of the calories in human milk is from protein. In contrast, whole cow milk has 21% calories as protein. Underwood was perhaps the first to suggest using diluted cow milk for infant feeding.[1]

In the 19th century, scientists accepted the need to dilute the protein content of cow milk and to increase the proportion of carbohydrate to prepare a formula that more closely resembled human milk. The German chemist Justus Von Liebig, a student of infant nutrition, proposed a recipe for an infant feeding consisting of one part malt flour, one part wheat flour, two parts water and ten parts cow milk along with some potassium chloride.[8]

Today, cow milk protein is the base for most of the routine infant formula sold. Cow milk is readily available, reasonably priced, and well accepted by the medical community. In addition, it contains a complete protein and all of the essential amino acids in approximate proportions needed by humans.

Milk proteins are divided into two classes based on relative solubility in acid: whey (soluble) and casein (insoluble). Unmodified cow milk protein is about

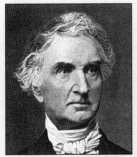

Justus von Liebig Ph.D.
(1803-1873) was a postdoctoral student of Gay-Lussac, a pupil of Lavoisier. Liebig was the father of the view that food proteins build the body and the non-proteins support respiration. He first envisioned the turnover of body tissues. Liebig developed the concept of minimal nutrient requirements for growth and health. In 1866, Liebig described the use of glucose oligomers (malzmehl) for the first artificial infant feeding using diluted cow milk designed to approximate human milk composition. J. Nutr. 7, 1-12,1934 (Etching courtesy of CNRC)

82% casein and 18% whey. When unheated casein-predominant cow milk protein enters the acidic environment of the stomach, it forms a relatively hard curd of casein and minerals that can be difficult for some infants to digest. In contrast, human milk protein is approximately 60 to 70% whey and 30 to 40% casein. It forms a very small, soft curd in acid. The differences in the whey-to-casein ratios between cow milk and human milk prompted some infant formula manufacturers to develop term infant formulas with higher proportions of whey than casein – termed whey-predominant or adapted formulas. The higher proportion of whey in whey-predominant formulas is achieved by combining equal amounts of demineralized whey protein with skim milk protein. Even though casein-predominant term infant formulas respond to acidity somewhat differently than do whey-predominant formulas, they result in equivalent growth and development. Commercial infant formulas made with cow milk proteins are heat-treated; as a result, they form smaller, softer curds than raw or pasteurized milk. Curd formation from infant formulas is similar to that of human milk (Figure 5).

Plasma and serum amino acid concentrations in infants fed formulas with whey-predominant or casein-predominant protein sources have been studied in several laboratories with varying results. Neither protein source results in amino acid patterns identical to those in human milk-fed infants, but the minor differences reported have been judged to be of little or no

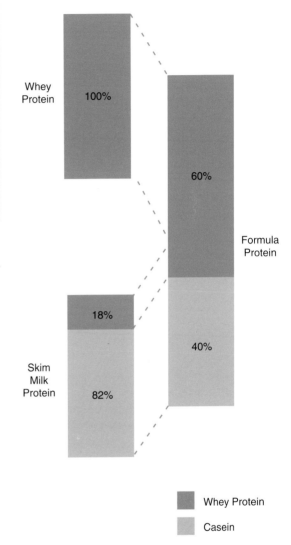

Figure 5: Approximating the whey:casein ratio of human milk.

physiological significance. Debate over which protein source results in serum amino acid patterns and concentrations closest to those in human milk-fed infants is difficult to resolve because of so many influential factors. These include the amount of protein fed; time of blood sampling after feeding; age of the infants; laboratory procedures and analytical equipment; and interpretation of the results.

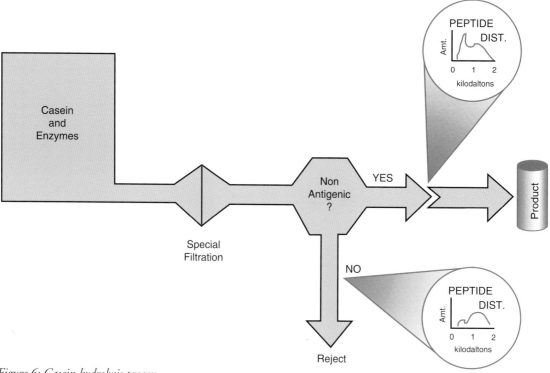

Figure 6: Casein hydrolysis process.

Heat treatment of cow milk protein during the manufacture of infant formula modifies the protein and reduces the allergenic properties of the protein to some extent. However, some infants remain sensitive to the cow milk protein in infant formulas. Alternate protein sources have been developed to meet the needs of these infants. The soybean contains an abundant amount of relatively high-quality protein, and some early cow milk-free formulas contained soy bean flour. However, the indigestible carbohydrate in the soy flour led to loose, bulky stools. A more satisfactory formula results when the soy protein is first isolated from the flour, then processed into a balanced formulation. The protein availability increases substantially because of the heat treatment required. However, the protein efficiency ratio (PER) of soy protein isolate alone does not quite equal that of casein. By supplementing the soy protein with the amino acid methionine, its protein quality improves to nearly equal that of milk protein. Therefore, most modern soy formulas are made with soy protein isolate supplemented with methionine.

In the 1940s, formulas containing extensively hydrolyzed casein were designed for infants who need to avoid intact protein. To manufacture an extensively hydrolyzed casein, casein is incubated with proteolytic enzymes until no intact protein remains. The crude hydrolysate is purified and tested for antigenicity before it is used in infant formula. The residual antigenicity of this casein hydrolysate is less than 1/100,000 (0.001%) of that of the starting material, intact casein. In other words, the antigenicity of casein is reduced by more than 99.99%. The pre-clinical and clinical trial section and the quality assurance section of this chapter further discuss the qualification of hypoallergenic proteins. During processing of the protein, levels of the amino acids cystine, tyrosine and tryptophan decrease. Adding these amino acids during product manufacturing ensures protein quality equal to or greater than that of casein. Some European manufacturers use extensively hydrolyzed whey to manufacture hypoallergenic formulas, even though many whey proteins are more resistant to hydrolysis (Figure 6).

Formulas containing extensively hydrolyzed casein sold in the U.S. meet the hypoallergenic criteria recommended by the American Academy of Pediatrics.[9] According to Sampson and colleagues, extensively hydrolyzed casein is not recognized as cow milk protein by most allergic infants, and formulas containing such protein can be used successfully.[10] These formulas should be considered hypoallergenic, not nonallergenic, however, since rare reactions have been documented.[11-13] There is no documentation of successful double-blind placebo-controlled food challenge trials with formulas containing extensively hydrolyzed whey. Anaphylactic reactions to formulas containing extensively hydrolyzed whey have been reported.[14]

Some manufacturers produce formulas with partially hydrolyzed proteins. In these formulas, the protein is not hydrolyzed as extensively and some large peptides remain. While the physical characteristics (taste, smell, color) of formulas made with partial hydrolysates may be more desirable than those in extensively hydrolyzed formulas, these formulas cannot be fed to cow milk-allergic infants because they do not meet the established criteria and may trigger anaphylaxis. In the United States at this time, the only indication for formula with partially hydrolyzed proteins is for routine feeding of healthy term infants (Figure 7).

Other Special Products

Inborn errors of amino acid metabolism require limiting dietary intake of one or more specific, essential amino acids. Products designed for patients with these disorders contain little or none of the offending amino acid. The "protein" component of such products consists of either selected crystalline amino acids or extensively hydrolyzed protein processed to reduce the amount of the offending amino acid(s). These products are generally made to address the needs of two groups: infants and older persons. They provide most of the protein along with vitamins and minerals according to the needs of the two groups. Some products also contain additional calories as carbohydrate and fat, providing patients and health care providers with a choice of the most convenient formulation to meet their needs.

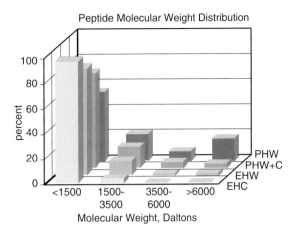

Peptide Molecular Weight Distribution

Figure 7: Typical cow milk protein hydrolysates include extensively hydrolyzed casein (EHC), extensively hydrolyzed whey (EHW), partially hydrolyzed whey and casein (PHW+C), and partially hydrolyzed whey (PHW).

The most common inborn error of metabolism is phenylketonuria (PKU). One of the earliest products made for this condition used protein hydrolysate processed to lower phenylalanine levels; this product is still in wide use today, especially in infants. Some other products for this condition are made with crystalline amino acids without including any phenylalanine. This permits patients to consume their entire phenylalanine requirement from normal foods and gives them the maximum flexibility possible in food choices. The remaining protein requirement is provided by the product.

Protein-free formulas were developed so that specific amino acid mixtures could be added to provide an appropriate infant formula for patients with inborn errors of amino acid metabolism for whom products are not available. They are also used as protein-free calorie supplements for infants and children on protein restricted diets.

Tube Feedings and Oral Supplements

Tube feeding, oral supplement products designed to meet the nutritional needs of children age one to ten years generally contain intact cow milk proteins such as caseinate, whey protein concentrate and/or milk protein isolate. Most recently, elemental formulas with

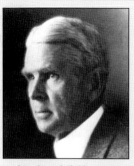

Emmett Holt, Sr., M.D.
(1855-1924) graduated from the College of Physicians and Surgeons, New York. Holt was appointed Professor of Pediatrics at New York Medical School in 1891. Responding to a need for the education of nurses, Holt wrote *The Care and Feeding of Children* in 1894. This book went through 12 revisions. Holt was the first recipient of funds from the Rockefeller Foundation which were used on studies of nutritional biochemistry in infants. Holt was a moderate in the debate about the percentage method of artificial feeding and complained, "would that the average physician knew how to use intelligently a half dozen formulas." *Pediatric Profiles* editor B. S. Veeder, Mosby, St. Louis, 1957, 33-60 (Photo courtesy of NLM)

protein from crystalline amino acids have been designed for children over the age of one year.

Protein Modules

Modular protein sources are available for supplementing infant feedings when more protein is desired. The protein sources for these modules include casein, calcium caseinate and cow milk whey protein. Some of the products contain significant levels of vitamins and minerals.

Fat

Experts agree that "...the profile of fatty acids in human milk is our best model at this time on which to base the fat composition of infant formula."[15] Fat provides about 50% of the energy in human milk. About 40% of the fatty acids are saturated with about half of the saturated fatty acids from palmitic acid. About 35 to 40% of the fatty acids are monounsaturated, primarily oleic acid and 10 to 20% are polyunsaturated, primarily linoleic acid. The fat in human milk is well absorbed. In contrast, fat from unmodified cow milk is poorly absorbed. Modern infant formulas contain one or more vegetable oils to improve fat absorption and provide essential fatty acids.

Linoleic acid (an omega 6 or n-6 fatty acid) and α-linolenic acid (an omega 3 or n-3 fatty acid) are essential fatty acids for infants because they cannot be made in the

body. The Infant Formula Act specifies that at least 2.7% of the calories in an infant formula come from linoleic acid. The Act does not specify an amount of α-linolenic acid, since it has only recently been recognized as essential for the infant. However, expert groups such as the European Society for Pediatric Gastroenterology and Nutrition recommend that the ratio of linoleic acid to α-linolenic acid be about 5:1-15:1.[16]

In recent years, much research on the fatty acid composition of human milk has been published. With improved technology and increased availability of a variety of oils, infant formula manufacturers can now more easily duplicate the fatty acid pattern of human milk by using combinations of oils. By blending oleo with vegetable oils, Wyeth was the first company to include a fat blend with a fatty acid pattern similar to human milk. Now 100% vegetable oil blends can be used to closely duplicate the major fatty acid pattern of human milk.

Oils in Infant Formulas

Oleo is an animal fat rich in saturated fatty acids but its use precludes a formula from Kosher certification. Coconut oil contributes low levels of the intermediate chain saturated fatty acids lauric and myristic, similar to levels found in human milk. Palm olein oil provides formulas with a level of palmitic acid similar to typical levels in human milk; it is made by fractionally crystallizing palm oil. The crystallization removes some of the longer chain saturated fatty acids. Thus, palm olein oil contains a higher proportion of unsaturated fatty acids, especially oleic acid, and lower proportions of longer chain saturated fatty acids (such as stearic and palmitic acids) compared to palm oil.

High oleic sunflower and high oleic safflower oils are major sources of oleic acid required to match human milk levels. Corn oil is an important source of the essential fatty-acid linoleic acid and soy oil provides both linoleic and α-linolenic acid.

Since palm oil is rather poorly absorbed by infants, some health care professionals have also questioned the absorption of palm olein oil. However, palm olein contains lower levels of palmitic and stearic acids, two fatty acids that are absorbed less well than others. Palm olein oil is also higher in better absorbed unsaturated fats. Some have also claimed that fat (and energy) absorption

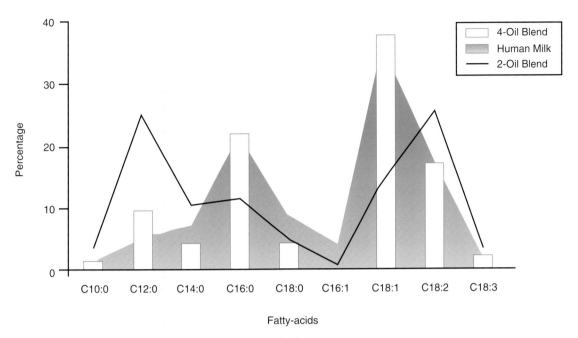

Figure 8: Fatty-acid profiles of fat blends used in infant feedings.

would be compromised since palmitic acid from vegetable oils is not enriched in the middle or beta-position in the triglyceride molecule as it is in human milk. However, when human milk and an infant formula with a vegetable oil blend mimicking human milk are compared, the difference of energy absorption due to the difference in palmitic acid position is estimated to be only about 2%.[17, 18] Furthermore, fat balance studies in growing premature infants show that formulations containing amounts of palm olein sufficient to mimic human milk palmitic acid levels are just as well absorbed as the human milk fat they emulate.[19]

Some consumers and health care professionals also question the practice of using tropical oils such as coconut oil and other highly saturated fats in infant formulas, since these fats have been associated with elevated serum lipids in adults. However, expert groups including the Expert Panel on Blood Cholesterol Levels in Children and Adolescents,[20] the American Academy of Pediatrics[21] and the American Heart Association[22] recommend that the diets of children under the age of two should not be modified in total or saturated fat content. Saturated fat is needed to duplicate the fatty acids in human milk and higher levels of fat are needed to ensure adequate energy intakes.

MCT (medium chain triglyceride) oil is made by saponifying coconut oil, separating the medium chain fatty acids, and then re-esterifying them. Medium chain triglycerides partially circumvent the hydrolysis, emulsification and micelle formation required to absorb typical food fats. MCTs typically do not require bile salts for digestion and absorption. After absorption, medium chain fatty acids are not generally incorporated into chylomicrons, but bypass the lymphatics and are transported in the blood as free fatty acids. Furthermore, they are largely metabolized as an immediate source of energy instead of being elongated and modified to form cholesterol or stored as fat.

Long Chain Polyunsaturated Fatty Acids

Recent data indicate that two long chain polyunsaturated fatty acids (LCP) found in human milk may be conditionally essential. These are docosahexaenoic acid (DHA, an omega 3 or n-3 fatty acid derived from α-linolenic acid) and arachidonic acid (ARA, an omega 6 or n-6 fatty acid derived from linoleic acid). Sources of LCP include marine oils (fish oil, a source of DHA) microbial oils (algal for DHA and fungal for ARA), egg lipids and animal organ fats. Egg lipids and animal organ fats can provide both ARA and DHA but in fairly low concentrations. Combinations of marine oils and/or microbial oils are needed to provide sources of both ARA and DHA. Each source of LCP is associated with safety issues.

Marine Oils

In one study, preterm infants fed formula supplemented with marine oil to nine months adjusted age had significantly poorer growth than infants who were not supplemented.[23] These infants also had lower plasma phospholipid ARA. The authors suggested that the poor growth may have been related to a high level of eicosapentaenoic acid (EPA, another omega 3 or n-3 LCP) in the marine oil. High levels of EPA may interfere with ARA synthesis and metabolism, causing depressed ARA levels which may affect growth. However, in a second study in which marine oil with lower EPA levels was fed until the adjusted age of two months, growth of the supplemented infants was again lower than growth of infants fed standard formula.[24] The plasma phospholipid ARA levels did not differ between the groups. The authors speculated that the higher DHA intake influenced the balance of n-6 to n-3 LCP in the infants' tissues causing growth to be negatively affected. Yet another study found no abnormalities in growth, clotting function, red blood cell membrane fluidity or plasma vitamin A or E levels in healthy, very-low-birth weight infants fed formula supplemented with marine oil (with relatively high EPA levels) up to four months adjusted age.[25] Although the exact reason for the poor growth in the first studies are unclear, scientists now suggest that LCP supplemented formulas should provide both DHA and ARA to ensure that both n-3 and n-6 LCP are available to the growing infant in sufficient amounts.

> *In discussing infant feeding Schick stressed the importance of the sterility of the formula rather than its composition. He enlarged on this subject in his reminiscences of "Pediatrics in Vienna at the Beginning of the Century". Schick quoted Kassowitz' excellent results using cow's milk in infant feeding. Kassowitz said, "The whole problem could be solved if cow's milk could flow from the breast of the mother." Schick commented, "This classic remark hit the nail on the head. Milk is an excellent culture medium for bacteria. If the infant cannot be breast-fed and no refrigeration is available, milk should be fed directly from the animal to the baby. The closer the baby is to the animal, the better, as in Italy, where the goat was driven into the courtyard to be milked for the baby's feeding.*
>
> *Aphorisms and Facetiae*
> *of Bela Schick*
> I.J. Wolf, M.D., Editor, 1965

DHA-rich marine oils with low EPA levels are now commercially available. These oils are refined to reduce concerns about potential contaminants such as pesticides and heavy metals.

Microbial Oils

Microbial oils high in DHA or ARA with essentially no EPA are available in limited quantities. Several companies are developing sources. These sources are undergoing extensive analytical, toxicological and clinical testing to confirm their safety.

Egg Lipids

Egg lipids contain both ARA and DHA. However, large amounts must be added to formulas to reach the desired concentrations. As a result, the phospholipid content of the formula increases to levels much greater than those found in human milk or typical infant formula.

Animal Organ Fats

There are no commercial sources of animal organ fats and their safety as food additives has not been documented.

Other Considerations

Because of the high degree of unsaturation of LCP, lipid autoxidation is a concern. Autoxidation can lead to rancidity and undesirable oxidation products. High-quality LCP oils and appropriate antioxidants and manufacturing processes should overcome these concerns.

No sources of LCP are currently generally regarded as safe (GRAS) or approved as additives for infant formulas in the United States. Consequently, before adding LCP to infant formulas in the U.S., infant formula manufacturers must be able to demonstrate that the source of LCP is safe. In other countries, however, some infant formula manufacturers already add sources of LCP.

Hypoallergenic Formulas

Highly refined and purified oils, such as those used in infant formulas, are nonallergenic because they do not contain protein. Therefore, oils such as corn and soy oil can be used in hypoallergenic formulas without concern for allergic reactions. In the past, it has been difficult for formula manufacturers to make hypoallergenic formulas with levels of fat as high as routine formulas because extensively hydrolyzed protein does not support the formula matrix and the physical characteristics of the formula are adversely affected. Consequently, the level of fat in some hypoallergenic formulas was lower than the level in routine formulas. Recently, these challenges have been overcome using specially modified starches and emulsifiers and the fat levels in such products have been increased nearly to levels found in human milk.

Other Special Formulas

The characteristics of MCT oil make it beneficial for patients with fat malabsorption. Fat malabsorption is common in disorders such as short gut syndrome, cystic fibrosis, biliary atresia, severe chronic diarrhea and monosaccharide intolerance. MCT oil-containing formulas are often used in patients with these conditions. It is important to remember that MCT oil contains no essential fatty acids. Infants with cholestatic disease who are fed formulas with 80% or more of the fat from MCT oil and only 3.5% of the fatty acids from linoleic acid may be at increased risk for essential fatty acid deficiency.[26, 27] In such patients, supplementation with linoleic acid and possibly α-linolenic acid should be considered.

Tube Feedings and Supplements

Thirty-seven to 44% of the calories in tube feedings and supplements designed for children come from fat. A significant proportion of the fat in these products often comes from MCT oil.

Carbohydrate

The carbohydrate in human milk is primarily lactose, a disaccharide composed of glucose and galactose. A minor but significant portion is composed of carbohydrate oligomers. Cow milk and cow milk-based formulas in the U.S. generally contain lactose as the carbohydrate source.

Some infants are born with congenital defects affecting lactose digestion or metabolism, while other infants may have transient problems with lactose. Congenital lactase deficiency can occur but is very rare. Infants with congenital lactase deficiency require lactose-free diets for life. Moderately severe diarrhea can depress intestinal lactase activity and otherwise healthy infants can become lactose intolerant following acute diarrheal illness. These babies may require lactose-free formulas for a period. Infants with the metabolic disorder galactosemia must follow galactose-free diets for life.

In the past, soy protein formulas and casein hydrolysate formulas without lactose were fed to lactose intolerant infants. The carbohydrate in these formulas is usually supplied by glucose polymers and/or sucrose. Soy and non-lactose-containing protein hydrolysate formulas remain appropriate choices for infants on lactose-free diets today. However, when these formulas are used, eliminating lactose is accompanied by a change in protein making an etiologic diagnosis difficult – it is unclear whether the improvement is due to the protein or the carbohydrate change. The alternate protein source can also affect the taste and increase the cost of the formula. Advances in technology have led to developing lactose-free formulas containing 100% cow milk protein; such products have a similar taste and price to milk-based formulas, yet are appropriate for infants who require a lactose-free diet (Figure 9). They are also helpful in diagnosing whether a problem with milk-based formula is related to the lactose or the protein.

Traces of lactose and galactose can be found in casein hydrolysate formulas and lactose-free milk-based formulas. Some practitioners do not feel that the small amounts of residual galactose in these products are a problem, and use these products for managing patients with galactosemia. Soy formulas are also used. Soybeans contain the oligosaccharides stachyose and raffinose. These oligosaccharides contain a small amount of galactose. Studies have shown, however, that these oligosaccharides are not digested; therefore,

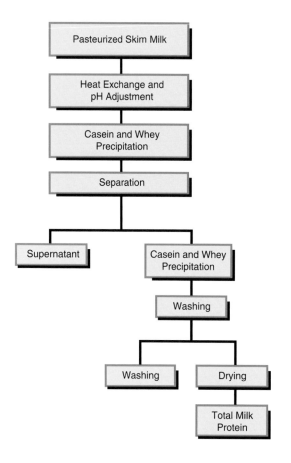

Figure 9: Extracting total milk protein from skim milk to make lactose-free cow milk formulas.

they are not a source of galactose. When subjects with galactosemia were given soy formula,[28] stachyose or raffinose[29] levels of galactose-1-phosphate in the erythrocyte did not increase.

In addition to lactose intolerance, some infants with diarrhea experience a significant reduction in intestinal sucrase activity with sucrose intolerance. Formulas with glucose polymers as the only carbohydrate can be fed to infants with sucrose intolerance as well as to those with lactose intolerance. Since sucrose intolerance is dose-dependent, some infants may also be able to tolerate a reduced sucrose intake.

Rarely, diarrhea can be so protracted and severe that it leads to disaccharide intolerance, glucose polymer intolerance and glucose intolerance. For infants with this problem, scientists developed formulas that are complete except that the carbohydrate is significantly

reduced or eliminated altogether. Some of these products are designed for infants who have carbohydrate intolerance accompanied by protein intolerance and/or fat malabsorption; they contain extensively hydrolyzed casein and MCT oil along with a balance of other essential nutrients. Others contain intact protein and no MCT oil. All of these formulas require added carbohydrate as indicated by the needs and tolerance of the patient.

Lactose and Calcium Absorption

Since lactose promotes calcium absorption, some health care professionals have questioned if calcium is adequately absorbed from lactose-free formulas. Researchers have found that glucose polymers also enhance calcium absorption in humans.[30-31] The results of metabolic balance studies of infants fed a milk-based, lactose-free formula showed that calcium absorption and retention were similar to the values reported by others for milk-based formulas.[32-34] In addition, no differences in calcium status as measured by bone mineral content were found when infants fed a cow milk-based lactose-free formula were compared to those fed a milk-based formula with lactose.[35] Soy formulas containing glucose polymers either with or without sucrose[36,37] also promote good bone mineral content.

Fiber and Starch

Since infant formula manufacturers strive to emulate human milk and human milk contains no fiber, fiber is not added to routine formulas. High fiber intakes may also interfere with adequate caloric intake and inhibit the absorption of minerals including trace elements.[38] Recently, however, Ross developed a soy-based infant formula with soy fiber, for short term feeding of infants with diarrhea. The added fiber holds water and the fiber-supplemented formula has been shown to reduce the number of watery stools during mild to severe diarrhea. Duration of the illness is not affected, however.[39]

Pediatricians often recommend feeding formula thickened with cereal to infants with simple regurgitation. Commercially thickened formulas have been introduced in several countries. The thickening agent in the formulas may be starch provided as a portion

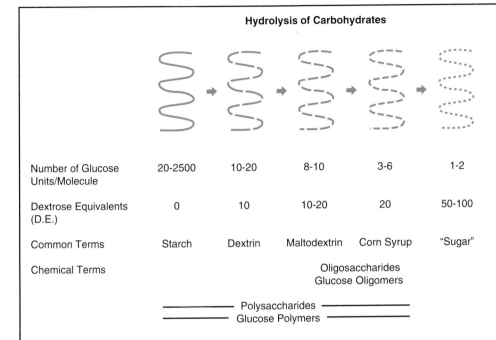

Hydrolysis of Carbohydrates

Number of Glucose Units/Molecule	20-2500	10-20	8-10	3-6	1-2
Dextrose Equivalents (D.E.)	0	10	10-20	20	50-100
Common Terms	Starch	Dextrin	Maltodextrin	Corn Syrup	"Sugar"

Chemical Terms — Oligosaccharides / Glucose Oligomers

Polysaccharides / Glucose Polymers

*D.E. reducing sugar content as per cost of d-glucose

Hydrolysis of Carbohydrates

The breakdown of large starch molecules into smaller and smaller glucose polymers is achieved via hydrolysis and is depicted in the figure above. Notice that this process can be interrupted at any point to yield the size of glucose polymer desired. This is important in infant formula manufacture because:
1. It allows the formulation of lactose-free products with small molecular weight carbohydrates that can be readily utilized by infants who cannot digest lactose.
2. By varying the amounts of the various glucose polymers in the formula, i.e., starch, dextrin, corn syrup, "sugar", etc. the osmolality of the finished product can be controlled while still providing the proper total amount of carbohydrates.
3. Starch molecules can be utilized to keep fats in a stabilized emulsion.

Figure 10: Modular carbohydrate products.

of the nutritional carbohydrate or non-absorbed gums or fibers. Compared to routine formulas, thickened formulas have higher viscosity which generally increases even further with acidification such as occurs in the stomach.

Modular Carbohydrate Products

Modular carbohydrate products provided by formula manufacturers are made with glucose polymers prepared by partial hydrolysis of corn starch. Their molecular size averages four to six glucose units. Lactose,

glucose and fructose are also available from pharmacies and sucrose (table sugar) from pharmacies and food stores. These mono- and disaccharides can be used as additional carbohydrate with low-carbohydrate or carbohydrate-free formulas (Figure 10).

Tube Feedings and Supplements

In general, formula manufacturers strive to make tube feedings and supplements lactose-free. This allows these products to be used and tolerated by individuals who are chronically or acutely sensitive to lactose. Tube feedings and supplements often contain glucose polymers (hydrolyzed cornstarch or corn syrup solids). Sucrose may be included to enhance acceptance of products consumed orally. Fiber may be included in some and/or added to others to help normalize bowel function if needed.

Vitamins

Vitamins are included in complete infant formulas in accordance with regulatory requirements (such as the Infant Formula Act in the U.S.) or recommendations of expert panels. In general, water-soluble vitamin needs are dependent upon caloric intake because most water-soluble vitamins are needed as coenzymes in energy metabolism reactions. Therefore, water-soluble vitamins can be incorporated in the formula according to caloric content. In contrast, recommendations for fat-soluble vitamins are more constant and independent of caloric intake. For example, 400 IU of vitamin D are recommended per day regardless of the level of energy consumed. Formula intakes of term infants tend to be relatively constant over time and the daily fat-soluble vitamin requirements can be incorporated in an appropriate amount of formula.

Minerals

Levels of most minerals in term formulas are within the ranges found in human milk. The safe range of sodium intakes for newborn infants is narrow compared with older individuals, due to their renal immaturity. For this reason, sodium content of infant formulas is closely monitored to keep it within a safe but adequate range.

Potassium content in formulas is kept within physiologic proportions of the sodium and chloride levels. Adequate chloride for normal metabolism of hydrogen ion is assured by ongoing monitoring of formula production (see quality control discussion). Molar equivalents of Na:K are generally kept in the range of 0.3:1 to 1:1, whereas (Na +K)/Cl molar ratio is usually between 1.5 and 2.5, consistent with ratios seen in human milk.

The bones of the rapidly-growing infant require abundant calcium and phosphorus to assure normal development. Formulas generally contain more of these minerals than does human milk; these minerals are more bioavailable from human milk than formulas. However, the relatively low solubility of these minerals in formulas creates challenges for incorporating large amounts into infant feedings. Nevertheless, the amounts of calcium and phosphorus provided by formulas generally result in formula-fed infants having bone mineral contents equaling or exceeding those of infants fed human milk.

In the U.S., cow milk formulas are available in low-iron and iron-fortified varieties. However, the American Academy of Pediatrics Committee on Nutrition recommends that infants who are not breast-fed receive iron-fortified formulas for the first year of life in order to prevent iron deficiency anemia and its consequences.[40] In the United States, iron-fortified formulas generally provide 12 mg iron per quart. The FDA specifies that the iron content of formulas in the U.S. range from 0.15 to 3.0 mg iron per 100 kcal (0.96 to 19.2 mg per quart). Most low-iron formulas in the U.S. contain 1-1.5 mg iron per quart, but one contains 4.5 mg iron per quart. Figure 11 illustrates how much iron would be consumed by infants on various formulas and compares the intakes to the Recommended Dietary Allowance for iron.[7] It is estimated that the amount of iron absorbed from low-iron formula with 4.5 mg per iron per quart is at least as much as the amount of iron absorbed from human milk. Only cow milk formulas come in low-iron and iron-fortified varieties. Other formulas such as soy, lactose-free cow milk formulas and hypoallergenic formulas are all iron-fortified.

The wide variety of fluoride levels in water across the United States led to uncertainty among some pediatricians regarding appropriate fluoride supplementation schedules for formula-fed infants. At one time, a number of manufacturing plants where infant formulas were made used water from municipal supplies that contained supplemental fluoride. In 1979, manufacturers decided to use only water that was low in fluoride to make infant formulas. Thus, the potential for undesirable fluoride intakes resulting from adding local fluoridated water to fluoride-containing formula was reduced. Health care professionals can now make informed decisions regarding fluoride supplementation based on the local water supplies and other relevant considerations.

Aluminum occurs naturally in food and water supplies. Consequently, infant formulas contain some aluminum. Infant formula manufacturers take steps to lower the aluminum content of infant formulas. Manufacturers specify maximum aluminum levels for raw ingredients such as water, mineral salts and protein sources, and they monitor the aluminum contents of formulas. Soy formulas and protein hydrolysates contain higher levels of aluminum than milk based formulas. The aluminum content of soy protein isolate reflects the aluminum content of the soil in which the soybean is grown. In addition, soy formulas and protein hydrolysate formulas contain more added mineral salts than milk-based formulas, causing the aluminum contents to be higher.

The Food and Agriculture Organization and the World Health Organization have established a provisional tolerable intake of aluminum. They suggest that infants consume no more than 1 mg aluminum per kg body weight per day.[41] An infant weighing 6 kg who consumes one quart of a typical milk, soy or casein hydrolysate formula per day would receive an amount of aluminum well below the provisional tolerable intake. In addition, a study by Litov and colleagues found no difference between serum aluminum concentrations in breast-fed and formula-fed infants.[42]

Other Factors Found in Human Milk

When scientific evidence indicates that a new substance may be needed in the infant's diet, it is generally incorporated quickly into infant formulas after appropriate testing for safety and tolerance. Such factors that have been added in the past have included choline, inositol, taurine and carnitine. Researchers have hypothesized there may be clinical benefits, such as better resistance to illness, from dietary nucleotide supplementation. However, these proposed benefit theories have not yet been clinically substantiated. Nevertheless, the presence of nucleotides in human milk suggests that they may have a role to play in infant feeding.

Fresh human milk does contain a number of non-nutritional factors not present in modern formulas. These include such things as living white blood cells, antibodies to organisms in the mother's environment, and hormones, as well as factors that encourage the growth of selective types of bacteria in the intestinal

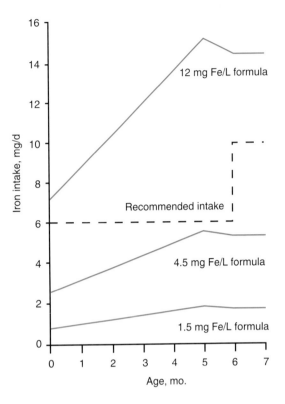

Figure 11: Daily iron intakes from infant formulas during the first six months of life.

tract and inhibit colonization by others. While some future formula may also contain some of these, many scientific and regulatory issues remain to be resolved.

Osmolality and Renal Solute Load
Osmolality

Human milk is iso-osmolar and infant formula manufacturers strive to make human milk substitutes iso-osmolar as well. Osmolality can be an important determinant of formula tolerance. If the osmolality is too high, it may draw water from the intestinal cells, interfere with nutrient and water absorption, and/or cause diarrhea. Figure 12 depicts how much each of the major components of a formula contributes to the total osmolality if the formula contains 20 kcal/oz, with 12% of the calories provided as protein, 45% of the calories as fat and 43% of the calories as carbohydrate. Clearly, the saccharides are the major contributors to formula

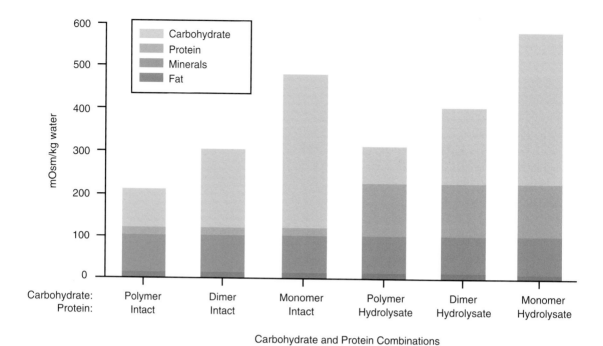

Figure 12: Contribution to osmolality.

osmolality. Selected saccharides can be used to produce a formula that will meet nutrient specifications and have an appropriate osmolality.

Renal Solute Load

The reserve renal capacity of the full-term newborn is limited. Hence, renal solute load is an important factor to consider in infant formula design. The following calculation compares renal solute factors of infant formulas computed as the Potential Renal Solute Load (PRSL):

$$PRSL(mOsm) = \frac{Protein\ (gms)}{0.175} + Na + K + Cl + P$$

where the mineral units are millimoles and all are expressed either per unit volume or per unit of energy.[43] The first term on the right calculates the potential number of millimoles of urea which could be formed from the protein. The actual renal solute load for the infant is normally somewhat less than the PRSL, since not all of the ingested nitrogen and minerals are excreted in the urine. Although there are some urinary constituents not included in the calculation for PRSL, the equation accounts for the major factors and serves as a basis for estimating potential renal stress. Thus, for an infant consuming a typical term infant formula at the rate of 100 kcal/kg/day, PRSL might be 20 mOsm/kg/day.

Preclinical and Clinical Evaluation of Infant Formulas

An essential part of establishing product safety, tolerance, and nutritional adequacy is through preclinical and clinical testing commensurate with changes in or development of infant formulas. Animal studies are useful for verifying protein quality, the bioavailability of selected nutrients, and characteristics of hypoallergenic formulas before clinical studies are started in human infants. A new product is released for general use in infants only after careful, controlled, clinical studies compare performance of the new formulation to human milk and/or formulas for which there is a substantial history of successful use in infants. Such clinical studies conform to rigorous scientific standards and follow scientific review and Institutional Review Board approval.[44]

Preclinical Studies

Protein Quality

The nutritional quality of any protein is related to the balance among the amino acids in the protein, the availability of those amino acids from the diet, and the needs of the test subject. There is no universally accepted test for comparing the quality of protein sources. However, a generally recognized compromise is the protein equivalency ratio (PER) assay.

In this test, young rats are fed a diet containing 10% control or test protein for a defined period, and the rat's growth is measured. Growth per gram of protein on the test is then compared to growth per gram of protein on the control. Growth on the test protein is expressed as a percentage of growth on the control protein. Casein is the official reference or control protein when the PER test is conducted as specified by the Association of Official Analytical Chemists.[45] The American Academy of Pediatrics Committee on Nutrition has recommended, and the FDA regulations on infant formula specify, that the PER of proteins used in infant formulas cannot be less than 70% of casein. Also, in 100 kcal of formula, the equivalent of at least 1.8 gm of protein with a PER of 100% casein must be supplied. Total protein content must not exceed 4.5 gm/100 kcal.[5]

Minerals

Animal studies also provide useful information on how minerals interact with each other and with other nutrients in infant formulas. In these studies, the amount of minerals ingested can be controlled and determined. Likewise, the amount excreted can be measured. From these measurements, scientists estimate relative mineral bioavailability. Results must be interpreted carefully, recognizing the limitations of the models used. However, these studies do provide information that help scientists assess the suitability of ingredients and/or the effects of processing on mineral bioavailability.

Hypoallergenic Formulas

Preclinical testing (physicochemical and immunochemical) of hypoallergenic formulas is needed to document that the protein source is consistent from batch to batch and that the antigenicity of the protein is significantly reduced. In these ways, preclinical testing helps assure consistent clinical performance of the product. Physicochemical tests provide information on the molecular weight profile of the protein. Formol titration or trinitrobenzenesulfonic acid can be used to estimate the percentage of peptide bonds broken during protein hydrolysis and to provide an estimate of the degree of hydrolysis.[46] The degree of hydrolysis of some hydrolyzed casein products for example is greater than 50%. This means that the protein is extensively hydrolyzed. Chromatographic analyses provide information on the molecular weight distribution of the peptides in the hydrolysate.

Immunochemical testing is used to estimate residual antigenicity and immunogenicity of the protein. Enzyme linked immunosorbent assay (ELISA) and radioimmunoassay are the preferred antigenicity tests. They measure the hydrolysate's ability to react with antibody obtained from animals that are sensitive to the protein from which the hydrolysate is derived. Animal models (such as the cow milk-sensitive guinea pig) can also be used for estimating residual antigenicity. The results from these tests are not as precise as ELISA. Nevertheless, tests of immunogenicity always include animal models during product development. However, only clinical trials in humans can document that a protein is hypoallergenic in humans. In any event, preclinical testing helps scientists predict how the protein will be tolerated with reasonable accuracy.[46]

Clinical Studies

Protein Utilization

New protein sources and/or new combinations of proteins may be evaluated in several ways. Evaluations include classical nitrogen balance studies and standard growth, acceptance and tolerance studies. These clinical studies may sometimes involve measuring of fasting and/or postprandial plasma amino acid profiles and urea nitrogen levels.

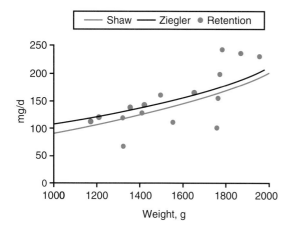

Figure 13: Calcium retention study. Smooth curves are estimates of intrauterine calcium accretion.

Fat Utilization

Careful fat balance studies determine the use of fat from a new fat source or new blend of fats or oils. Subsequent growth studies provide additional information on their utility as calorie sources.

Carbohydrate Utilization

A carbohydrate's suitability for use in infant formulas can be evaluated by the breath hydrogen, stool pH and stool characteristics of infants enrolled in clinical studies. Growth is also an indirect indicator of carbohydrate utilization, since the carbohydrate constitutes 40 to 50% of the calories in many formulas.

Mineral Balance/Availability

Several types of studies are used to evaluate mineral utilization. Balance studies indirectly measure infants' absorption of calcium, phosphorus, magnesium and other key minerals. In addition, stable isotope methods directly assess absorption of some minerals. Photon absorptiometry estimates the bone mineral content achieved while consuming various diets. It is another indicator of the relative availability of calcium and phosphorus from the feedings.

Serum mineral concentrations may document that the form and levels provided by the formulas support normal physiological function in infants. Careful attention to potential excesses as well as to potential deficiencies is important. A number of indirect para-

meters such as assays of alkaline phosphatase, parathyroid hormone and vitamin D metabolites (calcium/phosphorus/vitamin D), ferritin (iron stores) and ceruloplasmin (copper) may reflect the adequacy of provided minerals.

Figure 13 depicts a mineral retention study done in preterm infants.[47] In this example, calcium was evaluated, but similar studies are done for other minerals. The figure illustrates that as the preterm infant gains weight, the amount of retained calcium increases. The calcium accretion rates of the preterm infants are compared to intrauterine calcium accretion rates, e.g., as estimated by Ziegler[48] or Shaw.[49] Here, calcium retention is the difference between calcium consumed from formula and calcium excreted in the stools and urine.

Vitamins

Blood concentrations of selected vitamins are often monitored during clinical studies in infants to assure adequacy and safety. This is especially true when vitamin levels are changed or when new sources of vitamins are used.

Specific Growth Studies

Figure 14 illustrates the results of a typical growth study. Infants are observed over an extended period and their intake and growth noted. The two outside lines represent the range of normal growth and the middle dark line is the mean growth curve. Plots for individual infants are then made; in this case, all infants grew within the normal range.

Fomon, et al.[50] described a 112-day growth study that provides an excellent clinical evaluation of the nutritional adequacy of an infant formula in an integrated way. Studies involving very cooperative parents and infants of one sex (males and females have different growth patterns) accurately determine intake and growth. Results from infants consuming test and control formulas are compared with each other and with historical data from similar studies. Another more recent approach to growth studies is the use of a double-blind randomized trial comparing an experimental formula to an accepted commercial formula. Growth is carefully measured from eight days of age to 90 to 120 days of age, and the mean daily growth rate is calculated. To be acceptable, growth rates of infants on the experimental formula must be not more than three grams per day below those of infants on the control formula.

Acceptance, Tolerance and Growth

After a new formula is evaluated in a relatively small group of infants in metabolic balance studies, and somewhat larger groups in growth studies, large numbers of infants are then enrolled in controlled studies of general acceptance and tolerance in a "real world" setting. Infants in these studies consume the test product for several months. A similar number of infants consume a control product, usually a marketed formula. Care providers record the volume of formula consumed, the number and characteristics of the stools, any gastrointestinal disturbances, and any other pertinent observations. The infants' pediatricians may record the weight and length of the infant at regular intervals for additional data on growth. Depending on the study, physicians may collect a small blood and/or urine sample for laboratory evaluation. The results from the study groups are statistically analyzed and the two groups are compared to assure that the new product performs in a manner equal to or better than the control feeding.

Special Clinical Testing for Hypoallergenic Formulas

Before a formula is declared hypoallergenic, it must be evaluated in double-blind, placebo-controlled (DBPC) trials in infants or children with documented cow milk or infant formula hypersensitivity. The number of infants or children tested should be large enough to project with 95% confidence that 90% of milk-allergic infants will not react to the product. A formula containing extensively hydrolyzed casein is generally the placebo in such DBPC. The studies should be conducted in at least two centers and each center should contribute at least six subjects. A 24-hour supervised open challenge followed by a six-day home challenge should follow the DBPC trial. Extensively hydrolyzed casein formulas manufactured in the U.S. meet the criteria set forth by Kleinman, et al.[9] There is no documentation of successful DBPC food challenges with extensively hydrolyzed whey.

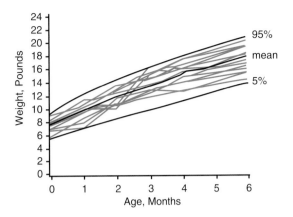

Figure 14: Clinical growth studies.

Product Forms

Routine infant formulas are usually available in three forms: powder, concentrated liquid, and ready-to-use liquid. When prepared according to package directions, the caloric and nutrient contents of the different forms are usually the same. Normal caloric content of infant formulas is 20 Calories per ounce (68 Calories per dL). The ingredients in the different forms may vary slightly due to the technical requirements for making some forms, particularly liquids. However, the slight differences in ingredients should not affect a baby's tolerance of a formula. A baby who tolerates a routine formula prepared from powder should also tolerate that same formula when prepared from concentrated liquid or ready-to-use liquid and vice versa.

The formulation for an infant formula brand sold in the U.S. may differ from the formulation of that same brand sold in another country. Consequently, the nutrients may also vary. Several factors contribute to the different nutrient levels such as the country's government regulations, cultural demands and the availability of formula ingredients. Consumers should not be surprised to learn that the ingredients and nutrients in a formula sold in the U.S. differ when compared to the ingredients and nutrients in that same formula sold in another country.

Powders

Powder forms require reconstitution with water and are usually the least expensive form with the longest shelf life. Routine infant formula powders are packaged in "reclosable" containers with measuring scoops provided. Normal dilution of most routine infant formulas sold in the U.S. and Canada is achieved by mixing one scoop of powder with two ounces of water (60 mL). In Europe, Latin America and Asia, consumers add one scoop of powder to 30 mL of water. Consumers should pay careful attention to the mixing instructions on the can of powder because some formulas require that the scoop be packed to provide the appropriate amount of powder and some formulas do not. The scoop provided with a can of routine formula powder is specifically designed to deliver the amount of powder required to make formula 20 Calories per ounce (68 Calories per dL) when mixed with the specified amount of water. Since the densities of powders vary among products, different products contain scoops of different sizes. In addition, when a product is reformulated, the density of the powder may change and the size of the scoop in the product may change as well. Therefore, consumers using infant formula powders should use only the scoop that comes with the product. When consumers change from formulas made in the U.S. to those made for Europe, Latin America and Asia (or vice versa), they should be made aware of the different standard mixing instructions to ensure that appropriately prepared formula is given to their babies.

Some specialty formulas, such as formulas for inborn errors of metabolism, are usually available only in the powder form. Since specialty formulas contain modified ingredients such as hydrolyzed proteins, amino acids and/or modified fats, the liquid forms are more difficult to manufacture and shelf life is reduced significantly. In addition, the sales volumes of such products are relatively low so they are manufactured less frequently than routine formulas. Consequently, it is important to manufacture the products in the most stable form possible.

Concentrated Liquids
Concentrated liquids require reconstitution with equal amounts of water. For every ounce (30 mL) of concentrated liquid used, one ounce (30 mL) of water should be added. Before water is added, concentrated liquids contain 40 Calories per ounce (136 Calories per dL) and twice the amount of nutrients found in properly diluted formula. After reconstitution, formulas made from concentrated liquids often have a different appearance than formulas prepared from powder. Formulas made from concentrated liquid appear slightly darker and slightly thicker. The color difference results from the heat processing the formula receives during manufacturing. The slightly thicker consistency results from the heat processing and ingredients that are added to the liquid to stabilize the emulsion. Since emulsifiers are needed to make concentrated liquids with acceptable consistency but are not needed for powders, the ingredient lists on powders and concentrated liquids may differ slightly. Infant formula manufacturers in the U.S. package concentrated liquids in 13-ounce cans; this is the only size can in which concentrated liquids are available.

> *Human milk vs. formula: Poor formula industry! The more they spend on research, the more it profits the competition!*
> Francis Mimouni, M.D.
> Maimonides Medical Center
> Brooklyn, New York

Ready-to-Use Liquids
Ready-to-use liquid formulas require no preparation and are the most expensive form of infant formula. They typically provide the same level of calories and other nutrients as their counterparts prepared from powder and concentrated liquid. Like concentrated liquids, ready-to-use liquids may appear darker and thicker than formula prepared from powder due to the addition of emulsifiers and the heat processing required during manufacturing. Ready-to-use liquid formulas are available in eight-ounce and 32-ounce cans in the U.S.

Nursettes
Individual nursettes (nursing bottles containing ready-to-use liquids) are often available from formula manufacturers. Hospitals are the primary users of nursettes, although individual consumers can also purchase nursettes containing routine infant formulas for convenience. Since hospitalized infants have a wide variety of nutritional needs, nursettes sold to hospitals may come in several different caloric strengths such as 13, 20

and 24 Calories per ounce (44, 68 and 82 Calories per dL). Some infant formula manufacturers prepare ready-to-use formula with different calorie levels simply by adjusting the amount of water used to make formula containing 20 Calories per ounce. The levels of nutrients decrease or increase in direct proportion to the amount of water added. Other formula manufacturers, however, may change the levels of nutrients in their formulas of varying caloric strengths. It is important to check the package label of infant formula nursettes of various caloric strengths to determine the nutrient levels.

Maintaining Quality
Quality Control of Infant Feedings

Natural physiological processes control the quality of human milk. It is limited primarily by the capacity of the mother to adapt to stresses of disease, malnutrition, environmental toxins, state of hydration, and hygiene. While such abilities are remarkable, when superimposed on genetic variability, the composition of human milk varies considerably from mother to mother. These wide variations, however, are usually within the range to which normal term infants can readily adapt.

Modern infant formulas undergo strict quality control procedures in compliance with applicable government regulations to assure product quality (i.e., the proper nutrients are supplied in acceptable amounts). As there are more than 30 quantitative descriptors of composition in an infant formula, this is a challenging task.

Quality assurance of a product requires coordinated interactions among many departments within the manufacturing firm. For consistent, high-quality infant formula, it is essential to integrate quality control considerations into all phases of product development and manufacturing including product planning, research testing, product development, pilot plant scale-up, purchasing of raw ingredients and containers and production. Quality control personnel may perform studies at each step. By being part of the development process, quality control personnel become knowledgeable about the raw materials used, the composition of the product during processing, and the effects of the process itself upon the product. This knowledge helps

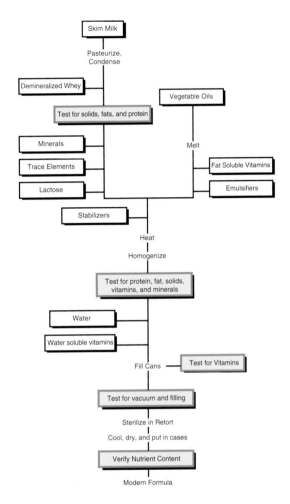

Figure 15: Infant formula production.

provide a smooth manufacturing process as quality control personnel can aid in trouble-shooting any problem that arises. The production process for an infant formula is outlined in Figure 15. Quality control checkpoints have been denoted by colored boxes. These and other checkpoints are summarized in Table 2.

Composition

Quality control starts with the acquisition of ingredients and containers. All suppliers must comply with "good manufacturing practices" and be qualified to assure that they can consistently provide the needed ingredients and containers within rigid tolerance limits of quality. The standards of quality are defined by the

Infant Formula Quality Control Checkpoints	
Specifications established by unanimous agreement of multidisciplinary panel of experts	✓
Ingredients analyzed for compliance with specifications	✓
Batch instructions compared to master instructions	✓
Certification that each instruction was followed	✓
Witness that each instruction was followed	✓
Analytical confirmation of nutrient composition	✓
Individual batch composition compared with trend analysis	✓
Appropriate container fill verified	✓
Processing temperatures verified by: a) On-line analysis of proper thermal processing	✓
b) Incubation test to assure proper thermal processing	✓
Comprehensive review of batch record and analytical	✓
Normal physical condition verified by infant caretaker	✓
Shelf-life assured by statistical sampling and analysis	✓

Table 2: Infant formula quality control checkpoints.

Food Chemicals Codex, the U.S. Pharmacopeia, the National Formulary or other official references. Emphasis is placed on properties determined to be critical in the product development steps. Usually manufacturers qualify and use multiple suppliers to assure an uninterrupted supply of quality ingredients for production. Each incoming shipment is evaluated upon receipt and must meet applicable compositional and microbiological specifications prior to acceptance for use in manufacturing infant formula.

The nutrient content of the formula is assured by numerous checks. The raw ingredients must meet stringent nutrient and quality specifications. The exact amount of each ingredient incorporated into each batch is recorded by a trained production worker, then confirmed by a second person.

Multiple nutrients are analyzed on every batch of the final product, and systems are in place to assure that

each specified ingredient is included in every batch of formula. Long-term trends in nutrient content of formulas and ingredients are closely monitored to assure that seasonal or other supply fluctuations do not affect product quality or consistency.

Multiple quality control checks are made, recorded and verified during the manufacturing of each batch of formula to assure that ingredient additions, processing temperatures, container filling and other aspects of product safety and quality are in compliance with all applicable federal and state regulations.

Microbiology

Several measures assure microbiological safety. Only processing procedures that are verified to be safe and effective are used. Liquid formulas always undergo heat treatment or aseptic processing and are commercially sterile. It is impossible to make powder products commercially sterile without destroying nutritional and organoleptic properties. Although they are not commercially sterile, they are of high microbiological quality. Finished powder products are cultured to assure that the total bacterial count is less than strict limits set by the U.S. government. No coliforms or other potential pathogens are permitted.

Special tests of the primary containers assure integrity of seals and surfaces that might be potential sites of contamination. The products are stored and shipped under controlled conditions. When used as directed, including dilution with boiled water in clean vessels and appropriate storage, these products are bacteriologically safe.

Shelf Life

Before an infant formula is marketed, the shelf life must be determined. Product samples are stored at ambient temperatures for varying time periods. The physical characteristics (such as color, consistency, homogeneity and mixability) and labile nutrient profiles of the samples are evaluated at the end of each period. The length of time that the formula maintains desirable physical characteristics and appropriate nutrient levels is the shelf life. Expiration dates are calculated from shelf life information. After the expiration date listed on a container, infant formula manufacturers can no longer guarantee that the nutrient levels in the product are as high as levels listed on the label. In addition, the physical characteristics of the formula may change. The color may darken and the formula may tend to separate and may not mix easily. Similar changes may occur before the formula's expiration date if the product is stored at extremely hot or cold (freezing) temperatures. Therefore, infant formula manufacturers recommend that unopened cans of product be stored at room temperature.

Manufacturers store sample packages or cans of product at room temperatures throughout the shelf-life of the product. They open representative packages periodically and evaluate product quality and nutrient content. Any departure from expectations is handled in an appropriate and expeditious manner.

Customer Evaluation

The ultimate quality assurance check is the evaluation of product appearance, odor, etc. that is done by the nurse, mother, or other infant caretaker before the product is fed. Occasionally, infant formulas reach consumers in a less than desirable condition. For example, extremely hot or cold temperatures during transit and storage can change the color of the formula or cause the formula to thicken. Rough treatment may dent the cans during transit. Understandably, consumers become concerned when the quality of formula they purchase is less than expected. Several infant formula manufacturers in the U.S. publish toll-free telephone numbers on their product labels. These numbers allow consumers to voice their questions and concerns about the product. In the U.S., the Infant Formula Act revision of 1992 mandates infant formula companies investigate all written and oral complaints about products. In addition, the potential for a hazard to health must be determined and documented. As part of the investigation, consumers may return formula to the company for analysis and the company may test the returned product. This provides formula manufacturers even more insight into how products perform outside of the controlled company environment and can help identify manufacturing changes that are needed.

Recalls

Infant formula manufacturers produce and sell millions of high quality feedings daily without mishap. However, manufacturers must maintain procedures on how they would remove product from the market if necessary. A recall or withdrawal may be warranted if the manufacturer determines that a formula may not provide the nutrients required by the Infant Formula Act, or that the formula is adulterated or misbranded. If the manufacturer and/or the Food and Drug Administration determines that the adulterated or misbranded formula poses a risk to human health, the manufacturer is required to recall the formula. If the product problem does not pose a threat to human health, the manufacturer may choose to voluntarily recall or withdraw the product from the market.

Manufacturers maintain production, distribution and sales records that document the total amount of product produced, how much has been shipped and how much is remaining in inventory. In addition, they document which distributors received which product, the batch numbers and the quantity. During a recall, company personnel analyze these records to identify how much of the affected product batch has been shipped and to whom. They then develop a plan for removing the product from the marketplace. The exact steps taken to remove the product depend on several factors such as the severity of the problem, the amount of product manufactured and the distribution of the product. For example, if the product in question is so highly specialized that only a small volume is manufactured and distributed to hospitals, sales representatives might visit the specific hospital and personally remove the product. However, if the product is a routine infant formula that is widely distributed to consumers, the media would be contacted with recall information. Consumers would receive special instructions on the product and batch in question, how to contact the company, how to return product and how replacement product would be provided. Manufacturers must maintain records of all activities associated with a recall and account for all recalled product, and the FDA will visit the facility to monitor recall activities. Fortunately, infant formula recalls are unusual as a result of the stringent quality control procedures maintained by infant formula manufacturers.

Summary

Modern infant formulas can meet the nutritional needs of infants when breast milk is not available. While they are not as complex as human milk, they are nutritious substitutes and often provide life-giving sustenance that would not otherwise be available to infants with special conditions. Infant formulas undergo preclinical and clinical testing to assure that nutrient quality, content and utilization are appropriate. The safety and accept- ability of products are also confirmed prior to market- ing. Infant formula manufacturers employ intensive quality assurance programs to assure that formulas meet nutrient content and microbiological safety specifica- tions. As more is learned about the science of infant nutrition, infant formula manufacturers will continue to use the latest information to provide for the nutri- tional needs of infants.

Historical Perspective...

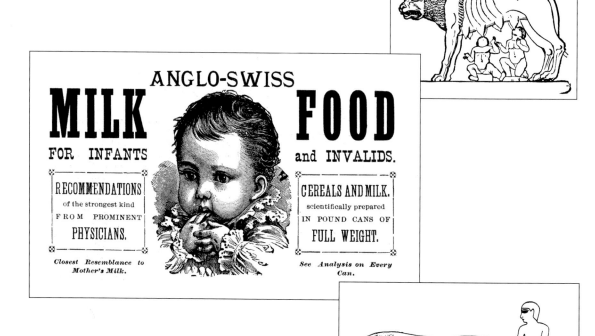

References

1. Cone TE Jr. History of infant and child feeding: from the earliest years through the development of scientific concepts. In: Bond JT, Filer LJ Jr, Leveille GA, et al, eds. *Infant and Child Feeding.* New York: Academic Press; 1981:4-34.

2. Greenberg MH. Neonatal feeding. In: Smith GF, Vidyasager D, eds. *Historical Review and Recent Advances in Neonatal and Perinatal Medicine,* Vol 1. Evansville, IN: Mead Johnson Nutritional Division; 1983:55-78.

3. Coursin DB. Convulsive seizures in infants with pyridoxine-deficient diet. *JAMA.* 1954;154:406-408.

4. Roy S, Arant BS. Alkalosis from chloride deficient Neo-Mull-Soy. *NEJM.* 1979;301:615.

5. *Nutrient Requirements for Infant Formulas, Final Rule, Federal Register.* 1985. Vol 50:45106-45108:21 CFR 107.

6. Kleinman RE, Baker SS, Bell EF, et al. Policy Statement. The Use of Whole Cow's Milk in Infancy. *AAP News.* May 1992:18-19.

7. Food and Nutrition Board, National Research Council. *Recommended Dietary Allowances.* Washington DC: National Academy Press; 1989.

8. Koch F. Uber die Pioniere der frühen Kinderheilkunde in und aus Giessen. *Der Kinderartz.* 1984;15:1623-1627.

9. Kleinman RE, Bahna S, Powell GF, Sampson HA. Use of infant formulas in infants with cow milk allergy. A review and recommendations. *Pediatr Allergy Immunol.* 1991;4:146-155.

10. Sampson HA, Bernhisel-Broadbent J, Yang E, Scanlon SM. Safety of casein hydrolysate formula in children with cow milk allergy. *J Pediatr.* 1991;118:520-525.

11. Lifschitz CH, Hawkins HF, Guerra C, Byrd H. Anaphylactic shock due to cow's milk protein hypersensitivity in a breast-fed infant. *J Pediatr Gastroenterol Nutr.* 1988;7:141-144.

12. Bock SA. Probable allergic reaction to casein hydrolysate formula [letter]. *J Allergy Clin Immunol.* 1990;84:272.

13. Amonette MS, Schwartz RH, Mattson L, Peers LB, Eldredge L. Double-blind, placebo-controlled food challenges (DBPCFC) demonstrating acute IgE medicated allergic reactions to Good Start, Ultra filtered Good Start, Alfare, Nutramigen and Alimentum in a seven-year-old. *Pediatr Asthma Allergy Immunol.* 1991;5:245-251.

14. Businco L, Cantani A, Longhi MA, Giampietro PG. Anaphylactic reactions to a cow's milk whey protein hydrolysate (Alfa-Ré, Nestlé) in infants with cow's milk allergy. *Ann Allergy.* 1989;62:333-335.

15. Innis SM. Human milk and formula fatty acids. *J Pediatr.* 1992;120:S56-S61.

16. ESPGAN Committee on Nutrition. Committee report. Comment on the content and composition of lipids in infant formulas. *Acta Paediatr Scand.* 1991;80:887-896.

17. Carnielli VP, Luijendijk IHT, van Goudoever JB, et al. Feeding premature newborn infants palmitic acid in amounts and stereoisomeric position similar to that of human milk: effects on fat and mineral balance. *Am J Clin Nutr.* 1995;61:1037-1042.

18. Jensen RG. *The lipids of human milk.* Boca Raton, FL: CRC Press Inc; 1989:70.

19. Data on file, Mead Johnson Research Center.

20. Expert Panel on Blood Cholesterol Levels in Children and Adolescents. National Cholesterol Education Program. Report of the Expert Panel on Blood Cholesterol Levels in Children and Adolescents. *Pediatrics.* 1992;89: Supplement.

21. American Academy of Pediatrics Committee on Nutrition. Prudent life-style for children: dietary fat and cholesterol. *Pediatrics.* 1986;78:521-525.

22. Weidman W, Kwiterovich P Jr, Jesse MJ, Nugent E. Diet in the healthy child. Task Force Committee of the Nutrition Committee and the Cardiovascular Disease in the Young Council of the American Heart Association. *Circulation.* 1983;67:1411A-1414A.

23. Carlson SE, Werkman SH, Peeples JM, Cooke RJ, Tolley EA. Arachidonic acid status correlates with first year growth in preterm infants. *Proc Natl Acad Sci.* 1993; 90:1073-1077.

24. Carlson SE, Werkman SH, Tolley EA. Effect of long-chain n-3 fatty acid supplementation on visual acuity and growth of preterm infants with and without bronchopulmonary dysplasia. *Am J Clin Nutr.* 1996;63: 687-697.

25. Uauy R, Hoffman DR, Birch EE, Birch DG, Jameson DDM, Tyson J. Safety and efficacy of omega-3 fatty acids in the nutrition of very low birth weight infants: soy oil and marine oil supplementation of formula. *J Pediatr.* 1994;124:612-620.

26. Kaufman SS, Scrivner DJ, Murray ND, et al. Influence of Portagen and Pregestimil on essential fatty acid status in infantile liver disease. *Pediatrics.* 1992;89:151-154.

27. Pettei MJ, Daftary S, Levine J. Essential fatty acid deficiency associated with the use of a medium-chain-triglyceride infant formula in pediatric hepatobiliary disease. *Am J Clin Nutr.* 1991;53:1217-1221.

28. Koch R, Acosta P, Ragsdale N, Donnell CN. Nutrition in the treatment of galactosemia. *J Am Diet Assoc.* 1963; 43:216-222.

29. Gitzelmann R, Auricchio S. The handling of soya alpha-galactosides by a normal and a galactosemic child. *Pediatrics.* 1965;36:231-235.

30. Wood RJ, Gerhardt A, Rosenberg IH. Effects of glucose and glucose polymers on calcium absorption in healthy subjects. *Am J Clin Nutr.* 1987;46:699-701.

31. Bei L, Wood RJ, Rosenberg IH. Glucose polymer increases jejunal calcium magnesium, and zinc absorption in humans. *Am J Clin Nutr.* 1986;44:244-247.

32. Data on file, Mead Johnson Research Center.

33. Fomon SJ, Nelson ES. Calcium, phosphorous, magnesium, and sulfur. In: Fomon SJ, ed. *Nutrition and Normal Infants.* St. Louis: Mosby-Year Book Inc; 1993: 192-218.

34. Bronner F, Salle BL, Putet G, Rigo J, Senterre J. Net calcium absorption in premature infants: results of 103 metabolic balance studies. *Am J Clin Nutr.* 1992;56: 1037-1044.

35. Ozolek JA, Cook LA, Mimouni FB, Moran JR, Doyle J, Sentipal-Walerius J. Bone mineralization over the first eight months of life in infants fed a lactose free formula. *Pediatr Res.* 1995;37:315A.

36. Mimouni F, Campaigne B, Neyean M, Tsang RC. Bone mineralization in the first year of life in infants fed human milk, cow milk, or soy-based formula. *J Pediatr.* 1993;122:348-354.

37. Hillman LS. Bone mineral content in term infants fed human milk, cow milk-based formula, or soy-based formula. *J Pediatr.* 1988;113:208-212.

38. Williams CL, Bollella M, Wynder EL. A new recommendation for dietary fiber in childhood. *Pediatrics.* 1995;96:985-988.

39. Brown KH, Perez F, Peerson JM, et al. Effect of dietary fiber (soy polysaccharide) on the severity, duration, and nutritional outcome of acute, watery diarrhea in children. *Pediatrics.* 1993;92:241-247.

40. American Academy of Pediatrics Committee on Nutrition. Iron-fortified infant formulas. *Pediatrics.* 1989; 84:1114-1115.

41. Joint Food and Agriculture Organization/World Health Organization Expert Committee on Food Additives. Geneva; March 21-30, 1988.

42. Litov RE, Sickels VS, Chan GM, Springer MA, Cordano A. Plasma aluminum measurements in term infants fed human milk or a soy-based infant formula. *Pediatrics.* 1989;84:1105-1106.

43. Ziegler EE, Fomon FJ. Fluid intake, renal solute load, and water balance in infancy. *J Pediatr.* 1971;78:561-568.

44. Cordano A. Pre-clinical and clinical evaluation of new infant formulas. *Nutr Res.* 1984;4:929-934.

45. Association of official analytical chemists. In: Hefrich K, ed. *Official methods of analysis of the association of official analytical chemists.* 15th Edition. Arlington, VA: Association of official analytical chemists Inc; 1990:1095.

46. Leary HL. Nonclinical testing of formulas containing hydrolyzed milk protein. *J Pediatr.* 1992;121:S42-S46.

47. Cordano A, Bancalari E, Hansen JW, Feller R. Nutritional balance studies: evaluation of a premature infant formula. *Arch Latinoamericanos de Nutr.* 1985;35:221-231.

48. Ziegler EE, O'Donnell AM, Nelson SE, Fomon SJ. Body composition of the reference fetus. *Growth.* 1976; 40:329-341.

49. Shaw JCL. Evidence for defective skeletal mineralizaiton in low birthweight infants. *Pediatr.* 1976;57:16-25.

50. Fomon SJ, Thomas LN, Filer LJ, Ziegler EE, Leonard MT. Food consumption and growth of normal infants fed milk-based formulas. *Acta Pediatr Scand (Suppl).* 1971;223:1-36.

Appendix 1 - Nutrient Composition of Infant Formulas

Product Type: First Age (Nutrient content per 100 kcal)							
Manufacturer:		**Mead Johnson**	**Mead Johnson**	**Mead Johnson**	**Nestle**	**Nestle**	**Milupa**
Product protein base		Cow milk	Cow milk	Cow milk	Cow milk, whey	Cow milk	Cow milk
Product name		Enfalac	Enfalac	Enfamil	NAN 1	LACTOGEN 1	Pre Aptamil Milupan (a)
Product form (concentration)	kcal/dL l pwd	Powder	Powder	Powder	67	67	Powder, liquid r.t.f.
Geographic distribution		E Europe	Latin America	Europe	Worldwide	Asia, Africa	Europe, Middle East
Protein	g	2.2	2.2	2.5	2.24	2.54	2.23
Source		Nonfat milk, whey protein concentrate	Nonfat milk, whey protein concentrate	Nonfat milk	Cow milk, whey	Cow milk	Milk
Type/whey:casein		60:40	60:40	18:82	60:40	23:77	60:40
Fat	g	5.5	5.5	5.3	5.1	5.1	5.36
C18:2ω6 Linoleic	mg	900	900	860	600	600	650
C18:3ω3 α-Linolenic	mg	94	94	90	52	52	61
C20:4ω6 Arachidonic	mg						18
C22:6ω3 Docosahexaenoic	mg						13
MCT added; % fat	%						
Sources		Palm olein, coconut, soy, high oleic sunflower	Palm olein, coconut, soy, high oleic safflower	Palm olein, coconut, soy, high oleic sunflower	Milk fat, corn oil	Milk fat, corn oil	Vegetable, milk, egg
Carbohydrate	g	10.4	10.4	10.5	11.4	11	10.7
Glucose	g						
Lactose	g	10.4	10.4	7.3	11.4	11	10.7
Sucrose	g						
Oligomers	g						
Maltodextrins	g			3.1			
Starch	g						
Fiber	g						
Source		Lactose	Lactose	Lactose, maltodextrin	Lactose	Lactose	Lactose
Vitamins							
Vitamin A Activity	IU	300	300	300	350	350	300
Vitamin D	µg	1.5	1.5	1.5	1.5	1.5	1.5
Vitamin E	IU	2.0	1.8	2	1.2	1.2	0.98
Vitamin K	µg	8	9	8	8	8	4.5
Thiamine (vitamin B1)	µg	80	75	80	70	70	60
Riboflavin (vitamin B2)	µg	140	180	90	150	150	75
Vitamin B6	µg	60	67	60	75	75	60
Vitamin B12	µg	0.3	0.4	0.3	0.3	0.3	0.3
Niacin	µg	1000	1200	1000	1000	1000	1040
Folic Acid (folacin)	µg	16	7.5	16	9	9	15
Pantothenic acid	µg	500	570	500	450	450	600
Biotin	µg	3.0	2.8	3	2.2	2.2	1.5
Vitamin C (ascorbic acid)	mg	12	11	12	10	10	12
Choline	mg	12	12	12	10	10	36
Inositol	mg		4.5		5	5	
Carnitine	mg				1.6	1.6	(b)
Taurine	mg	6	6	6	8	8	10
Minerals							
Calcium	mg	67	67	82	63	91	98
Phosphorus	mg	45	45	65	31	78	62
Magnesium	mg	8	8	8	7	8	7.4
Iron	mg	1.18	1.8	1.13	1.2	1.2	
Zinc	mg	1.0	0.6	1	0.75	0.75	0.74
Manganese	µg	10	11	10	7	7	15
Copper	µg	65	63	65	60	60	60
Iodine	µg	15	15	15	15	15	15
Selenium	µg						
Chromium	µg						
Molybdenum	µg						
Sodium	mg	26	26	35	24	37	34
Potassium	mg	110	110	125	98	119	122
Chloride	mg	70	70	80	65	85	79
Nucleotides	mg						
AMP	mg						
CMP	mg						
GMP	mg						
UMP	mg						
IMP	mg						
Recommended strength	kcal/L	676	676	710	670	670	672
Osmolarity	mosm/L	260	260		260	290	290

Product Type: First Age (Nutrient content per 100 kcal)						
Manufacturer:		**Milupa**	**Milupa**	**Nutricia**	**Nutricia**	**Nutricia**
Product protein base Product name Product form (concentration) Geographic distribution	kcal/dL I pwd	Cow milk Aptamil 1 Powder, liquid r.t.f. Europe, Middle East, Far East	Cow milk Milumil 1 Powder, liquid r.t.f. Europe, Middle East	Cow milk Nutrilon Premium (d) Powder, liquid r.t.f. Europe, Middle East, Far East, Middle & South America	Cow milk Plus (e) Powder, liquid r.t.f. Europe, Middle East, Far East, Middle & South America	Cow milk Bebelac 1 Powder Middle East, Far East, Middle & South America
Protein Source Type/whey:casein	g	2 Milk 60:40	2.41 Milk 50:50	2.09 Milk 60:40	2.56 Milk 20:80	2.2 Milk 60:40
Fat C18:2ω6 Linoleic C18:3ω3 α-Linolenic C20:4ω6 Arachidonic C22:6ω3 Docosahexaenoic MCT added; % fat Sources	g mg mg mg mg %	5 670 79 Vegetable, milk	4.81 610 71 Vegetable, milk	5.22 570 105 Vegetable, milk	5.12 590 110 Vegetable, milk	5 730 73 Vegetable, milk
Carbohydrate Glucose Lactose Sucrose Oligomers Maltodextrins Starch Fiber Source	g g g g g g g g	11.5 10.1 1.4 (c) Lactose, starch	11.8 9.8 0.8 1.2 (c) Lactose, starch, maltodextrin	11.2 11.2 Lactose	10.9 10.8 0.1 Lactose, maltodextrin	11.5 10 1.5 Lactose, maltodextrin
Vitamins Vitamin A Activity Vitamin D Vitamin E Vitamin K	IU µg IU µg	310 1.5 1.1 4	310 1.6 1 4	420 2.1 1.7 7.4	420 2.1 2.5 7.5	410 2 1.6 7.1
Thiamine (vitamin B1) Riboflavin (vitamin B2) Vitamin B6 Vitamin B12 Niacin Folic Acid (folacin) Pantothenic acid Biotin Vitamin C (ascorbic acid)	µg µg µg µg µg µg µg µg mg	60 80 60 0.3 1100 15 550 1.4 12	65 190 70 0.3 1100 16 670 1.3 12	60 180 60 0.33 590 15 450 2.3 12	60 210 60 0.23 540 15 460 2.2 12	80 200 60 0.2 610 10 390 2 10
Choline Inositol Carnitine Taurine	mg mg mg mg	 (b) 9.7	 (b) 8	15 (b) 8	12 (b) 8	13 4.5 2.7 6
Minerals Calcium Phosphorus Magnesium Iron Zinc	mg mg mg mg mg	104 61 8.3 0.97 0.69	88 52 9.4 1.1 0.8	80 40 7.4 0.74 0.74	120 72 8.5 0.75 0.75	80 40 8 0.8 0.65
Manganese Copper Iodine Selenium Chromium Molybdenum	µg µg µg µg µg µg	14 55 17	13 67 16	10 60 15 2.8	10 60 15 2.8	10 60 10
Sodium Potassium Chloride	mg mg mg	30 104 54	40 120 88	28 102 64	36 135 84	31 90 65
Nucleotides AMP CMP GMP UMP IMP	mg mg mg mg mg mg					
Recommended strength Osmolarity	kcal/L mosm/L	724 275	748 285	671 285	665 285	695 280

Product Type: First Age (Nutrient content per 100 kcal)					
Manufacturer:		**Wyeth**	**Wyeth**	**Wyeth**	**Wyeth**
Product protein base Product name Product form (concentration) Geographic distribution	kcal/dL I pwd	Cow milk SMA Gold 67.0 Europe	Cow milk S-26 65.5 Asia	Cow milk SMA 66.7 North America	Cow milk SMA 66.7 Latin America
Protein Source Type/whey:casein	g	2.2 Cow milk, whey 60:40	2.3 Cow milk, whey 60:40	2.2 Cow milk, whey 60:40	2.3 Cow milk 20:80
Fat C18:2ω6 Linoleic C18:3ω3 α-Linolenic C20:4ω6 Arachidonic C22:6ω3 Docosahexaenoic MCT added; % fat Sources	g mg mg mg mg %	5.4 1004(1) 72 Palm, coconut, oleic, soy, lecithin	5.5 891 125 9.9 Oleo, coconut, soy, oleic, lecithin	5.3 859(2) 121 9.5 Oleo, coconut, soy, oleic, lecithin	5.3 1762(2) 267 Soy, coconut, lecithin
Carbohydrate Glucose Lactose Sucrose Oligomers Maltodextrins Starch Fiber Source	g g g g g g g g	10.7 10.7 Cow milk	11.0 11.0 Cow milk	10.6 10.6 Cow milk	10.7 10.7 Cow milk
Vitamins Vitamin A Activity Vitamin D Vitamin E Vitamin K	IU µg IU µg	372 1.6 1.6 10.0	305 1.5 1.5 8.4	300 1.5 1.4 8.0	300 1.5 2.9 8.0
Thiamine (vitamin B1) Riboflavin (vitamin B2) Vitamin B6 Vitamin B12 Niacin Folic Acid (folacin) Pantothenic acid Biotin Vitamin C (ascorbic acid)	µg µg µg µg µg µg µg µg mg	149 223 89 0.3 1339 11.9 446 3.0 13.4	102 153 64 0.2 764 7.6 321 2.3 8.4	100 150 63 0.2 750 7.5 315 2.2 8.5	100 150 63 0.2 750 7.5 315 2.2 8.3
Choline Inositol Carnitine Taurine	mg mg mg mg	14.9		15.0 +	7.5 +
Minerals Calcium Phosphorus Magnesium Iron Zinc	mg mg mg mg mg	68.5 49.1 9.5 1.2 0.9	64.2 42.8 6.9 1.2 0.8	63.0 42.0 7.0 0.2 0.8	69.0 54.0 6.0 1.8 0.8
Manganese Copper Iodine Selenium Chromium Molybdenum	µg µg µg µg µg µg	 2.1	22.9 71.8 9.2	15.0 70.0 9.0	22.5 70.0 5.0
Sodium Potassium Chloride	mg mg mg	23.8 104.2 64.0	22.9 85.5 61.1	22.0 83.0 55.5	27.0 93.0 63.0
Nucleotides AMP CMP GMP UMP IMP	mg mg mg mg mg mg	None added	None added	+	None added
Recommended strength Osmolarity	kcal/L mosm/L	672 252	655 252	667 271	667 252

469

Product Type: Second Age (Nutrient content per 100 kcal)							
Manufacturer:		Mead Johnson	Mead Johnson	Mead Johnson	Mead Johnson	Mead Johnson	Nestle	Nestle
Product protein base		Cow milk	Cow milk	Cow milk	Cow milk	Cow milk	Cow milk	Cow milk
Product name		Enfalac 2	Enfamil 2	Enfamil 2	Enfapro	Enfapro	NAN 2	LACTO-GEN 2
Product form (concentration)	kcal/dL l pwd	67.6	Powder	Powder	Powder	Powder	67	
Geographic distribution		Europe	E Europe	Latin America, Europe, Asia	Latin America	Asia	Worldwide	Asia, Africa
Protein	g	3.3	3.3	3.3	4.1	4.1	3.34	
Source		Nonfat milk	Nonfat milk	Nonfat milk	Nonfat milk	Nonfat milk	Cow milk	Cow milk
Type/whey:casein		18:82	18:82	18:82	18:82	18:82	23:77	23:77
Fat	g	4.4	4.4	4.4	3.9	3.9	4.38	4.1
C18:2ω6 Linoleic	mg	720	720	720	930	930	560	480
C18:3ω3 α-Linolenic	mg	75	75	75	63	63	45	42
C20:4ω6 Arachidonic	mg							
C22:6ω3 Docosahaxaenoic	mg							
MCT added; % fat	%							
Sources		Palm olein, coconut, soy, high oleic sunflower	Palm olein, soy, coconut, high oleic safflower	Palm olein, soy, coconut, high oleic safflower	Palm, soy coconut, corn	Palm, soy coconut, corn	Milk fat, corn oil	Milk fat, corn oil
Carbohydrate	g	11.8	11.8	11.8	12.1	12.1	11.8	11.1
Glucose	g				1.1	1.1		
Lactose	g	4.7	8.3	4.7	8.8	8.8	11.8	6.8
Sucrose	g							2.6
Oligomers	g	7.1	3.5	7.1	2.2	2.2		
Maltodextrins	g							1.72
Starch	g							
Fiber	g							
Source		Corn syrup solids, lactose	Corn syrup solids, lactose	Corn syrup solids, lactose	Lactose, dextri-maltose	Lactose, dextri-maltose	Lactose	Lactose, sucrose, malto-dextrin
Vitamins								
Vitamin A Activity	IU	300	300	300	310	310	400	400
Vitamin D	µg	1.5	1.5	1.5	1.5	1.5	2.3	2.3
Vitamin E	IU	2	2	2	1.8	1.8	1.2	1.2
Vitamin K	µg	8	8	8	9	9	4.5	4.5
Thiamine (vitamin B1)	µg	80	80	80	90	90	150	150
Riboflavin (vitamin B2)	µg	150	150	150	220	220	240	240
Vitamin B6	µg	69	90	90	75	75	200	200
Vitamin B12	µg	0.3	0.3	0.3	0.6	0.6	0.2	0.2
Niacin	µg	1000	1000	1000	1200	1200	2700	2700
Folic Acid (folacin)	µg	16	16	16	9	9	30	30
Pantothenic acid	µg	500	500	500	750	750	700	700
Biotin	µg	3	3	3	3.7	3.7	3.4	3.4
Vitamin C (ascorbic acid)	mg	12	12	12	12	12	10	10
Choline	mg	12	12	12	12	12	10	10
Inositol	mg	5	5	5	6	6	5	5
Carnitine	mg							
Taurine	mg	6	6	6		6.5		
Minerals								
Calcium	mg	116	116	116	140	140	121	168
Phosphorus	mg	92	92	92	110	110	100	136
Magnesium	mg	11	11	11	13	13	11	15
Iron	mg	1.8	1.8	1.8	1.8	1.8	1.7	1.7
Zinc	mg	1	1	1	0.9	0.9	1.2	1.2
Manganese	µg	15	15	15	12	12	7	7
Copper	µg	75	75	75	60	60	120	120
Iodine	µg	8	8	8	9	9	21	21
Selenium	µg							
Chromium	µg							
Molybdenum	µg							
Sodium	mg	49	49	49	54	54	48	67
Potassium	mg	150	150	150	210	210	159	218
Chloride	mg	100	100	100	120	120	113	157
Nucleotides	mg							
AMP	mg							
CMP	mg							
GMP	mg							
UMP	mg							
IMP	mg							
Recommended strength	kcal/L	676	676	676	676	670	670	670
Osmolarity	mosm/L				290	290	360	

Product Type: Second Age (Nutrient content per 100 kcal)						
Manufacturer:		**Nestle**	**Milupa**	**Milupa**	**Nutricia**	**Nutricia**
Product protein base		Cow milk	Cow milk	Cow milk	Cow milk	Cow milk
Product name		Carnation	Aptamil 2	Milumil 2	Nutrilon Plus (g)	Follow-on
		Follow-up				
Product form	kcal/dL l pwd	136	Powder,	Powder,	Powder+liquid	Powder
(concentration)			liquid r.t.f.	liquid r.t.f.		
Geographic distribution		North America	Europe,	Europe,	Europe,	Middle East,
			Middle East	Far East	Far East	Far East,
						Middle & South
						America
Protein	g	2.6	2.72	2.81	2.59	3.9
Source		Milk	Milk	Milk	Milk	Milk
Type/whey:casein		23:77	50:50	20:80	20:80	20:80
Fat	g	4.1	4.77	4.42	4.86	4.05
C18:2ω6 Linoleic	mg	820	650	620	530	720
C18:3ω3 α-Linolenic	mg	90	75	70	95	12
C20:4ω6 Arachidonic	mg					
C22:6ω3	mg					
Docosahexaenoic						
MCT added; % fat	%					
Sources		Palm olein, soy,	Vegetable, milk	Vegetable, milk	Vegetable, milk	Milk, vegetable
		coconut, high oleic				
		safflower				
Carbohydrate	g	13.2	11.5	12.2	11.4	12
Glucose	g					
Lactose	g	4.9	9.9	10.3	11.2	5.5
Sucrose	g			(f)		
Oligomers	g	8.3				
Maltodextrins	g		1.6	0.7	0.2	6.5
Starch	g		(f)	1.2		
Fiber	g					
Source		Corn syrup	Lactose,	Lactose,	Lactose,	Lactose,
		solids, lactose	maltodextrin	maltodextrin	maltodextrin	maltodextrin
			(starch)	(starch, sucrose)		
Vitamins						
Vitamin A Activity	IU	250	270	280	310	380
Vitamin D	µg	1.6	1.4	1.3	2.7	1.7
Vitamin E	IU	2	0.9	0.9	2.4	1.4
Vitamin K	µg	8.1	4.1	4	7.2	8
Thiamine (vitamin B1)	µg	80	70	70	60	60
Riboflavin (vitamin B2)	µg	96	80	80	200	150
Vitamin B6	µg	66	60	60	60	60
Vitamin B12	µg	0.32	0.27	0.27	0.23	0.3
Niacin	µg	1280	950	1900	580	600
Folic Acid (folacin)	µg	16	14	15	14	15
Pantothenic acid	µg	480	540	540	420	400
Biotin	µg	2	1.4	1.3	2.2	2.3
Vitamin C (ascorbic acid)	mg	8	12	12	11	12
Choline	mg	12			12	10
Inositol	mg	18				
Carnitine	mg					
Taurine	mg	0.4			8	
Minerals						
Calcium	mg	135	146	116	126	135
Phosphorus	mg	90	89	83	72	110
Magnesium	mg	8.4	11	12	8.8	12
Iron	mg	1.9	1.6	1.6	1.9	1.8
Zinc	mg	0.63	1.6	1.6	1.3	0.7
Manganese	µg	7	27	10	20	10
Copper	µg	76	82	90	70	60
Iodine	µg	5.7	16	16	16	10
Selenium	µg				2.7	
Chromium	µg					
Molybdenum	µg					
Sodium	mg	39	42	46	39	55
Potassium	mg	135	137	154	136	190
Chloride	mg	90	68	88	85	115
Nucleotides	mg					
AMP	mg					
CMP	mg					
GMP	mg					
UMP	mg					
IMP	mg					
Recommended strength	kcal/L	680	734	750	700	720
Osmolarity	mosm/L	320	275	300	295	300

Product Type: Second Age (Nutrient content per 100 kcal)					
Manufacturer:		**Nutricia**	**Wyeth**	**Wyeth**	**Wyeth**
Product protein base		Cow milk	Cow milk	Cow milk	Cow milk
Product name		Bebelac 2	Progress	PROMIL	PROMIL
Product form	kcal/dL I pwd	Powder	67.0	65.0	66.7
(concentration)					
Geographic distribution		Europe, Middle East, Far East, Middle & South America	Europe	Asia	Latin America
Protein	g	3.7	3.3	4.5	3.3
Source		Cow milk protein	Skim milk powder	Nonfat milk	Skim milk
Type/whey:casein		30:70	20:80	20:80	20:80
Fat	g	4.53	4.5	4.0	4.2
C18:2ω6 Linoleic	mg	640	839	648(3)	1397(4)
C18:3ω3 α-Linolenic	mg	64	60	91	211
C20:4ω6 Arachidonic	mg			7.2	
C22:6ω3	mg				
Docosahexaenoic					
MCT added; % fat	%				
Sources		Vegetable, milk	Palm, coconut, oleic, soy, lecithin	Oleo, coconut, soy, oleic, lecithin	Soy, coconut, lecithin
Carbohydrate	g	11.1	11.6	12.3	12.3
Glucose	g	3			
Lactose	g	7.7	11.6	9.5	9.8
Sucrose	g				2.5
Oligomers	g				
Maltodextrins	g	0.4		2.8	
Starch	g				
Fiber	g				
Source		Lactose, glucose, maltodextrin	NONE Cow milk	Cow milk, corn syrup solids	Skim milk, sucrose
Vitamins					
Vitamin A Activity	IU	350	373	460	345
Vitamin D	µg	2	1.8	1.8	1.8
Vitamin E	IU	1.4	1.6	1.7	2.0
Vitamin K	µg	8		10.2	10.0
Thiamine (vitamin B1)	µg	60	149	125	122
Riboflavin (vitamin B2)	µg	130	224	185	180
Vitamin B6	µg	70	90	74	72
Vitamin B12	µg	0.23	0.3	0.2	0.2
Niacin	µg	720	1343	938	915
Folic Acid (folacin)	µg	8.4	11.9	9.2	9.0
Pantothenic acid	µg	390	448	369	360
Biotin	µg	2.3	3.0	2.6	2.6
Vitamin C (ascorbic acid)	mg	8.5	13.4	10.2	10.0
Choline	mg	13		7.3	7.1
Inositol	mg				
Carnitine	mg				
Taurine	mg				
Minerals					
Calcium	mg	145	134.3	176.9	105.0
Phosphorus	mg	99	92.5	144.6	75.0
Magnesium	mg	13	11.9	14.5	9.8
Iron	mg	1.9	1.9	1.2	1.8
Zinc	mg	1	0.9	0.7	0.8
Manganese	µg	10		26.2	15.0
Copper	µg	70	59.7	89.2	87.0
Iodine	µg	12	17.9	10.6	9.0
Selenium	µg				
Chromium	µg				
Molybdenum	µg				
Sodium	mg	45	49.3	75.4	41.0
Potassium	mg	150	159.7	204.6	131.0
Chloride	mg	99	92.5	156.9	86.0
Nucleotides	mg		None added	None added	None added
AMP	mg				
CMP	mg				
GMP	mg				
UMP	mg				
IMP	mg				
Recommended strength	kcal/L	691	670	650	667
Osmolarity	mosm/L	380	315	315	324

Product Type: Full Year (Nutrient content per 100 kcal)

Manufacturer:		Mead Johnson	Ross Labs	Ross Labs	Ross Labs	Wyeth	Wyeth
Product protein base		Cow milk		Cow milk		Cow milk	Cow milk
Product name		Enfamil w/Iron	Similac Advance	Similac with Iron	Similac PM 60/40	SMA WHITE	SMA
Product form (concentration)	kcal/dL I pwd	67.6	68	67.6	67.6	66.8	66.7
Geographic distribution		North America, Latin America	Canada†	†	††	Europe	Latin America
Protein	g	2.1	2.1	2.14	2.22	2.4	2.3
Source		Reduced minerals whey, nonfat milk		Nonfat milk	Whey protein concentrate, sodium caseinate	Skim milk powder	Cow milk
Type/whey:casein		60:40		18:82	60:40	20:80	20:80
Fat	g	5.3		5.4	5.59	5.4	5.3
C18:2ω6 Linoleic	mg	910	810	1300	1300	1010(1)	1762(2)
C18:3ω3 α-Linolenic	mg	90	110			73	267
C20:4ω6 Arachidonic	mg						
C22:6ω3 Docosahexaenoic	mg						
MCT added; % fat	%						
Sources		Palm olein, soy, coconut, high oleic sunflower		Soy, coconut	Corn, coconut, soy	Palm, coconut, oleic, soy, lecithin	Soy, coconut, lecithin
Carbohydrate	g	10.9	10.8	10.7	10.2	10.5	10.7
Glucose	g						
Lactose	g	10.9		10.7	10.2	10.5	10.7
Sucrose	g						
Oligomers	g						
Maltodextrins	g						
Starch	g						
Fiber	g					NONE	
Source		Lactose		Lactose	Lactose	Cow milk	Cow milk
Vitamins							
Vitamin A Activity	IU	300	300	300	300	374	300
Vitamin D	µg	1.5	1.5	1.5	1.5	1.6	1.5
Vitamin E	IU	2	3	3	2.5	1.7	2.9
Vitamin K	µg	8	8	8	8	10.0	8.0
Thiamine (vitamin B1)	µg	80	100	100	100	150	100
Riboflavin (vitamin B2)	µg	140	150	150	150	225	150
Vitamin B6	µg	60	60	60	60	90	63
Vitamin B12	µg	0.3	0.25	0.25	0.25	0.3	0.2
Niacin	µg	1000	1050	1050	1050	1347	750
Folic Acid (folacin)	µg	16	15	15	15	12.0	7.5
Pantothenic acid	µg	500	450	450	450	449	315
Biotin	µg	3	4.4	4.4	4.5	3.0	2.2
Vitamin C (ascorbic acid)	mg	12	9	9	9	13.5	8.3
Choline	mg	12	16	16	12	10.0	7.5
Inositol	mg	6	4.7	4.7	24		
Carnitine	mg	2					
Taurine	mg	6	5.5				+
Minerals							
Calcium	mg	78	78	73	56	83.8	69.0
Phosphorus	mg	53	42	56	28	65.9	54.0
Magnesium	mg	8	6.1	6	6	7.9	6.0
Iron	mg	1.8	1.77	1.8	0.22	1.2	1.8
Zinc	mg	1	0.75	0.75	0.75	0.9	0.8
Manganese	µg	15	5	5	5		22.5
Copper	µg	75	90	90	90	49.4	70.0
Iodine	µg	10	6.1	9	6	15.0	5.0
Selenium	µg	2.8	2.3	2.2	1.9	2.1	
Chromium	µg	None added					
Molybdenum	µg	None added					
Sodium	mg	27	24	27	24	32.9	27.0
Potassium	mg	108	105	105	86	119.8	93.0
Chloride	mg	63	64	64	59	82.3	63.0
Nucleotides	mg	3.85	10.1			+	None added
AMP	mg	0.74					
CMP	mg	1.63					
GMP	mg	0.59					
UMP	mg	0.89					
IMP	mg						
Recommended strength	kcal/L	676	680	676	676	668	667
Osmolarity	mosm/L	270		270	250	257	252

Product Type: Toddler (Nutrient content per 100 kcal)							
Manufacturer:		Mead Johnson	Mead Johnson	Mead Johnson	Mead Johnson	Mead Johnson	Mead Johnson
Product protein base		Cow milk	Soy		Cow milk		
Product name		Next Step	Next Step Soy	Kindercal	Enfagrow	Sustagen Mighty Drink, Chocolate	Sustagen Mighty Drink, Honeynut
Product form (concentration)	kcal/dL l pwd	67.6	67.6	106	Powder	Powder	Powder
Geographic distribution		North America	North America	North America	Asia	Asia	Asia
Protein	g	2.6	3	3.2	4.7	6.1	6.1
Source		Nonfat milk	Soy protein isolate, L-methionine	Calcium caseinate, sodium caseinate, milk protein conc	Whole milk, nonfat milk	Nonfat milk, whole milk	Nonfat milk, whole milk
Type/whey:casein		18:82		2:98	18:82	18:82	18:82
Fat	g	5	5.3	4.2	3.7	0.94	0.91
C18:2ω6 Linoleic	mg	860	910	870	690		
C18:3ω3 α-Linolenic	mg	90	90	190	54		
C20:4ω6 Arachidonic	mg						
C22:6ω3 Docosahexaenoic	mg				7.5	7.5	
MCT added; % fat	%			20			
Sources		Palm olein, soy, coconut, high oleic sunflower	Palm olein, soy, coconut, high oleic sunflower	Canola, MCT, corn, high oleic sunflower	Palm, soy, coconut, corn, DHA	Whole milk, DHA	Whole milk
Carbohydrate	g	11.1	10	12.8	12	16.9	16.9
Glucose	g				1.4		
Lactose	g	5.6			6.7	9	9.4
Sucrose	g		4.3	2.1		2.3	
Oligomers	g	5.5	5.6		2.8	5.6	7.5
Maltodextrins	g			10.6			
Starch	g						
Fiber	g			0.6			
Source		Lactose, corn syrup solids	Corn syrup solids, sugar	Maltodextrin, sucrose	Dextri-maltose, lactose, fructose (1.1)	Corn syrup solids, sucrose, lactose	Corn syrup solids, lactose
Vitamins							
Vitamin A Activity	IU	300	300	390	370	290	290
Vitamin D	µg	1.5	1.5	1.25	1.8	0.57	0.57
Vitamin E	IU	2	2	3.5	1.8	1.71	1.71
Vitamin K	µg	8	8	3	13		
Thiamine (vitamin B1)	µg	100	80	160	90	570	570
Riboflavin (vitamin B2)	µg	150	90	200	220	570	570
Vitamin B6	µg	60	60	200	75	290	290
Vitamin B12	µg	0.25	0.3	0.56	0.6	0.57	0.57
Niacin	µg	1050	1000	2000	1200	5700	5700
Folic Acid (folacin)	µg	15	16	15.2	13.5	5.7	5.7
Pantothenic acid	µg	450	500	1240	750	1140	1140
Biotin	µg	4.4	3	15.2	3.7	0.52	0.52
Vitamin C (ascorbic acid)	mg	9	12	23	12	23	23
Choline	mg	16	12	25	7.6	6.9	6.9
Inositol	mg	4.7	17	8	9.9	6.9	6.9
Carnitine	mg	2.5	2	6			
Taurine	mg	6	6	6			
Minerals							
Calcium	mg	120	105	80	198	230	230
Phosphorus	mg	84	83	80	130	143	143
Magnesium	mg	8	11	20	16	14.3	14.3
Iron	mg	1.8	1.8	1	1.8	1.04	1.04
Zinc	mg	0.9	1.2	1.2	0.9	0.57	0.57
Manganese	µg	7	25	160	12		
Copper	µg	90	75	120	60	15.6	15.6
Iodine	µg	8	15	12	14	8.1	8.1
Selenium	µg	2.8	2.8	3			
Chromium	µg	None added	None added	5			
Molybdenum	µg	None added	None added	5			
Sodium	mg	41	36	35	62	91	91
Potassium	mg	130	120	124	240	260	260
Chloride	mg	86	80	70	150	156	156
Nucleotides	mg						
AMP	mg						
CMP	mg						
GMP	mg						
UMP	mg						
IMP	mg						
Recommended strength	kcal/L	676	676	1060	676	837	837
Osmolarity	mosm/L	240	210	260			

Product Type: Toddler (Nutrient content per 100 kcal)

Manufacturer:		Mead Johnson	Mead Johnson	Nestle	Ross	Ross	Wyeth	Wyeth
Product protein base				Cow milk	Cow milk	Soy	Cow milk	Cow milk
Product name		Sustagen Mighty Drink, Orange	Sustagen Mighty Drink, Vanilla	NESLAC	Toddler's Best Milk-Based	Toddler's Best Soy-Based	Progress	Progress
Product form (concentration)	kcal/dL l pwd	Powder	Powder		67.6	67.6	65.0	100.0
Geographic distribution		Asia	Asia	Asia	†	†	Asia	Latin America
Protein	g	6.1	6.1	4.66	2.6	3	3.4	3.2
Source		Nonfat milk, whole milk	Nonfat milk, whole milk	Milk	Nonfat milk	Soy protein isolate	Nonfat milk	Nonfat milk, whey
Type/whey:casein		18:82	18:82	23:77			20:80	60:40
Fat	g	0.91	0.91	4.1	4.7	4.4	4.9	3.5
C18:2ω6 Linoleic	mg			520			1587 (3)	1164
C18:3ω3 α-Linolenic	mg			43			214	176
C20:4ω6 Arachidonic	mg							
C22:6ω3 Docosahexaenoic	mg							
MCT added; % fat	%							
Sources		Whole milk	Whole milk	Milk fat, corn oil	Soy	Soy	Soy, oleic, palm, lecithin	Soy, coconut, lecithin
Carbohydrate	g	16.9	16.9	11.1	11.9	11.8	11.1	14.5
Glucose	g							
Lactose	g	9.4	9.4	6.8			11.1	4.9
Sucrose	g	1.6		3.3				2.1
Oligomers	g	5.9	7.5					
Maltodextrins	g							7.5
Starch	g							
Fiber	g							
Source		Corn syrup solids, sucrose, lactose	Corn syrup solids, lactose	Lactose, sucrose, honey (1.0)	Sucrose, fructose	Corn syrup, sucrose	Cow milk	Nonfat milk, maltodextrin, sucrose
Vitamins								
Vitamin A Activity	IU	290	290	300	300	300	307	167
Vitamin D	µg	0.57	0.57	1.5	1.5	1.5	1.5	1.3
Vitamin E	IU	1.71	1.71	1.2	3	3	1.5	1.3
Vitamin K	µg			8.2	NA	NA	8.5	3.0
Thiamine (vitamin B1)	µg	570	570	60	113	100	103	90
Riboflavin (vitamin B2)	µg	570	570	280	250	250	154	160
Vitamin B6	µg	290	290	75	113	81	65	100
Vitamin B12	µg	0.57	0.57	0.32	0.56	0.56	0.2	0.2
Niacin	µg	5700	5700	750	1312	1312	769	1150
Folic Acid (folacin)	µg	5.7	5.7	9	31	31	11.5	5.0
Pantothenic acid	µg	1140	1140	450	769	769	323	300
Biotin	µg	0.52	0.52	2.2	NA	NA	2.3	2.0
Vitamin C (ascorbic acid)	mg	23	23	8	9.5	9.5	8.5	12.0
Choline	mg	6.9	6.9	19.2	NA	NA		
Inositol	mg	6.9	6.9	4.5	NA	NA		
Carnitine	mg							
Taurine	mg						+	
Minerals								
Calcium	mg	230	230	166	178	106	107.7	100.0
Phosphorus	mg	143	143	131	115	75	76.9	80.0
Magnesium	mg	14.3	14.3	15	7.5	7.5	10.0	10.0
Iron	mg	1.04	1.04	1.8	1.8	1.8	1.8	1.3
Zinc	mg	0.57	0.57	0.75	1.2	0.8	1.2	1.0
Manganese	µg			13	NA	NA	23.1	130.0
Copper	µg	15.6	15.6	60	156	156	72.3	90.0
Iodine	µg	8.1	8.1	5	NA	NA	9.2	19.0
Selenium	µg				NA	NA		
Chromium	µg							
Molybdenum	µg							
Sodium	mg	91	91	70	32	45	33.8	47.0
Potassium	mg	260	260	210	111	111	134.6	150.0
Chloride	mg	156	156	157	NA	NA	88.5	110.0
Nucleotides	mg						None added	None added
AMP	mg							
CMP	mg							
GMP	mg							
UMP	mg							
IMP	mg							
Recommended strength	kcal/L	837	837	670	676	676	650	1000
Osmolarity	mosm/L				NA	NA	383	383

475

Product Type: Thickened (Nutrient content per 100 kcal)

Manufacturer:		Mead Johnson	Mead Johnson	Nutricia	Nutricia	Wyeth	Nestle
Product protein base		Cow milk	Cow milk	Cow milk	Cow milk	Cow milk	Cow milk/whey
Product name		Enfamil AR 1	Enfamil AR 2	Nutrilon A.R. (h)	Nutrilon A.R. plus (h, i)	AR	AR‡
Product form (concentration)	kcal/dL I pwd	Powder	Powder	Powder	Powder	66.8	Powder
Geographic distribution		Europe, Latin America	Europe	Europe	Europe	Europe	Worldwide
Protein	g	2.5	3.3	2.6	3.61	2.4	2.6
Source		Nonfat milk	Nonfat milk	Milk	Milk	Skim milk powder	Nonfat milk demin, whey
Type/whey:casein		18:82	18:82	20:80	20:80	20:80	30:70
Fat	g	5.1	4.4	4.48	4.12	5.4	4.89
C18:2ω6 Linoleic	mg	860	720	840	730	1010(1)	730
C18:3ω3 α-Linolenic	mg	90	75	90	150	72.8(5)	92
C20:4ω6 Arachidonic	mg						
C22:6ω3 Docosahexaenoic	mg						
MCT added; % fat	%						
Sources		Palm olein, coconut, soy, high oleic sunflower	Palm olein, coconut, soy, high oleic safflower	Vegetable, milk	Vegetable, milk	Palm, coconut, oleic, soy, lecithin	Palm, olein, coco rapeseed (low erucic) sunflower
Carbohydrate	g	11	11.8	12.4	12.1	10.5	11.8
Glucose	g						
Lactose	g	6.2	5.3	9.2	9.8	7.5	9
Sucrose	g						
Oligomers	g		3.1				
Maltodextrins	g	1.4		2.56	1.66	0.3	
Starch	g	3.4	3.4			2.7	2.86
Fiber	g			0.64	0.64		
Source		Lactose, rice starch, malto-dextrin	Lactose, rice starch, corn syrup solids	Lactose, maltodextrin, locust bean gum	Lactose, maltodextrin, locust bean gum	Cow milk, precooked starch	Lactose cornstarch
Vitamins							
Vitamin A Activity	IU	300	300	380	290	374	350
Vitamin D	µg	1.5	1.5	2.1	2.6	1.6	1.5
Vitamin E	IU	2	2	1.8	1.8	1.7	1.2
Vitamin K	µg	8	8	7.5	8.1	10.0	8
Thiamine (vitamin B1)	µg	80	80	60	70	150	70
Riboflavin (vitamin B2)	µg	90	150	150	180	225	150
Vitamin B6	µg	60	90	60	70	90	75
Vitamin B12	µg	0.3	0.3	0.3	0.4	0.3	0.3
Niacin	µg	1000	1000	600	500	1347	1000
Folic Acid (folacin)	µg	16	16	15	16	12.0	9
Pantothenic acid	µg	500	500	450	480	449	450
Biotin	µg	3	3	2.3	2.4	3.0	2.2
Vitamin C (ascorbic acid)	mg	12	12	12	12	13.5	10
Choline	mg	12	12	11	11	10.5	10
Inositol	mg		5				5
Carnitine	mg			(b)			1.6
Taurine	mg	6	6	7		+	8
Minerals							
Calcium	mg	82	116	107	154	83.8	92
Phosphorus	mg	65	92	74	105	65.9	74
Magnesium	mg	8	11	8.7	13	7.9	8
Iron	mg	1.13	1.8	0.9	1.6	1.2	1.2
Zinc	mg	1	1	0.8	1.2	0.9	0.75
Manganese	µg	10	15	10	13	+	11
Copper	µg	65	75	65	65	49.4	60
Iodine	µg	15	8	15	15	15.0	15
Selenium	µg						
Chromium	µg						
Molybdenum	µg						
Sodium	mg	35	49	41	41	32.9	37
Potassium	mg	125	150	122	180	119.8	118
Chloride	mg	80	100	78	91	82.3	79
Nucleotides	mg					+	
AMP	mg						
CMP	mg						
GMP	mg						
UMP	mg						
IMP	mg						
Recommended strength	kcal/L	686	676	660	680	668	670
Osmolarity	mosm/L	210		270	270		

Product Type: Reduced Lactose Cow Milk Based (Nutrient content per 100 kcal)						
Manufacturer:		Mead Johnson	Mead Johnson	Mead Johnson	Mead Johnson	Mead Johnson	Nestle
Product protein base		Milk protein isolate	Cow milk	Milk protein	Milk protein	Milk protein	Casein
Product name		Lactofree	O-Lac Plus	O-Lac Follow-On	O-Lac	O-Lac	AL 110
Product form (concentration)	kcal/dL l pwd	67.6	Powder	Powder	Powder	Powder	
Geographic distribution		North America	Europe, Latin America	Asia	Europe, Asia, Latin America	Europe	Worldwide
Protein	g	2.1	2.28	4.1	2.2	2.28	2.8
Source		Milk protein isolate	Nonfat milk, whey protein concentrate, milk protein	Milk protein	Milk protein	Milk protein	Casein
Type/whey:casein		18:82	48:52	18:82	18:82	18:82	0:100
Fat	g	5.3	5.3	3.9	5.3	5.3	5.0
C18:2ω6 Linoleic	mg	910	900	600	900	900	670
C18:3ω3 α-Linolenic	mg	90	94	38	94	94	55
C20:4ω6 Arachidonic	mg						
C22:6ω3 Docosahexaenoic	mg						
MCT added; % fat	%						
Sources		Palm olein, soy, coconut, high oleic sunflower	Palm olein, soy, coconut, high oleic sunflower	Palm olein, soy, coconut, high oleic sunflower	Palm olein, coconut, soy, high oleic sunflower	Palm olein, coconut, soy, high oleic sunflower	Milk fat, corn oil
Carbohydrate	g	10.9	10.7	12.1	10.8	10.7	11
Glucose	g						
Lactose	g		5.2				
Sucrose	g						
Oligomers	g	10.9	5.5	12.1	10.8	10.7	
Maltodextrins	g						11
Starch	g						
Fiber	g						
Source		Corn syrup	Lactose, corn syrup solids	Corn syrup solids	Corn syrup solids	Corn syrup solids	Maltodextrin
Vitamins							
Vitamin A Activity	IU	300	300	300	300	300	300
Vitamin D	µg	1.5	1.5	1.25	1.5	1.5	1.5
Vitamin E	IU	2	2	0.75	2	2	1.2
Vitamin K	µg	8	8	4.5	11	8	8.2
Thiamine (vitamin B1)	µg	80	80	75	80	80	60
Riboflavin (vitamin B2)	µg	140	120	150	90	90	135
Vitamin B6	µg	60	60	60	60	60	75
Vitamin B12	µg	0.3	0.3	0.22	0.3	0.3	0.22
Niacin	µg	1000	1000	1200	1000	1000	750
Folic Acid (folacin)	µg	16	16	7.5	16	16	9
Pantothenic acid	µg	500	500	450	500	500	450
Biotin	µg	3	3	2.2	3	3	2.2
Vitamin C (ascorbic acid)	mg	12	12	8.2	12	12	8
Choline	mg	12	12	18	12	12	7.5
Inositol	mg	17	17	4.5	17	17	4.5
Carnitine	mg	2	0.92	1.5	1.8	2	1.6
Taurine	mg	6	6	6.5	6	6	8
Minerals							
Calcium	mg	82	75	138	82	82	90
Phosphorus	mg	55	50	109	55	55	60
Magnesium	mg	8	8	13	8	8	10
Iron	mg	1.8	1.2	1.8	1.8	1.2	1.2
Zinc	mg	1	1	0.6	1	1	0.75
Manganese	µg	15	15	5.2	27	15	7
Copper	µg	75	65	60	75	65	60
Iodine	µg	15	15	6.7	25	15	5
Selenium	µg	2.8					
Chromium	µg	None added					
Molybdenum	µg	None added					
Sodium	mg	30	30	53	30	30	34
Potassium	mg	110	110	182	110	110	120
Chloride	mg	67	70	85	67	67	74
Nucleotides	mg						
AMP	mg						
CMP	mg						
GMP	mg						
UMP	mg						
IMP	mg						
Recommended strength	kcal/L	676	676	676	676	676	670
Osmolarity	mosm/L	180	176				180

Product Type: Reduced Lactose Cow Milk Based (Nutrient content per 100 kcal)				
Manufacturer:		**Nutricia**	**Nutricia**	**Nutricia**
Product protein base Product name Product form (concentration) Geographic distribution	kcal/dL I pwd	Cow milk Nutrilon Low Lactose Powder Europe, Middle East, Far East, Middle & South America	Cow milk Nutrilon LF Powder Far East	Cow milk Bebelac FL Powder Europe, Middle East, Far East, Middle & South America
Protein Source Type/whey:casein	g	2.13 Milk 60:40	2.46 Milk 20:80	2.39 Casein 0:100
Fat C18:2ω6 Linoleic C18:3ω3 α-Linolenic C20:4ω6 Arachidonic C22:6ω3 Docosahexaenoic MCT added; % fat Sources	g mg mg mg mg %	5.42 600 115 Vegetable, milk	5.06 730 170 Vegetable, milk	5.26 750 80 Vegetable
Carbohydrate Glucose Lactose Sucrose Oligomers Maltodextrins Starch Fiber Source	g g g g g g g g	10.7 1.95 8.75 Maltodextrin, lactose	11.2 <0.04 11.1 Maltodextrin	10.8 10.8 Maltodextrin
Vitamins Vitamin A Activity Vitamin D Vitamin E Vitamin K	IU µg IU µg	380 2.1 1.9 8	380 1.6 1.9 7.3	410 2 1.6 7
Thiamine (vitamin B1) Riboflavin (vitamin B2) Vitamin B6 Vitamin B12 Niacin Folic Acid (folacin) Pantothenic acid Biotin Vitamin C (ascorbic acid)	µg µg µg µg µg µg µg µg mg	60 150 60 0.3 600 15 400 2.3 12	60 140 60 0.3 580 15 440 2.2 12	80 190 70 0.19 600 10 400 1.9 10
Choline Inositol Carnitine Taurine	mg mg mg mg	10 7	10 6.8	13 4.4 2.1 6
Minerals Calcium Phosphorus Magnesium Iron Zinc	mg mg mg mg mg	80 40 8 0.8 0.6	78 39 7.3 1.3 1	80 40 7.9 1.3 1
Manganese Copper Iodine Selenium Chromium Molybdenum	µg µg µg µg µg µg	10 60 15	10 70 22	20 80 10
Sodium Potassium Chloride	mg mg mg	27 100 60	25 100 69	31 90 64
Nucleotides AMP CMP GMP UMP IMP	mg mg mg mg mg mg			
Recommended strength Osmolarity	kcal/L mosm/L	660 195	690 200	700 190

Product Type: Alternate Protein (Nutrient content per 100 kcal)							
Manufacturer:		**Mead Johnson**	**Nestle**	**Ross Labs**	**Milupa**	**Nutricia**	**Nutricia**
Product protein base Product name		Soy ProSobee	Soy ALSOY	Soy Isomil	Soy SOM	Soy Nutrilon Soya (k)	Soy Nutrilon Soya Plus (i)
Product form (concentration)	kcal/dL I pwd	67.6		67.6	Powder	Powder	Powder
Geographic distribution		North America	Worldwide	North America	Europe	Europe, Middle East, Far East, Middle & South America	Europe, Far East, Middle & South America
Protein Source Type/whey:casein	g	3 Soy protein isolate, L-methionine Isolate	2.8 Soy isolate	2.45 Soy protein isolate, L-methionine	2.85 Soy protein isolate L-methionine	2.72 Soy protein isolate L-methionine	3.06 Soy protein isolate L-methionine
Fat C18:2ω6 Linoleic C18:3ω3 α-Linolenic C20:4ω6 Arachidonic C22:6ω3 Docosahexaenoic MCT added; % fat Sources	g mg mg mg mg %	5.3 910 90 Palm, soy, coconut, high oleic sunflower	5.0 1070 120 Palm olein, soybean oil	5.46 1300 Soy, coconut	5 650 60 Vegetable	5.42 630 110 Vegetable	5 950 180 Vegetable
Carbohydrate Glucose Lactose Sucrose Oligomers Maltodextrins Starch Fiber Source	g g g g g g g g	10 10 Corn syrup solids	11 11 Maltodextrin	10.3 Corn syrup, sucrose	10.9 4 6 0.9 Maltodextrin, glucose, starch	10.1 10.1 Maltodextrin	10.7 10.7 Maltodextrin
Vitamins Vitamin A Activity Vitamin D Vitamin E Vitamin K	IU µg IU µg	300 1.5 2 8	350 1.5 1.2 8	300 1.5 3 15	200 1.3 0.8 4	380 1.7 2 8	340 2.6 1.4 7.6
Thiamine (vitamin B1) Riboflavin (vitamin B2) Vitamin B6 Vitamin B12 Niacin Folic Acid (folacin) Pantothenic acid Biotin Vitamin C (ascorbic acid)	µg µg µg µg µg µg µg µg mg	80 90 60 0.3 1000 16 500 3 12	70 150 75 0.3 1000 9 450 2.2 16	60 90 60 0.45 1350 15 750 4.5 9	40 70 50 0.3 1000 8 600 8 9	60 150 60 0.3 600 15 400 2.3 12	60 140 60 0.4 600 14 400 2.2 12
Choline Inositol Carnitine Taurine	mg mg mg mg	12 17 2 6	10 5 3 8	8 5 	 2 9	10 5 2.3 7	
Minerals Calcium Phosphorus Magnesium Iron Zinc	mg mg mg mg mg	105 83 11 1.8 1.2	90 64 10 1.2 1.2	105 75 7.5 1.8 0.75	80 52 8 1.2 0.8	80 40 8 1.2 0.9	129 80 10 1.7 1.1
Manganese Copper Iodine Selenium Chromium Molybdenum	µg µg µg µg µg µg	25 75 15 2.8 None added None added	40 80 15 	30 75 15 2.1 	60 60 24 	50 60 20 	 60 24
Sodium Potassium Chloride	mg mg mg	36 120 80		44 108 62	38 112 66	27 100 60	32 139 80
Nucleotides AMP CMP GMP UMP IMP	mg mg mg mg mg mg						
Recommended strength Osmolarity	kcal/L mosm/L	676 182	670 170	676 205	700 255	663 180	719 210

Product Type: Alternate Protein (Nutrient content per 100 kcal)					
Manufacturer:		**Wyeth**	**Wyeth**	**Wyeth**	**Wyeth**
Product protein base		Soy	Soy	Soy	Soy
Product name		WYSOY	NURSOY	NURSOY	NURSOY
Product form	kcal/dL I pwd	67.2	65.6	66.7	66.7
(concentration)					
Geographic distribution		Europe	Asia	North America	Latin America
Protein	g	2.7	2.7	2.7	2.7
Source		Soy protein isolate	Soy protein isolate	Soy protein isolate	Soy protein isolate
Type/whey:casein					
Fat	g	5.4	5.5	5.3	5.3
C18:2ω6 Linoleic	mg	1004(1)	890	859(2)	1762(2)
C18:3ω3 α-Linolenic	mg	72	125	121	267
C20:4ω6 Arachidonic	mg		9.9	9.5	
C22:6ω3	mg				
Docosahexaenoic					
MCT added; % fat	%				
Sources		Palm, coconut, oleic, soy, lecithin	Oleo, coconut, soy, oleic, lecithin	Oleo, coconut, soy, oleic, lecithin	Soy, coconut, lecithin
Carbohydrate	g	10.3	10.5	10.2	10.2
Glucose	g				
Lactose	g				
Sucrose	g		2.6	2.0	2.0
Oligomers	g				
Maltodextrins	g	10.3	7.9	8.2	8.2
Starch	g				
Fiber	g	Trace			0.01
Source		Glucose syrup	Corn syrup solids, sucrose	Corn syrup solids, sucrose	Corn syrup solids, sucrose
Vitamins					
Vitamin A Activity	IU	372	305	300	300
Vitamin D	µg	1.6	1.5	1.5	1.5
Vitamin E	IU	1.6	1.4	1.4	2.85
Vitamin K	µg	14.9	15.3	15.0	15
Thiamine (vitamin B1)	µg	149	102	100	100
Riboflavin (vitamin B2)	µg	223	153	150	150
Vitamin B6	µg	89	64	63	63
Vitamin B12	µg	0.3	0.3	0.3	0.3
Niacin	µg	1339	763	750	750
Folic Acid (folacin)	µg	11.9	7.6	7.5	7.5
Pantothenic acid	µg	446	458	450	450
Biotin	µg	5.2	5.3	5.5	5.5
Vitamin C (ascorbic acid)	mg	13.4	8.4	8.3	8.3
Choline	mg	12.6		13.0	13
Inositol	mg	14.9		4.1	4.1
Carnitine	mg	+			+
Taurine	mg			+	+
Minerals					
Calcium	mg	99.7	91.5	90.0	90
Phosphorus	mg	74.4	64.1	63.0	63
Magnesium	mg	10.0	10.2	10.0	10
Iron	mg	1.2	1.8	1.8	1.8
Zinc	mg	0.9	0.8	0.8	0.8
Manganese	µg	49.1	30.5	30.0	30
Copper	µg	17.9	71.7	70.0	70
Iodine	µg	2.1	9.2	9.0	9
Selenium	µg				
Chromium	µg				
Molybdenum	µg				
Sodium	mg	28.3	30.5	30.0	30
Potassium	mg	107.1	106.8	105.0	105
Chloride	mg	64.0	61.0	56.0	56
Nucleotides	mg	None added	None added	None added	None added
AMP	mg				
CMP	mg				
GMP	mg				
UMP	mg				
IMP	mg				
Recommended strength	kcal/L	672	655	667	667
Osmolarity	mosm/L	198	198	197	198

Product Type: Reduced Antigen (Nutrient content per 100 kcal)					
Manufacturer:		**Mead Johnson**	**Nestle**	**Milupa**	**Milupa**
Product protein base Product name Product form (concentration) Geographic distribution	kcal/dL I pwd	Partial hydrolysate Enfastart Powder Europe	Partial hydrolysate Carnation Good Start Powder North America	Partial hydrolysate Aptamil 1 H.A. Milupan Powder, liquid r.t.f. Europe	Partial hydrolysate Aptamil H.A. 2 (i) Powder Europe
Protein Source Type/whey:casein	g	2.25 Nonfat milk, whey protein concentrate Partial hydrolysate	2.4 Whey protein Partial hydrolysate	2.32 Milk, enzym. hydrolysate 60:40	2.52 Milk, enzym. hydrolysate 50:50
Fat C18:2ω6 Linoleic C18:3ω3 α-Linolenic C20:4ω6 Arachidonic C22:6ω3 Docosahexaenoic MCT added; % fat Sources	g mg mg mg mg %	5.5 900 94 Palm olein, soy, coconut, high oleic sunflower	5.1 1030 110 Palm olein, soy, coconut, high oleic safflower	4.91 590 55 17 12 Vegetable, egg	4.84 620 60 Vegetable
Carbohydrate Glucose Lactose Sucrose Oligomers Maltodextrins Starch Fiber Source	g g g g g g g g	10.4 10.4 Lactose	11 7.7 3.3 Lactose, maltodextrins	11.6 10.1 1.5 Lactose, maltodextrin	11.6 8.1 1.9 1.6 Lactose, maltodextrin, starch
Vitamins Vitamin A Activity Vitamin D Vitamin E Vitamin K	 IU µg IU µg	 300 1.5 2 8	 300 1.5 2 8.2	 300 1.5 1 4.1	 270 1.4 0.8 4
Thiamine (vitamin B1) Riboflavin (vitamin B2) Vitamin B6 Vitamin B12 Niacin Folic Acid (folacin) Pantothenic acid Biotin Vitamin C (ascorbic acid)	µg µg µg µg µg µg µg µg mg	80 140 60 0.3 1000 16 500 3 12	60 135 75 0.22 750 9 450 2.2 8	50 80 50 0.3 1100 15 550 1.4 12	60 80 60 0.2 900 14 500 1.6 12
Choline Inositol Carnitine Taurine	mg mg mg mg	12 17 2 6	12 18 1.56 7.8	 2 9	
Minerals Calcium Phosphorus Magnesium Iron Zinc	 mg mg mg mg mg	 67 45 8 1.2 1	 64 36 6.7 1.5 0.75	 102 60 8 0.96 0.68	 113 71 9 1.1 0.8
Manganese Copper Iodine Selenium Chromium Molybdenum	µg µg µg µg µg µg	15 75 7	7 80 8	8 50 16	8 70 16
Sodium Potassium Chloride	mg mg mg	24 103 67	24 98 59	29 102 53	37 109 71
Nucleotides AMP CMP GMP UMP IMP	mg mg mg mg mg mg				
Recommended strength Osmolarity	kcal/L mosm/L	676	680 240	734 305	744 270

Product Type: Reduced Antigen (Nutrient content per 100 kcal)			
Manufacturer:		**Milupa**	**Milupa**
Product protein base		Partial hydrolysate	Partial hydrolysate
Product name		Milumil H.A. 1	Milumil H.A. 2 (i)
Product form	kcal/dL I pwd	Powder	Powder
(concentration)			
Geographic distribution		Germany	Europe
Protein	g	2.46	2.69
Source		Milk, enzym. hydrolysate	Milk, enzym. hydrolysate
Type/whey:casein		100:0	100:0
Fat	g	4.86	4.7
C18:2ω6 Linoleic	mg	630	610
C18:3ω3 α-Linolenic	mg	60	60
C20:4ω6 Arachidonic	mg		
C22:6ω3	mg		
Docosahexaenoic			
MCT added; % fat	%		
Sources		Vegetable	Vegetable
Carbohydrate	g	11.6	11.7
Glucose	g		
Lactose	g	4.9	5
Sucrose	g		
Oligomers	g		
Maltodextrins	g	5.1	5.1
Starch	g	1.6	1.6
Fiber	g		
Source		Maltodextrin, lactose, starch	Maltodextrin, lactose, starch
Vitamins			
Vitamin A Activity	IU	280	270
Vitamin D	µg	2	1.4
Vitamin E	IU	1.2	0.8
Vitamin K	µg	4.2	4
Thiamine (vitamin B1)	µg	80	60
Riboflavin (vitamin B2)	µg	160	160
Vitamin B6	µg	120	60
Vitamin B12	µg	0.2	0.2
Niacin	µg	2000	1000
Folic Acid (folacin)	µg	10	14
Pantothenic acid	µg	900	500
Biotin	µg	6	1.6
Vitamin C (ascorbic acid)	mg	10	12
Choline	mg		
Inositol	mg		
Carnitine	mg	2	
Taurine	mg	11	
Minerals			
Calcium	mg	99	113
Phosphorus	mg	58	71
Magnesium	mg	9	14
Iron	mg	1.1	1.6
Zinc	mg	0.8	0.8
Manganese	µg	160	10
Copper	µg	200	100
Iodine	µg	14	16
Selenium	µg		
Chromium	µg		
Molybdenum	µg		
Sodium	mg	48	67
Potassium	mg	131	184
Chloride	mg	71	109
Nucleotides	mg		
AMP	mg		
CMP	mg		
GMP	mg		
UMP	mg		
IMP	mg		
Recommended strength	kcal/L	744	766
Osmolarity	mosm/L	300	310

Product Type: Hypoallergenic (Nutrient content per 100 kcal)						
Manufacturer:		**Mead Johnson**	**Mead Johnson**	**Ross**	**Nestle**	**Nutricia**
Product protein base		Casein hydrolysate	Casein hydrolysate	Casein hydrolysate	Extensive hydrolysate	Extensive hydrolysate
Product name		Nutramigen	Pregestimil	Alimentum	Alfaré	Nutrilon Pepti
Product form (concentration)	kcal/dL I pwd	67.6	Powder	67.6	Powder	Powder, liquid r.t.f.
Geographic distribution		North America	North America	North America†	Worldwide	Europe
Protein	g	2.8	2.8	2.75	3.43	2.3
Source		Casein hydrolysate, amino acids	Casein hydrolysate, amino acids	Casein hydrolysate, amino acids	Whey protein	Milk, enzym. hydrolysate
Type/whey:casein					Extensive hydrolysate	100:0
Fat	g	5	5.6	5.54	5	5.4
C18:2ω6 Linoleic	mg	860	1120	1600	2938	600
C18:3ω3 α-Linolenic	mg	90	70		161	120
C20:4ω6 Arachidonic	mg					
C22:6ω3 Docosahexaenoic	mg					
MCT added; % fat	%		55	50	50	
Sources		Palm olein, soy, coconut, high oleic sunflower	MCT, corn, soy, high oleic safflower	MCT, safflower, soy	MCT, corn oil, milk fat, soy lecithin	Vegetable
Carbohydrate	g	11	10.3	10.2	10.8	10.4
Glucose	g		2			
Lactose	g					4
Sucrose	g					
Oligomers	g	8.1	5.9			
Maltodextrins	g				9.3	6.4
Starch	g	2.4	1.9		1.25	
Fiber	g					
Source		Corn syrup solids, modified corn starch	Corn syrup solids, dextrose, modified corn starch	Sucrose, modified tapioca starch	Maltodextrin, starch	Maltodextrin, lactose
Vitamins						
Vitamin A Activity	IU	300	380	300	300	380
Vitamin D	µg	1.5	1.88	1.13	1.5	3
Vitamin E	IU	2	3.8	3	1.2	1.8
Vitamin K	µg	8	18.8	15	8.2	8
Thiamine (vitamin B1)	µg	80	78	60	60	60
Riboflavin (vitamin B2)	µg	90	94	90	140	150
Vitamin B6	µg	60	63	60	75	60
Vitamin B12	µg	0.3	0.31	0.45	0.22	0.3
Niacin	µg	1000	1250	1350	750	1200
Folic Acid (folacin)	µg	16	15.6	15	9	15
Pantothenic acid	µg	500	470	750	450	450
Biotin	µg	3	7.8	4.5	2.2	2.3
Vitamin C (ascorbic acid)	mg	12	11.7	9	8	12
Choline	mg	12	13.3	8	7.5	11
Inositol	mg	17	4.7	5	4.5	5
Carnitine	mg	2	2		3	2.3
Taurine	mg	6	6		8	7
Minerals						
Calcium	mg	94	94	105	83	82
Phosphorus	mg	63	63	75	52	41
Magnesium	mg	11	10.9	7.5	12	8
Iron	mg	1.8	1.88	1.8	1.2	0.75
Zinc	mg	1	0.94	0.75	0.75	0.6
Manganese	µg	25	31	30	7	10
Copper	µg	75	94	75	60	60
Iodine	µg	15	7	15	5	15
Selenium	µg	2.8		2.8		
Chromium	µg	None added	None added			
Molybdenum	µg	None added	None added			
Sodium	mg	47	39	44	60	27
Potassium	mg	110	109	118	125	100
Chloride	mg	86	86	80	104	60
Nucleotides	mg					
AMP	mg					
CMP	mg					
GMP	mg					
UMP	mg					
IMP	mg					
Recommended strength	kcal/L	676	676	676	720	660
Osmolarity	mosm/L	290	290	330	200	260

Product Type: Hypoallergenic (Nutrient content per 100 kcal)						
Manufacturer:		**Nutricia**	**Nutricia**	**Milupa**	**SHS**	**Nutricia**
Product protein base		Extensive hydrolysate	Extensive hydrolysate	Extensive hydrolysate	Amino Acids	Amino acids
Product name		Nutrilon Pepti plus (i)	Pepti Junior	Pregomin	Neocate	Nutri-Junior
Product form (concentration)	kcal/dL I pwd	Powder	Powder	Powder, liquid r.t.f.	Powder, liquid r.t.f.	Powder
Geographic distribution		Europe	Europe, Middle East, Far East, Middle & South America	Europe, Middle East, Far East	Europe, North America	Europe
Protein	g	2.6	2.67	2.67	2.73	2.2
Source		Milk, enzym. hydrolysate	Milk, enzym. hydrolysate	Soy, beef enzym. hydrolysate	Amino acids	Amino acids
Type/whey:casein		100:0	100:0			
Fat	g	5.4	5.4	4.85	4.83	5.23
C18:2ω6 Linoleic	mg	1000	1200	630	850	590
C18:3ω3 α-Linolenic	mg	190	160	60	85	125
C20:4ω6 Arachidonic	mg					
C22:6ω3 Docosahexaenoic	mg					
MCT added; % fat	%		50			
Sources		Vegetable	Vegetable, MCT	Vegetable	Vegetable	Vegetable
Carbohydrate	g	10.2	10	11.4	11.3	11
Glucose	g					
Lactose	g	3.7	0.15			
Sucrose	g					
Oligomers	g					
Maltodextrins	g	6.5	9.8	9	11.3	11
Starch	g			2.4		
Fiber	g					
Source		Maltodextrin, lactose	Maltodextrin	Maltodextrin, starch	Maltodextrin	Maltodextrin
Vitamins						
Vitamin A Activity	IU	380	370	170	370	410
Vitamin D	µg	2.6	2	1.2	1.8	2
Vitamin E	IU	1.7	1.8	0.7	0.95	2.2
Vitamin K	µg	8	8	6.3	4.4	8
Thiamine (vitamin B1)	µg	60	60	60	80	60
Riboflavin (vitamin B2)	µg	160	160	100	130	150
Vitamin B6	µg	60	60	80	110	60
Vitamin B12	µg	0.3	0.3	0.26	0.26	0.3
Niacin	µg	560	580	900	950	600
Folic Acid (folacin)	µg	16	16	6	8	15
Pantothenic acid	µg	430	390	500	560	500
Biotin	µg	2.3	2.3	7	5.5	2.4
Vitamin C (ascorbic acid)	mg	12	12	4.5	8.4	13
Choline	mg	10	10		11	11
Inositol	mg		5		21	5
Carnitine	mg		2.3	2	2	2.3
Taurine	mg		7	8	4.2	7.1
Minerals						
Calcium	mg	125	81	68	68	83
Phosphorus	mg	71	41	42	48	42
Magnesium	mg	8.5	12	14	7	12
Iron	mg	1.8	1.4	2	1.5	0.8
Zinc	mg	1	0.6	1	1.1	0.6
Manganese	µg	20	10	20	130	11
Copper	µg	70	60	140	90	58
Iodine	µg	15	15	14	10	16
Selenium	µg		2		3.2	
Chromium	µg				3.2	
Molybdenum	µg			8	7.4	
Sodium	mg	33	30	50	25	31
Potassium	mg	122	100	110	88	100
Chloride	mg	72	59	54	61	58
Nucleotides	mg					
AMP	mg					
CMP	mg					
GMP	mg					
UMP	mg					
IMP	mg					
Recommended strength	kcal/L	700	668	750	710	650
Osmolarity	mosm/L	280	190	210	310	248

Footnotes - Nutricia

  (*)   due to local regulations or recommendations formula compositions may differ to some extent from country to country
  (a)   in some countries: Aptamil 1 Milupan
  (b)   carnitine derived from cows milk equal or in excess breast milk levels
  (c)   starch containing and starch free variants available on the market
  (d)   in some countries: Premium or Almiron 1
  (e)   in some countries: Babymilk Plus or Nutrilon Forte or Nutrilon Long Acting
  (f)   also variants available on the market with added starch or sucrose
  (g)   in some countries: Step Up or Almiron 2
  (h)   in some countries: Almiron 1 AR and Almiron 2 AR
  (i)   second age formula
  (j)   lactose restricted formula
  (k)   in some countries: Infasoy

Footnotes - Wyeth

  (1)   Typical value, Label claim = 580 mg/dl.
  (2)   Typical value, Label claim = 500 mg/100 Kcal.
  (3)   Typical value, Label claim = > 203 mg/dl.
  (4)   Typical value, Label claim = 300 mg/100 Kcal.
  (5)   Typical value, Label claim = 54 mg/dl.
  +   Added but no value claim.

Footnotes - Ross Labs

  †   Ross Labs international products may have slightly different nutrient levels based on local regulations.

Footnotes - Nestle

  ‡   several brands:Nldal AR, Nldina AR, Nestogeno AR, Nan AR

Appendix 2 - Growth Charts

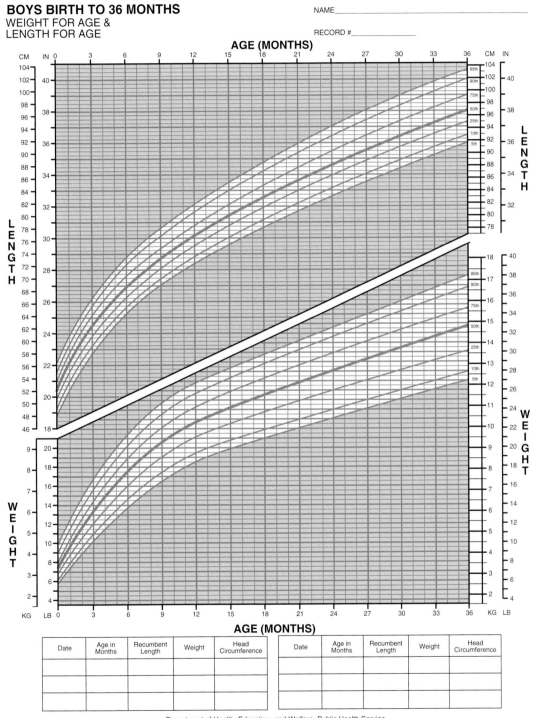

BOYS BIRTH TO 36 MONTHS
WEIGHT FOR AGE &
LENGTH FOR AGE

NAME_____

RECORD #_____

AGE (MONTHS)

Date	Age in Months	Recumbent Length	Weight	Head Circumference

Date	Age in Months	Recumbent Length	Weight	Head Circumference

Department of Health, Education, and Welfare, Public Health Service
Health Resources Administration, National Center for Health Statistics, and Center for Disease Control

Provided courtesy of Mead Johnson Company® and Enfamil™

BOYS: BIRTH TO 36 MONTHS
HEAD CIRCUMFERENCE FOR AGE &
WEIGHT FOR LENGTH

NAME_____

RECORD #_____

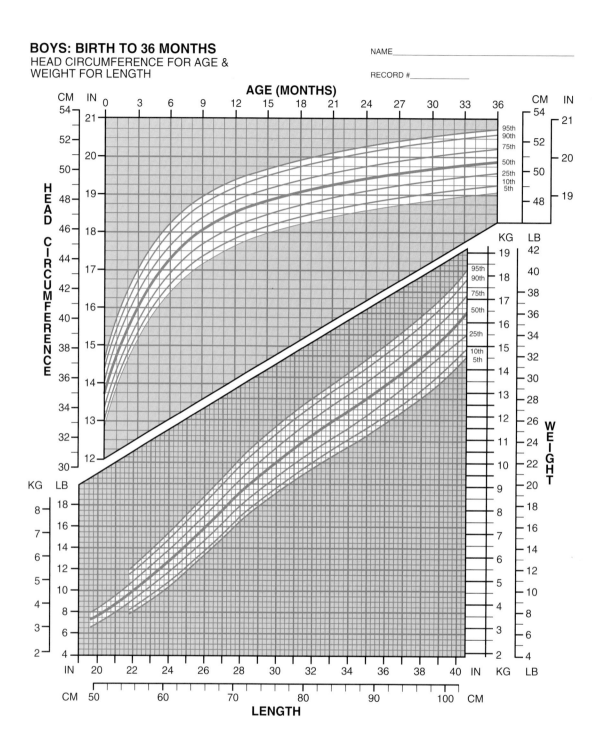

Provided courtesy of Mead Johnson Company® and Enfamil™

BOYS: 2 TO 18 YEARS

STATURE FOR AGE &
WEIGHT FOR AGE

NAME _____

RECORD # _____

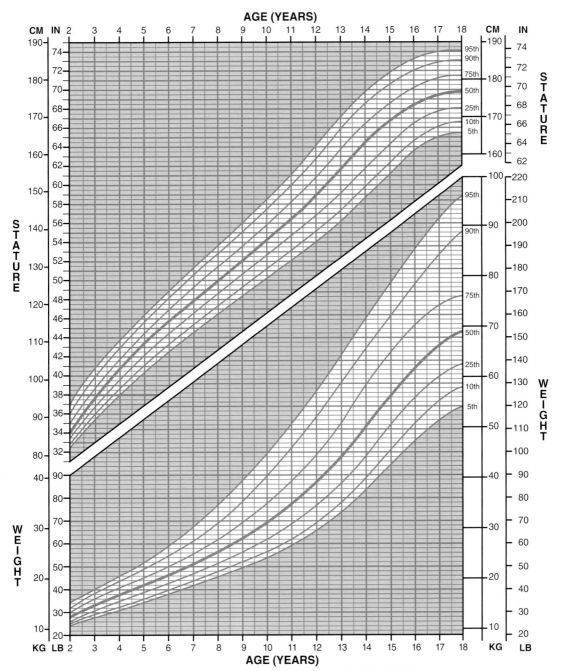

Department of Health, Education, and Welfare, Public Health Service
Health Resources Administration, National Center for Health Statistics, and Center for Disease Control

Provided courtesy of Mead Johnson Company® and Enfamil™

489

PRE-PUBERTAL BOYS: 2 TO 11-1/2 YEARS
WEIGHT FOR STATURE

NAME_____

RECORD #_____

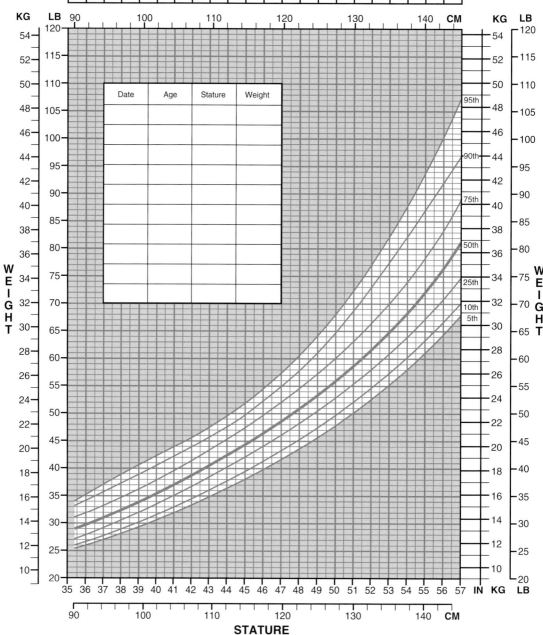

Date	Age	Stature	Weight

490

GIRLS BIRTH TO 36 MONTHS
WEIGHT FOR AGE &
LENGTH FOR AGE

NAME_____

RECORD #_____

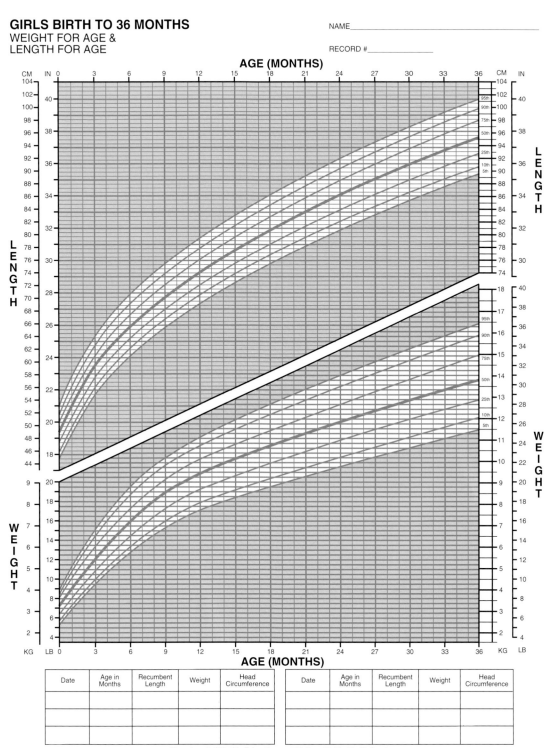

Date	Age in Months	Recumbent Length	Weight	Head Circumference		Date	Age in Months	Recumbent Length	Weight	Head Circumference

Department of Health, Education, and Welfare, Public Health Service
Health Resources Administration, National Center for Health Statistics, and Center for Disease Control

Provided courtesy of Mead Johnson Company® and Enfamil™

GIRLS: BIRTH TO 36 MONTHS
HEAD CIRCUMFERENCE FOR AGE & WEIGHT FOR LENGTH

NAME_____

RECORD #_____

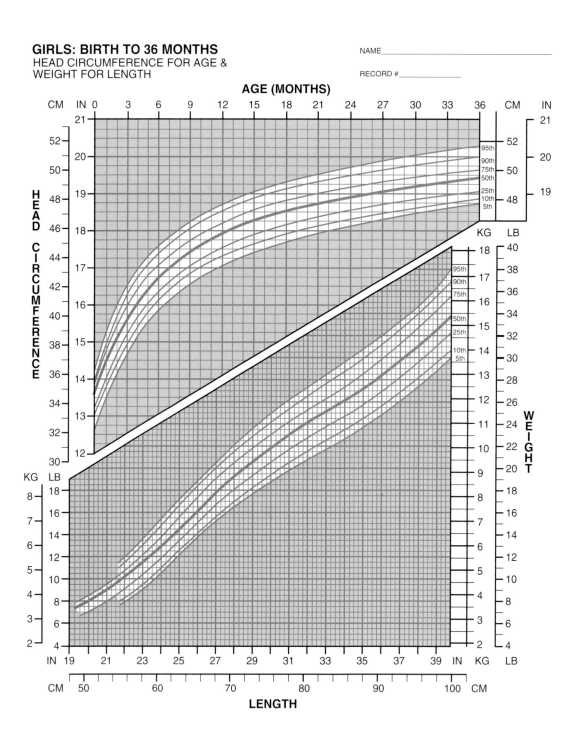

Provided courtesy of Mead Johnson Company® and Enfamil™

GIRLS: 2 TO 18 YEARS
STATURE FOR AGE &
WEIGHT FOR AGE

NAME _____

RECORD # _____

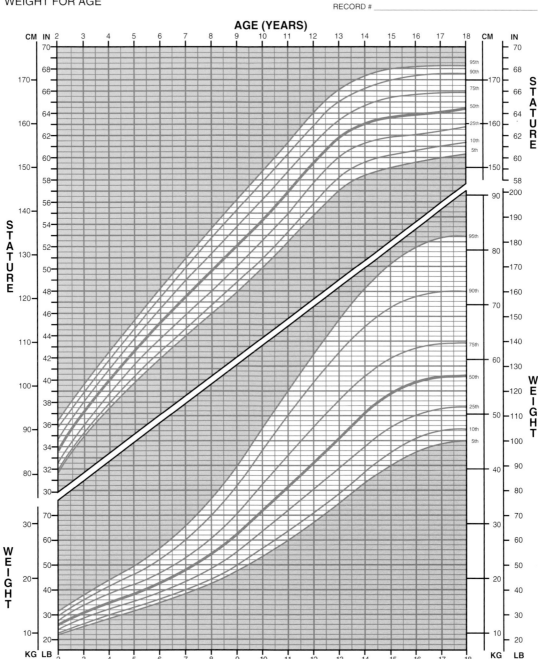

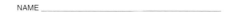

Department of Health, Education and Welfare, Public Health Resources Administration,
National Center for Health Statistics and Center for Disease Control

PRE-PUBERTAL GIRLS: 2 TO 10 YEARS
WEIGHT FOR STATURE

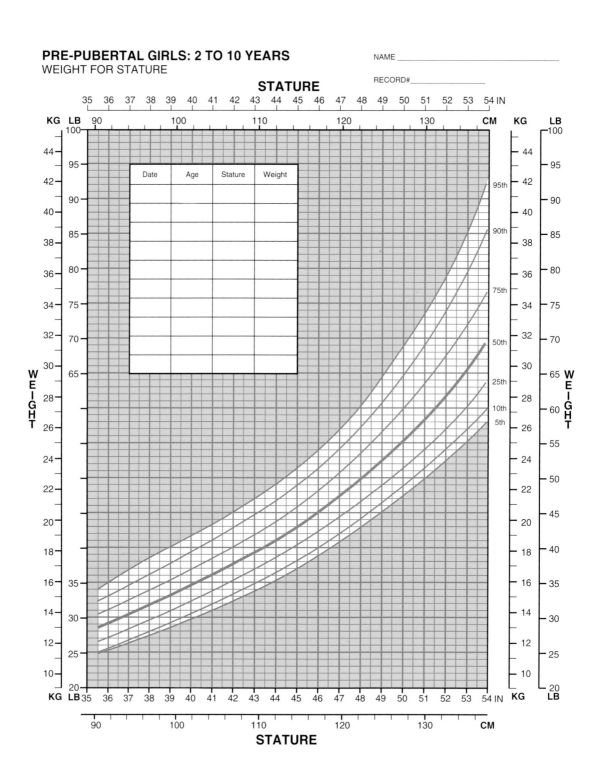

Date	Age	Stature	Weight

494

Appendix 3 - Arm Circumference and Skinfold Tables

MID-UPPER ARM CIRCUMFERENCE PERCENTILES (mm)							
AGE (yr)	5	10	25	50	75	90	95
Males							
1–1.9	142	146	150	159	170	176	183
2–2.9	141	145	153	162	170	178	185
3–3.9	150	153	160	167	175	184	190
4–4.9	149	154	162	171	180	186	192
5–5.9	153	160	167	175	185	195	204
6–6.9	155	159	167	179	188	209	228
7–7.9	162	167	177	187	201	223	230
8–8.9	162	170	177	190	202	220	245
9–9.9	175	178	187	200	217	249	257
10–10.9	181	184	196	210	231	262	274
11–11.9	186	190	202	223	244	261	280
12–12.9	193	200	214	232	254	282	303
13–13.9	194	211	228	247	263	286	301
14–14.9	220	226	237	253	283	303	322
15–15.9	222	229	244	264	284	311	320
16–16.9	244	248	262	278	303	324	343
Females							
1–1.9	138	142	148	156	164	172	177
2–2.9	142	145	152	160	167	176	184
3–3.9	143	150	158	167	175	183	189
4–4.9	149	154	160	169	177	184	191
5–5.9	153	157	165	175	185	203	211
6–6.9	156	162	170	176	187	204	211
7–7.9	164	167	174	183	199	216	231
8–8.9	168	172	183	195	214	247	261
9–9.9	178	182	194	211	224	251	260
10–10.9	174	182	193	210	228	251	265
11–11.9	185	194	208	224	248	276	303
12–12.9	194	203	216	237	256	282	294
13–13.9	202	211	223	243	271	301	338
14–14.9	214	223	237	252	272	304	322
15–15.9	208	221	239	254	279	300	322
16–16.9	218	224	241	258	283	318	334

Percentiles for mid-upper arm circumference (mm) for U.S. white persons aged one to seventeen years old. Data from the NHANES I (1971-1974) survey. From Frisancho (1981). © Am. J. Clin. Nutr. American Society for Clinical Nutrition.

\multicolumn{8}{c}{MID-UPPER ARM MUSCLE CIRCUMFERENCE PERCENTILES (mm)}							
AGE (yr)	5	10	25	50	75	90	95
Males							
1–1.9	110	113	119	127	135	144	147
2–2.9	111	114	122	130	140	146	150
3–3.9	117	123	131	137	143	148	153
4–4.9	123	126	133	141	148	156	159
5–5.9	128	133	140	147	154	162	169
6–6.9	131	135	142	151	161	170	177
7–7.9	137	139	151	160	168	177	190
8–8.9	140	145	154	162	170	182	187
9–9.9	151	154	161	170	183	196	202
10–10.9	156	160	166	180	191	209	221
11–11.9	159	165	173	183	195	205	230
12–12.9	167	171	182	195	210	223	241
13–13.9	172	179	196	211	226	238	245
14–14.9	189	199	212	223	240	260	264
15–15.9	199	204	218	237	254	266	272
16–16.9	213	225	234	249	269	287	296
Females							
1–1.9	105	111	117	124	132	139	143
2–2.9	111	114	119	126	133	142	147
3–3.9	113	119	124	132	140	146	152
4–4.9	115	121	128	136	144	152	157
5–5.9	125	128	134	142	151	159	165
6–6.9	130	133	138	145	154	166	171
7–7.9	129	135	142	151	160	171	176
8–8.9	138	140	151	160	171	183	194
9–9.9	147	150	158	167	180	194	198
10–10.9	148	150	159	170	180	190	197
11–11.9	150	158	171	181	196	217	223
12–12.9	162	166	180	191	201	214	220
13–13.9	169	175	183	198	211	226	240
14–14.9	174	179	190	201	216	232	247
15–15.9	175	178	189	202	215	228	244
16–16.9	170	180	190	202	216	234	249

Percentiles for mid-upper arm muscle circumference (mm) for U.S. white persons aged one to seventeen years old. Data from the NHANES I (1971-1974) survey. From Frisancho (1981). © Am. J. Clin. Nutr. American Society for Clinical Nutrition.

MID-UPPER ARM FAT AREA PERCENTILES (mm²)

AGE (yr)	5	10	25	50	75	90	95
Males							
1–1.9	452	486	590	741	895	1036	1176
2–2.9	434	504	578	737	871	1044	1148
3–3.9	464	519	590	736	868	1071	1151
4–4.9	428	494	598	722	859	989	1085
5–5.9	446	488	582	713	914	1176	1299
6–6.9	371	446	539	678	896	1115	1519
7–7.9	423	473	574	758	1011	1393	1511
8–8.9	410	460	588	725	1003	1248	1558
9–9.9	485	527	635	859	1252	1864	2081
10–10.9	523	543	738	982	1376	1906	2609
11–11.9	536	595	754	1148	1710	2348	2574
12–12.9	554	650	874	1172	1558	2536	3580
13–13.9	475	570	812	1096	1702	2744	3322
14–14.9	453	563	786	1082	1608	2746	3508
15–15.9	521	595	690	931	1423	2434	3100
16–16.9	542	593	844	1078	1746	2280	3041
Females							
1–1.9	401	466	578	706	847	1022	1140
2–2.9	469	526	642	747	894	1061	1173
3–3.9	473	529	656	822	967	1106	1158
4–4.9	490	541	654	766	907	1109	1236
5–5.9	470	529	647	812	997	1330	1536
6–6.9	464	508	638	827	1009	1263	1436
7–7.9	491	560	706	920	1135	1407	1644
8–8.9	527	634	769	1042	1383	1872	2482
9–9.9	642	690	933	1219	1584	2171	2524
10–10.9	616	702	842	1141	1608	2500	3005
11–11.9	707	802	1015	1301	1942	2730	3690
12–12.9	782	854	1090	1511	2056	2666	3369
13–13.9	726	838	1219	1625	2374	3272	4150
14–14.9	981	1043	1423	1818	2403	3250	3765
15–15.9	839	1126	1396	1886	2544	3093	4195
16–16.9	1126	1351	1663	2006	2598	3374	4236

Percentiles for mid-upper arm fat area (mm²) for U.S. white persons aged one to seventeen years old. Data from the NHANES I (1971-1974) survey. From Frisancho (1981). © Am. J. Clin. Nutr. American Society for Clinical Nutrition.

MID-UPPER ARM MUSCLE AREA PERCENTILES (mm²)

AGE (yr)	5	10	25	50	75	90	95
Males							
1–1.9	956	1014	1133	1278	1447	1644	1720
2–2.9	973	1040	1190	1345	1557	1690	1787
3–3.9	1095	1201	1357	1484	1618	1750	1853
4–4.9	1207	1264	1408	1579	1747	1926	2008
5–5.9	1298	1411	1550	1720	1884	2089	2285
6–6.9	1360	1447	1605	1815	2056	2297	2493
7–7.9	1497	1548	1808	2027	2246	2494	2886
8–8.9	1550	1664	1895	2089	2296	2628	2788
9–9.9	1811	1884	2067	2288	2657	3053	3257
10–10.9	1930	2027	2182	2575	2903	3486	3882
11–11.9	2016	2156	2382	2670	3022	3359	4226
12–12.9	2216	2339	2649	3022	3496	3968	4640
13–13.9	2363	2546	3044	3553	4081	4502	4794
14–14.9	2830	3147	3586	3963	4575	5368	5530
15–15.9	3138	3317	3788	4481	5134	5631	5900
16–16.9	3625	4044	4352	4951	5753	6576	6980
Females							
1–1.9	885	973	1084	1221	1378	1535	1621
2–2.9	973	1029	1119	1269	1405	1595	1727
3–3.9	1014	1133	1227	1396	1563	1690	1846
4–4.9	1058	1171	1313	1475	1644	1832	1958
5–5.9	1238	1301	1423	1598	1825	2012	2159
6–6.9	1354	1414	1513	1683	1877	2182	2323
7–7.9	1330	1441	1602	1815	2045	2332	2469
8–8.9	1513	1566	1808	2034	2327	2657	2996
9–9.9	1723	1788	1976	2227	2571	2987	3112
10–10.9	1740	1784	2019	2296	2583	2873	3093
11–11.9	1784	1987	2316	2612	3071	3739	3953
12–12.9	2092	2182	2579	2904	3225	3655	3847
13–13.9	2269	2426	2657	3130	3529	4081	4568
14–14.9	2418	2562	2874	3220	3704	4294	4850
15–15.9	2426	2518	2847	3248	3689	4123	4756
16–16.9	2308	2567	2865	3248	3718	4353	4946

Percentiles for mid-upper arm muscle area (mm²) for U.S. white persons aged one to seventeen years old. Data from the NHANES I (1971-1974) survey. From Frisancho (1981). © Am. J. Clin. Nutr. American Society for Clinical Nutrition.

TRICEPS SKINFOLD PERCENTILES (mm)

AGE (yr)	5	10	25	50	75	90	95
Males							
1–1.9	6	7	8	10	12	14	16
2–2.9	6	7	8	10	12	14	15
3–3.9	6	7	8	10	11	14	15
4–4.9	6	6	8	9	11	12	14
5–5.9	6	6	8	9	11	14	15
6–6.9	5	6	7	8	10	13	16
7–7.9	5	6	7	9	12	15	17
8–8.9	5	6	7	8	10	13	16
9–9.9	6	6	7	10	13	17	18
10–10.9	6	6	8	10	14	18	21
11–11.9	6	6	8	11	16	20	24
12–12.9	6	6	8	11	14	22	28
13–13.9	5	5	7	10	14	22	26
14–14.9	4	5	7	9	14	21	24
15–15.9	4	5	6	8	11	18	24
16–16.9	4	5	6	8	12	16	22
Females							
1–1.9	6	7	8	10	12	14	16
2–2.9	6	8	9	10	12	15	16
3–3.9	7	8	9	11	12	14	15
4–4.9	7	8	8	10	12	14	16
5–5.9	6	7	8	10	12	15	18
6–6.9	6	6	8	10	12	14	16
7–7.9	6	7	9	11	13	16	18
8–8.9	6	8	9	12	15	18	24
9–9.9	8	8	10	13	16	20	22
10–10.9	7	8	10	12	17	23	27
11–11.9	7	8	10	13	18	24	28
12–12.9	8	9	11	14	18	23	27
13–13.9	8	8	12	15	21	26	30
14–14.9	9	10	13	16	21	26	28
15–15.9	8	10	12	17	21	25	32
16–16.9	10	12	15	18	22	26	31

Percentiles for triceps skinfolds (mm) for U.S. white persons aged one to seventeen years old. Data from the NHANES I (1971-1974) survey. From Frisancho (1981). © Am. J. Clin. Nutr. American Society for Clinical Nutrition.

Appendix 4 - Growth Tables

	THE NCHS STANDARDS TABLE 2.1 LENGTH BY AGE OF BOYS 0-36 MONTHS							
	LENGTH							
AGE MONTHS	(-)3SD	(-)2SD	(-)1SD	MEDIAN	(+)1SD	(+)2SD	(+)3SD	AGE MONTHS
0	43.6	45.9	48.2	50.5	52.8	55.1	57.3	0
1	47.2	49.7	52.1	54.6	57	59.5	61.9	1
2	50.4	52.9	55.5	58.1	60.7	63.2	65.8	2
3	53.2	55.8	58.5	61.1	63.8	66.4	69	3
4	55.6	58.3	61	63.7	66.4	69.1	71.7	4
5	57.8	60.5	63.2	65.9	68.6	71.3	74	5
6	59.8	62.4	65.1	67.8	70.5	73.2	75.9	6
7	61.5	64.1	66.8	69.5	72.2	74.8	77.5	7
8	63	65.7	68.3	71.0	73.6	76.3	78.9	8
9	64.4	67	69.7	72.3	75	77.6	80.3	9
10	65.7	68.3	71	73.6	76.3	78.9	81.6	10
11	66.9	69.6	72.2	74.9	77.6	80.2	82.9	11
12	68	70.7	73.4	76.1	78.8	81.5	84.2	12
13	69	71.8	74.5	77.2	80	82.7	85.5	13
14	70	72.8	75.6	78.3	81.1	83.9	86.7	14
15	70.9	73.7	76.6	79.4	82.3	85.1	88	15
16	71.7	74.6	77.5	80.4	83.4	86.3	89.2	16
17	72.5	75.5	78.5	81.4	84.4	87.4	90.4	17
18	73.3	76.3	79.4	82.4	85.4	88.5	91.5	18
19	74	77.1	80.2	83.3	86.4	89.5	92.7	19
20	74.7	77.9	81.1	84.2	87.4	90.6	93.7	20
21	75.4	78.7	81.9	85.1	88.4	91.6	94.8	21
22	76.1	79.4	82.7	86	89.3	92.5	95.8	22
23	76.8	80.2	83.5	86.8	90.2	93.5	96.8	23
24	77.5	80.9	84.3	87.6	91	94.4	97.7	24

LENGTH BY AGE OF GIRLS 0-36 MONTHS

LENGTH

AGE MONTHS	(-)3SD	(-)2SD	(-)1SD	MEDIAN	(+)1SD	(+)2SD	(+)3SD	AGE MONTHS
0	43.4	45.5	47.7	49.9	52	54.2	56.4	0
1	46.7	49	51.2	53.5	55.8	58.1	60.4	1
2	49.6	52	54.4	56.8	59.2	61.6	64	2
3	52.1	54.6	57.1	59.5	62	64.5	67	3
4	54.3	56.9	59.4	62	64.5	67.1	69.6	4
5	56.3	58.9	61.5	64.1	66.7	69.3	71.9	5
6	58	60.6	63.3	65.9	68.6	71.2	73.9	6
7	59.5	62.2	64.9	67.6	70.3	72.9	75.6	7
8	60.9	63.7	66.4	69.1	71.8	74.5	77.2	8
9	62.2	65	67.7	70.4	73.2	75.9	78.7	9
10	63.5	66.2	69	71.8	74.5	77.3	80.1	10
11	64.7	67.5	70.3	73.1	75.9	78.7	81.5	11
12	65.8	68.6	71.5	74.3	77.1	80	82.8	12
13	66.9	69.8	72.6	75.5	78.4	81.2	84.1	13
14	67.9	70.8	73.7	76.7	79.6	82.5	85.4	14
15	68.9	71.9	74.8	77.8	80.7	83.7	86.6	15
16	69.9	72.9	75.9	78.9	81.8	84.8	87.8	16
17	70.8	73.8	76.9	79.9	82.9	86	89	17
18	71.7	74.8	77.9	80.9	84	87.1	90.1	18
19	72.6	75.7	78.8	81.9	85	88.1	91.2	19
20	73.4	76.6	79.7	82.9	86	89.2	92.3	20
21	74.3	77.4	80.6	83.8	87	90.2	93.4	21
22	75.1	78.3	81.5	84.7	87.9	91.2	94.4	22
23	75.9	79.1	82.4	85.6	88.9	92.1	95.4	23
24	76.6	79.9	83.2	86.5	89.8	93	96.3	24

AGE MONTHS	(-)3SD	(-)2SD	(-)1SD	MEDIAN	(+)1SD	(+)2SD	(+)3SD	AGE MONTHS
0	2	2.5	2.9	3.3	3.8	4.3	4.8	0
1	2.2	2.9	3.6	4.3	5	5.6	6.3	1
2	2.6	3.5	4.3	5.2	6	6.8	7.6	2
3	3.1	4.1	5	6	6.9	7.7	8.6	3
4	3.7	4.7	5.7	6.7	7.6	8.5	9.4	4
5	4.3	5.3	6.3	7.3	8.2	9.2	10.1	5
6	4.9	5.9	6.9	7.8	8.8	9.8	10.8	6
7	5.4	6.4	7.4	8.3	9.3	10.3	11.3	7
8	5.9	6.9	7.8	8.8	9.8	10.8	11.8	8
9	6.3	7.2	8.2	9.2	10.2	11.3	12.3	9
10	6.6	7.6	8.6	9.5	10.6	11.7	12.7	10
11	6.9	7.9	8.9	9.9	10.9	12	13.1	11
12	7.1	8.1	9.1	10.2	11.3	12.4	13.5	12
13	7.3	8.3	9.4	10.4	11.5	12.7	13.8	13
14	7.5	8.5	9.6	10.7	11.8	13	14.1	14
15	7.6	8.7	9.8	10.9	12	13.2	14.4	15
16	7.7	8.8	10	11.1	12.3	13.5	14.7	16
17	7.8	9	10.1	11.3	12.5	13.7	14.9	17
18	7.9	9.1	10.3	11.5	12.7	13.9	15.2	18
19	8	9.2	10.5	11.7	12.9	14.1	15.4	19
20	8.1	9.4	10.6	11.8	13.1	14.4	15.6	20
21	8.3	9.5	10.8	12	13.3	14.6	15.8	21
22	8.4	9.7	10.9	12.2	13.5	14.8	16	22
23	8.5	9.8	11.1	12.4	13.7	15	16.3	23
24	8.6	9.9	11.3	12.6	13.9	15.2	16.5	24

WEIGHT BY AGE OF GIRLS 0-36 MONTHS

WEIGHT

AGE MONTHS	(-)3SD	(-)2SD	(-)1SD	MEDIAN	(+)1SD	(+)2SD	(+)3SD	AGE MONTHS
0	1.7	2.2	2.7	3.2	3.6	4	4.3	0
1	2.2	2.8	3.4	4	4.5	5.1	5.6	1
2	2.7	3.3	4	4.7	5.4	6.1	6.8	2
3	3.2	3.9	4.7	5.4	6.2	7	7.7	3
4	3.7	4.5	5.3	6	6.9	7.7	8.6	4
5	4.1	5	5.8	6.7	7.5	8.4	9.3	5
6	4.6	5.5	6.3	7.2	8.1	9	10	6
7	5	5.9	6.8	7.7	8.7	9.6	10.5	7
8	5.3	6.3	7.2	8.2	9.1	10.1	11.1	8
9	5.7	6.6	7.6	8.6	9.6	10.5	11.5	9
10	5.9	6.9	7.9	8.9	9.9	10.9	11.9	10
11	6.2	7.2	8.2	9.2	10.3	11.3	12.3	11
12	6.4	7.4	8.5	9.5	10.6	11.6	12.6	12
13	6.6	7.6	8.7	9.8	10.8	11.9	13	13
14	6.7	7.8	8.9	10	11.1	12.2	13.2	14
15	6.9	8	9.1	10.2	11.3	12.4	13.5	15
16	7	8.2	9.3	10.4	11.5	12.6	13.7	16
17	7.2	8.3	9.5	10.6	11.8	12.9	14	17
18	7.3	8.5	9.7	10.8	12	13.1	14.2	18
19	7.5	8.6	9.8	11	12.2	13.3	14.5	19
20	7.6	8.8	10	11.2	12.4	13.5	14.7	20
21	7.8	9	10.2	11.4	12.6	13.8	15	21
22	7.9	9.1	10.3	11.5	12.8	14	15.2	22
23	8.1	9.3	10.5	11.7	13	14.2	15.5	23
24	8.2	9.4	10.7	11.9	13.2	14.5	15.8	24

				WEIGHT BY LENGTH OF BOYS 49-103 CM				
				WEIGHT				
LENGTH CM	(-)3SD	(-)2SD	(-)1SD	MEDIAN	(+)1SD	(+)2SD	(+)3SD	LENGTH CM
49	2.1	2.5	2.8	3.2	3.7	4.2	4.7	49
49.5	2.1	2.5	2.9	3.2	3.7	4.3	4.8	49.5
50	2.2	2.5	2.9	3.3	3.8	4.4	4.9	50
50.5	2.2	2.6	3	3.4	3.9	4.5	5	50.5
51	2.2	2.6	3.1	3.5	4	4.6	5.1	51
51.5	2.3	2.7	3.1	3.6	4.1	4.7	5.2	51.5
52	2.3	2.8	3.2	3.7	4.2	4.8	5.4	52
52.5	2.4	2.8	3.3	3.8	4.4	4.9	5.5	52.5
53	2.4	2.9	3.4	3.9	4.5	5	5.6	53
53.5	2.5	3	3.5	4	4.6	5.2	5.8	53.5
54	2.6	3.1	3.6	4.1	4.7	5.3	5.9	54
54.5	2.6	3.2	3.7	4.2	4.8	5.4	6	54.5
55	2.7	3.3	3.8	4.3	5	5.6	6.2	55
55.5	2.8	3.3	3.9	4.5	5.1	5.7	6.3	55.5
56	2.9	3.4	4	4.6	5.2	5.9	6.5	56
56.5	3	3.6	4.1	4.7	5.4	6	6.6	56.5
57	3.1	3.7	4.3	4.8	5.5	6.1	6.8	57
57.5	3.2	3.9	4.4	5	5.6	6.3	7	57.5
58	3.3	3.9	4.5	5.1	5.8	6.4	7.1	58
58.5	3.4	4	4.6	5.2	5.9	6.6	7.3	58.5
59	3.5	4.1	4.8	5.4	6.1	6.7	7.4	59
59.5	3.6	4.2	4.9	5.5	6.2	6.9	7.6	59.5
60	3.7	4.4	5	5.7	6.4	7.1	7.8	60
60.5	3.8	4.5	5.1	5.8	6.5	7.2	7.9	60.5
61	4	4.6	5.8	5.9	6.7	7.4	8.1	61
61.5	4.1	4.8	5.4	6.1	6.8	7.5	8.3	61.5
62	4.2	4.5	5.6	6.2	7	7.7	8.4	62
62.5	4.3	5	5.7	6.4	7.1	7.9	8.6	62.5
63	4.5	5.2	5.8	6.5	7.3	8	8.8	63
63.5	4.6	5.3	6	6.7	7.4	8.2	8.9	63.5
64	4.7	5.4	6.1	6.8	7.6	8.3	9.1	64
64.5	4.9	5.6	6.3	7	7.7	8.5	9.3	64.5
65	5	5.7	6.4	7.1	7.9	8.7	9.4	65
65.5	5.1	5.8	6.5	7.3	8	8.8	9.6	65.5
66	5.3	6	6.7	7.4	8.2	9	9.8	66
66.5	5.4	6.1	6.8	7.6	8.3	9.1	9.9	66.5
67	5.5	6.2	7	7.7	8.5	9.3	10.1	67
67.5	5.7	6.4	7.1	7.8	8.6	9.5	10.3	67.5
68	5.8	6.5	7.2	8	8.8	9.6	10.4	68
68.5	5.9	6.6	7.4	8.1	8.9	9.8	10.6	68.5
69	6	6.8	7.5	8.3	9.1	9.9	10.8	69
69.5	6.2	6.9	7.7	8.4	9.2	10.1	10.9	69.5
70	6.3	7	7.8	8.5	9.4	10.2	11.1	70
70.5	6.4	7.2	7.9	8.7	9.5	10.4	11.2	70.5
71	6.5	7.3	8.1	8.8	9.7	10.5	11.4	71
71.5	6.7	7.4	8.2	8.9	9.8	10.7	11.5	71.5

WEIGHT BY LENGTH OF BOYS 49-103 CM CONT'D.D293							
WEIGHT							
LENGTH CM	(-)3SD	(-)2SD	(-)1SD	MEDIAN	(+)1SD	(+)2SD	(+)3SD	LENGTH CM
72	6.8	7.5	8.3	9.1	9.9	10.8	11.7	72
72.5	6.9	7.7	8.4	9.2	10.1	11	11.8	72.5
73	7	7.8	8.6	9.3	10.2	11.1	12	73
73.5	7.1	7.9	8.7	9.5	10.3	11.2	12.1	73.5
74	7.2	8	8.8	9.6	10.5	11.4	12.3	74
74.5	7.3	8.1	8.9	9.7	10.6	11.5	12.4	74.5
75	7.4	8.2	9	9.8	10.7	11.6	12.5	75
75.5	7.5	8.3	9.1	9.9	10.8	11.8	12.7	75.5
76	7.6	8.4	9.2	10	11	11.9	12.8	76
76.5	7.7	8.5	9.3	10.2	11.1	12	12.9	76.5
77	7.8	8.6	9.4	10.3	11.2	12.1	13.1	77
77.5	7.9	8.7	9.5	10.4	11.3	12.3	13.2	77.5
78	8	8.8	9.7	10.5	11.4	12.4	13.3	78
78.5	8.1	8.9	9.8	10.6	11.6	12.5	13.5	78.5
79	8.2	9	9.9	10.7	11.7	12.6	13.6	79
79.5	8.2	9.1	10	10.8	11.8	12.7	13.7	79.5
80	8.3	9.2	10.1	10.9	11.9	12.9	13.8	80
80.5	8.4	9.3	10.1	11	12	13	14	80.5
81	8.5	9.4	10.2	11.1	12.1	13.1	14.1	81
81.5	8.6	9.5	10.3	11.2	12.2	13.2	14.2	81.5
82	8.7	9.6	10.4	11.3	12.3	13.3	14.3	82
82.5	8.8	9.6	10.5	11.4	12.4	13.4	14.4	82.5
83	8.8	9.7	10.6	11.5	12.5	13.5	14.6	83
83.5	8.9	9.8	10.7	11.6	12.6	13.7	14.7	83.5
84	9	9.9	10.8	11.7	12.7	13.8	14.8	84
84.5	9.1	10	10.9	11.8	12.9	13.9	14.9	84.5
85	9.2	10.1	11	11.9	13	14	15	85
85.5	9.3	10.2	11.1	12	13.1	14.1	15.1	85.5
86	9.3	10.3	11.2	12.1	13.2	14.2	15.3	86
86.5	9.4	10.4	11.3	12.2	13.3	14.3	15.4	86.5
87	9.5	10.5	11.4	12.3	13.4	14.4	15.5	87
87.5	9.6	10.5	11.5	12.4	13.5	14.5	15.6	87.5
88	9.7	10.6	11.6	12.5	13.6	14.7	15.7	88
88.5	9.8	10.7	11.7	12.7	13.7	14.8	15.8	88.5
89	9.9	10.8	11.8	12.8	13.8	14.9	16	89
89.5	10	10.9	11.9	12.9	13.9	15	16.1	89.5
90	10	11	12	13	14	15.1	16.2	90
90.5	10.1	11.1	12.1	13.1	14.2	15.2	16.3	90.5
91	10.2	11.2	12.2	13.2	14.3	15.3	16.4	91
91.5	10.3	11.3	12.3	13.3	14.4	15.5	16.5	91.5
92	10.4	11.4	12.4	13.4	14.5	15.6	15.7	92
92.5	10.5	11.5	12.5	13.5	14.6	15.7	16.8	92.5
93	10.6	11.6	12.6	13.7	14.7	15.8	16.9	93
93.5	10.7	11.7	12.8	13.8	14.9	15.9	17	93.5
94	10.8	11.9	12.9	13.9	15	16.1	17.1	94
94.5	10.9	12	13	14	15.1	16.2	17.3	94.5

LENGTH CM	(-)3SD	(-)2SD	(-)1SD	MEDIAN	(+)1SD	(+)2SD	(+)3SD	LENGTH CM
				WEIGHT				
49	2.2	2.6	2.9	3.3	3.6	4	4.3	49
49.5	2.2	2.6	3	3.3	3.7	4.1	4.5	49.5
50	2.3	2.6	3	3.4	3.8	4.2	4.6	50
50.5	2.3	2.7	3.1	3.5	3.9	4.3	4.7	50.5
51	2.3	2.7	3.1	3.5	4	4.4	4.9	51
51.5	2.4	2.8	3.2	3.6	4.1	4.5	5	51.5
52	2.4	2.8	3.3	3.7	4.2	4.7	5.1	52
52.5	2.5	2.9	3.4	3.8	4.3	4.8	5.3	52.5
53	2.5	3	3.4	3.9	4.4	4.9	5.4	53
53.5	2.6	3.1	3.5	4	4.5	5	5.6	53.5
54	2.7	3.1	3.6	4.1	4.6	5.2	5.7	54
54.5	2.7	3.2	3.7	4.2	4.7	5.3	5.9	54.5
55	2.8	3.3	3.8	4.3	4.9	5.4	6	55
55.5	2.9	3.4	3.9	4.4	5	5.6	6.2	55.5
56	3	3.5	4	4.5	5.1	5.7	6.3	56
56.5	3	3.6	4.1	4.6	5.3	5.9	6.5	56.5
57	3.1	3.7	4.2	4.8	5.4	6	6.6	57
57.5	3.2	3.8	4.3	4.9	5.5	6.2	6.8	57.5
58	3.3	3.9	4.4	5	5.7	6.3	7	58
58.5	3.4	4	4.6	5.1	5.8	6.5	7.1	58.5
59	3.5	4.1	4.7	5.3	5.9	6.6	7.3	59
59.5	3.6	4.2	4.8	5.4	6.1	6.8	7.4	59.5
60	3.7	4.3	4.9	5.5	6.2	6.9	7.6	60
60.5	3.8	4.4	5.1	5.7	6.4	7.1	7.7	60.5
61	3.9	4.6	5.2	5.8	6.5	7.2	7.9	61
61.5	4	4.7	5.3	6	6.7	7.4	8.1	61.5
62	4.1	4.8	5.4	6.1	6.8	7.5	8.2	62
62.5	4.2	4.9	5.6	6.2	7	7.7	8.4	62.5
63	4.4	5	5.7	6.4	7.1	7.8	8.5	63
63.5	4.5	5.2	5.8	6.5	7.3	8	8.7	63.5
64	4.6	5.3	6	6.7	7.4	8.1	8.9	64
64.5	4.7	5.4	6.1	6.8	7.6	8.3	9	64.5
65	4.8	5.5	6.3	7	7.7	8.4	9.2	65
65.5	4.9	5.7	6.4	7.1	7.9	8.6	9.3	65.5
66	5.1	5.8	6.5	7.3	8	8.7	9.5	66
66.5	5.2	5.9	6.7	7.4	8.1	8.9	9.6	66.5
67	5.3	6	6.8	7.5	8.3	9	9.8	67
67.5	5.4	6.2	6.9	7.7	8.4	9.2	9.9	67.5
68	5.5	6.3	7.1	7.8	8.6	9.3	10.1	68
68.5	5.6	6.4	7.2	8	8.7	9.5	10.2	68.5
69	5.8	6.5	7.3	8.1	8.9	9.6	10.4	69
69.5	5.9	6.7	7.5	8.2	9	9.8	10.5	69.5
70	6	6.8	7.6	8.4	9.1	9.9	10.7	70
70.5	6.1	6.9	7.7	8.5	9.3	10.1	10.8	70.5
71	6.2	7	7.8	8.6	9.4	10.2	11	71
71.5	6.3	7.1	8	8.8	9.5	10.3	11.1	71.5

WEIGHT BY LENGTH OF GIRLS 49-101 CM

LENGTH CM	(-)3SD	(-)2SD	(-)1SD	MEDIAN	(+)1SD	(+)2SD	(+)3SD	LENGTH CM
72	6.4	7.2	8.1	8.9	9.7	10.5	11.2	72
72.5	6.5	7.4	8.2	9	9.8	10.6	11.4	72.5
73	6.6	7.5	8.3	9.1	9.9	10.7	11.5	73
73.5	6.7	7.6	8.4	9.3	10	10.8	11.6	73.5
74	6.8	7.7	8.5	9.4	10.2	11	11.8	74
74.5	6.9	7.8	8.6	9.5	10.3	11.1	11.9	74.5
75	7	7.9	8.7	9.6	10.4	11.2	12	75
75.5	7.1	8	8.8	9.7	10.5	11.3	12.1	75.5
76	7.2	8.1	8.9	9.8	10.6	11.4	12.3	76
76.5	7.3	8.2	9	9.9	10.7	11.6	12.4	76.5
77	7.4	8.3	9.1	10	10.8	11.7	12.5	77
77.5	7.5	8.4	9.2	10.1	11	11.8	12.6	77.5
78	7.6	8.5	9.3	10.2	11.1	11.9	12.7	78
78.5	7.7	8.6	9.4	10.3	11.2	12	12.9	78.5
79	7.8	8.7	9.5	10.4	11.3	12.1	13	79
79.5	7.9	8.7	9.6	10.5	11.4	12.2	13.1	79.5
80	8	8.8	9.7	10.6	11.5	12.3	13.2	80
80.5	8	8.5	9.8	10.7	11.6	12.4	13.3	80.5
81	8.1	9	9.9	10.8	11.7	12.6	13.4	81
81.5	8.2	9.1	10	10.9	11.8	12.7	13.5	81.5
82	8.3	9.2	10.1	11	11.9	12.8	13.7	82
82.5	8.4	9.3	10.2	11.1	12	12.9	13.8	82.5
83	8.5	9.4	10.3	11.2	12.1	13	13.9	83
83.5	8.6	9.5	10.4	11.3	12.2	13.1	14	83.5
84	8.7	9.6	10.5	11.4	12.3	13.2	14.1	84
84.5	8.7	9.6	10.6	11.5	12.4	13.3	14.2	84.5
85	8.8	9.7	10.6	11.6	12.5	13.4	14.3	85
85.5	8.9	9.8	10.7	11.7	12.6	13.5	14.5	85.5
86	9	9.9	10.8	11.8	12.7	13.6	14.6	86
86.5	9.1	10	10.9	11.8	12.8	13.7	14.7	86.5
87	9.2	10.1	11	11.9	12.9	13.9	14.8	87
87.5	9.3	10.2	11.1	12	13	14	14.9	87.5
88	9.4	10.3	11.2	12.2	13.1	14.1	15	88
88.5	9.4	10.4	11.3	12.3	13.2	14.2	15.2	88.5
89	9.5	10.5	11.4	12.4	13.3	14.3	15.3	89
89.5	9.6	10.6	11.5	12.5	13.4	14.4	15.4	89.5
90	9.7	10.7	11.6	12.6	13.6	14.5	15.5	90
90.5	9.8	10.8	11.7	12.7	13.7	14.7	15.7	90.5
91	9.9	10.9	11.8	12.8	13.8	14.8	15.8	91
91.5	10	11	11.9	12.9	13.9	14.9	15.9	91.5
92	10.1	11.1	12.1	13	14	15	16	92
92.5	10.2	11.2	12.2	13.1	14.2	15.2	16.2	92.5
93	10.3	11.3	12.3	13.3	14.3	15.3	16.3	93
93.5	10.4	11.4	12.4	13.4	14.4	15.4	16.5	93.5
94	10.5	11.5	12.5	13.5	14.5	15.6	16.6	94
94.5	10.6	11.6	12.6	13.6	14.7	15.7	16.7	94.5

508

Appendix 5 - Growth Velocity and Skinfold Charts

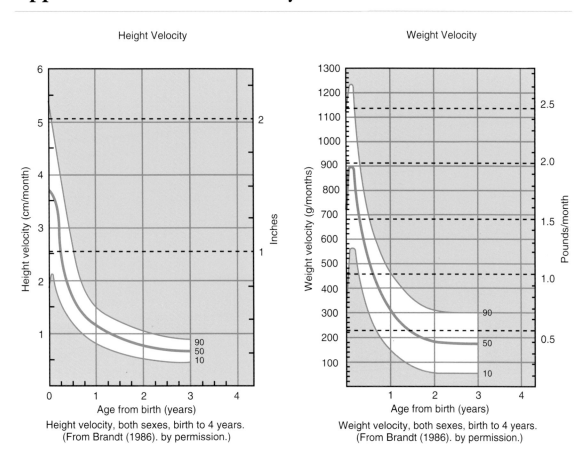

Height Velocity

Weight Velocity

Height velocity, both sexes, birth to 4 years.
(From Brandt (1986). by permission.)

Weight velocity, both sexes, birth to 4 years.
(From Brandt (1986). by permission.)

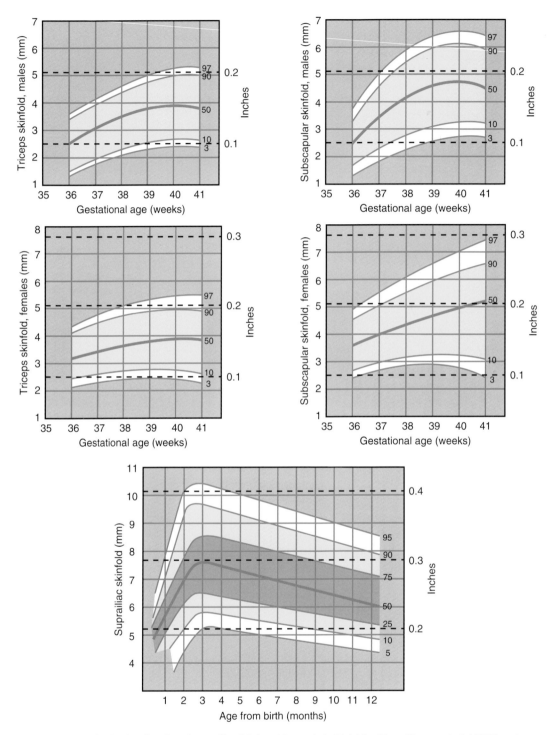

Triceps and subscalpular (newborn) and suprailiac (birth to 12 months) skinfolds. (From Maaser et al. (1972) and Schlueter et al. (1976), by permission.)

Index

Abscess, breast, 400
Absorptive function, 45, 159
Acid excretion, 273, 276, 278, 322
Acidosis, metabolic, carbohydrate and, 29, 43
Acids, fatty. *See* Fatty acids
Acrodermatitis enteropathica, zinc and, 14
Activity, energy requirements and, 66-67
Acute gastroenteritis, lactose malabsorption and, 93, 95
Adiposity, determinants of, 75
Allergy, milk-protein, 95, 100, 432
Allowances, nutrient, 67, 71
Aluminum, 175, 195, 221-222
Alveoli, 401
Amino acids. *See also* Protein entries; specific amino acid
    absorption of, 84-86
    milk protein synthesis and, 86-87
    in MSUD treatment formulas, 322
    parenteral solutions of, 93
    serum concentrations of, protein adequacy, 89
    toxicity to, 95-96
Ammonia, 88
Amphipathic lipids, 124
Amylase, 106-112, 426
Amylase activity development of, 108-109
Amylopectin, 106
Amylose, 106
Anatomic ontogeny. *See also* Ontogeny
Anemia, 241-254
    definition of, 241
    folate deficiency in, 249
    iron deficiency in, 244-245, 247
    prevention of, 248
    iron excess and, 248
    iron needs during development and, 243-244
    megaloblastic, 250
    treatment of, 247
    vitamin B_{12} deficiency in, 250
Antigens, milk sIgA and, 361, 366
Anxiety maternal breast-feeding and, 364-365
Appetite spurts, breast-feeding and, 75
Arachidonic acid, 129, 136, 138, 142, 358, 449
Areola, 370, 385, 390, 392, 394-396, 399, 402, 408
Arignase, 86
Ariboflavinosis, 260
Ascorbic acid,
    availability of, needs and, 273-274
    deficiency of, 275

in milk, 274
    iron absorption and, 242-243
    physiology and, 273-274
    recommended intake of, 274-275
    toxicity associated with, 276
Atwater's fuel values, 64

Basal metabolic rate (BMR), 58
    definition of, 58, 77
    energy requirements and, 58-60
        marasmus and, 73, 74
Beriberi, 236, 254, 256-257, 277, 364
Bile secretion, development of, 294
Bilirubin,
    breast-feeding and, 368-370, 387, 396, 397
Biotin, 255, 267-268, 278
    availability of, needs and, 267
    deficiency of, 267
    in formulas, 267
    in milk, 267
    physiology and, 267
    preterm infants and, 267
    recommended intake of, 267-268
    TPN and, 268, 278
Blood urea nitrogen (BUN), protein intake and, 86, 88, 98-99
BMI (body mass index), 11
BMR. *See* Basal metabolic rate
Body water, 40, 60-61
    potassium and, 15, 31, 47
Bolus feeding, intermittent, 31, 42, 94, 116, 160, 165
Bone demineralization, 156, 190-191, 194, 369
Bone disease,
    parenteral nutrition and, 191
    vitamin D deficiency and, 190
BPD. *See* Bronchopulmonary dysplasia
Brain, ascorbic acid in, 284, 323
Breast,
    abscess of, 400
    anatomy of, 387
Breast engorgement, 395-396, 399-400
Breast examination, 385
Breast-fed infants, iron in, 423-424
Breast-feeding. *See also* Lactation
    abscess and, 400
    breast engorgement and, 395-396
    breast pumps and, 371-372, 406-407
    consultation services for, 409, 415
    discharge planning and, 406-407

thermic effect of, 59
   definition of, 77
Feeding tubes, 47
Ferritin,
   serum, iron deficiency diagnosis and, 246-247
Ferrous sulfate, iron deficiency treatment with, 247
Fiber, 452-453
Fish oils, 131, 140, 161
Flavin adenine dinucleotide (FAD), riboflavin
   and, 260
Fluoride, 215-216
   dental health and, 215-216
   requirements for, 216
   toxicity associated with, 216
Fluorosis, 216-217, 237
Folate 268-271
   dietary lack of, 268
   vitamin B_{12} deficiency and, 270
Folate deficiency, 270-271
Folic acid, 268-271
Football hold, 390-391
Formula(s), 441-508
   aluminum in, 455
   carbohydrate content of, 451-452
   cow milk, 444
   preterm infant and, 445
   soy, 442, 446
   composition of, 443
   energy intake and, 449
   evaluation of,
      clinical, 456-457
      preclinical, 456-457
   evolution of, fat content of, 448
   sources of, 446
   oils in, 448-450
   high-energy, 448
   inborn errors of metabolism and, 447
      See also Inborn errors of metabolism; 313-328
   iron-fortified, 454
   lactose-free, 451
   microbiology of, 462
   milk versus,
      fat percentage in, 445
      preterm infants and, 445
   non-nutritional factors in, 455
   nutrient characteristics of, 443-444
      carbohydrate, 451-452
      fat, 448
      minerals, 454
      protein, 444-447
      vitamins, 454
   osmolality of, 455-456
      glucose and, 451-452

product forms, 459-460
   production process for, 461
   protein requirements and, 444-445
   quality control of, 461
   recalls of, 463
   renal solute load and, 456
   sanitation and, 462
   shelf-life of, 462-463
   supplementary, 453-454
   vitamin A in, 450
   vitamin D in, 454
   water-soluble vitamins in, 454
Fructose, 108-112
Furosemide, calciuric effect of, 194

Galactose, 318
Galactosemia, 318, 320, 451-452
   deficiency in, 318
   physiology and, 318-319
   toxicity in, 319
   treatment of, 319-320
Gastric residual volumes, 365
Gastrin, 84-85
Gastrointestinal disorders, 155-168
   Celiac disease, 156-157
   short-bowel syndrome, 157-161
   Inflammatory bowel disease, 161-165
   nutritional therapy and, 165-166
Gastrointestinal tract, 83-85
   circulating hormones of, 83-84
   digestion and absorption in,
      adult, 85
      neonatal, 84-85
   functional development of, 83
      digestive/absorptive, 84-85
      immaturity and, 84
      secretion in, 84
   ontogeny of, 83-85
Gavage feeding, 305
Glomerular filtration rate (GFR), 180
Glucoamylase, 106-109
Gluconeogenesis, 86
Glucose,
   absorption of, 106-118
   energy metabolism and, 63
   fuel source, 71-72
Glucose metabolism, chromium and, 218-219
Goiter, iodine and, 219-221
Gross energy, definition of, 77
Growth faltering, 21-36
   diagnosis, 21-26
   management, 30-32
   milk intolerance, 28-29